O'Flynn

Prenatal Diagnosis of Congenital Anomalies

PRENATAL DIAGNOSIS OF CONGENITAL ANOMALIES

Roberto Romero, M.D.
Associate Professor of Obstetrics and Gynecology
Director of Perinatal Research
Yale University School of Medicine
New Haven, Connecticut

Gianluigi Pilu, M.D.
Attending Physician
Section of Prenatal Pathophysiology
Second Department of Obstetrics and Gynecology
University of Bologna School of Medicine
Bologna, Italy

Philippe Jeanty, M.D.
Assistant Professor
Department of Radiology
Vanderbilt University
Nashville, Tennessee

Alessandro Ghidini, M.D.
Research Fellow
Department of Obstetrics and Gynecology
Yale University School of Medicine
New Haven, Connecticut

John C. Hobbins, M.D.
Professor of Obstetrics and Gynecology
and Diagnostic Imaging
Yale University School of Medicine
Director of Obstetrics
Yale–New Haven Hospital
New Haven, Connecticut

APPLETON & LANGE
Norwalk, Connecticut/San Mateo, California

0-8385-7921-3

88 89 90 91 92 / 10 9 8 7 6 5 4 3 2 1

Prentice-Hall of Australia, Pty. Ltd., Sydney
Prentice-Hall Canada, Inc.
Prentice-Hall Hispanoamericana, S.A., Mexico
Prentice-Hall of India Private Limited, New Delhi
Prentice-Hall International (UK) Limited, London
Prentice-Hall of Japan, Inc., Tokyo
Prentice-Hall of Southeast Asia (Pte.) Ltd., Singapore
Whitehall Books Ltd., Wellington, New Zealand
Editora Prentice-Hall do Brasil Ltda., Rio de Janeiro

Library of Congress Cataloging-in-Publication Data

Prenatal diagnosis of congenital anomalies.

Includes index.
1. Prenatal diagnosis. 2. Fetus—Abnormalities—
Diagnosis. I. Romero, Roberto. [DNLM: 1. Abnormalities
—diagnosis. 2. Fetal Diseases—diagnosis.
3. Prenatal Diagnosis—methods. QS 675 P926]
RG628.P74   1987   618.2'2   87-14557
ISBN 0-8385-7921-3

Production Editor: Donald L. Delauter
Design: M. Chandler Martylewski

To my parents and the memory of Angela Galue. They made it all possible
Roberto Romero

To Antonella, with love

Gianluigi Pilu

To Dominique, Cerine, and Cedric, who mean so much to me
Philippe Jeanty

To my family, with love and gratitude

Alessandro Ghidini

To Toni, with love

John C. Hobbins

Contents

Preface

This book was born out of a clinical need. In the past, when the diagnosis of an anatomic congenital anomaly was made with ultrasound in our practice, multiple concerns and issues were raised for both patients and physicians. Patients typically wanted to know the prognosis for the fetus and the likelihood of recurrence in future pregnancies. In addition, physicians wanted to understand the mechanisms for the anomaly, the genetic basis, and the differential diagnosis. Colleagues were also faced with making obstetrical management decisions and wanted help in deciding timing and route of delivery. The information required to assist us and our colleagues in practice was not available in a single source. We had to consult journals and books in the fields of pediatrics, pediatric surgery, genetics, pathology, radiology, and obstetrics. Often when we told parents that their fetus had a serious congenital anomaly, further discussion was delayed to allow us to make a trip to the library. It was clear that we had not been trained for this task. Ultrasound diagnosis of congenital anomalies had created a new field. It was this very problem that moved us to write this book. The book is intended to provide the practicing sonographer and obstetrician with a source to be used in the clinical setting.

This book is organized by organ systems. For each anomaly we have tried to provide information about the frequency, etiology, genetic basis, pathology, associated anomalies, diagnosis, prognosis, and obstetrical management. Although each chapter has a brief introduction in which some anatomic considerations are discussed, these are overviews (with the exception of the chapters on the central nervous system and the heart). Recently, excellent texts on fetal sectional anatomy have become available, and we encourage their use.* Our text is not a basic book on obstetrical ultrasound; it has been written for the experienced sonographer.

In writing this book, several sections were challenging. We designed the prognosis sections to provide information about the outcome of the disorders. At this time, a paucity of outcome data exists for cases identified in utero. Therefore, we had to use the information available in the pediatric literature regarding neonates born with anomalies. The reader should keep in mind that there may be important differences between fetuses and newborns. Also, there are limitations in extrapolating data from pediatric and autopsy studies, rather than from the live fetus.

The obstetrical management sections were written in response to the need for guidance in the management of anomalies. They reflect our opinions and experiences. They conform to the reality of the practice of medicine in the United States today. In a country where pregnancy termination is available for social as well as medical reasons, we believe that this option must be offered to parents carrying an anomalous fetus. Placing limits on the gestational age at which termination can be offered was avoided because this varies from state to state and among institutions. The term "viability" has been employed to refer to such a limit in full recognition of its changing meaning. After this point in gestation, we subscribe to the view that the option of pregnancy termination can be offered if an anomaly is uniformly lethal (e.g., anencephaly, alobar holoprosencephaly). Regarding time and route of delivery, we have advocated a nonaggressive management approach in those cases where the prognosis is dismal. The term "nonaggressive management" means that our analysis of the risk:benefit ratio is slanted toward maternal

---

*These texts are: (1) Bowerman RA: Atlas of Normal Fetal Ultrasonographic Anatomy. Chicago, Year Book, 1986. (2) Isaacson G, Mintz MC, Crelin ES: Atlas of Fetal Sectional Anatomy: With Ultrasound and Magnetic Resonance Imaging. New York, Springer-Verlag, 1986. (3) Staudach A: Fetal Anatomie im Ultraschall. Berlin, Springer-Verlag, 1986.

well-being and, therefore, we would be reluctant to recommend a cesarean section if fetal distress should arise.

We have also advocated liberal use of karyotype determination for fetuses with congenital anomalies. The method for obtaining material for these studies has not been defined throughout the text. Amniocentesis has been the standard, but the rapid development of percutaneous umbilical cord sampling may evolve as the method of choice in some cases where a rapid answer is desirable. Delivery of infants with congenital anomalies should ideally occur in a center where a newborn special care unit is available. This has been referred to throughout the text as a tertiary care center.

The illustrations used throughout the book are from our own collections or from other authors, who have kindly agreed to the use of their material. We are grateful to them. In those cases where an anomaly is particularly rare and has not been diagnosed recently, we had no choice but to include a picture that may not be "state of the art."

The field of prenatal diagnosis is rapidly expanding. Because of this, we have made every effort to include the most recent, up-to-date references available.

Fetal biometry is an important part of the diagnosis of congenital anomalies. Tables and figures have been placed throughout the text where we thought they were relevant. There is a separate index for tables and figures on page 448 for easy access to this material.

We welcome input from our readers and would be happy to provide our opinion in the diagnosis and management of unusual congenital anomalies. It is only through the sharing of this information that the field can advance. We would be grateful to those giving us the opportunity to learn.

If this book renders the task of prenatal diagnosis and counseling of our patients easier, more precise, and more informed, we feel that our efforts will have accomplished a purpose.

Roberto Romero
Gianluigi Pilu
Philippe Jeanty
Alessandro Ghidini
John C. Hobbins

Acknowledgments

The writing of this book would not have been possible without the help of many people. Prof. Luciano Bovicelli, Chairman of the Cattedra di Fisiopatologia Prenatale at Bologna University, has been a constant source of enthusiasm and support to us and to the field of prenatal diagnosis. Prof. Costantino Mangioni, Chairman of the 5th Clinica Ostetrica e Ginecologica at Milan University, provided encouragement and assistance in promoting the value of research in prenatal diagnosis of congenital anomalies.

The editorial help of Carmen Habeck, who worked through many changes and revisions, is gratefully acknowledged. Sonographers Carole Burdine and Jackie Green have assisted us in acquiring some of the illustrations for this book. Barbara Coster also helped us in the initial stages of this book. We are also grateful to our colleagues for their input, particularly Nicole Rizzo, L. Filippo Orsini, Giovanna Baccarani, Patricia Stewart, and Charles Lockwood.

Special recognition is due to Dr. M.J. Mahoney, Professor of Human Genetics, Obstetrics and Gynecology, and Pediatrics at Yale University. Through many years of fertile collaboration, he has provided support and enthusiasm for clinical research in fetal disease and has stimulated us to push the limits of ultrasound in prenatal diagnosis.

PRENATAL DIAGNOSIS OF CONGENITAL ANOMALIES

The Central Nervous System

Normal Sonographic Anatomy of the Fetal Central Nervous System

INTRACRANIAL ANATOMY

The objective of the sonographic examination of the fetal central nervous system (CNS) is to reconstruct with a two-dimensional tool a complex three-dimensional structure. In this effort, the larger the number of scanning planes obtained, the more accurate the representation will appear. The three planes traditionally used for such an evaluation are the axial, sagittal, and coronal (Fig. 1–1). The sonographer should be aware that important developmental changes occur in the fetal brain well after the end of embryogenesis and up to the third trimester. The lateral ventricles and subarachnoid cisterns decrease steadily in size throughout gestation, resulting not only in a geometric modification of the cerebral structures but also in important changes in the sonographic appearance of the fetal brain. During the early second trimester, the fluid-filled lateral ventricles are large. This causes enhancement of sound transmission, and the distal cerebral cortex appears more echoic than later in gestation. Familiarity with the normal ultrasound appearance of the fetal brain in different scanning planes and at different gestational ages is critical for the recognition of congenital anomalies.

Axial Planes

Axial planes are obtained by scanning the head of the fetus at an angle of about 20 degrees to the canthomeatal line.[9] Four different levels are commonly used (Fig. 1–2). The first scanning plane passes through the bodies of the lateral ventricles. In Figure 1–3A, the different appearances of this view throughout gestation can be seen. At 16 weeks, the lateral ventricles occupy most of the relative hemispheres and are partially filled with the echogenic choroid plexuses. At midgestation, the size of the lateral ventricles has considerably diminished, but in many cases it is still possible to observe the two walls that line the ventricular cavity on both sides. During the third trimester, only the lateral wall can be visualized. The distance between the midline echo and the lateral wall of the ventricle is now approximately one third of the hemispheric width. This value will remain constant throughout life (Fig. 1–3B).

The axial view has been used to derive nomograms for the normal size of the ventricles.[2,5,7,8] The

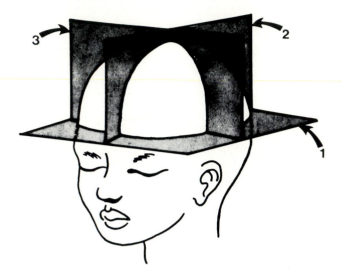

Figure 1–1. Schematic representation of the scanning planes used for the study of fetal cerebral anatomy: (1) axial, (2) sagittal, and (3) coronal.

ratio between the distance from the midline echo to the lateral ventricular wall (lateral ventricular width, LVW) and the hemispheric width (HW) measured from the midline echo to the inner echo of the calvarium is illustrated in Figure 1–4. Tables 1–1 and 1–2 are the corresponding nomograms.

It should be stressed that after the 20th week of gestation, the choroid plexus is considerably reduced in size. It is no longer observed in the previously described axial plane and can only be imaged in a lower section (Fig. 1–5A,B). Because the lateral ventricles diverge inferiorly and posteriorly, the measurement of the LVW:HW ratio at this level would result in a falsely elevated value. Therefore, this measurement should not be taken in a section that displays the choroid plexus later than 20 weeks of gestation. Furthermore, in normal fetuses, it is usually possible with current high-resolution ultrasound equipment to visualize both the lateral and medial walls of the lateral ventricle. This observation is important because it has been suggested that simultaneous demonstration of both ventricular walls in the third trimester is an early sign of hydrocephaly.[4] The sonographer should be aware that such findings may be entirely normal in this scanning plane.

The second scanning plane passes through the frontal horns, atria, and occipital horns of the lateral ventricles (Fig. 1–6). At 18 weeks, the atria are round and are entirely filled with the echogenic choroid plexus. Later in gestation, the atria decrease in size and assume a convex shape due to the development of the calcar avis. The occipital horns appear as a fluid-filled posterior prolongation of the atria. In this scanning plane, it is possible to appreciate the progressive opercularization of the insula. Until the 18th

or 19th week, the temporal lobe is convex and the lobe of the insula is apposed to the calvarium. In the following weeks, the insula deepens medially while the adjacent frontal and temporal lobes (so-called opercula) move progressively closer to each other, forming the sylvian fissure. The beginning of sylvian fissure demarcation is already visible at 22 weeks of gestation. However, it is not until 32 to 34 weeks of gestation that the opercularization is complete[3] (Fig. 1–7).

The third axial section corresponds to the biparietal diameter level (Fig. 1–8A,B). In this scanning plane, the thalami appear as two triangular echo-free areas. Between the thalami, the slitlike third ventricle can be seen. It is sometimes possible to visualize a cross-section of the aqueductus of Sylvius posterior to the third ventricle. On both sides of the thalami, the hippocampal gyrus appears as a circular space delineated medially by the ambient cistern and laterally by the atrium of the lateral ventricle. Anterior to the thalami, it is possible to visualize the frontal horns of the lateral ventricles. During the

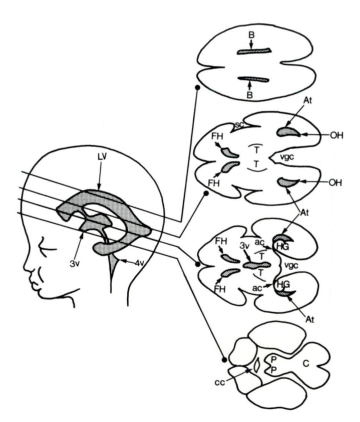

Figure 1–2. Schematic representation of the axial examination of the fetal head. In the four scanning planes (from rostral to caudal), the following structures can be recognized: bodies of the lateral ventricles (B), frontal horns (FH), atria (At), and occipital horns (OH) of the lateral ventricles, thalami (T), sylvian and vein of Galen cisterns (sc, vgc), third ventricle (3v), ambient cistern (ac), hippocampal gyrus (HG), cerebral peduncles (P), chiasmatic cistern (cc), and cerebellum (C). LV, lateral ventricles; 4v, fourth ventricle.

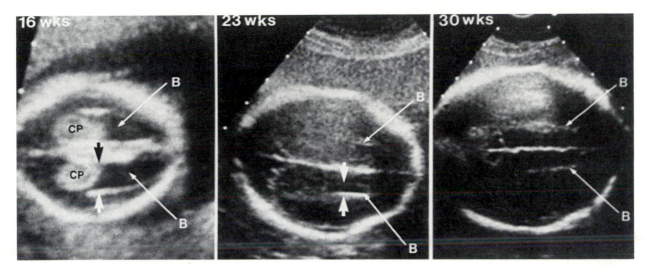

Figure 1–3. A. Axial scans at the level of the bodies (B) of the lateral ventricles at 16, 23, and 30 weeks. Note the prominent choroid plexus (CP) in the 16-week fetus and the progressive shrinking of the ventricular cavity. The arrowheads indicate the medial and lateral walls of the ventricle.

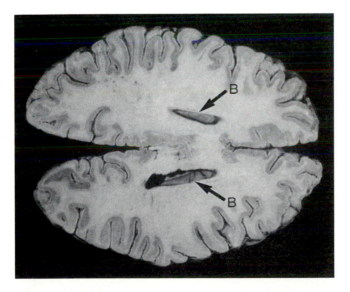

Figure 1–3. B. Anatomic specimen from an adult brain corresponding to the axial section shown in Figure 1–3A. Note the similarity in ventricular versus hemispheric size with the ultrasound image of the 30-week fetus. *(Reproduced with permission from Matsui, Irano: An Atlas of the Human Brain for Computed Tomography. Tokyo, Igaku Shoin, 1978.)*

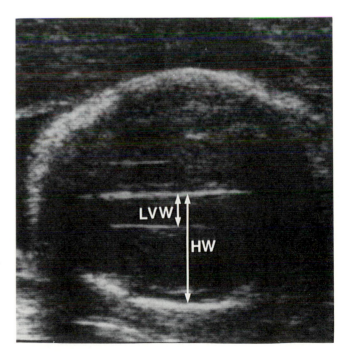

Figure 1–4. A. Measurement of the LVW:HW ratio.

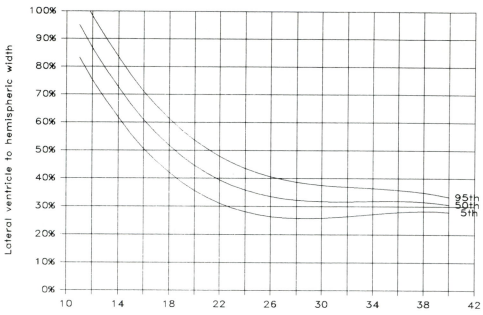

Figure 1–4. B. Relationship between the LVW:HW ratio and gestational age.

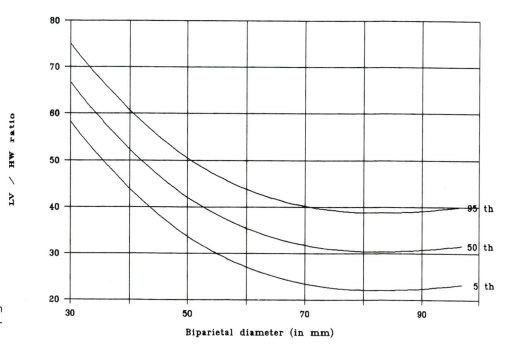

Figure 1–4. C. Relationship between the LVW:HW ratio and biparietal diameter (BPD).

TABLE 1–1. NOMOGRAM FOR EVALUATION OF LVW:HW RATIO AGAINST GESTATIONAL AGE

Age (weeks)	LVW:HW (%) 5th	50th	95th	Age (weeks)	LVW:HW (%) 5th	50th	95th
11	83	95	107	26	26	34	41
12	75	87	98	27	26	33	40
13	68	79	91	28	26	32	39
14	62	73	83	29	26	32	38
15	56	66	77	30	26	32	38
16	51	61	71	31	26	32	37
17	46	56	66	32	26	32	37
18	42	52	61	33	27	32	37
19	39	48	57	34	27	32	36
20	36	45	54	35	28	32	36
21	33	42	50	36	28	32	36
22	31	39	48	37	28	32	35
23	29	37	45	38	28	32	35
24	28	36	44	39	28	31	34
25	27	35	42	40	28	31	33

TABLE 1–2. LATERAL VENTRICLE HEMISPHERIC WIDTH RATIO VERSUS BIPARIETAL DIAMETER

BPD (mm)	Percentile 5th	50th	95th	BPD (mm)	Percentile 5th	50th	95th
30	58	67	75	67	24	33	41
31	57	65	73	68	24	32	41
32	55	63	72	69	24	32	40
33	54	62	70	70	23	32	40
34	52	60	69	71	23	32	40
35	51	59	67	72	23	31	40
36	49	57	66	73	23	31	40
37	48	56	65	74	23	31	39
38	46	55	63	75	23	31	39
39	45	54	62	76	22	31	39
40	44	52	61	77	22	31	39
41	43	51	59	78	22	31	39
42	42	50	58	79	22	31	39
43	40	49	57	80	22	30	39
44	39	48	56	81	22	30	39
45	38	47	55	82	22	30	39
46	37	46	54	83	22	30	39
47	36	45	53	84	22	30	39
48	35	44	52	85	22	30	39
49	35	43	51	86	22	30	39
50	34	42	50	87	22	31	39
51	33	41	50	88	22	31	39
52	32	40	49	89	22	31	39
53	31	40	48	90	22	31	39
54	31	39	47	91	22	31	39
55	30	38	47	92	23	31	39
56	29	38	46	93	23	31	39
57	29	37	45	94	23	31	40
58	28	37	45	95	23	31	40
59	28	36	44	96	23	31	40
60	27	35	44	97	23	32	40
61	27	35	43	98	23	32	40
62	26	35	43	99	24	32	40
63	26	34	42	100	24	32	40
64	25	34	42				
65	25	33	42				
66	25	33	41				

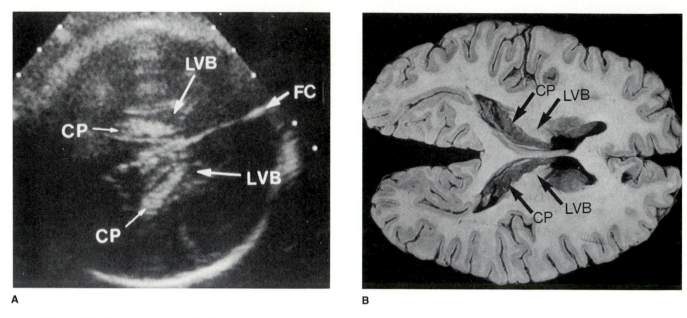

A   **B**

Figure 1–5. A. Axial scan at a slightly lower level than shown in Figure 1–3A in a third trimester fetus. This plane passes through the floor of the body of the lateral ventricle (LVB) and shows the choroid plexus (CP) arising from the foramen of Monro. FC, falx cerebri. **B.** Anatomic specimen from an adult brain corresponding to the axial section shown in Figure 1–5A. *(Figure B reproduced with permission from Matsui, Irano: An Atlas of the Human Brain for Computed Tomography. Tokyo, Igaku Shoin, 1978.)*

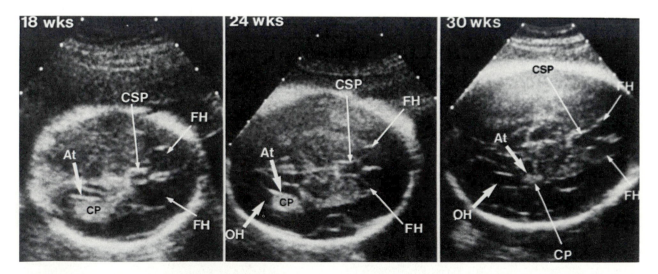

Figure 1–6. A. Axial scan passing through the frontal horns (FH), atria (At), and occipital horns (OH) of the lateral ventricles. At the same level, the superior portion of the cavum septi pellucidum (CSP) and thalami (unlabeled) are seen. Note the brightly echogenic choroid plexus (CP), which entirely fills the atria.

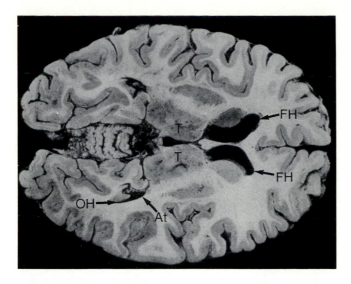

Figure 1–6. B. Anatomic specimen from an adult brain corresponding to the axial section shown in Figure 1–6A. T, thalami. *(Reproduced with permission from Matsui, Irano: An Atlas of the Human Brain for Computed Tomography. Tokyo, Igaku Shoin, 1978.)*

second trimester and early third trimester, the frontal horns are usually separated by a widely patent cavum septi pellucidi. During the late third trimester, the cavum septi pellucidi may decrease in size and appear as either one or two lines internal to the frontal horns (Fig. 1–9). Halfway between the thalami and the calvarium, a linear echo representing the insula is seen. This structure should not be confused with the lateral wall of the lateral ventricles, because this would obviously lead to the erroneous diagnosis

of hydrocephaly. A useful hint for the recognition of this structure is the demonstration of a pulsating echo corresponding to the middle cerebral artery.

The biparietal diameter (BPD) is one of the most frequently used fetal biometric parameters. It is measured from the outer echo of the superior parietal bone to the inner echo of the inferior parietal bone (Fig. 1–10). Tables 1–3 and 1–4 and Figures 1–11 and 1–12 are used to predict gestational age and to assess the normality of a BPD for a given gestational age. Tables 1–3 and 1–4 should be used only after verifying that the size of the BPD is not affected by molding of the fetal head. This is achieved by obtaining an occipitofrontal diameter (OFD) and calculating the cephalic index. The OFD can be imaged in the same section used for the BPD and is measured from midecho to midecho (Fig. 1–10). Figure 1–13 and Table 1–5 illustrate the growth of the OFD. The cephalic index is calculated by dividing the BPD by the OFD. Normal values are between 75 and 85 percent. Dolicocephaly is diagnosed by cephalic indices below 75 percent and brachycephaly by cephalic indices above 85 percent.

The circumference of the head either can be measured directly with a mapreader or, alternatively, can be calculated from the BPD and OFD. The formula used to calculate the head circumference is:

$$\text{Head circumference} = 1.62 \, (\text{BPD} + \text{OFD})$$

We have compared the results of these calculations with actual measurements of the fetal head circumference and found them acceptable for clinical use. Similar comparisons have been made by others.[1,6]

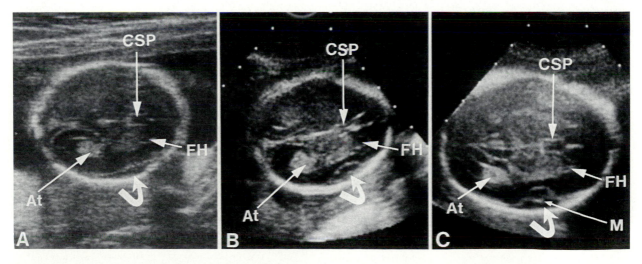

Figure 1–7. Axial scans at the level of the insula (*curved arrow*) throughout gestation. **A.** At 18 weeks, the cerebral hemisphere is convex, and only a thin, fluid layer separates the insula from the calvarium. **B.** At 22 weeks, the insula is deepened, beginning the formation of the sylvian cistern. **C.** At 28 weeks, growth of the opercula and deepening of the insula result in the formation of a square-shaped, fluid-filled area. At this time, a thin membrane (M), probably representing the arachnoid, is seen bridging between the opercula. CSP, cavum septi pellucidum; At, atria of the lateral ventricles; FH, frontal horns of the lateral ventricles.

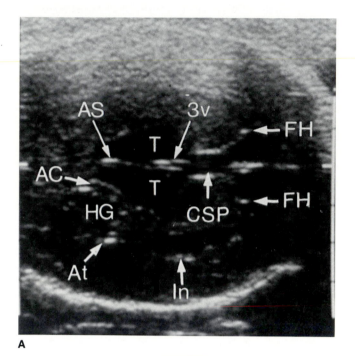

A

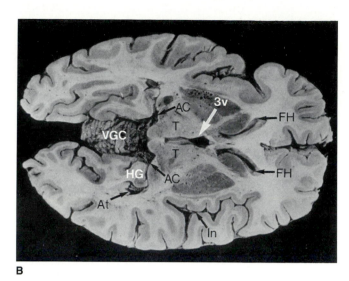

B

Figure 1–8. A. Axial scan at the level of the thalami (T) and third ventricle (3v). Anterior to the thalami, the frontal horns (FH) of the lateral ventricles, which are separated by a widely patent cavum septi pellucidi (CSP), can be seen. The hippocampal gyrus (HG) can be recognized by the presence of the medial ambient cistern (AC) and lateral atrium of the lateral ventricle (At). The linear echo that can be seen lateral to the thalamus corresponds to the insula (In). On real-time examination, the active pulsation of the middle cerebral artery distinguishes it from the wall of the lateral ventricle. **B.** Anatomic specimen corresponding to the axial section shown in Figure A. This specimen was obtained from the brain of an adult, and the cavum septi pellucidi is obliterated. VGC, vein of Galen cistern. *(Figure B reproduced with permission from Matsui, Irano: An Atlas of the Human Brain for Computed Tomography. Tokyo, Igaku Shoin, 1978.)*

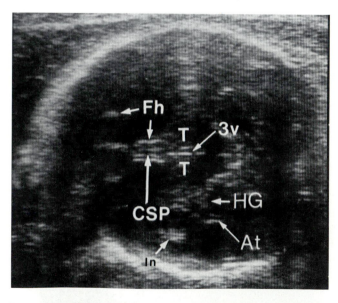

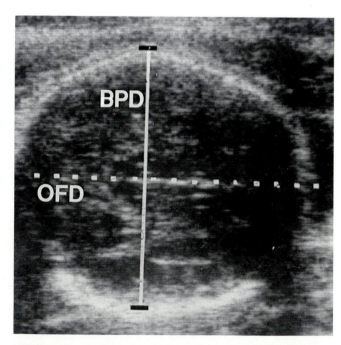

Figure 1–9. Axial scan at the same level as in Figure 1–8A in a late third trimester fetus. The two lines that are seen medial to the frontal horns (Fh) of the lateral ventricles are thought to represent the walls of a patent but small cavum septi pellucidi (CSP). At, atria; HG, hippocampal gyrus; In, insula; T, thalami; 3v, third ventricle.

Figure 1–10. Measurement of the biparietal diameter (BPD) and occipitofrontal diameter (OFD).

TABLE 1–3. GESTATIONAL AGE FROM THE BIPARIETAL DIAMETER (BPD)

BPD (mm)	Age (weeks) 5th	Age (weeks) 50th	Age (weeks) 95th	BPD (mm)	Age (weeks) 5th	Age (weeks) 50th	Age (weeks) 95th
10	7	10 + 1	13 + 1	55	19	22	25 + 1
11	7 + 2	10 + 2	13 + 3	56	19 + 2	22 + 3	25 + 3
12	7 + 3	10 + 4	13 + 4	57	19 + 5	22 + 5	25 + 6
13	7 + 5	10 + 5	13 + 5	58	20	23 + 1	26 + 1
14	7 + 6	10 + 6	14	59	20 + 3	23 + 3	26 + 3
15	8 + 1	11 + 1	14 + 1	60	20 + 5	23 + 6	26 + 6
16	8 + 2	11 + 2	14 + 3	61	21 + 1	24 + 1	27 + 1
17	8 + 4	11 + 4	14 + 4	62	21 + 3	24 + 4	27 + 4
18	8 + 5	11 + 5	14 + 6	63	21 + 6	24 + 6	27 + 6
19	9	12	15	64	22 + 1	25 + 2	28 + 2
20	9 + 1	12 + 2	15 + 2	65	22 + 4	25 + 4	28 + 5
21	9 + 3	12 + 3	15 + 3	66	22 + 6	26	29
22	9 + 4	12 + 5	15 + 5	67	23 + 2	26 + 2	29 + 3
23	9 + 6	12 + 6	16	68	23 + 5	26 + 5	29 + 5
24	10 + 1	13 + 1	16 + 1	69	24	27 + 1	30 + 1
25	10 + 2	13 + 3	16 + 3	70	24 + 3	27 + 3	30 + 4
26	10 + 4	13 + 4	16 + 5	71	24 + 6	27 + 6	30 + 6
27	10 + 6	13 + 6	17	72	25 + 1	28 + 2	31 + 2
28	11	14 + 1	17 + 1	73	25 + 4	28 + 5	31 + 5
29	11 + 2	14 + 3	17 + 3	74	26	29	32 + 1
30	11 + 4	14 + 4	17 + 5	75	26 + 3	29 + 3	32 + 4
31	11 + 6	14 + 6	18	76	26 + 6	29 + 6	32 + 6
32	12 + 1	15 + 1	18 + 1	77	27 + 1	30 + 2	33 + 2
33	12 + 3	15 + 3	18 + 3	78	27 + 4	30 + 5	33 + 5
34	12 + 4	15 + 5	18 + 5	79	28	31 + 1	34 + 1
35	12 + 6	16	19	80	28 + 3	31 + 3	34 + 4
36	13 + 1	16 + 2	19 + 2	81	28 + 6	31 + 6	35
37	13 + 3	16 + 4	19 + 4	82	29 + 2	32 + 2	35 + 3
38	13 + 5	16 + 6	19 + 6	83	29 + 5	32 + 5	35 + 6
39	14	17 + 1	20 + 1	84	30 + 1	33 + 1	36 + 2
40	14 + 2	17 + 3	20 + 3	85	30 + 4	33 + 4	36 + 5
41	14 + 4	17 + 5	20 + 5	86	31	34	37 + 1
42	14 + 6	18	21	87	31 + 3	34 + 3	37 + 4
43	15 + 1	18 + 2	21 + 2	88	31 + 6	35	38
44	15 + 3	18 + 4	21 + 4	89	32 + 2	35 + 3	38 + 3
45	15 + 6	18 + 6	21 + 6	90	32 + 5	35 + 6	38 + 6
46	16 + 1	19 + 1	22 + 1	91	33 + 2	36 + 2	39 + 2
47	16 + 3	19 + 3	22 + 4	92	33 + 5	36 + 5	39 + 6
48	16 + 5	19 + 5	22 + 6	93	34 + 1	37 + 1	40 + 2
49	17	20 + 1	23 + 1	94	34 + 4	37 + 5	40 + 5
50	17 + 3	20 + 3	23 + 3	95	35	38 + 1	41 + 1
51	17 + 3	20 + 5	23 + 6	96	35 + 4	38 + 4	41 + 4
52	18	21	24 + 1	97	36	39	42 + 1
53	18 + 2	21 + 3	24 + 3	98	36 + 3	39 + 4	42 + 4
54	18 + 5	21 + 5	24 + 5	99	37	40	43

TABLE 1–4. NOMOGRAM TO EXAMINE COMPATIBILITY OF BIPARIETAL DIAMETER FOR GIVEN GESTATIONAL AGE

Age (weeks)	Biparietal Diameter			Age (weeks)	Biparietal Diameter		
	5th	*50th*	*95th*		*5th*	*50th*	*95th*
11	13	17	22	27	65	70	74
12	16	21	25	28	68	72	77
13	20	24	29	29	70	75	79
14	23	28	32	30	73	77	82
15	27	31	36	31	75	79	84
16	30	35	39	32	77	82	86
17	34	38	43	33	79	84	88
18	37	42	46	34	81	86	90
19	40	45	49	35	83	87	92
20	44	48	53	36	84	89	93
21	47	51	56	37	86	90	95
22	50	55	59	38	87	91	96
23	53	58	62	39	88	93	97
24	56	61	65	40	89	93	98
25	59	64	68	41	89	94	99
26	62	67	71	42	90	94	99

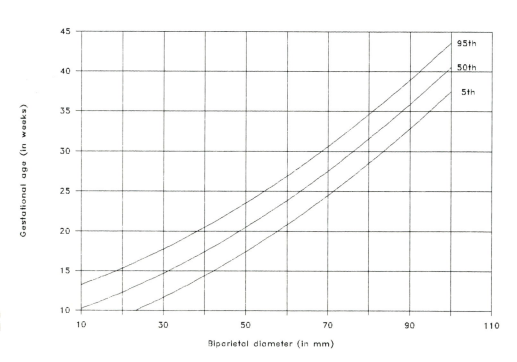

Figure 1–11. Relationship between gestational age and biparietal diameter.

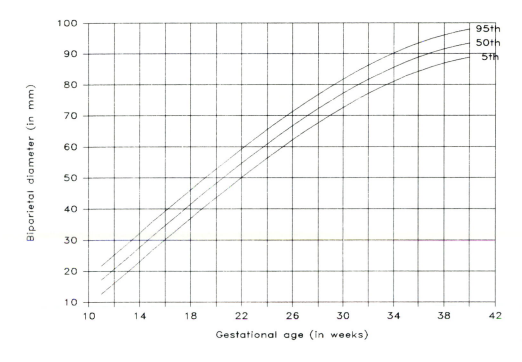

Figure 1–12. Relationship between biparietal diameter and gestational age.

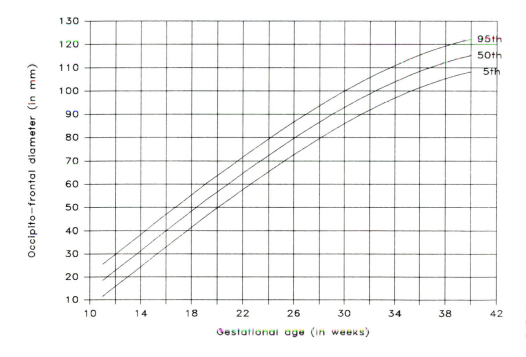

Figure 1–13. Relationship between gestational age and occipitofrontal diameter.

TABLE 1–5. NOMOGRAM FOR EVALUATION OF GROWTH OF OCCIPITOFRONTAL DIAMETER

Age (weeks)	Occipitofrontal Diameter		
	5th	50th	95th
11	11	18	25
12	16	23	30
13	20	27	34
14	24	31	38
15	29	36	43
16	33	40	47
17	37	44	51
18	41	48	55
19	46	53	60
20	50	57	64
21	54	61	68
22	58	65	72
23	62	69	76
24	65	72	79
25	69	76	83
26	73	80	87
27	76	83	90
28	80	87	94
29	83	90	97
30	86	93	100
31	89	96	103
32	92	99	106
33	95	102	108
34	97	104	111
35	99	106	113
36	102	109	116
37	104	111	118
38	105	112	119
39	107	114	121
40	108	115	122
41	109	116	123
42	110	117	124

until the cerebellar hemispheres come into view. The corresponding ultrasound image is shown in Figure 1–17. The cerebellar hemispheres can be seen joining in the midline at the superior cerebellar vermis (Fig. 1–17A,B). This view of the fetal brain can be used for the measurement of the cerebellar transverse diameter, a new parameter useful for both evaluating fetal growth and development and diagnosing posterior fossa abnormalities (Fig. 1–17C).

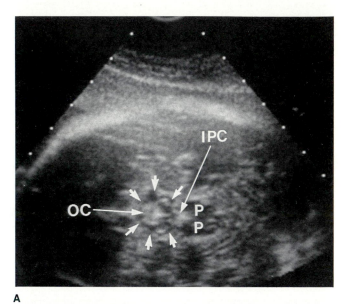

A

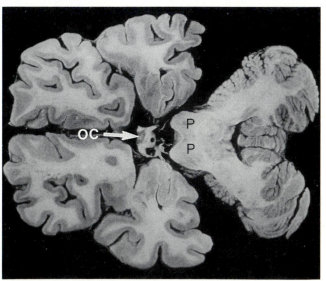

B

Figure 1–14. A. Axial scan of the fetal head at the level of the cerebral peduncles (P). The interpeduncular cistern (IPC) can be recognized on real-time examination by the presence of the pulsating basilar artery. The chiasmatic cistern (*arrows*) is seen surrounding the optic chiasma (OC). **B.** Anatomic specimen from an adult brain corresponding to the axial section shown in Figure A. *(Figure B reproduced with permission from Matsui, Irano: An Atlas of the Human Brain for Computed Tomography. Tokyo, Igaku Shoin, 1978.)*

The fourth axial plane passes through the midbrain and the chiasmatic cistern. The cerebral peduncles are seen as an echo-free, heart-shaped structure posterior to the active pulsation of the basilar artery, which is found in the interpeduncular cistern. Anterior to the interpeduncular cistern, a quadrangular, echo-free area is seen corresponding to the chiasmatic cistern. Within these cysternae, the pulsations of the arteries of the circle of Willis are seen surrounding the echogenic optic chiasma (Fig. 1–14).

At a lower level, the bony structures forming the base of the skull are visualized. The petrous ridges of the temporal bones and the anterior wings of the sphenoid bones converge to delineate the anterior, middle, and posterior fossae (Fig. 1–15).

Evaluation of the posterior fossa is most easily accomplished by a methodical plan of examination (Fig. 1–16). To obtain section 1, the transducer is first placed axially in the same plane used to obtain a BPD measurement and subsequently rotated posteriorly

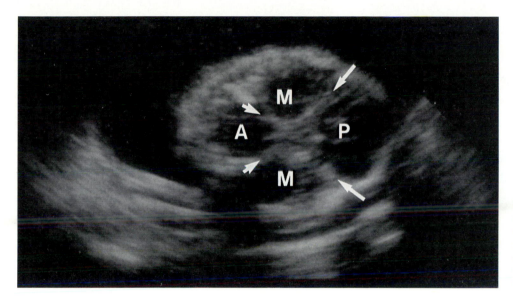

Figure 1–15. Axial scan at the level of the skull base. The anterior (A), middle (M), and posterior (P) fossae are delineated by the anterior wings of the sphenoid bones (*short arrows*) and petrous ridges of the temporal bones (*long arrows*).

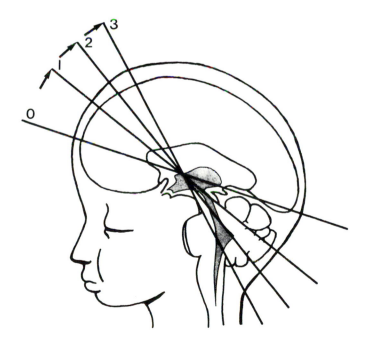

Figure 1–16. Schematic representation of the ultrasound examination of the fetal posterior fossa. At first, the transducer is positioned to obtain a BPD measurement (0). Subsequently, the transducer is rotated posteriorly. The ultrasound images corresponding to levels 1, 2, and 3 are shown in Figures 1–17, 1–18, and 1–19, respectively.

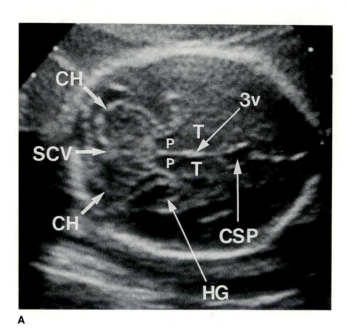

A

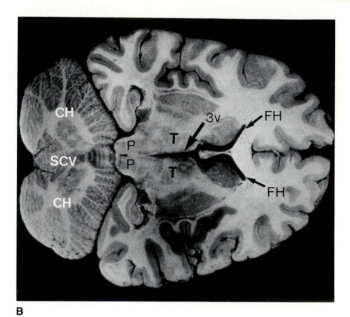

B

Figure 1–17. A. Axial scan directed posteriorly, corresponding to scanning plane 1 shown in Figure 1–16. The two cerebellar hemispheres (CH) connect on the midline in the superior cerebellar vermis (SCV). T, thalami; 3v, third ventricle; P, cerebral peduncles; CM, cisterna magna. **B.** Anatomic specimen from an adult brain corresponding to the axial section shown in Figure A. **C.** The relationship between cerebellar transverse diameter and gestational age. *(Figure B reproduced with permission from Matsui, Irano: An Atlas of the Human Brain for Computed Tomography. Tokyo, Igaku Shoin, 1978.)*

CEREBELLAR TRANSVERSE DIAMETER

GESTATIONAL AGE IN WEEKS

C

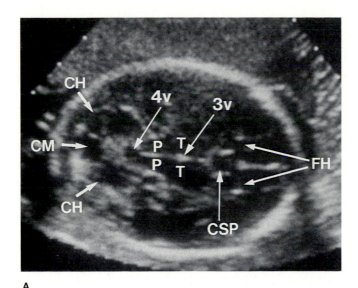

A

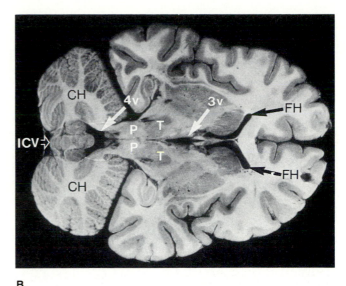

B

Figure 1–18. A. Axial scan directed posteriorly corresponding to scanning plane 2 shown in Figure 1–16. The echogenic inferior cerebellar vermis separates the fourth ventricle (4v) from the posterior cisterna magna (CM). CH, cerebellar hemispheres; T, thalami; 3v, third ventricle; P, cerebral peduncles; CSP, cavum septi pellucidi; FH, frontal horns. **B.** An anatomic specimen from an adult brain corresponding to the axial section shown in Figure A. *(Figure B reproduced with permission from Matsui, Irano: An Atlas of the Human Brain for Computed Tomography. Tokyo, Igaku Shoin, 1978.)*

At the level of section 2, the fourth ventricle appears as a square anechoic area lined inferiorly by the echogenic inferior vermis (Fig. 1–18). Between the cerebellum and the occipital bone lies the anechoic cisterna magna. Finally, movement of the transducer to section 3 will occasionally show the cerebellar tonsils (Fig. 1–19).

Sagittal Planes

Sagittal views are obtained by scanning the head along the anteroposterior axis (Fig. 1–1). These views are very informative, but they are difficult to obtain, since the fetus must be in either a breech or a transverse presentation. Two sagittal planes should be considered. The first passes through the brain at the level of the midline structures. It reveals the third ventricle, which appears as a square, echo-spared area, and the fourth ventricle, which indents the cerebellar vermis posteriorly (Fig. 1–20). The corpus callosum can be visualized superiorly to the cavum septi pellucidum and the triangular velum cistern (Fig. 1–21).

By laterally tilting the transducer, it is possible to visualize the entire lateral ventricle coursing around the thalamus (Fig. 1–22).

Since the fetal spine is not completely calcified, it is usually possible, in a posterior sagittal scan, to visualize the spinal cord as it enters the brain stem (Fig. 1–23).

Coronal Planes

Coronal views are obtained by scanning the fetal head along the laterolateral axis (Fig. 1–1). In the

anterior coronal scan (Fig. 1–24), the corpus callosum can be seen as an echo-spared area interposed between the roof of the frontal horns of the lateral ventricles and the interhemispheric fissure. In Figure 1–25, a more posterior scan passing through the brain stem is shown. In the fetus younger than 32 to 34

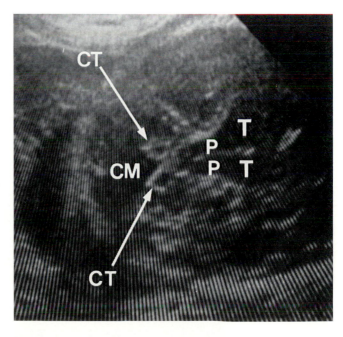

Figure 1–19. Because of the large cisterna magna (CM), the cerebellar tonsils (CT) that lie between the posterior aspect of the medulla oblongata and the cerebellar vermis are clearly defined in this view of the fetal head.

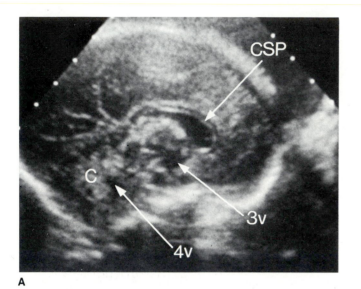

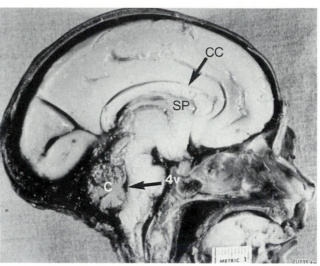

A   **B**

Figure 1–20. A. A midsagittal scan of the fetal brain at 30 weeks of gestation, demonstrating the third ventricle (3v) and the fourth ventricle (4v). A widely patent cavum septi pellucidi (CSP) is seen above the roof of the third ventricle. Note the echogenic cerebellar vermis (C). **B.** Anatomic specimen from a 30-week-old fetus corresponding to the sagittal section shown in Figure A. CC, corpus callosum; SP, septum pellucidum. *(Figure B reproduced with permission from Keir: In Newton, Potts (eds): Radiology of the Skull and Brain. Anatomy and Pathology. St. Louis, CV Mosby, 1977, pp 2787–2913.)*

Figure 1–21. A midsagittal scan of the fetal brain at 26 weeks. The corpus callosum is the thin anechoic area interposed between the hyperechogenic triangular velum cistern (TVC) and the large cavum septi pellucidum (CSP), which is posteriorly continuous with a patent cavum vergae (unlabeled). The arrows indicate the continuity between the triangular velum cistern and the posteroinferior vein of Galen cistern within which the vein of Galen is seen (VG). 3v, 3rd ventricle; Ant, anterior; Post, posterior.

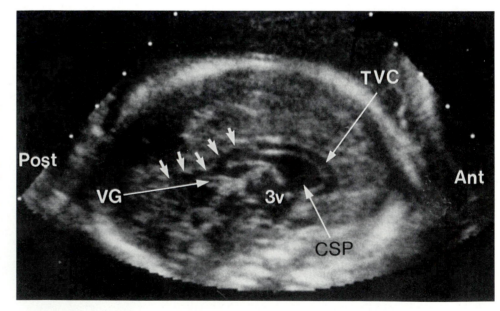

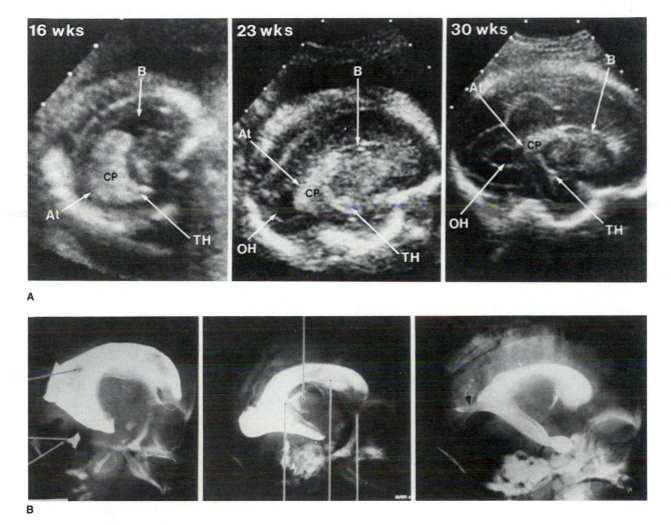

Figure 1–22. A. Developmental changes of the lateral ventricles during gestation. At 16 weeks, the ventricle occupies most of the hemisphere. The occipital horn has not yet developed, and the atrium (At) is posteriorly blunt. The prominent choroid plexus (CP) fills most of the ventricular cavity. Note the high roof of the body (B) of the lateral ventricle. At 23 weeks, the ventricle is reduced considerably in size, and the occipital horn (OH) starts to develop. At 30 weeks, the occipital horn is fully developed. TH, temporal horns. **B.** Barium casts of the fetal lateral ventricles at 16, 23, and 30 weeks of gestation. Note the similarity to the ultrasound images. *(Figure B reproduced with permission from Keir: In Newton, Potts (eds): Radiology of the Skull and Brain. Anatomy and Pathology. St. Louis, CV Mosby, 1977, pp 2787–2913.)*

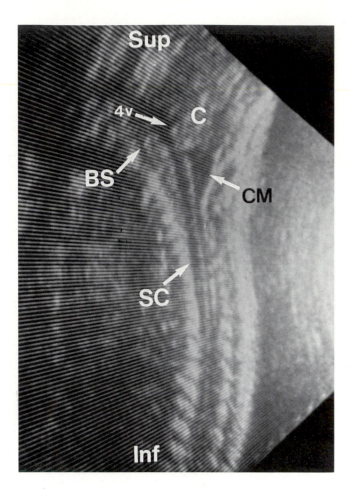

Figure 1–23. Sagittal scan of the upper fetal spine. Because of incomplete calcification of the vertebrae, the spinal cord (SC) can be seen clearly and followed superiorly to the brain stem (BS) and cerebellum (C). The cisterna magna (CM) appears as a triangular, echo-spared area interposed between the brain stem and the cerebellar vermis. The fourth ventricle (4v) is seen indenting the cerebellar vermis posteriorly. Sup, superior; Inf, inferior.

weeks, the opercularization of the insula is incomplete. Therefore, the sylvian cistern extends as a square-shaped, fluid-filled area between the lobe of the insula and the inner layer of the calvarium.

SCANNING THE FETAL SPINE

There are three main scanning planes used in the evaluation of the spine: sagittal, transverse, and coronal (Fig. 1–26).

In the sagittal plane, the spine appears as two parallel lines converging caudally in the sacrum. The lines correspond to the posterior elements of the vertebrae and the vertebral body (Fig. 1–27). Between the two lines, the spinal cord can be seen. This plane is useful for evaluating spinal curvatures; exaggeration of the curvature may be an indirect sign of spina bifida. A useful hint in the evaluation of the integrity

of the fetal spine is the presence of a normal thickness of subcutaneous tissue overlying the vertebrae.

In the coronal plane, the normal spine appears as either two or three parallel lines. The two lines are seen when the scanning plane is more dorsal. Moving the transducer anteriorly, a third line comes into view (Fig. 1–28). There is disagreement about the precise nature of these images. The two parallel lines have been attributed to the echo created by the complex formed by the articular elements and the

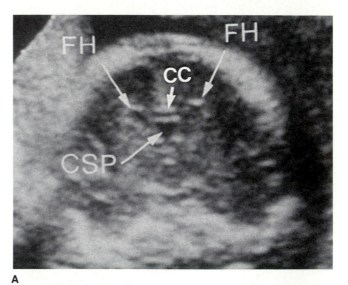

A

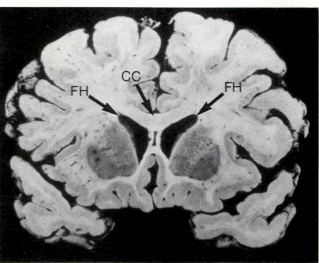

B

Figure 1–24. A. Anterior coronal scan in a second trimester fetus. The frontal horns (FH) of the lateral ventricles are separated by the patent cavum septi pellucidi (CSP). The corpus callosum (CC) appears as an anechoic band interposed between the cavum septi pellucidi and the interhemispheric fissure. **B.** Anatomic specimen corresponding to the coronal section shown in Figure A obtained from the brain of an adult. The cavum septi pellucidi is obliterated. *(Figure B reproduced with permission from Matsui, Irano: An Atlas of the Human Brain for Computed Tomography. Tokyo, Igaku Shoin, 1978.)*

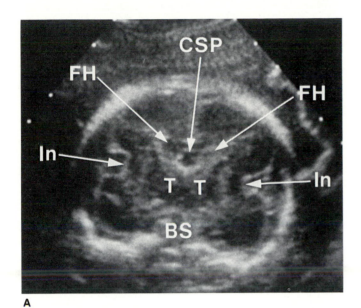

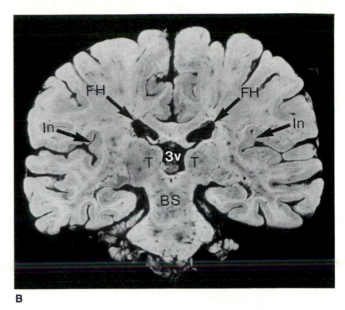

A   **B**

Figure 1–25. A. Midcoronal scan in a second trimester fetus passing through the frontal horns (FH), cavum septi pellucidi (CVS), thalami (T), and brain stem (BS). Because of the incomplete opercularization of the insula (In), the sylvian cistern appears as a prominent, fluid-filled area extending to the inner layer of the calvarium. **B.** Anatomic specimen corresponding to the coronal section shown in Figure A. This specimen was obtained from the brain of an adult, and the insula is normally covered by the opercula. 3v, third ventricle. *(Figure B reproduced with permission from Matsui, Irano: An Atlas of the Human Brain for Computed Tomography. Tokyo, Igaku Shoin, 1978.)*

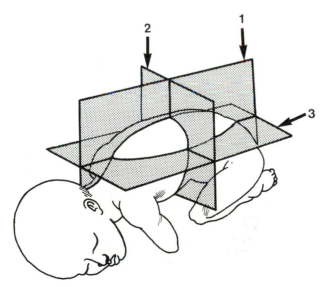

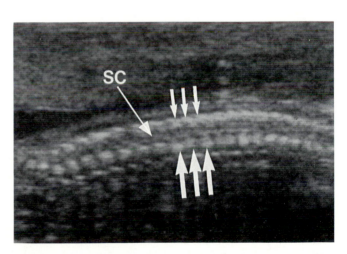

Figure 1–27. Sagittal scan of the fetal spine. The vertebral bodies (*large arrows*) and the posterior processes of the vertebrae (*small arrows*) delineate on both sides the neural canal, within which the spinal cord (SC) can be seen. Note the normal amount of soft tissue overlying the spine.

Figure 1–26. Schematic representation of the evaluation of the fetal spine: (1) sagittal plane, (2) transverse plane, and (3) coronal plane.

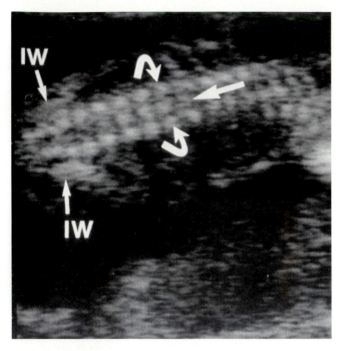

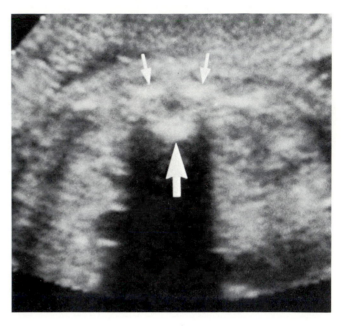

Figure 1–28. Coronal scan of the fetal spine. Note the typical three-lined appearance of the vertebrae (*arrows*). The iliac wings (IW) are seen on both sides of the sacrum.

Figure 1–29. A. A cross-section of the fetal spine on the lumbar area. The neural canal is lined by the two posterior ossification centers of the laminae (*small arrows*) and by the vertebral body (*large arrow*). Note the normal amount of soft tissue overlying the spine.

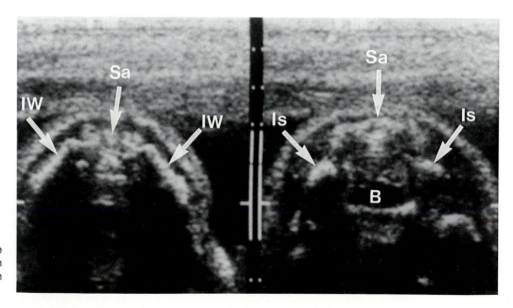

Figure 1–29. B. Cross-section of the fetal spine at the level of the sacrum (Sa), iliac wings (IW), and ischium (Is). B, bladder.

lamina of the vertebrae. The third line probably corresponds to the vertebral body.

Coronal planes should not be confused with oblique sections. A helpful hint in this regard is to examine the amount of tissue on both sides of the fetus. A correct coronal plane requires equal amounts of soft tissue on both sides of the spine. Oblique sections can be recognized by the asymmetry of the fetal trunk.

In transverse sections, the neural canal appears as a closed circle. It is lined anteriorly by the ossification center in the body of the vertebrae and posteriorly by the two ossification centers of the laminae (Fig. 1–29).

REFERENCES

1. Christenson D, McCown RB: The elusive ellipse. Am J Obstet Gynecol 152:114, 1985.
2. Denkhaus H, Winsberg F: Ultrasonic measurement of the fetal ventricular system. Radiology 131:781, 1979.
3. Dorovini-Zis K, Dolman CL: Gestational development of brain. Arch Pathol Lab Med 101:192, 1977.
4. Fiske CE, Filly RA, Callen PW: Sonographic measurement of lateral ventricular width in early ventricular dilation. J Clin Ultrasound 9:303, 1981.
5. Hadlock FP, Deter RL, Park SK: Real-time sonography: Ventricular and vascular anatomy of the fetal brain in utero. AJR 136:133, 1981.
6. Hadlock FP, Kent WR, Loyd JL, et al.: An evaluation of two methods for measuring fetal head and body circumferences. J Ultrasound Med 1:359, 1982.
7. Jeanty P, Dramaix-Wilmet M, Delbeke D, et al.: Ultrasonic evaluation of fetal ventricular growth. Neuroradiology 21:127, 1981.
8. Johnson ML, Dunne MG, Mack LA, et al.: Evaluation of fetal intracranial anatomy by static and real-time ultrasound. J Clin Ultrasound 8:311, 1980.
9. Shepard M, Filly RA: A standarized plane for biparietal diameter measurement. J Ultrasound Med 1:145, 1982.

HYDROCEPHALUS

Hydrocephalus is commonly defined as an increased intracranial content of cerebrospinal fluid (CSF). Even though many disorders of the CNS share this condition, the term "hydrocephalus" is generally used to refer to a situation in which an abnormal accumulation of CSF results in enlargement of the ventricular system. Figure 1–30 shows the origin, circulation, and drainage of CSF. CSF is formed mainly at the level of the choroid plexuses inside the ventricular system and flows slowly from the lateral ventricles to the third ventricle and from there to the fourth ventricle. At this level, CSF passes through the foramina of Luschka and Magendie inside the subarachnoid space that externally bathes the cerebral structures. Flowing along the subarachnoid cisterns, the fluid is then reabsorbed by the granulations of Pacchioni that are mainly distributed along the superior sagittal sinus.

In the majority of cases, congenital hydrocephalus is the consequence of an obstruction along the normal pathway of the CSF (obstructive hydrocephaly). Hydrocephalus is one of the most common congenital anomalies, with an incidence of 0.3 to 0.8 per 1000 births.[12]

The diagnosis of hydrocephalus has traditionally relied on the demonstration of enlarged lateral ventricles (Fig. 1–31). Several nomograms have been developed to quantify the dimensions of the lateral ventricles.[9,13–15] As previously described (see p. 2), the LVW:HW ratio is the parameter most frequently used for this assessment. However, several false negative diagnoses in early pregnancy have been reported[4,10,14] and they raise questions about the sensitivity of the measurement of the LVW:HW ratio in diagnosing early or mild ventricular dilatation. Morphologic, rather than purely biometric, criteria have been suggested for the early detection of hydrocephalus, including the simultaneous visualization of the medial and lateral wall of the lateral ventricle[10] and the anterior displacement of the choroid plexus[7] (Fig. 1–32). Recently, measurement of the atria of the lateral ventricle has been suggested.[2] At present, the problem of early detection of hydrocephalus remains unsolved. We have found that from 16 to 20 weeks of pregnancy, a combination of morphologic and biometric criteria allows for either a specific diagnosis or a questionable diagnosis in the majority of cases.

Associated Anomalies

Hydrocephalus is commonly associated with other congenital anomalies. Associated intracranial anomalies have been reported in 37 percent of hydrocephalus cases. They include hypoplasia of the corpus callosum, cephalocele, arteriovenous malformation, and arachnoid cyst. Extracranial anomalies were pres-

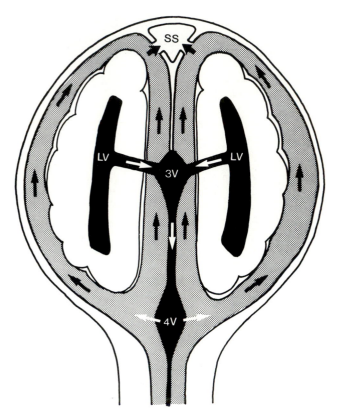

Figure 1–30. Schematic representation of the circulation and turnover of cerebrospinal fluid. The fluid is formed mainly inside the ventricular system by the choroid plexuses. It then flows slowly from the lateral ventricles (LV) to the third ventricle (3V) and fourth ventricle (4V). At this level, it escapes into the subarachnoid space (shaded area) and flows toward the superior sagittal sinus (SS), where it is reabsorbed.

ent in 63 percent of cases and included meningomyelocele, renal anomalies (bilateral or unilateral renal agenesis, dysplastic kidneys), cardiac anomalies (ventricular septal defect, tetralogy of Fallot), gastrointestinal anomalies (colon and anal agenesis,

malrotation of the bowel), cleft lip and palate, Meckel syndrome, gonadal dysgenesis, sirenomelia, arthrogryposis, and dysplastic phalanges. Chromosomal anomalies were present in 11 percent of cases, including trisomy 21, balanced translocation, and mosaicism.[3] Table 1–6 displays the associated anomalies found in a different obstetrical series.

Prognosis

The three major forms of hydrocephalus are aqueductal stenosis, communicating hydrocephalus, and Dandy-Walker syndrome.[1,11] Because the sonographic appearance[18] and prognosis of each variety differ, they are discussed separately.

Prognostic figures reported in each section are derived from pediatric series, and therefore they should be used with caution in counseling obstetric patients. Furthermore, because it is not always possible to identify the specific type of hydrocephalus, some general information about prognosis and obstetrical management guidelines will be addressed.

There is only one study that examimes the prognosis of infants with hydrocephalus diagnosed in utero. In this report, 37 infants with a heterogeneous group of disorders having ventriculomegaly in common (uncomplicated hydrocephaly, myelomeningocele, intracranial teratoma, Meckel syndrome) were followed for 7 to 60 months.[6] Immediate neonatal death (in less than 24 hours) was associated with the presence of other congenital anomalies, namely intracranial teratoma, thanatophoric dysplasia with cloverleaf skull, cebocephaly, sirenomelia, Meckel syndrome, tetralogy of Fallot, and arthrogryposis multiplex congenita. Among the survivors, a poor mental score (Bayley mental or Stanford-Binet <65) was associated with the presence of other anomalies, such as cephalocele, intraventricular cyst with agenesis of corpus callosum, arachnoid cyst with

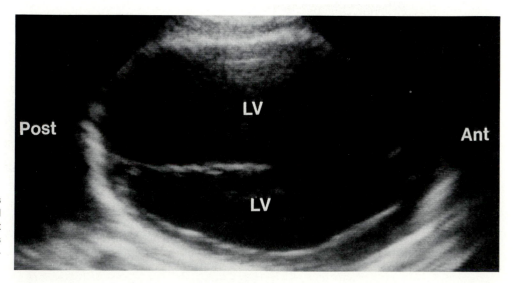

Figure 1–31. Severe hydrocephalus in a third trimester fetus. An axial scan reveals important enlargement of the bodies of the lateral ventricles (LV) and thinning of the cerebral mantle. Ant, anterior; Post, posterior.

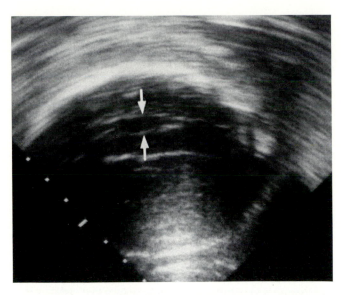

Figure 1–32. A. In this 30-week fetus, both medial and lateral walls of the body of the lateral ventricle (*arrows*) are simultaneously visualized. The fetus was found to have spina bifida and subsequently developed marked ventriculomegaly.

agenesis of corpus callosum, microcephaly, and ring chromosome 18. On the other hand, all cases with normal intelligence (Bayley mental or Stanford-Binet score >80) did not have associated anomalies or they had meningomyelocele. Therefore, the most important prognostic consideration is the presence and nature of the associated anomalies.

Pediatric data suggest that a correlation exists between cortical mantle thickness before shunting and long-term intellectual performances. Thickness of less than 1 cm has been associated with a poor outcome.[19] However, this correlation is imperfect and excellent neurologic outcomes have been observed

after early shunting with mantle thickness of less than 1 cm. This parameter, therefore, should not be used for obstetrical management decisions.

Obstetrical Management

A search for associated congenital anomalies and a workup for congenital infections associated with hydrocephaly (i.e., toxoplasmosis, cytomegalovirus, rubella) is indicated. Amniocentesis should be performed for alphafetoprotein, fetal karyotype, and viral cultures. Before viability, the option of pregnancy termination should be offered to the parents. After viability, the management issues are the role of intrauterine treatment with ventriculo-amniotic shunt, time and mode of delivery, and cephalocentesis.

Little data exist to support any specific management plan. Our general recommendations include delaying delivery until fetal lung maturity is documented, avoiding cephalocentesis, and using cesarean section for obstetrical indications only. Fetal lung maturity is determined by performing weekly amniocenteses beginning at 36 weeks of gestation. Cephalocentesis is associated with a perinatal mortality in excess of 90 percent[5,6] and its use should be limited to those instances in which hydrocephaly is associated with anomalies carrying a dismal prognosis (e.g., thanatophoric dysplasia and Meckel syndrome). This procedure should be performed under sonographic guidance. Macrocrania or overt hydrocephaly (head circumference above the 98th percentile for gestational age) in the absence of any other associated anomaly suggesting poor prognosis is not an indication for cephalocentesis. Most infants with hydrocephaly do not have macrocrania, and therefore a trial of labor is indicated in vertex presentation. Cesarean section should be reserved for stan-

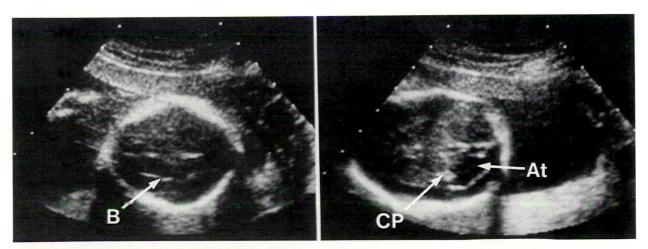

Figure 1–32. B. Early hydrocephalus in an 18-week fetus with spina bifida. Although the LVW:HW ratio is within normal limits, ventriculomegaly is inferred by the anterior displacement of the choroid plexus (CP), which does not entirely fill the atrium (At). The body of the lateral ventricle (B) is within normal limits.

TABLE 1–6. SYSTEMIC ANOMALIES IN 30 HYDROCEPHALIC FETUSES

Anomaly	No.
Trisomy 18	2
Trisomy 21	1
Complete atrioventricular canal	1
Pulmonary atresia with intact ventricular septum	1
Duodenal atresia	1
Obstructive uropathy	1
Unilateral renal agenesis and rectovesical fistula	1
Thanatophoric dysplasia	1
TOTAL	9

Modified from Pilu et al.: Ultrasound Med Biol 12:319, 1986.

dard obstetrical indications (e.g., fetal distress, failure to progress in labor, and malpresentations).

Intrauterine treatment for hydrocephaly, consisting of the implantation of a ventriculoamniotic shunt for the relief of intracranial pressure during gestation, has been attempted.[5,8] Although experience in animal models appears encouraging,[17] the clinical application of these procedures remains undetermined. In a group of 39 treated fetuses, the perinatal mortality rate was 18 percent, and 66 percent of the survivors were affected by moderate to severe handicaps.[16]

REFERENCES

1. Burton BK: Recurrence risks for congenital hydrocephalus. Clin Genet 16:47, 1979.
2. Campbell S, Pearce JM: Ultrasound visualization of congenital malformations. Br Med Bull 39:322, 1983.
3. Chervenak, FA, Berkowitz RL, Romero R, et al.: The diagnosis of fetal hydrocephalus. Am J Obstet Gynecol 147:703, 1983.
4. Chervenak, FA, Berkowitz RL, Tortora M, et al.: Diagnosis of ventriculomegaly before fetal viability. Obstet Gynecol 64:652, 1984.
5. Chervenak, FA, Berkowitz RL, Tortora M, et al.: The management of fetal hydrocephalus. Am J Obstet Gynecol 151:933, 1985.
6. Chervenak, FA, Duncan C, Ment LR, et al.: Outcome of fetal ventriculomegaly. Lancet 2:179, 1984.
7. Chinn DH, Callen PW, Filly RA: The lateral cerebral ventricle in early second trimester. Radiology 148:529, 1983.
8. Clewell WH, Johnson ML, Meier PR, et al.: A surgical approach to the treatment of fetal hydrocephalus. N Engl J Med 306:1320, 1982.
9. Denkhaus H, Winsberg F: Ultrasonic measurement of the fetal ventricular system. Radiology 131:781, 1979.
10. Fiske CE, Filly RA, Callen PW: Sonographic measurement of lateral ventricular width in early ventricular dilation. J Clin Ultrasound 9:303, 1981.
11. Guidetti B, Giuffre R, Palma L, et al.: Hydrocephalus in infancy and childhood. Childs Brain 2:209, 1976.
12. Habib Z: Genetics and genetic counseling in neonatal hydrocephalus. Obstet Gynecol Surv 36:529, 1981.
13. Hadlock FP, Deter RL, Park SK: Real-time sonography: Ventricular and vascular anatomy of the fetal brain in utero. AJR 136:133, 1981.
14. Jeanty P, Dramaix-Wilmet M, Delbeke D, et al.: Ultrasound evaluation of fetal ventricular growth. Neurology 21:127, 1981.
15. Johnson ML, Dunne MG, Mack LA, et al.: Evaluation of fetal intracranial anatomy by static and real-time ultrasound. J Clin Ultrasound 8:311, 1980.
16. Manning FA: International fetal surgery registry: 1985 update. Clin Obstet Gynecol 29:551, 1986.
17. Michejda M, Hodgen GD: In utero diagnosis and treatment of non-human primate fetal skeletal anomalies. I. Hydrocephalus. JAMA 246:1093, 1981.
18. Pilu G, Rizzo N, Orsini LF, et al.: Antenatal detection of fetal cerebral anomalies. Ultrasound Med Biol 12:319, 1986.
19. Vintzileos AM, Ingardia CJ, Nochimson, DJ: Congenital hydrocephalus: A review and protocol for perinatal management. Obstet Gynecol 62:539, 1983.

Aqueductal Stenosis

Synonyms
Stenosis of the aqueduct of Sylvius and aqueduct stenosis.

Definition
Aqueductal stenosis is a form of obstructive hydrocephalus caused by narrowing of the aqueduct of Sylvius.

Incidence
Aqueductal stenosis is the most frequent cause of congenital hydrocephaly. It has been reported to account for 43 percent of the cases studied. Male to female ratio is 1.8.[3]

Etiology
Aqueductal stenosis is a heterogeneous disease for which genetic,[2,3,5,6,8,14,17–19,21,22] infectious,[1,9,11,20] teratogenic,[18] and neoplastic[13,18] causes have been implicated. The relative contributions of these factors have been determined from autopsy studies. Histologic evi-

dence of inflammation (gliosis) has been found in approximately 50 percent of the cases studied.[13] Toxoplasmosis, syphilis, cytomegalovirus, mumps, and influenza virus have caused aqueductal stenosis in animals.[18] In cases without evidence of inflammation, the disease appears to be the consequence of maldevelopment for an unknown reason. This maldevelopment is histologically expressed by forking (see Pathology) or simple narrowing of the aqueduct. Genetic transmission has been postulated to account for some of these cases. Many familial studies have demonstrated that aqueductal stenosis can be inherited as an X-linked recessive trait.[2,3,5,6,8,14,17,19,21,22] Sex-linked transmission was thought to be a rare cause of the disease, because only 1 case was found among 200 siblings of probands with hydrocephalus.[6] However, it has been suggested that this mode of inheritance involves 25 percent of affected male infants.[3] The possibility of a coexistent polygenic pattern of inheritance has been suggested by case reports of families in which both females and males were affected.[3]

Teratogenic agents, such as radiation, have been implicated in animal models, but the relevance of these observations to humans is uncertain.[18] Such tumors as gliomas, pinealomas, meningiomas, and other conditions (neurofibromatosis and tuberous sclerosis) may cause aqueductal stenosis by a compressive mechanism.[13] However, the prevalence of these entities in the prenatal period is extremely low.

It has also been suggested that communicating hydrocephalus may lead to secondary aqueductal stenosis, causing white matter edema and extrinsic compression.[15]

Embryology
The aqueduct of Sylvius is the portion of the ventricular system that connects the third and fourth ventricles (Fig. 1–30). The aqueduct develops from a narrowing of the primitive ventricular cavity between the prosencephalon and rhomboencephalon at about the sixth week (conceptional age).

Pathology
Aqueductal stenosis may result from an inflammatory process or a developmental anomaly. "Gliosis" is the term used to describe the inflammatory reaction seen in the CNS. This reaction is characterized by a mononuclear–microglial response and a repair process conducted by astrocytes.[13] Malformations include forking, narrowing, and the presence of a transverse septum.[18] Forking describes the substitution of the aqueduct by multiple narrow channels. Narrowing may be of variable degree and is usually accompanied by an irregular outline of the ependymal wall. When a septum is responsible for the stenosis of the aqueduct, it is usually located in its posterior portion.

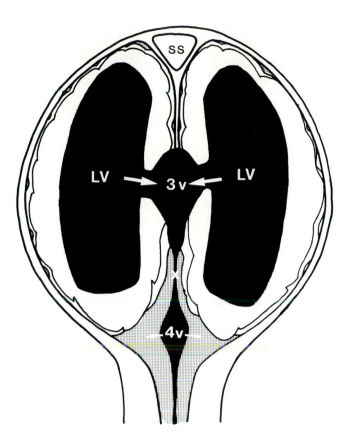

Figure 1–33. Schematic representation of aqueductal stenosis. Narrowing of the aqueduct of Sylvius leads to enlargement of the lateral and third ventricles. LV, lateral ventricles; 3v, third ventricle; 4v, fourth ventricle; SS, superior sagittal sinus.

Narrowing is the most common finding in hereditary cases. Aqueductal stenosis is associated with a variable degree of dilatation of the lateral and third ventricles (Fig. 1–33).

Knowledge about the pathogenesis of congenital obstructive hydrocephaly is largely incomplete. Studies performed in experimental animals and based on biopsies of brain tissue obtained in children at the time of shunting seem to demonstrate the following sequence of events. Initially, there is disruption of the ependymal lining, followed by edema of the white matter. This phase has been considered reversible. Later, there is astrocyte proliferation and fibrosis of the white matter. The gray matter seems to be spared during the initial phase of the process.

Associated Anomalies
Other congenital anomalies occur in 16 percent of infants with aqueductal stenosis.[3] Bilateral thumb deformities of flexion and adduction have been seen in 17 percent of the sex-linked inherited type.[18]

Diagnosis
A diagnosis of aqueductal stenosis is suggested by enlargement of the lateral ventricles (which can be

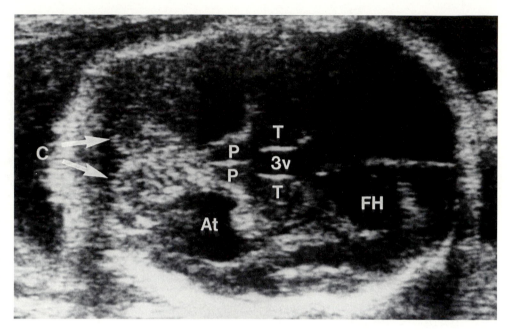

Figure 1–34. Axial scan angled posteriorly of the head of a fetus that was found at birth to have aqueductal stenosis. There is enlargement of the frontal horns (FH) and atria (At) of the lateral ventricles and of the third ventricle (3v). The fourth ventricle is not visualized. T, thalami; C, cerebellum; P, peduncles.

either symmetrical or slightly asymmetrical) and of the third ventricle in the presence of a normal fourth ventricle (Figs. 1–34, 1–35).[16] Unfortunately, this finding is nonspecific, since many cases of communicating hydrocephaly may have similar appearances, and the differential diagnosis between these two conditions may be impossible. Careful scanning of the fetal spine is recommended in order to rule out a coexistent spinal defect.

Prognosis
Data about survival are not complete, because a significant number of infants with this condition have been reported to die either in utero or in the very early neonatal period, thereby escaping epidemio-

logic surveillance. Data concerning intellectual development come mainly from two neurosurgical series of overt hydrocephaly. Guthkelch and Riley[7] reported a mortality rate of 30 percent and normal intellectual development (IQ >70) in 50 percent of treated infants. In contrast, McCullough and Balzer-Martin[12] found a mean IQ of 71 (SD = 23) among all treated neonates and a mortality rate of 11 percent. From these figures, it is clear that there is a possibility for intellectual normality.

Obstetrical Management
An amniocentesis for chromosomal determination is always recommended. The approach to obstetrical management varies depending on the time of the

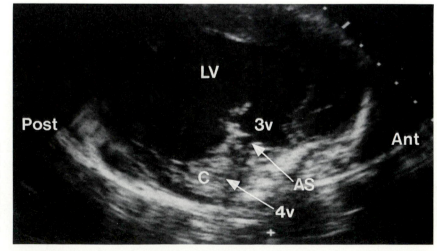

Figure 1–35. Midsagittal scan in the same patient as in Figure 1–34. The lateral ventricle (LV), third ventricle (3v), and proximal aqueduct of Sylvius (AS) are dilated. The fourth ventricle (4v) appears to be of normal size. It should be stressed that these findings may indicate aqueductal stenosis and communicating hydrocephalus as well. Ant, anterior; Post, posterior.

diagnosis. Before viability, the option of pregnancy termination should be offered to the mother. The mode of delivery depends purely on obstetrical indications. Cephalocentesis should not be used in cases of isolated aqueductal stenosis. Cesarean section is only indicated for macrocephaly, fetal distress, or other obstetrical indications. If another congenital anomaly invariably associated with neonatal death is present, cesarean section should be avoided.[4] The role of intrauterine shunting is experimental at the present time (see also p. 23).

REFERENCES

1. Adams RD, Kubik CS, Bonner FJ: The clinical and pathological aspects of influenzal meningitis. Arch Pediatr 65:354, 1948.
2. Bickers DS, Adams RD: Hereditary stenosis of the aqueduct of Sylvius as a cause of congenital hydrocephalus. Brain 72:246, 1949.
3. Burton BK: Recurrence risks for congenital hydrocephalus. Clin Genet 16:47, 1979.
4. Chervenak FA, Berkowitz RL, Tortora M, et al.: The management of fetal hydrocephalus. Am J Obstet Gynecol 151:933, 1985.
5. Edwards JH: The syndrome of sex-linked hydrocephalus. Arch Dis Child 36:486, 1961.
6. Edwards JH, Norman RM, Roberts JM: Sex-linked hydrocephalus: Report of a family with 15 affected members. Arch Dis Child 36:481, 1961.
7. Guthkelch AN, Riley NA: Influence of aetiology on prognosis in surgically treated infantile hydrocephalus. Arch Dis Child 44:29, 1969.
8. Holmes LB, Nash A, ZuRhein GM, et al.: X-linked aqueductal stenosis: Clinical and neuropathological findings in two families. Pediatrics 51:697, 1973.
9. Johnson RT, Johnson KP, Edmonds CJ: Virus-induced hydrocephalus: Development of aqueductal stenosis in hamsters after mumps infection. Science 157:1066, 1967.
10. Lorber J: Results of treatment of myelomeningocele: An analysis of 524 unselected cases, with special reference to possible selection for treatment. Dev Med Child Neurol 13:279, 1971.
11. Margolis G, Kilham L: Hydrocephalus in hamsters, ferrets, rats and mice following inoculations with reovirus Type I. J Clin Invest 21:183, 1969.
12. McCullough DC, Balzer-Martin LA: Current prognosis in overt neonatal hydrocephalus. J Neurosurg 57:378, 1982.
13. Milhorat TH: Hydrocephalus and the Cerebrospinal Fluid. Baltimore, Williams & Wilkins, 1972.
14. Needleman HL, Root AW: Sex-linked hydrocephalus. Report of 2 families with chromosomal study of 2 cases. Pediatrics 31:396, 1963.
15. Nugent GR, Al-Mefty O, Chou S: Communicating hydrocephalus as a cause of aqueductal stenosis. J Neurosurg 51:812, 1979.
16. Pilu G, Rizzo N, Orsini CF, et al.: Antenatal detection of cerebral anomalies. Ultrasound Med Biol 12:319, 1986.
17. Price JR, Horne BM: Family history indicating hereditary factors in hydrocephalus. Ment Retard 6:40, 1968.
18. Salam MZ: Stenosis of the aqueduct of Sylvius. In: Vinken PJ, Bruyn GW (eds): Handbook of Clinical Neurology. Amsterdam, Elsevier/North Holland Biomedical Press, 1977, Vol 30, pp 609–622.
19. Shannon MW, Nadler HL: X-linked hydrocephalus. J Med Genet 5:326, 1968.
20. Timmons GD, Johnson KP: Aqueductal stenosis and hydrocephalus after mumps encephalitis. N Engl J Med 283:1505, 1970.
21. Warren MC, Lu AT, Ziering WH: Sex-linked hydrocephalus with aqueductal stenosis. J Pediatr 63:1104, 1963.
22. Williamson EM: Incidence and family aggregation of major congenital malformations of central nervous system. J Med Genet 2:161, 1965.

Communicating Hydrocephalus

Synonym
External hydrocephalus.

Definition
Communicating hydrocephalus is a form of enlargement of the ventricles and subarachnoid system caused by an obstruction to CSF flow outside the ventricular system.

Incidence
Communicating hydrocephalus is the second major form of congenital hydrocephalus. It accounts for 38 percent of all cases.[1]

Etiology

In most cases, the etiology is unknown. Communicating hydrocephalus is found in infants with spinal defects and has also been seen in association with obliteration of the superior sagittal sinus,[3] subarachnoid hemorrhage,[2] absence of Pacchioni granulations,[4] and choroid plexus papilloma.[8] Subarachnoid hemorrhage is probably the most common cause of infantile communicating hydrocephalus, but it is probably rare in the prenatal period. Familial transmission is rare; only 1 affected individual was found among 154 siblings of 77 probands.[1] However, the recurrence rate quoted for this condition is 1 to 2 percent, which is higher than the incidence in the general population.[1]

Pathology

The basic cause of communicating hydrocephalus is either a mechanical obstruction outside the ventricular system or an impaired reabsorption of cerebrospinal fluid.[6] This leads to dilatation of the subarachnoid space and later to the dilatation of the ventricular system[12] (Fig. 1–36). Over time, the enlargement of the subarachnoid space may become less prominent, and ventriculomegaly may be the only finding. In fact, most patients with communicating hydrocephalus show only triventricular hydrocephalus without overt enlargement of the subarachnoid space and fourth ventricle.[11] The pathophysiology of the disappearance of cisternal dilatation is not clear. However, it has been suggested that the increased intracranial pressure may eventually lead to obstruction of the aqueduct, resulting in hydrocephalus.[9]

Diagnosis

Communicating hydrocephalus causes tetraventricular enlargement (dilatation of the lateral, third, and fourth ventricles). However, because the enlargement of the fourth ventricle is often minimal (Fig. 1–37A), the main problem arises with the differential diagnosis from aqueductal stenosis. The dilatation of the subarachnoid cistern is pathognomonic of communicating hydrocephaly. This is most easily demonstrated at the level of the subarachnoid space overlying the cerebral convexities (Fig. 1–37B) and interhemispheric fissure (Fig. 1–37C).[10] Unfortunately, in a large number of cases, this image is rarely detected, making it impossible to differentiate it from aqueductal stenosis. In one longitudinal study of infants developing communicating hydrocephaly, isolated dilatation of the subarachnoid space was seen prior to ventriculomegaly.[12] Therefore, the visualization of such a finding in a fetus is an indication for follow-up examinations.

The natural history of communicating hydrocephalus is unknown. Some cases are diagnosed in utero,[10] whereas others are not recognized until infancy.[12]

Prognosis

Data concerning the survival and intellectual performance of infants with isolated congenital communicating hydrocephaly are limited, since many studies are probably biased because of the inclusion of infantile forms. The outcome appears to be much better than with other types of hydrocephaly. In an old series of 35 treated infants, the mortality rate was 11 percent. Eighty-four percent of the survivors developed a normal intelligence (IQ > 70).[5] In a more recent series of 9 treated infants, no deaths were observed, and the mean IQ was 101 (SD = 19).[7] If communicating hydrocephaly is associated with either a neural tube defect or a choroid plexus papilloma, the prognosis is different (see Spina Bifida and Choroid Plexus Papilloma).

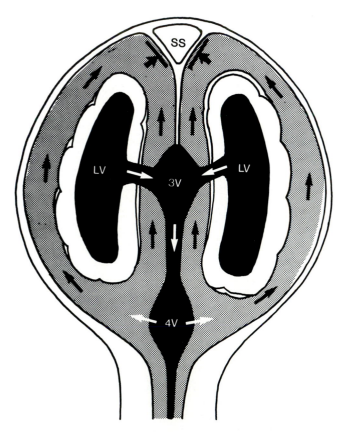

Figure 1–36. Schematic representation of communicating hydrocephalus resulting from a block of the reabsorption of the CSF at the level of the superior sagittal sinus (SS). Accumulation of fluid results in simultaneous enlargement of the ventricular and subarachnoid compartments. LV, lateral ventricles; 3v, third ventricle; 4v, fourth ventricle; shaded area corresponds to the subarachnoid space.

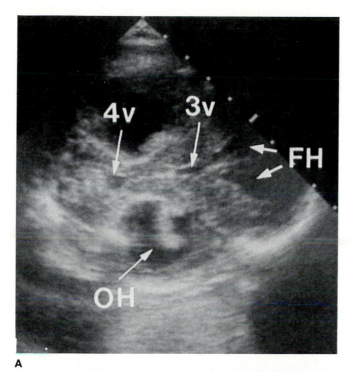

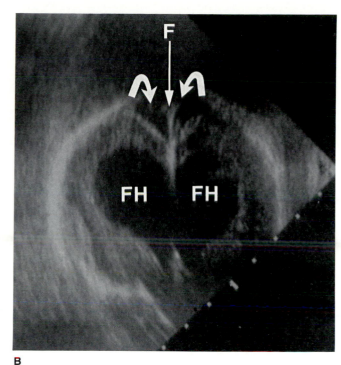

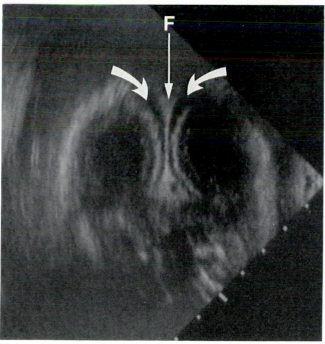

Figure 1–37. Communicating hydrocephaly in a 30-week-old fetus. **A.** An axial scan angled posteriorly reveals the dilatation of the frontal horns (FH) and occipital horns (OH) of the lateral ventricles and of the third ventricle (3v). There is a questionable enlargement of the fourth ventricle (4v). **B.** An anterior coronal scan reveals the simultaneous enlargement of the frontal horns (FH) and of the supracortical cisterns (*curved arrows*). F, falx cerebri. **C.** A slightly posterior coronal scan reveals a prominent interhemispheric fissure (*arrows*). F, falx cerebri. *(Figures B and C reproduced with permission from Pilu et al.: J Ultrasound Med 5:365, 1986.)*

Obstetrical Management
The approach does not differ from that outlined for aqueductal stenosis (see pp. 23, 27).

REFERENCES

1. Burton BK: Recurrence risks for congenital hydrocephalus. Clin Genet 16:47, 1979.
2. Ellington E, Margolis G: Block of arachnoid villus by subarachnoid hemorrhage. J Neurosurg 30:651, 1969.
3. Emery JL, Zachary RB: Hydrocephalus associated with obliteration of the longitudinal sinus. Arch Dis Child 31:288, 1956.
4. Gutierrez Y, Friede RL, Kaliney WJ: Agenesis of arachnoid granulations and its relationship to communicating hydrocephalus. J Neurosurg 43:553, 1975.
5. Guthkelch AN, Riley NA: Influence of aetiology on prognosis in surgically treated infantile hydrocephalus. Arch Dis Child 44:29, 1969.
6. McComb JG: Recent research into the nature of cerebrospinal fluid formation and absorption. J Neurosurg 59:369, 1983.
7. McCullough DC, Balzer-Martin LA: Current prognosis in overt neonatal hydrocephalus. J Neurosurg 57:378, 1982.
8. Milhorat TH, Hammock MK, Davis DA, et al.: Choroid plexus papilloma. I. Proof of cerebrospinal fluid overproduction. Childs Brain 2:273, 1976.
9. Nugent GR, Al-Mefty O, Chou S: Communicating hydrocephalus as a cause of aqueductal stenosis. J Neurosurg 51:812, 1979.
10. Pilu G, DePalma L, Romero R, et al.: The fetal subarachnoid cisterns: An ultrasound study. With report of a case of communicating hydrocephalus. J Ultrasound Med 5:365, 1986.
11. Raybaud C, Bamberger-Bozo C, Laffont J, et al.: Investigation of nontumoral hydrocephalus in children. Neuroradiology 16:24, 1978.
12. Robertson WC, Gomez MR: External hydrocephalus. Early finding in congenital communicating hydrocephalus. Arch Neurol 35:541, 1978.

Dandy-Walker Malformation

Synonym
Dandy-Walker syndrome.

Definition
Dandy-Walker malformation (DWM) is characterized by the association of (1) hydrocephalus of variable degree, (2) a cyst in the posterior fossa, and (3) a defect in the cerebellar vermis through which the cyst communicates with the fourth ventricle.

Incidence
DWM accounts for 12 percent of all cases of congenital hydrocephalus.[5] However, this figure may represent an underestimation of the real incidence because cases without hydrocephalus and without significant symptoms have also been reported.[23]

Etiology
Unknown. DWM may occur as a part of mendelian disorders, such as Meckel syndrome and Warburg syndrome. It has been found in chromosomal aberrations, such as Turner syndrome, 6p−, 9qh+, trisomy 9, and triploidy. Environmental factors, such as viral infection, alcohol, and diabetes, have been suggested as playing a role in its etiology.[29] When DWM is not associated with mendelian disorders, the recurrence risk is 1 to 5 percent.[29] In rare cases, the disease is probably inherited as an autosomal recessive trait, with a recurrence risk of 25 percent.[23] A cerebral anomaly similar to DWM, Joubert syndrome, is also inherited as an autosomal recessive trait.[24]

History
DWM was formally described by Dandy and Blackfan at the beginning of the century.[7,8] They postulated this condition to be secondary to congenital atresia of the foramina of Luschka and Magendie, which provide an exit to the CSF from the fourth ventricle to the subarachnoid space. Walker was the physician who described the first surgical treatment.[35] Although Benda[2] proved that the pathogenetic hypothesis suggested by these authors was untenable, he suggested the eponym, Dandy-Walker syndrome.

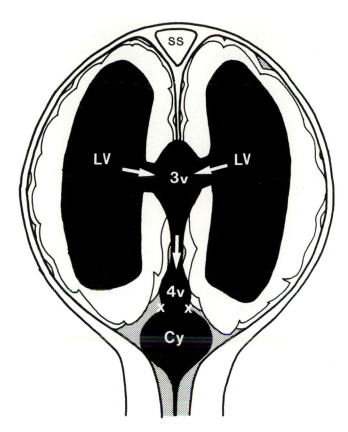

Figure 1–38. Schematic representation of Dandy-Walker syndrome. The fourth ventricle (4v) communicates with a posterior fossa cyst (Cy). An exit block of the CSF at the level of the foramina of Luschka and Magendie (X) results in enlargement of the fourth, third (3v), and lateral ventricles (LV). SS, superior sagittal sinus.

Embryology

According to the original theory of Dandy[7,8] and Walker,[35] atresia of the foramina of Luschka and Magendie would lead to dilatation of the ventricular system. However, Benda[2] subsequently observed that (1) the foramina of Luschka and Magendie are not atretic in all cases and (2) it is difficult to understand how atresia of these foramina (which are not normally patent until the fourth month of gestation) would lead to cerebellar vermis hypoplasia. It is now commonly accepted that DWM is a more complex developmental abnormality of the rhomboencephalic midline structures. Gardner et al.[14] have proposed that the malformation is due to an imbalance between the CSF production in the lateral and third ventricles and in the fourth ventricle. The overproduction of CSF at the level of the fourth ventricle would lead to early dilatation and herniation of the rhomboencephalic roof. Dilatation would be maximal at the level of the fourth ventricle, resulting in compression and secondary hypoplasia of the cerebellar vermis. The enlargement of the fourth ventricle would be responsible for the cyst seen in the posterior fossa.

Pathology

The three pathologic features are hydrocephalus, a cerebellar vermis defect, and a retrocerebellar cyst (Fig. 1–38). The vermian defect is variable, ranging from complete aplasia to a small fissure. The retrocerebellar cyst is internally lined by ependyma and is of variable size.[2-4,20] Although hydrocephalus has been classically considered to be an essential diagnostic element of DWM, recent evidence suggests that it is not present at birth in most patients, but it develops usually in the first months of life.[23] This is relevant for prenatal diagnosis because the only detectable signs in these fetuses would be the posterior fossa abnormalities. Depending on whether the foramina of Luschka and Magendie are open or closed, the malformation would be classified as "communicating" or "noncommunicating." This classification is relevant because the noncommunicating forms are associated with variable degrees of hydrocephaly.

TABLE 1–7. DWM ASSOCIATION WITH OTHER ABNORMALITIES

Mendelian	Chromosomal	Environmental	Multifactoral	Sporadic
Warburg* (AR)	45, X	Rubella*	Congenital heart disease*	Holoprosencephaly
Aase-Smith (arthrogryposis) (AD)	6p−	Coumadin	Neural tube defects*	Cornelia de Lange
Ruvalcaba syndrome (AD/XL)	9qh+*	Alcohol	Cleft lip/palate*	Goldenhar
Coffin-Siris syndrome* (AR)	dup 5p*	CMV		Kidney abnormalities*
Oral–facial digital syndrome, type II* (AR)	dup 8p*	Diabetes		Facial hemangiomas*
	dup 8q*			
Meckel-Gruber syndrome* (AR)	trisomy 9*	Isotretinoin*		Klippel-Feil*
Aicardi syndrome* (XL)	triploidy*			Polysyndactyly*
Joubert-Boltshauser syndrome* (AR)	dup 17q			
X-linked cerebellar hypoplasia* (XL)				
Ellis van Creveld (AR)				
Fraser cryptophthalmos (AR)				

AD, autosomal dominant; AR, autosomal recessive; XL, X-linked.
* Reported in more than one unrelated child.
Modified from Murray et al.: Clin Genet 28:272, 1985.

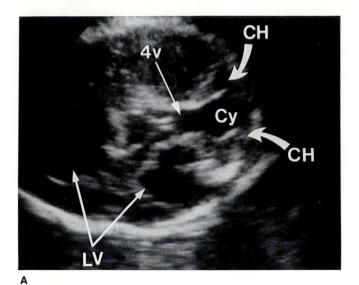

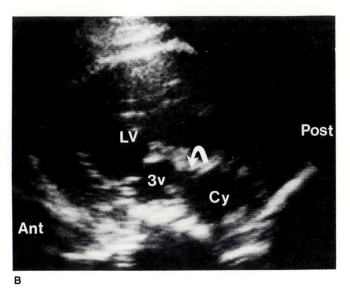

A

B

Figure 1–39. A. In this fetus with hydrocephaly, an axial scan directed posteriorly demonstrates the pathognomonic findings of Dandy-Walker syndrome: A posterior fossa cyst (Cy) is seen to communicate with the grossly enlarged fourth ventricle (4v) through a vermian defect. CH, cerebellar hemispheres; LV, enlarged lateral ventricle. **B.** In this midsagittal scan of fetus in Figure A, the enlarged third ventricle (3v) communicates through a typically dilated and kinked aqueduct (*curved arrow*) with the posterior fossa cyst (Cy). LV, lateral ventricle; Ant, anterior; Post, posterior. *(Reproduced with permission from Pilu et al.: J Reprod Med 31:1017, 1986.)*

Associated Anomalies

DWM is frequently associated with other CNS abnormalities. Clinical studies have found an incidence of 50 percent of associated anomalies.[34] Agenesis of the corpus callosum has been reported to occur in between 7[23] and 17[34] percent of patients studied. Pathologic studies have demonstrated an incidence of cerebral defects as high as 68 percent.[20] However, it should be stressed that most of these anomalies (polymicrogyria, agyria, microgyria, malformation of the inferior olives) are not sonographically detectable in utero. Other anomalies include encephaloceles, polycystic kidneys, and cardiovascular de-

fects (mainly ventricular septal defects).[4,23,31,34] A detailed list of genetic and nongenetic conditions associated with DWM is given in Table 1–7.

Diagnosis

The diagnosis of DWM should be considered whenever a cystic mass is seen in the posterior fossa.[9–11,22,25,26,30,32,36] The differential diagnosis includes an arachnoid cyst and dilatation of the cisterna magna. A defect in the vermis, through which the cyst communicates with the fourth ventricle, is pathognomonic of DWM. Such a finding is well documented in both computed tomo-

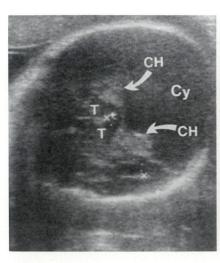

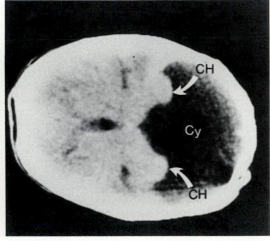

Figure 1–40. Dandy-Walker syndrome with a large posterior fossa cyst (Cy). Note the widely separated cerebellar hemispheres (CH). The prenatal ultrasound study is compared with a postnatal computed tomographic scan. T, thalami. *(Reproduced with permission from Pilu et al.: J Reprod Med 31:1017, 1986.)*

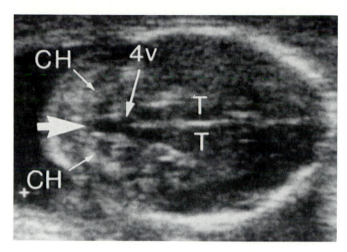

Figure 1–41. In this 21-week fetus, Dandy-Walker syndrome is revealed only by the presence of a defect of the inferior vermis (*arrow*) at the level of the 4th ventricle (4v). CH, cerebellar hemispheres; T, thalami. (*Reproduced with permission from Pilu et al.: J Reprod Med 31:1017, 1986.*)

graphic[13,17,21,23,27,34] and ultrasound studies[15–17,36] in the postnatal period, and it can be demonstrated in the fetus as well[32] (Fig. 1–39). The defect may vary in size from a small fissure to a large tunnel with widely separated cerebellar hemispheres (Fig. 1–40). Extreme care is necessary because, in some cases, the superior vermis is intact and the defect can only be demonstrated by careful examination of the inferior vermis (Fig. 1–41).

Differentiation from an arachnoid cyst or enlarged cisterna magna may be difficult, however. This difficulty can be encountered even in the neonatal period despite the use of computed tomography. There is controversy in the radiologic literature about the optimal means of making a diagnosis. Some authors are concerned about the limitations of computed tomography and recommend that a pneumoencephalogram be performed.[1] Other authors believe that pneumoencephalography may be misleading and recommend contrast studies (metrimazide, radionucleotides) when noncontrast computed tomography is equivocal.[27,34]

Traditionally, DWM has been considered a cause of intrauterine hydrocephalus. However, the evidence indicates that this association is not frequent in the fetus.[23,32] Therefore, we recommend a careful study of the posterior fossa as part of a routine survey of the intracranial anatomy.[32]

Prognosis and Obstetrical Management

Data on the prognosis of DWM are controversial. The first in-depth large series concerning the treatment of infants affected by DWM indicated a uniformly poor prognosis.[12,18,19,33] The mortality rate was about 50 percent, and 50 to 60 percent of the survivors were intellectually impaired. In two recent series, survival rates of 74 percent[34] and 88 percent,[23] with an IQ above 80 in 30 and 60 percent of survivors, respectively, have been reported. Consequently, we believe that if a positive diagnosis is made before viability, the option of pregnancy termination should be offered to the parents. It is difficult to provide guidelines for the management of fetuses diagnosed in the third trimester. Fetal karyotyping is indicated because of the occasional association with chromosomal aberrations.[29] Depp et al.[10] reported intrauterine shunting in a case of DWM. The role of intrauterine treatment for this disease is experimental, and its efficacy is yet to be proven.

REFERENCES

1. Archer CR, Darwish H, Smith K: Enlarged cisternae magnae and posterior fossa cysts simulating Dandy-Walker syndrome on computed tomography. Radiology 127:681, 1978.
2. Benda CE: The Dandy-Walker syndrome or the so-called atresia of the foramen Magendie. J Neuropathol Exp Neurol 13:14, 1954.
3. Brodal A, Hauglie-Hanssen E: Congenital hydrocephalus with defective development of the cerebellar vermis (Dandy-Walker syndrome): Clinical and anatomical findings in two cases with particular reference to the so-called atresia of the foramina of Magendie and Luschka. J Neurol Neurosurg Psychiatry 22:99, 1959.
4. Brown JR: The Dandy-Walker syndrome. In: Vinken PJ, Bruyn GW (eds): Handbook of Clinical Neurology. Amsterdam, Elsevier/North Holland Biomedical Press, 1977, Vol 30, pp 623–646.
5. Burton BK: Recurrence risks for congenital hydrocephalus. Clin Genet 16:47, 1979.
6. Chervenak FA, Romero R: Is there a role for fetal cephalocentesis in modern obstetrics? Am J Perinatol 1:170, 1984.
7. Dandy WE: The diagnosis and treatment of hydrocephalus due to occlusion of the foramina of Magendie and Luschka. Surg Gynecol Obstet 32:112, 1921.
8. Dandy WE, Blackfan KD: Internal hydrocephalus: an experimental, clinical and pathological study. Am J Dis Child 8:406, 1914.
9. Dempsey PJ, Koch HJ: In utero diagnosis of the Dandy-Walker syndrome: Differentiation from extra-axial posterior fossa cyst. J Clin Ultrasound 9:403, 1981.
10. Depp R, Sabbagha RE, Brown T, et al.: Fetal surgery for hydrocephalus: Successful in utero ventriculoamniotic shunt for Dandy-Walker syndrome. Obstet Gynecol 61:710, 1983.
11. Fileni A, Colosimo C, Mirk P, et al.: Dandy-Walker syndrome: Diagnosis in utero by means of ultrasound and CT correlations. Neuroradiology 24:233, 1983.
12. Fischer EG: Dandy-Walker syndrome: An evaluation of surgical treatment. J Neurosurg 39:615, 1973.
13. Fitz CR: Midline anomalies of the brain and spine. Radiol Clin North Am 20:95, 1982.
14. Gardner E, O'Rahilly R, Prolo D: The Dandy-Walker

and Arnold-Chiari malformations: Clinical, developmental and teratological considerations. Arch Neurol 32:393, 1975.

15. Goodwin V, Quisling RG: The neonatal cisterna magna: Ultrasonic evaluation. Radiology 149:691, 1983.
16. Grant EG, Schellinger D, Richardson JD: Real-time ultrasonography of the posterior fossa. J Ultrasound Med 2:73, 1983.
17. Groenhout CM, Gooskens RH, Veiga-Pires JA, et al.: Value of sagittal sonography and direct sagittal CT of the Dandy-Walker syndrome. AJNR 5:476, 1984.
18. Guidetti B, Giuffre R, Palma L, et al.: Hydrocephalus in infancy and childhood. Childs Brain 2:209, 1976.
19. Guthkelch AN, Riley NA: Influence of aetiology on prognosis in surgically treated infantile hydrocephalus. Arch Dis Child 44:29, 1969.
20. Hart MN, Malamud N, Ellis WG: The Dandy-Walker syndrome: A clinicopathological study based on 28 cases. Neurology 22:771, 1972.
21. Harwood-Nash DC, Fitz CR: Congenital anomalies of the brain. In: Neuroradiology in Infants and Children. St. Louis, Mosby, 1976, Vol 3, pp 998–1053.
22. Hatjis CG, Horbar JD, Anderson GG: The in utero diagnosis of a posterior fossa intracranial cyst (Dandy-Walker cyst). Am J Obstet Gynecol 140:473, 1981.
23. Hirsch JF, Pierre-Kahn A, Renier D, et al.: The Dandy-Walker malformation: A review of 40 cases. J Neurosurg 61:515, 1984.
24. Joubert M, Eisenring JJ, Robb JP, et al.: Familial agenesis of the cerebellar vermis: A syndrome of episodic hyperpnea, abnormal eye movements, ataxia and retardation. Neurology 19:813, 1969.

25. Kirkinen P, Jouppila P, Valkeakari T, et al.: Ultrasonic evaluation of the Dandy-Walker syndrome. Obstet Gynecol 59:18S, 1982.
26. Mahony BS, Callen PW, Filly RA, et al.: The fetal cisterna magna. Radiology 153:773, 1984.
27. Masdeu JC, Dobben GD, Azar-Kia B: Dandy-Walker syndrome studied by computed tomography and pneumoencephalography. Radiology 147:109, 1983.
28. McCullough DC, Balzer-Martin LA: Current prognosis in overt neonatal hydrocephalus. J Neurosurg 57:378, 1982.
29. Murray JC, Johnson JA, Bird TD: Dandy-Walker malformation: Etiologic heterogeneity and empiric recurrence risks. Clin Genet 28:272, 1985.
30. Newman GC, Buschi AI, Sugg NK, et al.: Dandy-Walker syndrome diagnosed in utero by ultrasonography. Neurology 32:180, 1982.
31. Olson GS, Halpe DC, Kaplan AM, et al.: Dandy-Walker malformation and associated cardiac anomalies. Childs Brain 8:173, 1981.
32. Pilu G, Romero R, DePalma L, et al.: Antenatal diagnosis and obstetrical management of Dandy-Walker syndrome. J Reprod Med 31:1017, 1986.
33. Raimondi AJ, Samuelson G, Yarzagaray L, et al.: Atresia of the foramina of Luschka and Magendie: The Dandy-Walker cyst. J Neurosurg 31:202, 1969.
34. Sawaya R, McLaurin RL: Dandy-Walker syndrome: Clinical analysis of 23 cases. J Neurosurg 55:89, 1981.
35. Taggart JK, Walker AE: Congenital atresia of the foramens of Luschka and Magendie. AMA Arch Neurol Psychiatr 48:583, 1942.
36. Taylor GA, Sanders RC: Dandy-Walker syndrome: Recognition by sonography. AJNR 4:1203, 1983.

Choroid Plexus Papilloma

Definition
Choroid plexus papilloma (CPP) is a generally benign tumor of the choroid plexus.

Incidence
CPP is an exceedingly rare intracranial neoplasm that accounts for 0.6 percent of all brain tumors found in adults and 3 percent in children.[6,7]

Etiology
Unknown. This tumor has been reported in four patients with Aicardi syndrome, an X-linked disorder characterized by agenesis of the corpus callosum, chorioretinal lacunae, vertebral abnormalities, seizure disorder, and mental retardation.[2,13,15]

Pathology
Choroid plexuses are the main source of CSF. They are normally located inside the lateral, third, and fourth ventricles. Papillomas may occur in any of these sites,[1,4,11] but they occur most frequently at the level of the atria of the lateral ventricles.[7,16] The lesion is unilateral in the overwhelming majority of cases. Only a few cases of bilateral papilloma have been reported.[18] In most instances, these tumors are benign and are formed by villi that are histologically similar to normal choroid plexus. Malignancy may occur and can be recognized by invasion of adjacent nervous tissue and histologic departure from the normal cellular pattern, with mitosis and pleomorphism.[6-8]

CPPs are usually associated with hydrocephalus. This may be caused either by overproduction of CSF, leading to communicating hydrocephalus, or by an obstruction to the flow of CSF, resulting in dilatation of different portions of the ventricular system.[3,6,7,9,14]

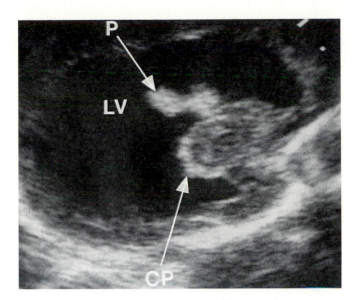

Figure 1–42. Parasagittal scan in a 30-week fetus with hydrocephalus secondary to a choroid plexus papilloma. The papilloma (P) is seen as an echogenic mass attached to the normal choroid plexus (CP) and protruding inside the dilated lateral ventricle (LV). *(Reproduced with permission from Pilu et al.: Ultrasound Med Biol 12:319, 1986.)*

Diagnosis

The diagnosis is usually made in hydrocephalic infants using radiologic techniques[7,17,18] or ultrasound,[18] and it relies on the demonstration of a mass protruding inside the ventricular system. The diagnostic technique of choice is contrast computed tomography. Other techniques, such as angiography and ventriculography, have missed this lesion in the past.[10] Intrauterine diagnosis was made in one case.[12]

Ultrasound often demonstrates a bright echogenic mass located at the level of the atrium of one lateral ventricle. In many cases of fetal hydrocephalus, the choroid plexuses may appear echogenic and prominent because of the fluid-filled lateral ventricles, often raising the suspicion of a papilloma. We believe that the most important hints are (1) comparison of the size and shape of the two choroid plexuses, because papillomas are generally unilateral, and (2) demonstration by either coronal or sagittal scans (Fig. 1–42) that an echogenic mass is adjacent to the normal choroid plexus. Prenatal diagnosis of CPP of the third and fourth ventricles has not yet been reported. However, the condition should be suspected if a hyperechogenic image is seen in this site.

Prognosis

The treatment of choice is surgical removal of the tumor.[7] The benign form of CPP may be extirpated with good results. However, this procedure is not easy and may be associated with significant hemorrhage. Temporarization with a CSF shunt is not advised.[5–7] The development of significant ascites after a ventriculoperitoneal shunt has been reported. Malignancy, reported in 20 percent of cases studied,[6] has a dismal prognosis even after surgical intervention and radiotherapy.[7] In a series of 17 treated infants, the operative mortality was 24 percent. There were 2 late deaths (11 percent), and 4 of the survivors were moderately mentally handicapped.[5] Mental retardation was found in 4 of 11 successfully treated infants.[7]

Obstetrical Management

The optimal mode of delivery of fetuses with CPP has not been established. There is no evidence suggesting that vaginal delivery is harmful. However, we believe that an operative vaginal delivery (vacuum or forceps) is contraindicated. The choice of a cesarean section may be offered to reduce the risk of birth trauma that could cause intracranial hemorrhage. These infants should be delivered in a center where both a neonatologist and a pediatric neurosurgeon are immediately available.

REFERENCES

1. Chan RC, Thompson GB, Durity FA: Primary choroid plexus papilloma of the cerebellopontine angle. Neurosurgery 12:334, 1983.
2. De Jong JGY, Delleman JW, Houben M, et al.: Agenesis of the corpus callosum, infantile spasms, ocular anomalies (Aicardi's syndrome). Neurology 26:1152, 1976.
3. Eisenberg HM, McComb JG, Lorenzo AV: Cerebrospinal fluid overproduction and hydrocephalus associated with choroid plexus papilloma. J Neurosurg 40:381, 1974.
4. Gradin WC, Taylon C, Fruin AH: Choroid plexus papilloma of the third ventricle: Case report and review of the literature. Neurosurgery 12:217, 1983.
5. Hawkins JC: Treatment of choroid plexus papillomas in children: A brief analysis of twenty years' experience. Neurosurgery 6:380, 1980.
6. Laurence KM: The biology of choroid plexus papilloma in infancy and childhood. Acta Neurochir 50:79, 1979.
7. Matson DD, Crofton FDL: Papilloma of the choroid plexus in childhood. J Neurosurg 17:1002, 1960.
8. Matsushima T: Choroid plexus papillomas and human choroid plexus: A light and electron microscopic study. J Neurosurg 59:1054, 1983.
9. Milhorat TH, Hammock MK, Davis DA, et al.: Choroid plexus papilloma. I. Proof of cerebrospinal fluid overproduction. Childs Brain 2:273, 1976.
10. Pascual-Castroviejo I, Roche MC, Villarejo F, et al.: Choroid plexus papillomas of the fourth ventricle. Childs Brain 9:373, 1982.
11. Piguet V, de Tribolet N: Choroid plexus papilloma of the cerebellopontine angle presenting as a subarachnoid hemorrhage: Case report. Neurosurgery 15:114, 1984.

12. Pilu G, De Palma L, Romero R, et al.: The fetal subarachnoid cisterns: An ultrasound study with report of a case of congenital communicating hydrocephalus. J Ultrasound Med 5:365, 1986.
13. Robinow M, Johnson FG, Minella PA: Aicardi syndrome, papilloma of the choroid plexus, cleft lip, and cleft of the posterior palate. J Pediatr 104:404, 1984.
14. Sahar A, Feinsod M, Beller AJ: Choroid plexus papilloma: Hydrocephalus and cerebrospinal fluid dynamics. Surg Neurol 13:476, 1980.
15. Tachibana H, Matsui A, Takeshita K: Aicardi's syndrome with multiple papilloma of choroid plexus. Arch Neurol 39:194, 1982.
16. Turcotte JF, Copty M, Bedard F, et al.: Lateral ventricle choroid plexus papilloma and communicating hydrocephalus. Surg Neurol 13:143, 1980.
17. Veiga-Pires JA, Dossetor RS, van Nieuwenhuizen O: CT scanning for papilloma of choroid plexus. Neuroradiology 17:13, 1978.
18. Welch K, Strand R, Bresnan M, et al.: Congenital hydrocephalus due to villous hypertrophy of the telencephalic choroid plexuses. J Neurosurg 59:172, 1983.

NEURAL TUBE DEFECTS

The term "neural tube defects" refers to a group of malformations including anencephaly, cephaloceles, and spina bifida.

Spina Bifida

Synonyms
Spinal dysraphism, rachischisis, meningocele, and myelomeningocele.

Definition
Spina bifida can be defined as a midline defect of the vertebrae resulting in exposure of the contents of the neural canal. In the vast majority of cases, the defect is localized to the posterior arch (dorsal) of the vertebrae. In rare cases, the defect consists of a splitting of the vertebral body.

Incidence
Spina bifida is the most common malformation of the CNS. The incidence varies according to many factors, such as geographical area, ethnic differences, and seasonal variation.[2,11,15,21,40,43] Typically, these anomalies are very common in the British Isles and uncommon in the eastern world (Table 1–8). Spinal defects are more frequent in Caucasians than in Orientals or blacks. These differences seem to persist even after migration, suggesting a genetic rather than an environmental effect.

Etiology
Neural tube defects are most commonly inherited with a multifactorial pattern. They could also occur as part of a mendelian syndrome or chromosomal anomalies, or result from teratogenic exposure. Table 1–9 lists the recognized causes of neural tube defects.[3,6,38] Table 1–10 describes the recurrence risk for neural tube defects according to different risk factors.

Embryology
Most of the CNS derives from the neural plate by means of a process called "neurulation." The chronology of this event is depicted in Figure 1–43. The

TABLE 1–8. INCIDENCE OF NEURAL TUBE DEFECTS IN VARIOUS GEOGRAPHICAL AREAS

	Spina Bifida Incidence per 1000 Births	Anencephaly Incidence per 1000 Births
South Wales[15]	4.1	3.5
Southampton[43]	3.2	1.9
Birmingham, UK[21]	2.8	2.0
Charleston[2]		
White	1.5	1.2
Black	0.6	0.2
Alexandria[40]	2.0	3.6
Japan[23]	0.3	0.6

Modified from Brocklehurst. In: Vinken, Bruyn (eds): Handbook of Clinical Neurology. Amsterdam, Elsevier/North Holland Biomedical Press, 1978, Vol 32, pp 519–578.

TABLE 1–9. RECOGNIZED CAUSES OF NEURAL TUBE DEFECTS

Multifactorial inheritance—anencephaly, meningomyelocele, meningocele, and encephalocele

Single mutant genes
    Meckel syndrome—autosomal recessive (phenotype includes occipital encephalocele and rarely anencephaly)
    Median-cleft face syndrome—possible autosomal dominant (phenotype includes anterior encephalocele)
    Robert syndrome—autosomal recessive (phenotype includes anterior encephalocele)
    Syndrome of anterior sacral meningomyelocele and anal stenosis—dominant, either autosomal or X-linked
    Jarco-Levin syndrome—autosomal recessive (phenotype includes meningomyelocele)
    HARDE syndrome—autosomal recessive (phenotype includes encephalocele)

Chromosome abnormalities
    13 trisomy
    18 trisomy
    Triploidy
    Other abnormalities, such as unbalanced translocation and ring chromosome

Probably hereditary, but mode of transmission not established
    Syndrome of occipital encephalocele, myopia, and retinal dysplasia
    Anterior encephalocele among Bantus and Thais

Teratogens
    Valproic acid (phenotype includes spina bifida)
    Aminopterin/amethopterin (phenotype includes anencephaly and encephalocele)
    Thalidomide (phenotype includes, rarely, anencephaly and meningomyelocele)

Maternal predisposing factors
    Diabetes mellitus (anencephaly more frequent than spina bifida)

Specific phenotypes, but without known cause
    Syndrome of craniofacial and limb defects secondary to aberrant tissue bands (phenotype includes multiple encephaloceles)
    Cloacal exstrophy (phenotype includes myelocystocele)
    Sacrococcygeal teratoma (phenotype includes meningomyelocele)

Reproduced with permission from Main, Mennuti: Obstet Gynecol 67:1, 1986.

neural plate is derived from dorsal ectoderm. At about the 16th day after conception, an invagination occurs, leading to the formation of the neural groove. About the 21st day, the neural groove begins to close in the midportion of the embryo and advances both rostrally and caudally. The rostral opening (anterior neuropore) of the spine closes at about 24 days, and the caudal neuropore, which corresponds to the lumbar area, closes at about 28 days (Fig. 1–43).[3,12]

The two main theories concerning the origin of neural tube defects are the arhaphic theory and the hydromyelic theory. The first proposes a primary failure of closure of the caudal neuropore.[27] The second suggests an imbalance between the production and reabsorption rate of CSF in the embryonic period. This causes excessive accumulation of fluid in the normally closed neural tube (hydromyelia) and

secondary separation of the dorsal wall.[10] The absence of skin and muscle directly above the defect results from failure of induction of the ectodermal and mesodermal tissues.

Pathology

Spina bifida encompasses a broad spectrum of abnormalities. Lesions are commonly subdivided into ventral and dorsal defects. Ventral defects are extremely rare and are characterized by the splitting of the vertebral body and the occurrence of a cyst that is neuroenteric in origin. The lesion is generally seen in the lower cervical or upper thoracic vertebrae. Dorsal defects are by far the most common. They are subdivided into two types: spina bifida occulta and spina bifida aperta. Spina bifida occulta represents approximately 15 percent of the cases and is characterized by a small defect completely covered by skin. In many cases, this condition is completely asymptomatic and is diagnosed only incidentally at radiographic examination of the spine. In other instances, there is an area of hypertrichosis, pigmented or dimpled skin, or the presence of subcutaneous lipomas.[8] A dermal sinus connecting the skin to the vertebrae and to the dura mater can occasionally be seen. The clinical importance of this lesion is its frequent association with infection of the neural contents.

Spina bifida aperta is the most frequent lesion, resulting in 85 percent of dorsal defects. The neural canal may be exposed, or the defect may be covered

TABLE 1–10. ESTIMATED INCIDENCE OF NEURAL TUBE DEFECTS BASED ON SPECIFIC RISK FACTORS IN THE UNITED STATES

Population	Incidence per 1000 Live Births
Mother as reference	
General incidence	1.4–1.6
Women undergoing amniocentesis for advanced maternal age	1.5–3.0
Women with diabetes mellitus	20
Women on valproic acid in first trimester	10–20
Fetus as reference	
1 sibling with NTD	15–30
2 siblings with NTD*	57
Parent with NTD	11
Half sibling with NTD	8
First cousin (mother's sister's child)	10
Other first cousins	3
Sibling with severe scoliosis secondary to multiple vertebral defects	15–30
Sibling with occult spina dysraphism	15–30
Sibling with sacrococcygeal teratoma or hamartoma	≤15–30

NTD = neural tube defect.
*Risk is higher in British studies. Risk increases further for three or more siblings or combinations of other close relatives.
Reproduced with permission from Main, Mennuti: Obstet Gynecol 67:1, 1986.

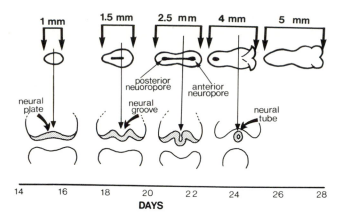

Figure 1–43. Chronology of neurulation.

by a thin meningeal membrane. More often, the lesion appears as a cystic tumor (spina bifida cystica). If the tumor contains purely meninges, the lesion is referred to as a "meningocele." More frequently, neural tissue is part of the mass, and the name "myelomeningocele" is used.[3]

The term "myeloschisis" is sometimes used to refer to a condition in which the spinal cord is widely opened dorsally and is part of the wall of the myelomeningocele. The vertebrae are lacking the dorsal arches, and the pedicles are typically spread apart.[3]

Associated Anomalies

The two main categories of anomalies associated with spina bifida are other CNS defects and foot deformities. In almost all cases of spina bifida aperta, a typical abnormality of the posterior fossa is found.[41] The lesion is Arnold-Chiari malformation type II, and it is characterized by a herniation of the cerebellar vermis through the foramen magnum. The fourth ventricle is displaced downward inside the neural canal. The posterior fossa is shallow and the tentorium is displaced downward. Displacement and kinking of the medulla are also observed. Arnold-Chiari malformation is almost invariably associated with obstructive hydrocephalus.[17] The genesis of hydrocephalus seems to be related to the low position of the exit

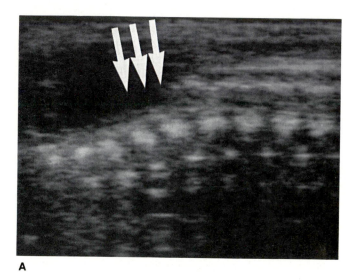

A

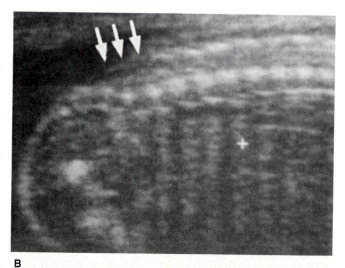

B

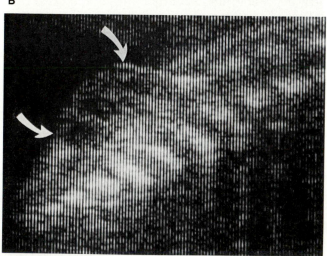

C

Figure 1–44. A. Sagittal scan of the spine of a fetus demonstrating a large defect running from the upper lumbar area to S5. Note the interruption in the posterior processes and soft tissues (*arrows*). **B.** A sagittal scan of the spine in an 18-week fetus revealing a small sacral defect (S2–S5) (*arrows*). **C.** Sagittal scan of the spine revealing a meningocele (*arrows*) overlying a spinal defect.

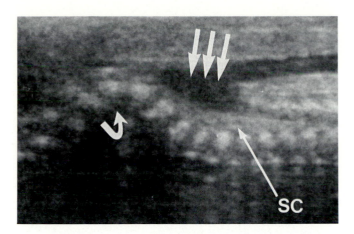

Figure 1–45. Sagittal scan of the spine of a fetus affected by a large spina bifida (*triple arrow*) and severe kyphoscoliosis (*curved arrow*). SC, spinal cord.

Diagnosis

The criteria for the diagnosis of spina bifida are based upon soft tissue and bony signs. The soft tissue signs include absence of skin covering the defect and presence of a bulging sac that may correspond to a meningocele or myelomeningocele. The bony signs are derived from the vertebral abnormalities associated with spina bifida. A clear understanding of the normal anatomy of the spine in different scanning planes is absolutely essential to the diagnosis.

There are three main scanning planes used in the evaluation of the spine: sagittal, transverse, and coronal (Fig. 1–26).

In the sagittal plane, the normal spine appears as two parallel lines converging in the sacrum.[4,5] The lines correspond to the posterior elements of the vertebrae and the vertebral body (Fig. 1–27). In the presence of spina bifida, the disappearance of the posterior line and of the overlying soft tissues is evident[4] (Fig. 1–44). Sagittal scans are also useful for evaluating the spinal curvatures of which exaggeration may be an indirect sign of spina bifida (Fig. 1–45).

In the coronal plane, the normal spine appears as either two or three parallel lines (Fig. 1–28). The two lines are seen when the scanning plane is more dorsal. Moving the transducer anteriorly, a third line comes into view. Spina bifida is typically characterized by a widening of the two external lines due to a divergent separation of the lateral processes of the vertebrae (Fig. 1–46).

In the transverse section, the neural canal appears as a closed circle. It is lined anteriorly by the ossification center in the body of the vertebra and posteriorly by the two ossification centers of the lamina. In the presence of a defect, the posteri-

foramen of the fourth ventricle, which drains the CSF inside the spinal canal. Reentry of the fluid to the intracranial cavity is then blocked by the cerebellum that obstructs the foramen magnum.[34,35] In many cases, deformities of the aqueduct are found, and these are believed to be secondary to ventricular enlargement and brain stem compression.[42] Another frequently encountered CNS abnormality is polymicrogyria.

Dislocation of the hip and foot deformities (clubfoot, rockerbottom foot) are frequently seen in association with spina bifida. The pathogenesis of the malformation is related to the unopposed action of muscle groups because of a defect of the peripheral nerve corresponding to the involved myotomes.[36]

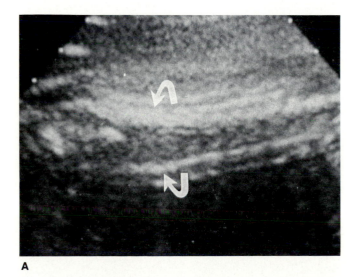
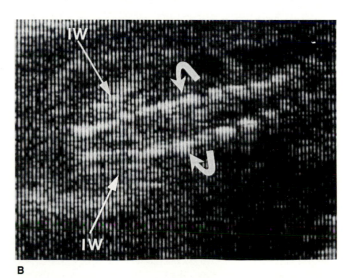

A   **B**

Figure 1–46. A. Coronal scan of the spine of a fetus affected by a large lumbosacral defect, appearing as a widening of the spinal echoes (*curved arrows*). **B.** A similar scan in a second-trimester fetus with spina bifida (*curved arrows*). IW, iliac wings.

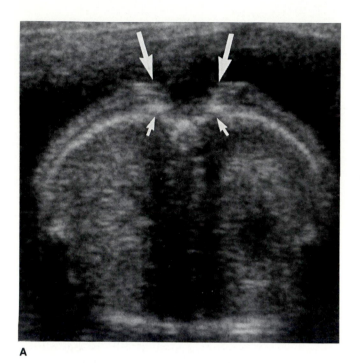

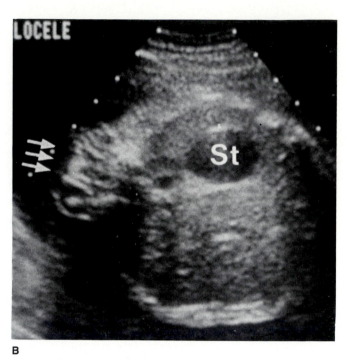

A   **B**

Figure 1–47. A. Transverse scan of the body of a fetus affected by a large spinal defect. Note the absence of the soft tissue overlying the spine in the area of the defect (*large arrows*) and the typical separation of the articular elements (*small arrows*). **B.** Transverse scan of the body of a fetus with a large thoracolumbar spinal defect at the level of the stomach (St). The irregular echoes arising posteriorly from the defect suggest the presence of a myelomeningocele (*triple arrows*).

or laminae are typically absent, and the lateral processes are set apart.[4] The skin and muscles above the defect are absent (Fig. 1–47). In our opinion, this is the most important section for the diagnosis of spinal defects. We find the most informative image to be the one in which the posterior process is up. Otherwise, shadowing from the ribs and limited lateral resolution may result in a false positive diagnosis. Closed spinal defects are extremely difficult to diagnose.

It is a common belief that indirect signs of spina bifida, such as paralysis of the lower extremities and bladder distention, can be useful in the diagnosis of the lesion. The reader is alerted to the unreliability of such signs. We have seen apparently normal motion of the lower extremities in many fetuses with severe defects. The presence of a clubfoot, which is frequently associated with this defect, increases the

index of suspicion in a patient at risk, as does the observation of hydrocephaly.

Accuracy of Ultrasound in the Prenatal Diagnosis of Spina Bifida

The detection of spina bifida is one of the most difficult tasks required of a sonographer. These examinations are known in the United States as level II scans and should only be performed by very experienced operators.

Several authors have reported their experience in the prenatal diagnosis of spina bifida. When evaluating this literature, it is extremely important to know the criteria for patient admission into a given study. For example, the risk of having a neural tube defect is very different if a patient is referred with a history of a previously affected child (recurrence rate 2 to 5

TABLE 1–11. ACCURACY OF ULTRASOUND IN THE PRENATAL DIAGNOSIS OF SPINA BIFIDA

	n	Prevalence (%)	Sensitivity (%)	Specificity (%)	PPV	NPV
Allen et al.[1]	374	2.1	87	99	87	99
Persson et al.[29]	10.147	0.1	40	100	100	99
Roberts et al.[33]	1261	1.4	30	96	92	99
Roberts et al.[33]	1991	1.7	80	99	80	99

PPV, positive predictive value; NPV, negative predictive value.

percent) or if the patient has an elevated amniotic fluid alpha-fetoprotein.[1,5,13,14,29,30,37]

Several authors have reported on the accuracy of the prenatal diagnosis of spina bifida by ultrasound. Table 1–11 shows the results of the three largest series available for study. Allen et al.[1] reported that in a group of patients at risk because of a positive family history, ultrasound was able to identify 87 percent of the affected cases. Roberts et al.[33] reported two different studies. The first study covered a 3-year period between 1977 and 1980 and exhibited a sensitivity of only 30 percent. During the next 3 years, the sensitivity increased to 80 percent. This is a clear demonstration of the value of experience in diagnostic accuracy. Pearce et al.[28] have reported that in over 1500 patients at risk, 92 defects were correctly identified, 7 were missed, and 2 false positive diagnoses were made.

Our own experience at Yale indicates that ultrasound is 94 percent sensitive and 98 percent specific for the diagnosis of spina bifida when used in a population at risk (amniotic fluid alphafetoprotein 3 standard deviations above the mean). The experience of the operator and the quality of the equipment are important factors in the accurate prenatal diagnosis of these defects. However, a finite number of cases will not be diagnosable with sonography. Small sacral defects are probably the major diagnostic problem. The reason for this difficulty is that the interrogation of the sacral area is difficult because of its normal curvature and its flat shape.

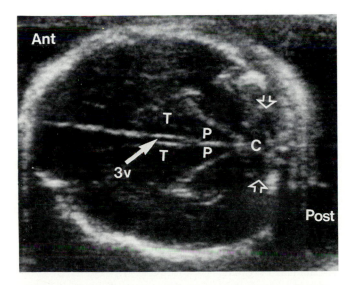

Figure 1–48. A suboccipitobregmatic scan of the head of a fetus with spina bifida reveals a shallow posterior fossa and an abnormally small cerebellar transverse diameter (*open arrows*). The cisterna magna is obliterated. T, thalami; P, peduncles; C, cerebellum; 3v, third ventricle; Ant, anterior; Post, posterior.

Sonographic Evaluation of Intracranial Anatomy in Fetuses with Spina Bifida

Spina bifida is associated with a variety of typical intracranial abnormalities,[3,17,41,42] including ventriculomegaly and hypoplasia of the posterior fossa structures. As the fetal head is easily accessible to sonographic examination, identifying alterations of the cerebral architecture predictive of spina bifida would assist both targeted examinations of fetuses at risk and screening programs of the general population.

Nicolaides et al.[25] have recently reported a retrospective study of the intracranial anatomy in fetuses with spina bifida. They described a typical abnormality of the cerebellum, which appeared on sonography as a crescent with the concavity pointing anteriorly ("banana sign"). They also found that fetuses with spina bifida usually have enlarged atria of the lateral ventricles and a frontal deformity in a cross section of the head at the level of the BPD ("lemon sign").

In our own series of 18 cases with spina bifida prospectively examined, we have found that abnormalities of the posterior fossa or lateral ventricles (or both) were present in all fetuses, starting from as early as 18 weeks of gestation. In 16 cases (88.8 percent), either the cerebellum was impossible to visualize or the cerebellar transverse diameter was abnormally small (Figs. 1–17C, 1–48). In none of our 18 cases could we document the presence of the banana sign. Conversely, all fetuses had some degree of frontal deformity. In only 14 cases (77.7 percent), ventriculomegaly was attested by an abnormal LVW: HW ratio. However, 17 fetuses (94.4 percent) had a disproportion between the atrial lumen and the corresponding choroid plexus (Fig. 1–32).

These preliminary data seem to support the hypothesis that examination of the fetal cerebral structures (skull, ventricles, and cerebellum) are extremely useful for the prenatal identification of spina bifida.

Prognosis

Spina bifida is a serious congenital anomaly. The stillbirth rate is widely quoted to be 25 percent.[3] The majority of untreated infants die within the first few months of life.[18] Survival of infants treated in the early neonatal period is only 40 percent at 7 years.[18] Twenty-five percent of these infants are totally paralyzed, 25 percent are almost totally paralyzed, 25 percent require intense rehabilitation, and only 25 percent have no significant lower limb dysfunction. Seventeen percent of infants at late follow-up have normal continence.[3,18] At present, it is impossible to predict in utero the outcome of these infants. Prognostic factors include the level and extent of the lesion (cervical and high thoracic lesions are frequently fatal) and kyphoscoliosis (see Table 1–12). The presence of severe hydrocephaly has always

TABLE 1–12. RESULTS OF AGGRESSIVE TREATMENT OF 171 CONSECUTIVE INFANTS WITH MENINGOMYELOCELES IN THE 1960s*

Level of Lesion	Percent With This Level of Lesion	Mortality (%)	IQ >80 (%)	Able to Walk† (%)	Able to Walk Without Appliances (%)
Thoracolumbar	37	35	44	71	0
Lumbosacral	59	11	65	81	16
Sacral	4	0	100	100	83

* 3- to 8-year follow-up.
† Many of the children, particularly those with higher lesions, can walk with braces and other supports in the first decade of life, but lose this ability in adolescence.
Reproduced with permission from Main, Mennuti: Obstet Gynecol 67:1, 1986.

been considered a poor prognostic sign.[18] Early neonatal shunting has significantly improved the intellectual development of these infants.[16,20] Mapstone et al.[19] reported that in a group of 75 infants with spina bifida, the mean IQ of those not requiring shunting procedures was 104, whereas those shunted in the absence of complications had a mean IQ of 91. The occurrence of complications, such as ventriculitis, lowers the mean IQ to 70.

All infants with spina bifida have some degree of Arnold-Chiari type II malformation. This condition is symptomatic (e.g., dyspnea, swallowing difficulties, opisthotonos) and represents a potentially fatal complication only in a small number of cases. Death is usually related to respiratory failure. In a series, 45 infants with symptomatic Arnold-Chiari malformation underwent laminectomy for relief of brain stem compression. The mortality rate was 38 percent in a follow-up period ranging from 6 months to 6 years.[26]

Obstetrical Management

When the diagnosis is made in the second trimester, the option of pregnancy termination should be offered to the parents. In the third trimester, patients should be counseled (see Prognosis). The most important issues of obstetrical management are the timing and mode of delivery. Infants with spina bifida ideally should be delivered at term. An indication for preterm delivery could be the rapid development of severe ventriculomegaly and macrocrania. In this case, delivery should be accomplished when there is fetal lung maturity. There are inadequate data regarding the optimal mode of delivery. The vaginal route could traumatize the defect and expose the neural tissue to bacteria normally present in the birth canal.[7,31,32,39] Furthermore, it has been postulated that birth injury in these infants may lead to delayed onset of syringomyelia.[24] Because of these

considerations, it has been suggested that the preferable mode of delivery is cesarean section.[7]

Intrauterine treatment of fetuses with spina bifida has been suggested by some authors, the primary purpose being to achieve cerebral decompression when there is associated ventriculomegaly. This would be done with a ventriculoamniotic shunt. However, such an approach may carry significant risks to both the mother and fetus, and the benefits are unclear, while recent data suggest an acceptable mean IQ when these infants are treated in the neonatal period.[19] It has been postulated that the spinal lesion has a progressive course in utero.[9] On the basis of these considerations, fetal allogeneic bone paste has been used in primate models to close the defect in utero.[22] However, the results of these efforts are yet to be published.

REFERENCES

1. Allen LC, Doran TA, Miskin M, et al.: Ultrasound and amniotic fluid alpha-fetoprotein in the prenatal diagnosis of spina bifida. Obstet Gynecol 60:169, 1982.
2. Alter M: Anencephalus, hydrocephalus, and spina bifida. Epidemiology with special reference to a survey in Charleston, S.C. Arch Neurol 7:411, 1962.
3. Brocklehurst G: Spina bifida. In: Vinken PJ, Bruyn GW (eds): Handbook of Clinical Neurology. Amsterdam, Elsevier/North Holland Biomedical Press, 1977, Vol 30, pp 519–578.
4. Campbell S: Early prenatal diagnosis of neural tube defects by ultrasound. Clin Obstet Gynecol 20:351, 1977.
5. Campbell S, Allan L, Griffin D, et al.: The early diagnosis of fetal structural abnormalities. In: Lerski RA, Morley P (eds): Ultrasound '82. Oxford, Pergamon Press, 1983, pp 547–563.
6. Carter CO: Clues to the aetiology of neural tube malformations. Dev Med Child Neurol [Suppl] 32:3, 1974.
7. Chervenak FA, Duncan C, Ment L, et al.: Perinatal management of meningomyelocele. Obstet Gynecol 63:376, 1984.
8. Emery JL, Lendon RG: Lipomas of the cauda equina and other fatty tumours related to neurospinal dysraphism. Dev Med Child Neurol [Suppl] 20:62, 1969.
9. Epstein F, Marlin A, Hochwald G, et al.: Myelomeningocele: A progressive intra-uterine disease. Dev Med Child Neurol [Suppl] 37:12, 1976.
10. Gardner WJ: Myelomeningocele, the result of rupture of the embryonic neural tube. Cleve Clin Q 27:88, 1960.
11. Guthkelch AN: Studies in spina bifida cystica. III. Seasonal variation in the frequency of spina bifida births. Br J Prev Soc Med 16:159, 1962.
12. Hamilton WJ, Boyd JD, Mossman HW: Human Embryology, 2d ed. Baltimore, Williams & Wilkins, 1952.
13. Hashimoto BE, Mahony BS, Filly RA, et al.: Sonography, a complementary examination to alpha-fetoprotein testing for fetal neural tube defects. J Ultrasound Med 4:307, 1985.

14. Hobbins JC, Venus I, Tortora M, et al.: Stage II ultrasound examination for the diagnosis of fetal abnormalities with an elevated amniotic fluid alpha-fetoprotein concentration. Am J Obstet Gynecol 142:1026, 1982.

15. Laurence KM, Carter CO, David PA: Major central nervous system malformations in South Wales. I. Incidence, local variations and geographical factors. Br J Prev Soc Med 22:146, 1968.

16. Leonard CO, Freeman JM: Spina bifida: A new disease. Pediatrics 68:136, 1981.

17. Lorber J: Systematic ventriculographic studies in infants born with meningomyelocele and encephalocele. The incidence and development of hydrocephalus. Arch Dis Child 36:381, 1961.

18. Lorber J: Results of treatment of myelomeningocele. An analysis of 524 unselected cases, with special reference to possible selection for treatment. Dev Med Child Neurol 13:279, 1971.

19. Mapstone TB, Rekate HL, Nulsen FE, et al.: Relationship of CSF shunting and IQ in children with myelomeningocele: A retrospective analysis. Childs Brain 11:112, 1984.

20. McCullough DC, Balzer-Martin LA: Current prognosis in overt neonatal hydrocephalus. J Neurosurg 57:378, 1982.

21. McKeown T, Record RG: Malformations in a population observed for 5 years after birth. In: Wolstenholme GEW, O'Connor CM (eds): Ciba Foundation Symposium on Congenital Malformations. London, Churchill, 1960, pp 2–14.

22. Michejda M, McCullough D, Bacher J, et al.: Investigational approaches in fetal neurosurgery. Concepts Pediatr Neurosurg 4:44, 1983.

23. Neel JV: A study of major congenital defects in Japanese infants. Am J Hum Genet 10:398, 1958.

24. Newman PW, Terenty TR, Foster JB: Some observations on the pathogenesis of syringomyelia. J Neurol Neurosurg Psychiatry 44:964, 1981.

25. Nicolaides KH, Campbell S, Gabbe SG, et al.: Ultrasound screening for spina bifida: Cranial and cerebellar signs. Lancet 2:72, 1986.

26. Park TS, Hoffman HJ, Hendrick EB, et al.: Experience with surgical decompression of the Arnold-Chiari malformation in young infants with myelomeningocele. Neurosurgery 13:147, 1983.

27. Patten BM: Embryological stages in the establishing of myeloschisis with spina bifida. Am J Anat 93:365, 1953.

28. Pearce JM, Little D, Campbell S: The diagnosis of abnormalities of the fetal central nervous system. In: Sanders RC, James AE (eds): The Principles and Practice of Ultrasonography in Obstetrics and Gynecology, 3d ed. Norwalk, CT, Appleton-Century-Crofts, 1985, pp 243–256.

29. Persson PH, Kullander S, Gennser G, et al.: Screening for fetal malformations using ultrasound and measurements of alpha-fetoprotein in maternal serum. Br Med J 286:747, 1983.

30. Polanska N, Burgess DE, Hill P, et al.: Screening for neural tube defect: False positive findings on ultrasound and in amniotic fluid. Br Med J 287:24, 1983.

31. Ralis ZA: Traumatizing effect of breech delivery on infants with spina bifida. J Pediatr 87:613, 1975.

32. Ralis Z, Ralis HM: Morphology of peripheral nerves in children with spina bifida. Dev Med Child Neurol [Suppl] 27:109, 1972.

33. Roberts CJ, Hibbard BM, Roberts EE, et al.: Diagnostic effectiveness of ultrasound in detection of neural tube defect. The South Wales experience of 2509 scans (1977–1982) in high-risk mothers. Lancet 2:1068, 1983.

34. Russell DS: Observations on the pathology of hydrocephalus. Med Res Counc Spec Sev 265:1, 1949.

35. Russell DS, Donald C: The mechanism of internal hydrocephalus in spina bifida. Brain 58:203, 1935.

36. Sharrard WJW: The mechanism of paralytic deformity in spina bifida. Dev Med Child Neurol 4:310, 1962.

37. Slotnick N, Filly RA, Callen PW, et al.: Sonography as a procedure complementary to alpha-fetoprotein testing for neural tube defects. J Ultrasound Med 1:319, 1982.

38. Smith C: Computer programme to estimate recurrence risks for multifactorial familial disease. Br Med J 1:495, 1972.

39. Stark G, Drummond M: Spina bifida as an obstetric problem. Dev Med Child Neurol [Suppl] 22:157, 1970.

40. Stevenson AC, Johnston HA, Stewart MIP, et al.: Congenital malformations. A report study of a series of consecutive births in 24 centres. Bull WHO 34 [Suppl 9]:127, 1966.

41. Variend S, Emery JL: The weight of the cerebellum in children with myelomeningocele. Dev Med Child Neurol 15 [Suppl 29]:77, 1973.

42. Williams B: Is aqueduct stenosis a result of hydrocephalus? Brain 96:399, 1973.

43. Williamson EM: Incidence and family aggregation of major congenital malformations of central nervous system. J Med Genet 2:161, 1965.

Anencephaly

Synonyms

Pseudoencephaly, extracranial disencephaly, and acleidencephaly.

Definition

Anencephaly is an anomaly characterized by the absence of cerebral hemispheres and cranial vault.

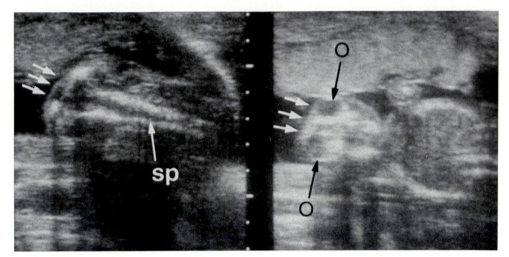

Figure 1–49. A. Anencephaly at 15 weeks of gestation. The absence of the cranial vault is obvious (*triple arrows*). O, orbits; sp, spine.

Incidence

The epidemiology of anencephaly is very similar to that of spina bifida. There is considerable variation in the prevalence of this condition in different parts of the world (Table 1–8). In neonates, the anomaly is more frequent in females than in males. The incidence of anencephaly in abortion material has been found to be five times greater than that observed at birth.[6]

Etiology

Anencephaly, as well as spina bifida, has a recognized multifactorial etiology. The recurrence risks are depicted in Table 1–9. A number of teratogenic agents, including radiation,[11] trypan blue,[7] salicylates,[10] sulfonamides,[9] and CO_2 excess and anoxia,[4] etc., have induced this anomaly in experimental animals.

Embryology

There are two main theories regarding the origin of anencephaly. The first proposes that the defect is due to failure of closure of the anterior neuropore,[6] and the second suggests that an excess of CSF causes disruption of the normally formed cerebral hemispheres.[2,5,8]

Pathology

Most of the cranial vault is absent. The frontal bone is defective above the supraorbital region, and the parietal bones, as well as the squamous portion of the occipital bone, are absent. The crown of the head is covered by a vascular membrane known as "area cerebrovasculosa." Beneath the mass, few remnants of the cerebral hemispheres can be found. The diencephalic and mesencephalic structures are either completely or par-

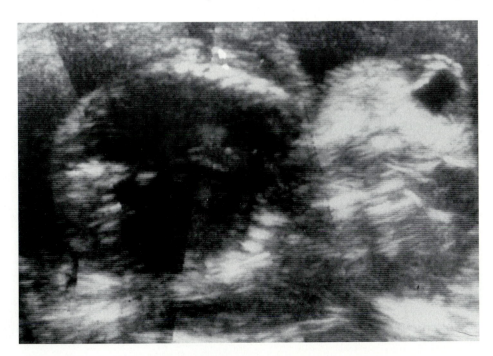

Figure 1–49. B. Typical froglike appearance of an anencephalic fetus. The head is to the right, caudal end to the left. (*Reproduced with permission from Jeanty, Romero: Obstetrical Ultrasound. New York, McGraw-Hill, 1984.*)

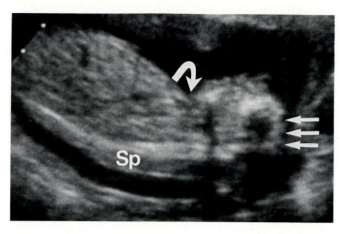

Figure 1–49. C. A longitudinal view of a second trimester anencephalic fetus revealing the absence of the cranial vault (*triple arrows*) and the typical shortness of the neck (*curved arrow*). Sp, spine.

tially destroyed. The hypophysis and the rhomboencephalic structures are generally preserved.[6]

Other features that are quite characteristic of anencephalic infants include bulging eyes, a large tongue, and a very short neck.

Associated Malformations

Spina bifida is present in 17 percent of patients (craniorachischisis), cleft lip or palate in 2 percent, and clubfoot in 1.7 percent. Omphaloceles have also been described in some cases.[3,6]

Diagnosis

Anencephaly was the first congenital anomaly identified in utero with ultrasound.[1] The diagnosis relies on the failure to demonstrate the cranial vault. The anencephalic fetus has a typical froglike appearance and usually has a short neck (Fig. 1–49). The diagnosis can probably be made as early as the 12th to the 13th week. In the third trimester, the diagnosis is quite obvious when the fetus is in transverse or breech presentation. However, difficulties can be encountered when a fetus is in vertex presentation because the base of the skull is often seen deep in the maternal pelvis, and there is only a perception that there is not enough room for a normal head in the lower uterine segment. The differential diagnosis between anencephaly and severe forms of microcephaly can be difficult.

Polyhydramnios is frequently associated with anencephaly. The mechanism is unclear, and several hypotheses have been suggested, including failure to swallow because of a brain stem lesion, excessive

micturition, and failure of reabsorption of CSF.[6] A frequent accompanying phenomenon is increased fetal activity. The explanation remains unknown, but irritation of the meninges and neural tissue by CSF has been proposed.

Prognosis

This disease is uniformly fatal within the first hours or days of life. Fifty-three percent are premature births, and 15 percent are postterm infants.[3] Only 32 percent of these fetuses are live births.[6]

Obstetrical Management

Termination of pregnancy can be offered to the patient at any time in gestation when this diagnosis is made. Anencephalic infants are a potential source of organs for transplantation.[6a,8a]

REFERENCES

1. Campbell S, Johnstone FD, Holt EM, et al.: Anencephaly: Early ultrasonic diagnosis and active management. Lancet 2:1226, 1972.
2. Frazer JE: Report on an anencephalic embryo. J Anat 56:12, 1921.
3. Frezal J, Kelley J, Guillemot ML, et al.: Anencephaly in France. Am J Hum Genet 16:336, 1964.
4. Gallera J: Influence de l'atmosphere artificiellement modifiee sur le developpement embryonnaire du poulet. Acta Anat 11:549, 1951.
5. Gardner WJ: The Dysraphic States from Syringomyelia to Anencephaly. Amsterdam, Excerpta Medica, 1973.
6. Giroud A: Anencephaly. In: Vinken GW, Bruyn PW (eds): Handbook of Clinical Neurology. Amsterdam, Elsevier/North Holland Biomedical Press, 1977, Vol 30, pp 173–208.
6a. Holzgreve W, Beller FK, Buchholz B, et al.: Kidney transplantation from anencephalic donors. N Engl J Med 316:1069, 1987.
7. Katsunuma S, Murakami U: La periode critique ou apparait la malformation des embryons produite par diverses agressions au cours de la grossesse. C R Soc Biol 148:1309, 1954.
8. Keen JA: The genesis of spina bifida. Clin Proc 7:162, 1948.
8a. McCullagh P: The Foetus as Transplant Donor: Scientific, Social and Ethical Perspectives. Chichester, Wiley, 1987.
9. Tuchmann-Duplessis H, Mercier-Parot L: Sur l'action teratogene d'un sulfamide hypoglycemiant, etude experimentale chez la ratte. J Physiol 51:65, 1959.
10. Warkany J, Takacs E: Experimental production of congenital malformations in rats by salicylate poisoning. Am J Pathol 35:315, 1959.
11. Wilson JG, Karr JW: Effects of irradiation on embryonic development. I. X-rays on the 10th day of gestation in the rat. Am J Anat 88:1, 1951.

Cephalocele

Synonyms
Encephalocele, cranial or occipital meningocele, and cranium bifidum.

Definition
Cephalocele is a protrusion of the intracranial contents through a bony defect of the skull. The term "cranial meningocele" is used when only meninges are herniated. The term "encephalocele" defines the presence of brain tissue in the herniated sac. Encephalocele is commonly but incorrectly used to refer to both conditions.

Incidence
Rare. Occipital cephaloceles are by far the most frequent form in the Western world. In England, the frequency of this condition has been estimated to be 0.3 to 0.6 in 1000 births.[10]

Etiology
Other neural tube defects are often found in siblings of infants with cephalocele, implying a familial tendency.[10,12] Besides the conditions associated with neural tube defects listed in Table 1–9, cephaloceles are frequent components of a number of genetic (e.g., Meckel syndrome) and nongenetic (e.g., amniotic band syndrome) syndromes (Table 1–13). They have also been reported in association with maternal rubella, diabetes, and hyperthermia and can be produced experimentally in animals by the administration of several teratogens, such as x-ray radiation, trypan blue, and hypervitaminosis A.[12]

Embryology
The basic disorder responsible for the defect is unknown. It has been suggested that overgrowth of the rostral portion of the neural tube may interfere with the closure of the skull. Alternatively, the defect may result from failure of closure induction by the mesoderm.[9] Most cephaloceles are, therefore, located in the midline. An exception to this occurs in cases of amniotic band syndrome, in which cephaloceles may be multiple, irregular, or asymmetrical (see p. 411).

Pathology
According to the bone in which the defect is located, cephaloceles are commonly subdivided into occipital, parietal, and frontal. By far the most common location is the occipital bone.[11] The lesion may vary in size from a few millimeters to a mass larger than the cranial vault. It may contain only meninges (meningocele) or variable amounts of brain tissue (encephalocele). In some cases, most of the brain tissue is

contained in the herniated sac. Frontal cephaloceles occur more frequently between the frontal and ethmoidal bones (frontonasal cephalocele). Not all cephaloceles are externally evident. Some occur through a defect located in the base of the skull and protrude inside the orbits, nasopharynx, or

TABLE 1–13. CONDITIONS ASSOCIATED WITH CEPHALOCELES

Amniotic band syndrome (sporadic)
  Multiple cephaloceles, predominantly anterior
  Amputations of digits or limbs
  Bizarre oral clefts
Chemke syndrome (AR)
  Hydrocephaly
  Agyria
  Cerebellar dysgenesis
Cryptophtalmos syndrome (AR)
  Forehead skin covers one or both eyes
  Ear abnormalities
  Soft tissue syndactyly
Dyssegmental dysplasia (AR)
  Short limb dysplasia
  Metaphyseal widening
  Small thorax
  Micrognathia
Frontonasal dysplasia (sporadic, some cases are familial)
  Frontal cephalocele
  Ocular hypertelorism
Meckel syndrome (AR)
  Polycystic kidneys
  Polydactyly
  Microphthalmia
  Orofacial clefting
  Ambiguous genitalia
von Voss syndrome (?)
  Agenesis of the corpus callosum
  Phocomelia
  Urogenital anomalies
  Thrombocytopenia
Warfarin syndrome
  Nasal hypoplasia
  Bone stippling
  Limb shortening
  Hydrocephaly

Associations
  Absence of corpus callosum
  Cleft lip or palate
  Cleft lip-palate
  Craniostenosis
  Dandy-Walker syndrome
  Ectrodactyly
  Hemifacial microsomia (see microphthalmia section)
  Iniencephaly
  Meningomyelocele

Modified from Cohen, Lemire:Teratology 25:161, 1982.

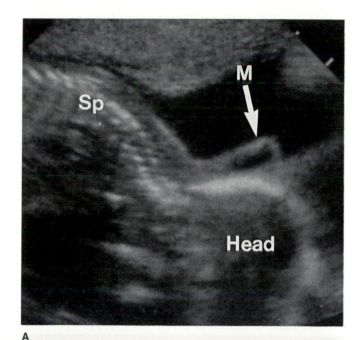

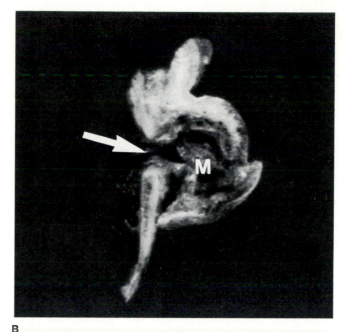

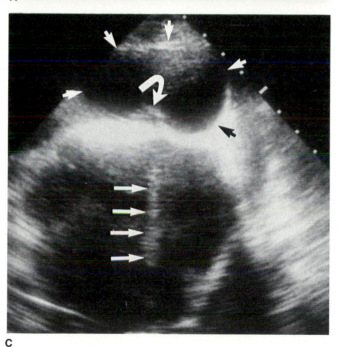

Figure 1–50. A. Longitudinal scan of the upper torso and head in a 21-week fetus with a small occipital meningocele (M). Sp, spine. **B.** Pathologic specimen obtained from the same fetus. The arrow points to the bony defect in the skull that connected the intracranial cavity to the meningocele (M). The diameter of the orifice was 2 mm. **C.** Occipital meningocele (*arrowheads*). A small amount of neural tissue is seen protruding inside the meningeal sac (*curved arrow*). A small bony defect is inferred by the presence of a pencil-like sound enhancement (*straight arrows*).

oropharynx. Frontal cephaloceles almost always contain brain tissue.[12]

Associated Anomalies

As previously mentioned, cephaloceles can be found as part of a number of specific syndromes (Table 1–13). In addition, both meningoceles and encephaloceles are associated with other CNS abnormalities. Hydrocephalus has been reported in 80 percent of occipital meningoceles, 65 percent of occipital encephaloceles,[10] and 15 percent of frontal cephaloceles.[5] Spina bifida is found in 7 to 15 percent of all cephaloceles.[1] Microcephaly was observed in 20

percent of cases studied.[10] By definition, the herniation of the cerebellum inside the cephalocele is termed "Chiari type III deformity." This deformity, combined with aqueductal stenosis, is the major cause of hydrocephalus in these infants.[12] Frontal cephaloceles are often associated with the median cleft face syndrome, characterized by hypertelorism and median cleft lip or palate.[3]

Diagnosis

Traditionally, the diagnosis of cephalocele relies on the demonstration of a paracranial mass.[1,4,6,8,13,14] However, this criterion is insufficient to distinguish

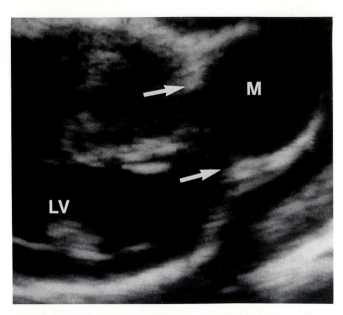

Figure 1–51. Occipital meningocele. Note the fluid-filled para-cranial mass (M) and the enlargement of the lateral ventricle (LV). The lack of continuity of the calvarium indicated by the arrows is an artifactual dropout of echoes. At autopsy, a bony defect of a few millimeters in diameter was found.

them from other nonneural masses, such as cystic hygromas, and soft tissue masses, such as scalp edema.[4,13] For this reason, an effort should be made to identify the skull defect.[1] This may be difficult, since the bony defect is usually smaller than the herniated mass and sometimes falls below the resolutive power of current ultrasound equipment (Fig.

1–50). In axial scans, the complete contour of the occipital and frontal bones is not adequately visualized because of sound refraction. Furthermore, the normal sutures can be confused with a defect.

Hints for a proper differential diagnosis are: (1) cephaloceles are often associated with hydrocephaly (Fig. 1–51), (2) brain tissue can be seen in some cephaloceles (Fig. 1–52), (3) cystic hygromas usually have multiple septa, are often associated with other signs of hydrops, and have a paracervical origin (see p. 117), and (4) severe scalp edema can be confused with a cephalocele, but usually a sagittal scan can identify an intact skull and the diffuse nature of the condition (Fig. 1–53).

Amniotic fluid alpha-fetoprotein (AFAFP) is usually elevated when the brain tissue or meninges are exposed. However, we have seen one case with a defect covered by skin in which the level of AFAFP was normal.

Whenever the diagnosis of a cephalocele is made, a careful examination of the fetus is indicated to search for other associated anomalies (Table 1–13).

Prognosis

The prognosis of cephaloceles depends on three factors: (1) the presence of brain in the herniated sac, (2) hydrocephalus, and (3) microcephaly. The most important prognostic factor is the herniation of the brain. The mortality rate in these cases has been reported to be 44 percent versus no deaths observed in cases of simple meningocele.[10] Intellectual development was normal in only 9 percent of patients in the former group and 60 percent in the latter.[10]

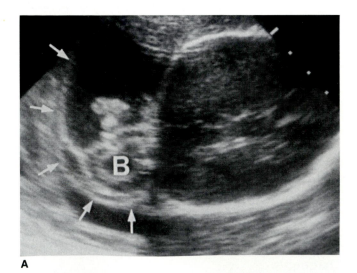

A

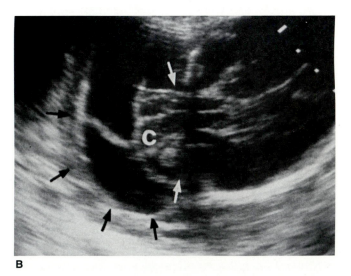

B

Figure 1–52. A. True encephalocele. Inside the meningeal sac (*arrows*), there is clear evidence of brain tissue (B). Head biometry revealed severe microcephaly. **B.** A different angulation of the transducer reveals the displacement of the entire cerebellum (C) inside the meningeal sac (*black arrows*) and the bony defect (*white arrows*).

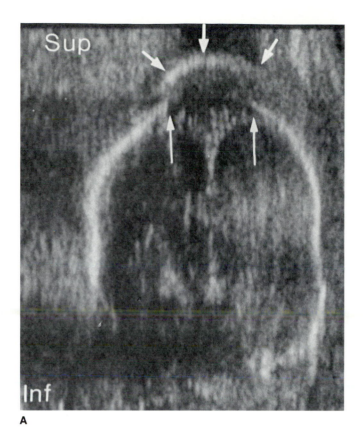
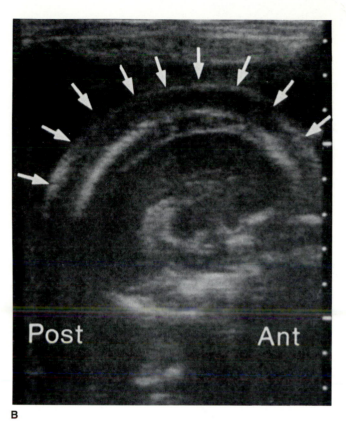

Figure 1–53. A. In this fetus with nonimmune hydrops, a coronal scan revealed a paracranial mass located along the sagittal suture (*short arrows*) and a corresponding dropout of echoes at the level of the calvarium (*long arrows*). The diagnosis of cephalocele was entertained. Inf, inferior; Sup, superior. **B.** A parasagittal scan reveals that the paracranial mass (*arrows*) extends all the way from the forehead to the occiput, suggesting that it is scalp edema. Ant, anterior; Post, posterior.

The influence of hydrocephalus on intellectual development is controversial. Lorber observed no significant difference in the groups of infants with and without ventriculomegaly.[10] In another series reported by Guthkelch, 86 percent of patients with meningocele without hydrocephalus had an IQ higher than 70, whereas only 50 percent of those with hydrocephalus had IQs above this level.[7]

The effect of microcephaly has been reported in a limited number of infants. Lorber[10] observed that 3 of 8 infants with microcephaly died, and the remaining five were intellectually impaired.

Obstetrical Management

Termination of pregnancy should be offered before viability. In the third trimester, obstetrical management depends on the size of the defect, the amount of herniated brain tissue, and associated anomalies. If associated anomalies incompatible with life are present (e.g., iniencephaly or Meckel syndrome), termination in the third trimester can be undertaken. In the absence of such findings, patients should be counseled (see Prognosis). Theoretically, a cesarean section could improve prognosis by avoiding birth trauma and contamination of brain tissue with

vaginal flora. Nonaggressive management is recommended in case of microcephaly.[1]

REFERENCES

1. Chervenak FA, Isaacson G, Mahoney MJ, et al.: Diagnosis and management of fetal cephalocele. Obstet Gynecol 64:86, 1984.
2. Cohen MM, Lemire RJ: Syndromes with cephaloceles. Teratology 25:161, 1982.
3. DeMyer W: The median cleft face syndrome: Differential diagnosis of cranium bifidum occultum, hypertelorism, and median cleft nose, lip, and palate. Neurology 17:961, 1967.
4. Fiske CE, Filly RA: Ultrasound evaluation of the normal and abnormal fetal neural axis. Radiol Clin North Am 20:285, 1982.
5. Fitz CR: Midline anomalies of the brain and spine. Radiol Clin North Am 20:95, 1982.
6. Graham D, Johnson TR, Winn K, et al.: The role of sonography in the prenatal diagnosis and management of encephalocele. J Ultrasound Med 1:111, 1982.
7. Guthkelch AN: Occipital cranium bifidum. Arch Dis Child 45:104, 1970.
8. Herzog KA: The detection of fetal meningocele and meningoencephalocele by B-scan ultrasound: A case report. J Clin Ultrasound 3:307, 1975.

9. Leong AS, Shaw CM: The pathology of occipital encephalocele and a discussion of the pathogenesis. Pathology 11:223, 1979.
10. Lorber J: The prognosis of occipital encephalocele. Dev Med Child Neurol [Suppl] 13:75, 1966.
11. Matson DD: Neurosurgery of Infancy and Childhood. Springfield, IL, Charles C Thomas, 1969.
12. McLaurin RL: Cranium bifidum and cranial cephaloceles. In: Vinken GW, Bruyn PW (eds): Handbook of Clinical Neurology. Amsterdam, Elsevier/North Holland Biomedical Press, 1977, Vol 30, pp 209–218.
13. Nicolini U, Ferrazzi E, Massa E, et al.: Prenatal diagnosis of cranial masses by ultrasound: Report of five cases. JCU 11:170, 1983.
14. Pilu, G, Rizzo N, Orsini LF, et al.: Antenatal recognition of cerebral anomalies. Ultrasound Med Biol 12:319, 1986.

Porencephaly

Synonyms
Porencephalic cyst, schizencephaly, and congenital brain clefts.

Definition
The term "porencephaly" describes an intracerebral, CSF-containing cystic cavity, which may or may not communicate with the ventricular system and the subarachnoid space.

Incidence
True porencephaly is an extremely rare disease. In an autopsy study of 1000 cases of infantile brain damage, 25 infants (2.5 percent) had this condition.[5] The prevalence of congenital pseudoporencephaly is unknown.

Etiopathogenesis
Porencephalic disorders are generally subdivided into two types: true porencephaly and pseudoporencephaly. True porencephaly (schizencephaly) is a developmental anomaly caused by a failure in the migration of cells destined to form the cerebral cortex. This anomaly causes a local defect in both gray and white matter. In the absence of neural tissue, the subarachnoid space expands to fill the void, and, hence, the appearance of a porous cyst occurs. The designation "porous" alludes to the frequently seen communication of the brain with the subarachnoid space.

Pseudoporencephaly is a consequence of local destruction of the cerebral parenchyma by a vascular, infectious, or traumatic cause that may occur either in utero or any time after birth.[1,2,5] Examples of this acquired pseudoporencephaly are the cysts that developed after repeated needling of the ventricular system in hydrocephalic infants before early neonatal shunting procedures were introduced.[7] There is no evidence of familial occurrence of porencephaly.

The cytoarchitectural disorders due to failure of migration comprise a broad spectrum from microgyria to porencephaly.[6] In the former, the migration disorder is mild, and there are small cerebral gyri. The spectrum continues through macrogyria (large and fewer cerebral gyri), lissencephaly or agyria (absence of cerebral gyri), to porencephaly, where the defect is so severe that it affects a local portion of both cortex and white matter.[5,10,11]

Pathology
True porencephaly is characterized by cystic cavities of variable size usually localized around the Sylvian fissure and, in many cases, symmetrical in shape. They are frequently associated with other localized cytoarchitectural disorders, such as micropolygyria

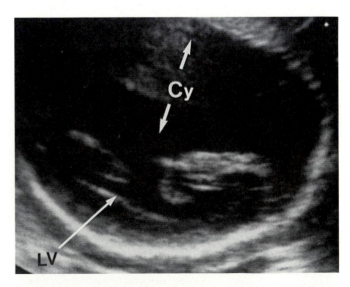

Figure 1–54. Axial scan of the head of a 32-week fetus with severe porencephaly. The cerebral hemisphere that is closer to the transducer is entirely replaced by a cystic structure (Cy). Note the marked shift of the midline and the mildly enlarged contralateral ventricle (LV). *(Reproduced with permission from Pilu et al.: Ultrasound Med Biol 12:319, 1986.)*

and heterotopias of gray matter. The corpus callosum may be hypoplastic or absent.[4,5,10,11]

Pseudoporencephaly differs from true porencephaly in that it is almost always unilateral and associated with histologic evidence of inflammation or ischemic injury.[4,5]

True porencephaly is frequently seen in association with microcephaly. Ventriculomegaly is seen in both porencephaly and pseudoporencephaly and is, in most cases, asymmetrical. Although the most frequent locations for porencephalic cysts are the cerebral hemispheres, these lesions can occur in the cerebellum and the spinal cord as well.

Diagnosis

The diagnosis depends on the demonstration of intracranial cystic areas. They may be either bilateral in cases of true porencephaly or, more frequently, unilateral.[8] A marked asymmetrical dilatation of the lateral ventricles with a shift of the midline is a common finding (Fig. 1–54) Porencephaly should always be considered whenever a marked asymmetrical ventriculomegaly is found.[3] The most valuable

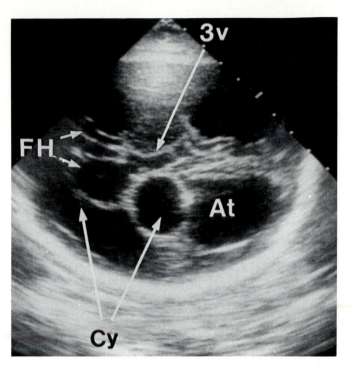

Figure 1–56. Multiple cystic lesions (Cy) are seen within the cerebral parenchyma in this third trimester fetus with infectious pseudoporencephaly. An asymmetrical enlargement of the lateral ventricles is seen. At, atria of lateral ventricles; FH, frontal horns of lateral ventricle; 3v, third ventricle.

information is provided by coronal scans, which clearly demonstrate loss of cerebral tissue (Fig. 1–55).

Differential diagnosis includes other congenital cystic lesions of the brain, such as arachnoid cyst[3] and cystic tumors.[9] If the cystic lesion is on the base of the skull, porencephaly is not the most likely diagnosis. Consequently, arachnoid cysts or other tumors should be considered first. A positive diagnosis can be made in most cases in which extensive destruction of a brain hemisphere has occurred (Figs. 1–54, 1–55, 1–56). In milder forms, the differentiation between arachnoid cysts and cystic tumors may prove impossible.

Prognosis

The prognosis largely depends on the size of the lesion. Infants with true porencephaly have an extremely poor outcome, with invariable, severe intellectual impairment and neurologic sequelae. In a series of 22 cases reported by Gross and Simanyi,[5] 81.8 percent of infants had idiocy and 18.2 percent imbecility. Furthermore, signs of severe neurologic compromise, such as spastic tetraplegia (95.4 percent), and blindness (40.8 percent), were found. The development of speech was absent or poor with this lesion. The clinical course for severe pseudoporencephaly is similar to that of true porencephaly. Milder lesions may result in fewer neurologic disabilities.

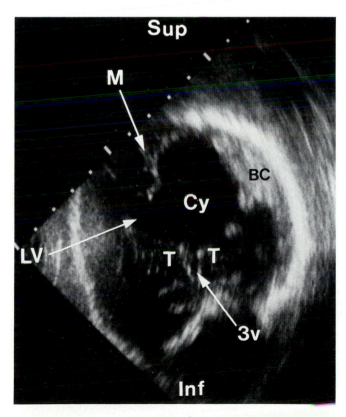

Figure 1–55. Coronal scan of the head of a 30-week fetus with severe porencephaly. A large cystic cavity (Cy) occupying most of one hemisphere and amply communicating with the contralateral lateral ventricle (LV) is seen. The hyperechoic area seen close to the parietal bone was found at birth to be a large blood clot (BC). Inf, inferior; Sup, superior; T, thalami; M, midline.

Parents and physicians should be aware that porencephaly is an untreatable anomaly because the basic defect is a localized absence of cerebral mass.

Obstetrical Management

Termination of pregnancy should be offered before viability. After viability, nonaggressive management is recommended. Macrocephaly has been reported to occur in 9.1 percent of infants studied.[5] Cephalocentesis may be used under these circumstances to avoid a cesarean section caused by failure of progress in labor.

REFERENCES

1. Benda CE: The late effects of cerebral birth injuries. Medicine 24:71, 1945.
2. Cantu RC, LeMay M: Porencephaly caused by intracerebral hemorrhage. Radiology 88:526, 1967.
3. Chervenak FA, Berkowitz RL, Romero R, et al.: The diagnosis of fetal hydrocephalus. Am J Obstet Gynecol 147:703, 1983.
4. Gross H, Jellinger K: Morphologische aspekte cerebraler Midbildungen. Wien Z Nervenheilk 27:6, 1969.
5. Gross H, Simanyi M: Porencephaly. In: Vinken PJ, Bruyn GW (eds): Handbook of Clinical Neurology. Amsterdam, Elsevier/North Holland Biomedical Press, 1977, Vol 30, pp 681–692.
6. Larroche JC: Cytoarchitectonic abnormalities (abnormalities of cell migration). In: Vinken PJ, Bruyn GW (eds); Handbook of Clinical Neurology. Amsterdam, Elsevier/North Holland Biomedical Press, 1977, Vol 30, pp 479–506.
7. Lorber J, Grainger RG: Cerebral cavities following ventricular punctures in infants. Clin Radiol 14:98, 1963.
8. Mori K: Porencephaly and schizencephaly. In: Anomalies of the Central Nervous System. Neuroradiology and Neurosurgery. New York, Thieme Stratton, 1985, pp 35–38.
9. Sauerbrei EE, Cooperberg PL: Cystic tumors of the fetal and neonatal cerebrum: Ultrasound and computed tomographic evaluation. Radiology 147:689, 1983.
10. Yakovlev PI, Wadsworth RC: Schizencephalies: A study of the congenital clefts in the cerebral mantle. I. Clefts with fused lips. J Neuropathol Exp Neurol 5:116, 1946.
11. Yakovlev PI, Wadsworth RC: Schizencephalies: A study of the congenital clefts in the cerebral mantle. II. Clefts with hydrocephalus and lips separated. J Neuropathol Exp Neurol 5:169, 1946.

Hydranencephaly

Synonyms
Hydrocephalic anencephaly, hydroencephalodysplasia, hydromerencephaly, and cystencephaly.

Definition
Hydranencephaly describes a condition in which most of the cerebral hemispheres are absent and are replaced by CSF.

Epidemiology
Hydranencephaly is found in 0.2 percent of infant autopsies. Approximately 1 percent of infants thought to have hydrocephalus by clinical examination are later found to have hydranencephaly.[4]

Etiology
Hydranencephaly does not seem to be a developmental anomaly but rather the result of a destructive intrauterine insult of vascular or infectious origin. Vascular occlusion of the internal carotid artery cuts the blood supply to the cerebral hemispheres and causes extensive necrosis. Myers[10] has successfully created hydranencephaly in monkeys by either bilateral occlusion of the carotid artery and jugular vein in

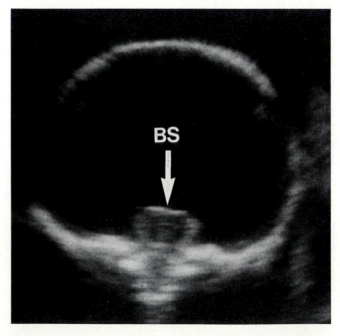

Figure 1–57. Coronal scan in a fetus with hydranencephaly and macrocrania. Note the typical appearance of the brain stem (BS) that bulges inside an entirely fluid-filled intracranial cavity. *(Reproduced with permission from Pilu et al.: Ultrasound Med Biol 12:319, 1986.)*

utero or by incomplete placental abruption. This view is supported by observations of absence,[6] thrombosis,[11] and vasculitis[7] of the cerebral vessels in hydranencephalic infants. Infection[1] may cause hydranencephaly either by a necrotizing vasculitis or by local destruction of brain tissue. In these cases, dilatation of the ventricular system will occur, filling the intracranial cavity. Some authors have expressed the view that hydranencephaly may be considered as an extreme form of pseudoporencephaly. Familial cases are rare.[5,15]

Pathology

There is variability in the extent of destruction of the cerebral hemispheres. Destruction may be complete[5] or may spare portions of the temporal and occipital cortex.[4,5,9] The brain stem is present, although the thalami and cerebellum may be smaller than normal. The head is filled with CSF, which is contained in a cavity lined by leptomeninges. Macrocrania may develop.[5,14] The falx cerebri may be absent or incomplete.

Diagnosis

A positive diagnosis can be made by identifying a large cystic mass filling the entire intracranial cavity or by detecting the absence or discontinuity of the cerebral cortex and of the midline echo.[2,3,8,13] The ultrasound appearance of the brain stem protruding inside the cystic cavity is quite characteristic[12] (Fig. 1–57).

The most common diagnostic problem is the differentiation among hydranencephaly, extreme hydrocephalus, and porencephaly. In porencephaly, some spared cortical mantle is usually seen. Extreme hydrocephalus may be difficult to differentiate from those cases of hydranencephaly in which the falx is present, even in the neonatal period.[14] The most important clue is the typical appearance of the thalami and brain stem, which bulge inside the fluid-filled intracranial cavity when hydranencephaly is present. In extreme hydrocephalus, these structures are surrounded by cortex and do not acquire such an appearance. The presence of even minimal frontal cerebral cortex indicates extreme hydrocephalus instead of hydranencephaly.

Pathologists can make a differential diagnosis between hydranencephaly and hydrocephalus by examining the lining of the cystic structures. While leptomeninges will be found in hydranencephaly, ependyma lines the ventricular system in hydrocephalus.

Prognosis

Data on the neurologic performance of hydranencephalic infants is scanty. Some infants with hydranencephaly have severe neurologic abnormalities at birth and die. Abnormalities include seizures, myoclonus, and respiratory failure. Chronic survival (up to 3.5 years) occurs in some cases and seems to depend on an intact hypothalamus capable of thermoregulation.[5] These infants have no intellectual function.[4]

Obstetrical Management

The option of pregnancy termination before viability should be offered. In those cases where a clear differentiation from extreme hydrocephaly cannot be made (e.g., a normal midline echo), the pregnancy should be managed as if the fetus had hydrocephaly. If macrocephaly is present in a fetus with a confident diagnosis of hydranencephaly, cephalocentesis is indicated to allow vaginal delivery. Cesarean section for fetal distress does not seem justifiable.

REFERENCES

1. Altshuler G: Toxoplasmosis as a cause of hydranencephaly. Am J Dis Child 125:251, 1973.
2. Carrasco CR, Stierman ED, Harnsberger HR, et al.: An algorithm for prenatal ultrasound diagnosis of congenital central nervous system abnormalities. J Ultrasound Med 4:163, 1985.
3. Fiske CE, Filly RA: Ultrasound evaluation of the normal and abnormal fetal neural axis. Radiol Clin North Am 20:285, 1982.
4. Halsey JH, Allen N, Chamberlin HR: Hydranencephaly. In: Vinken PJ, Bruyn GW (eds): Handbook of Clinical Neurology. Amsterdam, Elsevier/North Holland Biomedical Press, 1977, Vol 30, pp 661–680.
5. Hamby WB, Krauss RF, Beswick WF: Hydranencephaly: Clinical diagnosis. Presentation of 7 cases. Pediatrics 6:371, 1950.
6. Johnson EE, Warner M, Simonds JP: Total absence of the cerebral hemispheres. J Pediatr 38:69, 1951.
7. Lange-Cossack H: Die Hydranencephalie (Blasenhirn) als Sonderform der grosshirnlosigkeit. Arch Psychiatr Nervenkr 117:1, 1944.
8. Lee TG, Warren BH: Antenatal diagnosis of hydranencephaly by ultrasound: Correlation with ventriculography and computed tomography. JCU 5:271, 1977.
9. Lindenberg R, Swanson PD: "Infantile hydranencephaly": A report of five cases of infarction of both cerebral hemispheres in infancy. Brain 90:839, 1967.
10. Myers RE: Brain pathology following fetal vascular occlusion: An experimental study. Invest Ophthalmol 8:41, 1969.
11. Norman RM: Malformations of the central nervous system, birth injury, and diseases of early life. In: Greenfield JG, Blackwood W, McMenemey WH, et al. (eds): Neuropathology. London, Edward Arnold, 1958, pp 300–407.
12. Pilu G, Rizzo N, Orsini LF, et al.: Antenatal recognition

of cerebral anomalies. Ultrasound Med Biol 12:319, 1986.

13. Strauss S, Bouzouki M, Goldfarb H, et al.: Antenatal ultrasound diagnosis of an unusual case of hydranencephaly. JCU 12:420, 1984.

14. Sutton LN, Bruce DA, Schut L: Hydranencephaly versus maximal hydrocephalus: An important clinical distinction. Neurosurgery 6:35, 1980.

15. Williamson EM: Incidence and family aggregation of major congenital malformations of central nervous system. J Med Genet 2:161, 1965.

Microcephaly

Synonym
Microencephaly.

Definition
Microcephaly is a clinical syndrome characterized by a head circumference below the normal range. It is associated with abnormal neurologic findings and subnormal mental development.[18]

Historically, the interest in microcephaly arose from the observation that infants with ape-shaped heads were mentally retarded. Autopsy findings demonstrated that they had a small brain (microencephaly), and this was thought to be the cause of the intellectual handicap. The diagnosis has been based on measurement of the head circumference at the level of the occipitofrontal plane.[4,16] Different thresh-

TABLE 1–14. CLASSIFICATION OF MICROCEPHALY

I. Microcephaly with associated malformations

A. Genetic
1. Chromosomal aberrations
   Down syndrome
   Trisomy 13 syndrome
   Trisomy 18 syndrome
   Trisomy 22 syndrome
   4p− syndrome
   Cat cry (5p−) syndrome
   18p− syndrome
   18q− syndrome
2. Single gene defects
   Bloom syndrome (AR)
   Borjeson-Forssman-Lehmann syndrome (XLR)
   Cockayne syndrome (AR)
   DeSanctis-Cacchione syndrome (AR)
   Dubowitz syndrome (AR)
   Fanconi pancytopenia (AR)
   Focal dermal hypoplasia (XLD)
   Incontinentia pigmenti (XLD)
   Lissencephaly syndrome (AR)
   Meckel-Gruber syndrome (AR)
   Menkes syndrome (XLR)
   Roberts syndrome (AR)
   Seckel bird-headed dwarfism (AR)
   Smith-Lemli-Opitz syndrome (AR)

B. Environmental
1. Prenatal infections
   Rubella syndrome
   Cytomegalovirus disease
   Herpesvirus hominis
   Toxoplasmosis
2. Prenatal exposure to drugs or chemicals
   Fetal alcohol syndrome
   Fetal hydantoin syndrome
   Aminopterin syndrome
3. Maternal phenylketonuria

C. Unknown etiology
1. Recognized syndromes
   Coffin-Siris syndrome
   DeLange syndrome
   Johanson-Blizzard syndrome
   Langer-Giedion syndrome
   Rubenstein-Taybi syndrome
   Williams syndrome
2. Undefined combinations

II. Microcephaly without associated malformations

A. Genetic
1. Primary microcephaly (AR)
2. Paine syndrome (XLR)
3. Alpers disease (AR)
4. Inborn errors of metabolism
   Disorders of folic acid metabolism (AR)
   Hyperlysinemia (AR)
   Methylmalonic acidemia (AR)
   Phenylketonuria (AR)

B. Environmental
1. Prenatal exposure to radiation
2. Fetal malnutrition
3. Perinatal trauma or hypoxia
4. Postnatal infections

C. Unknown etiology
   Happy puppet syndrome

Adapted from Ross, Frias: In: Vinken, Bruyn (eds.): Handbook of Clinical Neurology. Amsterdam, Elsevier/North Holland Biomedical Press, 1977, Vol 30, pp 507–524.

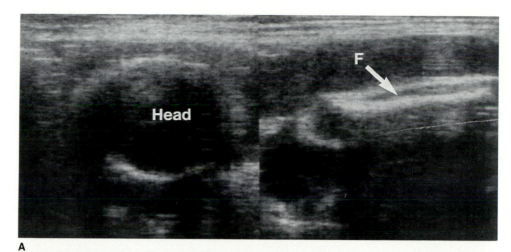

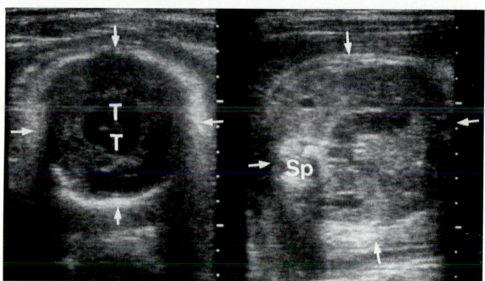

Figure 1–58. Severe microcephaly. **A.** The size of the head of a full-term fetus is compared to the length of the femur (F). Intracranial structures cannot be visualized. **B.** In a 35-week fetus, the size of the head is compared to the size of the abdomen. The fetus was found to have holoprosencephaly. T, thalami; Sp, spine.

olds have been proposed. Some authors have used a head circumference 2 SD below the mean[1,17] as a diagnostic criterion, whereas others require 3 SD.[2,3,7,10,19] The prevalence of the condition is different according to the chosen threshold. If 2 SD below the mean is used, 2.5 percent of the general population are considered microcephalic. A significant number of intellectually normal infants would be included in this group.[18] If 3 SD below is employed, the incidence of the condition is 0.1 percent, a figure more in keeping with the epidemiologic observations and the intention of the definition—to identify infants at risk for mental retardation. Although the head circumference in a normally shaped head correlates with brain weight (volume), this may not be true in cases of true microcephaly, since the cranial deficit is above the base of the skull.[20] This problem may explain the difficulties and pitfalls in diagnosing microcephaly purely on the basis of a head circumference. Therefore, we believe that the shape of the head should also be taken into account.

Incidence

The incidence is estimated to be 1.6 per 1000 single-birth deliveries. Only 14 percent of all microcephalic infants diagnosed by the first year of age had been detected at birth.[15]

Etiology and Associated Malformations

Microcephaly is classified into two categories: (1) microcephaly without associated anomalies and (2) microcephaly with associated malformations. Table 1–14 presents a classification of microcephaly and etiologic causes.

Pathology

When microcephaly is present, the most affected part is the forebrain. Associated anomalies are frequent and include asymmetries, macrogyria, pachygyria, and atrophy of the basal ganglia.[8] In some instances, the lateral ventricles are enlarged due to the atrophy of the cortex.[18] The basal ganglia appear disproportionately large.[14] A decrease in dendritic arborization has also been described.[9]

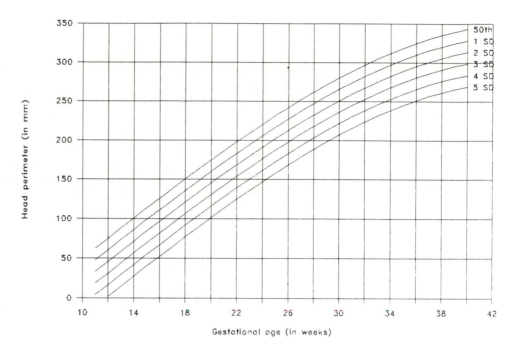

Figure 1–59. Relationship between head perimeter and gestational age. SD, standard deviation.

TABLE 1–15. HEAD PERIMETER

Age (weeks)	Head Perimeter (mm)					
	50th	−1SD	−2SD	−3SD	−4SD	−5SD
11	63	48	33	19	4	—
12	75	61	46	31	17	2
13	88	73	59	44	29	15
14	101	86	71	57	42	27
15	113	99	84	69	55	40
16	126	111	96	82	67	52
17	138	124	109	94	80	65
18	151	136	121	107	92	77
19	163	148	133	119	104	89
20	175	160	145	131	116	101
21	187	172	157	143	128	113
22	198	184	169	154	140	125
23	210	195	180	166	151	136
24	221	206	191	177	162	147
25	232	217	202	188	173	158
26	242	227	213	198	183	169
27	252	238	223	208	194	179
28	262	247	233	218	203	189
29	271	257	242	227	213	198
30	281	266	251	236	222	207
31	289	274	260	245	230	216
32	297	283	268	253	239	224
33	305	290	276	261	246	232
34	312	297	283	268	253	239
35	319	304	289	275	260	245
36	325	310	295	281	266	251
37	330	316	301	286	272	257
38	335	320	306	291	276	262
39	339	325	310	295	281	266
40	343	328	314	299	284	270

SD = standard deviation.

Diagnosis

The diagnosis should be suspected if the head perimeter is 3 SD below the mean for gestational age (Figs. 1–58, 1–59, Table 1–15). Although other authors have proposed the use of the biparietal diameter as a diagnostic parameter, this measurement can be modified by intrauterine molding, whereas the head perimeter is not. Interpretation of the head perimeter assumes a precise knowledge of the gestational age. Because this information is not always available, an alternative is to use noncephalic biometric parameters instead of gestational age.[6] Table 1–16 and Figure 1–60 show the head perimeter and femur length relationships. Caution is advised in the use of the nomogram as it assumes that skeletal growth of the limbs is not affected in microcephaly, although it is known that growth impairment of the long bones occurs in some cases. Another alternative is to use the head to abdomen perimeter ratio (Fig. 1–61). However, head to body disproportion could be caused by intrauterine growth retardation. We discourage making a diagnosis of microcephaly based solely on this parameter.

A potentially helpful diagnostic hint is the shape of the fetal head. Microcephalic fetuses have a sloping forehead that can be demonstrated by ultrasound[13] (Fig. 1–62). The index of suspicion should be raised also when dilatation of the lateral ventricles is seen in association with a head with borderline dimensions (e.g., head perimeter between 2 SD and 3 SD below the mean). Kurtz et al.[11] have suggested that in some instances of severe microcephaly, the intracranial contents may not be visible (Fig. 1–58). A

TABLE 1–16. FEMUR LENGTH/HEAD CIRCUMFERENCE

Age (weeks)	SD Below Mean					Mean	SD Above Mean				
	−5	−4	−3	−2	−1		+1	+2	+3	+4	+5
20	0.107	0.122	0.137	0.152	0.167	0.180	0.197	0.212	0.227	0.242	0.257
21	0.111	0.126	0.141	0.156	0.171	0.190	0.201	0.216	0.231	0.246	0.261
22	0.115	0.130	0.145	0.160	0.175	0.190	0.205	0.220	0.235	0.250	0.265
23	0.118	0.133	0.148	0.163	0.178	0.190	0.208	0.223	0.238	0.253	0.268
24	0.121	0.136	0.151	0.166	0.181	0.200	0.211	0.226	0.241	0.256	0.271
25	0.123	0.138	0.153	0.168	0.183	0.200	0.213	0.228	0.243	0.258	0.273
26	0.125	0.140	0.155	0.170	0.185	0.200	0.215	0.230	0.245	0.260	0.275
27	0.127	0.142	0.157	0.172	0.187	0.200	0.217	0.232	0.247	0.262	0.277
28	0.129	0.144	0.159	0.174	0.189	0.200	0.219	0.234	0.249	0.264	0.279
29	0.130	0.145	0.160	0.175	0.190	0.200	0.220	0.235	0.250	0.265	0.280
30	0.131	0.146	0.161	0.176	0.191	0.210	0.224	0.236	0.251	0.266	0.281
31	0.132	0.147	0.162	0.177	0.192	0.210	0.222	0.237	0.252	0.267	0.282
32	0.134	0.149	0.164	0.179	0.194	0.210	0.224	0.239	0.254	0.269	0.284
33	0.135	0.150	0.165	0.180	0.195	0.210	0.225	0.240	0.255	0.270	0.285
34	0.136	0.151	0.166	0.181	0.196	0.210	0.226	0.241	0.256	0.271	0.286
35	0.138	0.153	0.168	0.183	0.198	0.210	0.228	0.243	0.258	0.273	0.288
36	0.140	0.155	0.170	0.185	0.200	0.210	0.230	0.245	0.260	0.275	0.290
37	0.142	0.157	0.172	0.187	0.202	0.220	0.232	0.247	0.262	0.277	0.292
38	0.144	0.159	0.174	0.189	0.204	0.220	0.234	0.249	0.264	0.279	0.294
39	0.147	0.162	0.177	0.192	0.207	0.220	0.237	0.252	0.267	0.282	0.297
40	0.151	0.166	0.181	0.196	0.211	0.230	0.241	0.256	0.271	0.286	0.301
41	0.155	0.170	0.185	0.200	0.215	0.230	0.245	0.260	0.275	0.290	0.305
42	0.160	0.175	0.190	0.205	0.220	0.230	0.250	0.265	0.280	0.295	0.310

SD = standard deviation.

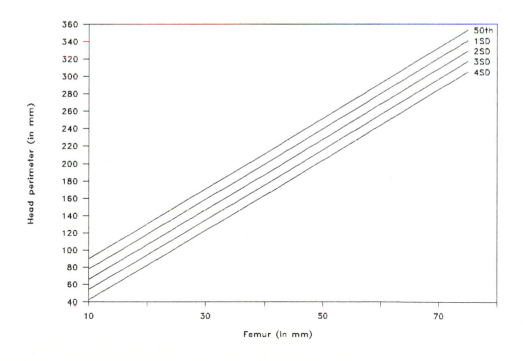

Figure 1–60. Relationship between femur length and head perimeter. SD, standard deviation.

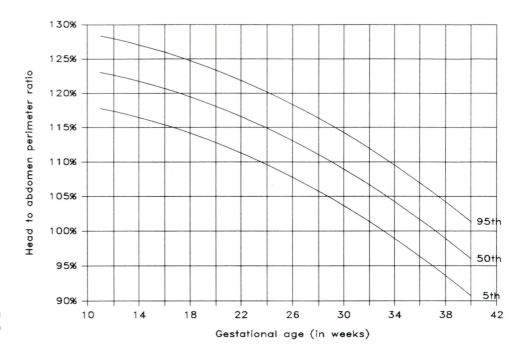

Figure 1–61. Relationship between the head to abdomen perimeter ratio and gestational age.

major problem with the antenatal diagnosis of microcephaly is that the natural history is unknown. The onset and course of head growth impairment in utero have not been established, and it has been suggested that in some cases the diagnosis is not possible in the second trimester.[5]

The problem of the differential diagnosis between microcephaly and craniosynostosis cannot be solved in utero at the present time because closure of the sutures cannot be identified. Potential clues include (1) the shape of the head, (2) association with congenital anomalies suggesting specific syndromes

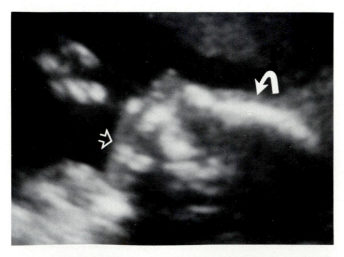

Figure 1–62. Profile of a second trimester fetus with microcephaly and multiple anomalies, demonstrating sloping forehead (*curved arrow*) and striking micrognathia (*open arrow*).

seen with microcephaly (e.g., polycystic kidney, Meckel syndrome), (3) a family history of microcephaly or other genetic syndromes including this anomaly, and (4) occurrence of a viral or parasitic infection or exposure to other agents (e.g., alcohol, diphenylhydantoin) known to be associated with microcephaly.

Prognosis

The prognosis is different for infants with or without associated anomalies. For the latter group, the outlook is related to the severity of the associated anomalies. Trisomy 13, trisomy 18, Meckel syndrome, and alobar holoprosencephaly are all fatal conditions. For infants without associated malformations, the prognosis is dependent on head size. The available information was obtained in the postnatal period, and it is not known if these figures are applicable to antenatally diagnosed cases, because the natural history of this condition is unknown. Avery et al.[1] have addressed the issue of the clinical relevance of biometrically diagnosed microcephaly and found that infants with head circumferences between 2 and 3 SD below the mean had an incidence of moderate to severe mental retardation of 33 percent. The remainder were either normal or mildly retarded. Infants with head circumferences below 3 SD had a 62 percent incidence of moderate to severe mental retardation. These observations were made in infants diagnosed during the first year of life with a Bailey mental development index. Pryor and Thelander[17] reported that infants with head circumferences between 4 SD and 7 SD below the mean had a mean IQ of 35.6, and those with head circumferences below 7 SD had a mean IQ of 20.

Obstetrical Management

Microcephaly is an untreatable disease. A very serious attempt should be made to identify associated congenital anomalies. Both a detailed ultrasound evaluation and an amniocentesis for fetal karyotype are mandatory. In the absence of associated anomalies, patients are counseled only on the basis of the head perimeter. If this is between 2 SD and 3 SD below the mean for gestational age, there is a very good chance that the infant will be normal. Below 4 SD, the prognosis is guarded. The relationship between the femur to head perimeter ratio and intellectual development is unknown and should not be used to predict mental handicaps. Therefore, if the diagnosis is made before viability, the option of termination of pregnancy should be considered.

REFERENCES

1. Avery GB, Meneses L, Lodge A: The clinical significance of "measurement microcephaly." Am J Dis Child 123:214, 1972.
2. Book JA, Schut JW, Reed SC: A clinical and genetical study of microcephaly. Am J Ment Defic 57:637, 1953.
3. Brandon MWG, Kirman BH, Williams CE: Microcephaly. J Ment Sci 105:721, 1959.
4. Bray PF, Shields WD, Wolcott GJ, et al.: Occipitofrontal head circumference—An accurate measure of intracranial volume. J Pediatr 75:303, 1969.
5. Campbell S, Allan LD, Griffin D, et al.: The early diagnosis of fetal structural abnormalities. In: Lerski RA, Morley P (eds): Ultrasound '82. Oxford, Pergamon Press, 1983, pp 547–563.
6. Chervenak FA, Jeanty P, Cantraine F, et al.: The diagnosis of fetal microcephaly. Am J Obstet Gynecol 149:512, 1984.
7. Daniel WL: A genetic and biochemical investigation of primary microcephaly. Am J Ment Defic 75:653, 1971.
8. Davies H, Kirman BH: Microcephaly. Arch Dis Child 37:623, 1962.
9. Huttenlocher PR: Dendritic development in neocortex of children with mental defect and infantile spasms. Neurology 24:203, 1974.
10. Komai T, Kishimoto K, Ozaki Y: Genetic study of microcephaly based on Japanese material. Am J Hum Genet 7:51, 1955.
11. Kurtz AB, Wapner RJ, Rubin CS, et al.: Ultrasound criteria for in utero diagnosis of microcephaly. J Clin Ultrasound 8:11, 1980.
12. Lenke RR, Platt LD, Koch R: Ultrasonographic failure of early detection of fetal microcephaly in maternal phenylketonuria. J Ultrasound Med 2:177, 1983.
13. Pearce JM, Little D, Campbell S: The diagnosis of abnormalities of the fetal central nervous system. In: Sanders RC, James EA (eds): The Principles and Practice of Ultrasonography in Obstetrics and Gynecology, 3d ed. Norwalk, CT, Appleton-Century-Crofts, 1985, pp 243–256.
14. Ludwin KS, Malamud N: Pathology of congenital anomalies of the brain. In: Newton TH, Potts DG (eds): Radiology of the Skull and Brain, Anatomy and Pathology. St. Louis, CV Mosby, 1977, pp 2979–3015.
15. Myrianthopoulos NC, Chung CS: Congenital malformations in Singletons: Epidemiologic survey. Birth Defects 10:1, 1974.
16. Nellhaus G: Head circumference from birth to eighteen years. Practical composite international and interracial graphs. Pediatrics 41:106, 1968.
17. Pryor HB, Thelander H: Abnormally small head size and intellect in children. J Pediatr 73:593, 1968.
18. Ross JJ, Frias JL: Microcephaly. In: Vinken GW, Bruyn PW (eds): Handbook of Clinical Neurology. Amsterdam, Elsevier/North Holland Biomedical Press, 1977, Vol 30, pp 507–524.
19. Van Den Bosch J: Microcephaly in the Netherlands: A clinical and genetical study. Ann Hum Genet 23:91, 1959.
20. Warkany J: Congenital Malformations. Chicago, Year Book, 1971.

Holoprosencephaly

Definition

Holoprosencephaly is a complex developmental abnormality of the brain arising from failure of cleavage of the prosencephalon. The condition termed "holoprosencephaly" includes cyclopia, cebocephaly, ethmocephaly, median cleft, and holotelencephaly (see Table 1–17).

Epidemiology

The incidence of holoprosencephaly is not known because milder forms without facial defects may be unrecognized unless appropriate diagnostic investigation is undertaken. Cyclopia has been reported to occur in 1:40,000 births, whereas cebocephaly and median cleft lip occur at a rate of 1:16,000 births.[10, 24] The disease may be more frequent in abortuses; Matsunaga and Shiota[21] report an incidence of 0.4 percent of induced abortions. This observation suggests a high fatality rate.

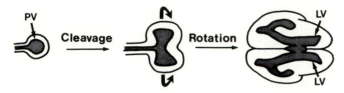

Figure 1–63. Normal development of the prosencephalon. PV, primitive ventricular cavity; LV, lateral ventricles.

Etiology

Chromosomal abnormalities (primarily trisomy 13, trisomy 18, and trisomy 13/15) are found in association with holoprosencephaly.[8,10] Other abnormalities include deletions (18p−) and ring chromosomes (mainly 18).[10] Teratogenic agents, such as veratrum alkaloids and radiation, have induced holoprosencephaly in animals.[10] Ingestion of salicylates in pregnancy has also been reported in relation to holoprosencephaly.[4] Several studies have indicated a familial tendency, with both autosomal dominant with variable penetrance and autosomal recessive transmission.[8,10,24] An association with diabetes and maternal infections during pregnancy has been suggested but not proven.[10] The empirical recurrence risk in the absence of chromosomal abnormalities has been estimated to be 6 percent.[8,10,24] In the presence of an abnormal karyotype, the recurrence risk depends on the chromosomal aberration. A primary trisomy is associated with a less than 1 percent chance of recurrence. If the parents are carriers of a balanced translocation, the recurrence risks are much greater.

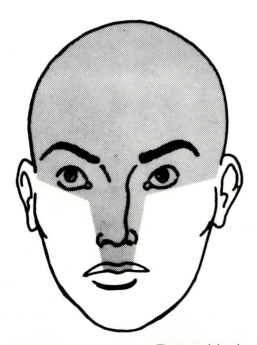

Figure 1–64. Median facial structures. The normal development of these areas is induced by the prechordal mesenchyma.

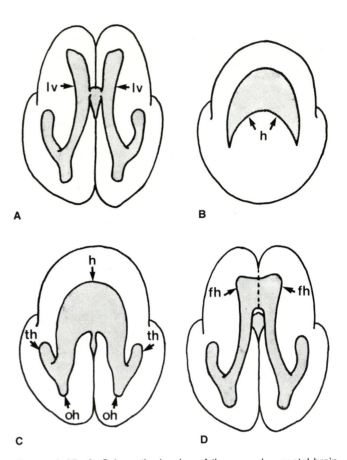

Figure 1–65. A. Schematic drawing of the normal neonatal brain seen from above. Both cerebral hemispheres and lateral ventricles are completely separated. **B.** Alobar holoprosencephaly. There is absence of division of the cerebral hemispheres and a single primitive ventricular cavity. **C.** Semilobar holoprosencephaly. There is an incipient separation of the hemispheres in the occipital area and partial development of the occipital and temporal horns of the ventricles. **D.** Lobar holoprosencephaly. Note the almost complete separation of the cerebral hemispheres. The ventricles are almost totally separated, except for the frontal portion, and are generally mildly dilated. The antenatal differential diagnosis between lobar holoprosencephaly and some forms of hydrocephaly may be very difficult. lv, lateral ventricles; h, holoventricle; oh, occipital horns; th, temporal horns; fh, frontal horns). *(Reproduced with permission from Pilu et al.: Am J Perinatol 4:41, 1987.)*

Embryology

Holoprosencephaly is the result of a failure of cleavage of the prosencephalon. The prosencephalon is the most rostral of the three primitive cerebral vesicles and gives rise to the cerebral hemispheres and diencephalic structures (including neurohypophysis, thalami, third ventricle, and optic bulbs) (Fig. 1–63). This differentiation process is thought to be induced by the prechordal mesenchyma interposed between the roof of the mouth and the prosencephalon. The same tissue is responsible for the normal development of the median facial structures (forehead, nose, interorbital structures, and upper lip) (Fig. 1–64).

An interference with the activity of the prechordal mesenchyma would lead to defects in both areas, brain

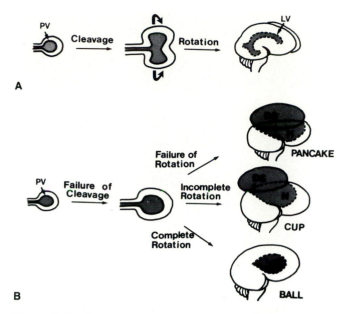

Figure 1–66. Comparative development of normal and holoprosencephalic brain. **A.** The primitive prosencephalon undergoes cleavage, and, subsequently, the two hemispheres rotate medially to form the interhemispheric fissure. From the primitive ventricular cavity (PV), two separated lateral ventricles (LV) are formed. **B.** In alobar holoprosencephaly, failure of cleavage results in a single ventricular cavity (H). The degree of subsequent inward rotation of the cortex determines the morphologic type. Absence of rotation results in the pancake type, in which the membranous diencephalic roof bulges to form the so-called dorsal sac (DS). In the intermediate form (cup type), the cortex rolls over to partially cover the diencephalic roof. In the ball type, full rotation has occurred, and the single ventricle is completely covered.

and face.[9,10,12] The cerebral anomalies are due to varying degrees of failure of cleavage of the prosencephalon, with incomplete division of the cerebral hemispheres and underlying structures.[9,10]

The facial anomalies encompass a broad range of defects that are due to aplasia or varying degrees of hypoplasia of the median central structures.[12]

Pathology

The most relevant classification of holoprosencephaly for antenatal diagnosis is that suggested by DeMyer, which recognizes three types: alobar, semilobar, and lobar according to the degree of incomplete division of the prosencephalic derivatives[9–12] (Fig. 1–65).

In the most severe form (alobar holoprosencephaly), there is an absence of the interhemispheric fissure, a single primitive ventricle, fused thalami, absence of the third ventricle, neurophypophysis, and olfactory bulbs. Failure of inward rotation of the primitive cerebral hemispheres prevents the thin membranous roof of the ventricular cavity from being enfolded within the brain. Because of an increase in CSF, the membrane may balloon out to form a cyst between the cerebral convexity and the calvarium (so-called dorsal sac). According to the degree of failure of rotation, alobar holoprosencephaly is commonly subdivided into three types: pancake, cup, and ball varieties (Fig. 1–66).

In semilobar holoprosencephaly, the two cerebral hemispheres are partially separated posteriorly, but there is still a single ventricular cavity. Alobar and semilobar holoprosencephaly might be associated with either microcephaly or macrocephaly.

In lobar holoprosencephaly, the interhemispheric fissure is well developed anteriorly and posteriorly, but there is a certain degree of fusion of structures, such as the lateral ventricles and the cingulate gyrus and absence of the cavum septum pellucidum.

The facial defects have been categorized into five different types.[12] Table 1–17 describes the diagnostic criteria and the associated brain anomaly.

Diagnostic Criteria

The antenatal diagnosis of holoprosencephaly has been reported on several occasions.[35–7,13,16,17,19,20,22,23] Diagnostic criteria vary depending on the type of

TABLE 1–17. FACIAL DEFECTS IN HOLOPROSENCEPHALY

Type of Face	Facial Features	Cranium–Brain
Cyclopia	Single eye or partially divided eye in single orbit	Microcephaly
	Arhinia with proboscis	Alobar holoprosencephaly
Ethmocephaly	Extreme hypotelorism	Microcephaly
	Arhinia with proboscis	Alobar holoprosencephaly
Cebocephaly	Orbital hypotelorism	Microcephaly
	Proboscislike nose but no median cleft or lip	Usually alobar holoprosencephaly
With median cleft lip	Orbital hypotelorism	Sometimes trigonocephaly
	Flat nose	Usually alobar holoprosencephaly
With median philtrum–premaxilla anlage	Orbital hypotelorism	Sometimes trigonocephaly
	Bilateral cleft lip with median process representing philtrum–premaxilla anlage	Semilobar or lobar holoprosencephaly
	Flat nose	

Adapted from DeMyer et al.: Pediatrics 34:256, 1964.

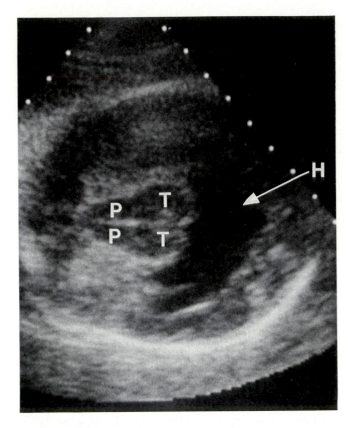

Figure 1–67. Axial scan in a fetus with alobar holoprosencephaly, revealing the sickle-shaped holoventricle (H) lined anteriorly by the undivided cortex and posteriorly by the prominent uncleft thalami (T). Both the midline echo and the third ventricle are absent. P, cerebral peduncles. *(Reproduced with permission from Pilu et al.: Am J Perinatol 4:41, 1987.)*

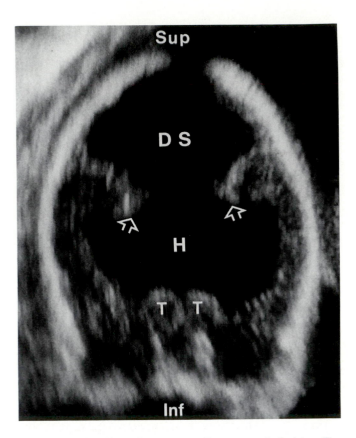

Figure 1–69. Midcoronal scan in a holoprosencephalic fetus. The cortex *(arrows)* is only partially enfolded over the holoventricle (H), which amply communicates with the superior dorsal sac (DS). Note the uncleft thalami (T) on the floor of the ventricular cavity. Sup, superior; Inf, inferior. *(Reproduced with permission from Pilu et al.: Am J Perinatol 4:41, 1987.)*

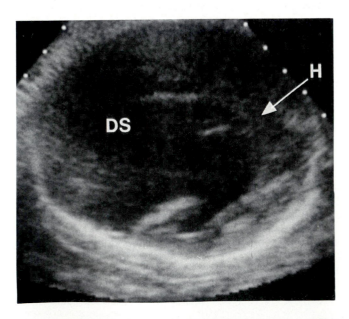

Figure 1–68. Axial scan at the level of the large dorsal sac (DS) in a fetus with alobar holoprosencephaly, cup variety. Note the crescent-shaped cortex and the absence of the midline echo. H, holoventricle. *(Reproduced with permission from Pilu et al.: Am J Perinatol 4:41, 1987.)*

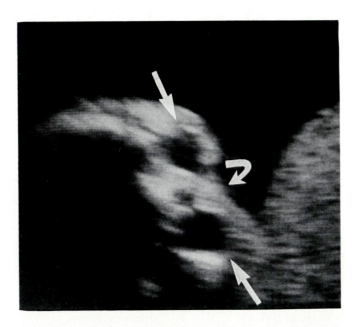

Figure 1–70. Axial scans at the level of the orbits in a holoprosencephalic fetus, revealing hypotelorism and absence of the nasal bridge. *(Reproduced with permission from Pilu et al.: Am J Perinatol 4:41, 1987.)*

holoprosencephaly. In the alobar and semilobar varieties, the single most valuable finding is the identification of a single sickle-shaped ventricle. In an axial scan, this primitive ventricular cavity is lined anteriorly by a crescent-shaped cortex with no discernible interhemispheric fissure and posteriorly by the bulblike undivided thalami[13,23] (Fig. 1–67). In the alobar variety, the presence of a dorsal sac can be easily recognized either in an axial scan above the level of the thalami or in a coronal scan, which would demonstrate the continuity between this structure and the single ventricle (Figs. 1–68, 1–69). The semilobar variety is recognized in the neonatal period by observing well-developed occipital horns and an incomplete interhemispheric fissure,[1,2,14,15] but it is yet to be demonstrated that ultrasound can differentiate the

semilobar from the alobar type of holoprosencephaly in utero. The lobar form is a serious diagnostic challenge because the interhemispheric fissure is well formed and the lateral ventricles are separated, with the exception of the frontal portions.[14,15] It has not been identified in the fetus. Fusion of the frontal horns could probably be recognized by ultrasound. In all forms of holoprosencephaly, the posterior fossa contents are normal.[17a]

The facial findings are further diagnostic hints. The presence of hypotelorism,[7,22,23] cyclopia,[3,5,13] absence of orbits and nose,[23] identification of a proboscis,[13,19,23] and cleft palate or lip[23] strengthens the diagnosis based on CNS findings (Figs. 1–70, 1–71, 1–72). On the other hand, if any of the aforementioned facial features are serendipitously encoun-

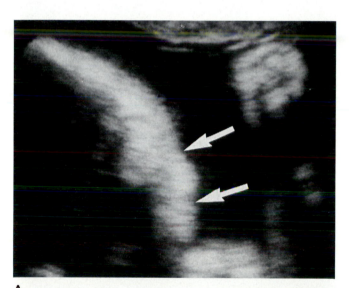

A

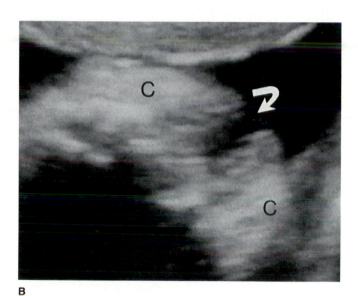

B

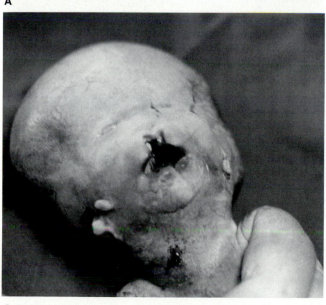

C

Figure 1–71. A. Axial scan at the presumed level of the orbits in a holoprosencephalic fetus, revealing anophthalmia (*arrows*). **B.** A slightly lower scan in the same fetus reveals a large median defect of the lip and palate (*curved arrow*). C, cheeks. **C.** Postnatal appearance of the infant, revealing the classic stigmata of holoprosencephaly with median cleft face. (*Reproduced with permission from Pilu et al.: Am J Perinatol 4:41, 1987.*)

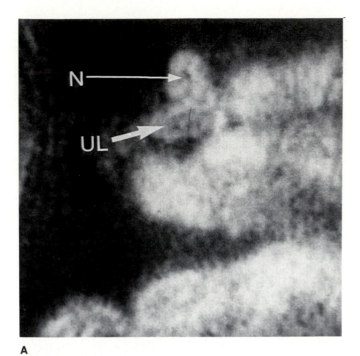

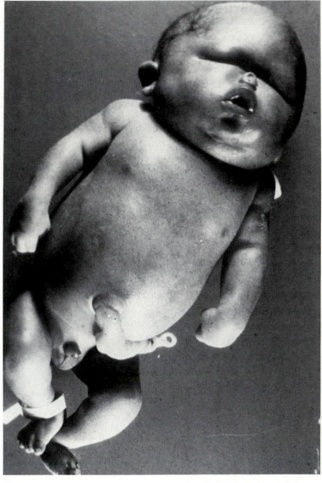

Figure 1–72. A. Coronal scan of the face of a fetus with holoprosencephaly. The presence of a single central nostril (N) within the nasal appendage allows the identification of a proboscis. UL, upper lip. **B.** Postnatal appearance of the infant, revealing the typical stigmata of cebocephaly.

tered, a careful examination of the intracranial contents is indicated.

Prognosis

The prognosis depends on the type of holoprosencephaly. Infants with the alobar form usually die within the first year of life. An exception to this, an infant who survived for 9 years, was reported by DeMyer.[10] Infants with semilobar holoprosencephaly may reach childhood, but they will have amentia.[10,11] Lobar holoprosencephaly may be compatible with a normal lifespan. The affected individuals are usually intellectually impaired, but some may have enough intelligence "to live free in society."[10,11]

Obstetrical Management

When the diagnosis of alobar or semilobar holoprosencephaly is made before viability, the option of pregnancy termination should be offered to the patient. Fetal karyotype is indicated. In the third trimester, we believe that this diagnosis is one of the few in which the option of late termination of pregnancy should be offered, and premature labor should not be

arrested. Every attempt should be made to accomplish a vaginal delivery. If macrocephaly is present, a cephalocentesis is recommended. Decision making in lobar holoprosencephaly is difficult, because data concerning outcome are not available.

REFERENCES

1. Altman NR, Altman DH, Sheldon JJ, et al.: Holoprosencephaly classified by computed tomography. AJNR 5:433, 1984.
2. Babcock DS, Han BK: Cranial ultrasonography of Infants. Baltimore, Williams & Wilkins, 1981.
3. Benacerraf BR, Frigoletto FD, Bieber FR: The fetal face. Ultrasound examination. Radiology 153:495, 1984.
4. Benawra R, Mangurten HH, Duffell DR: Cyclopia and other anomalies following maternal ingestion of salicylates. J Pediatr 96:1069, 1980.
5. Blackwell DE, Spinnato JA, Hirsch G, et al.: Antenatal ultrasound diagnosis of holoprosencephaly: A case report. Am J Obstet Gynecol 143:848, 1982.
6. Cayea PD, Balcar I, Alberti O, et al.: Prenatal diagnosis of semilobar holoprosencephaly. AJR 142:401, 1984.

7. Chervenak FA, Isaacson G, Mahoney MJ, et al.: The obstetric significance of holoprosencephaly. Obstet Gynecol 63:115, 1984.
8. Cohen MM: An update on the holoprosencephalic disorders. J. Pediatr 101:865, 1982.
9. DeMyer W: Classification of cerebral malformations. Birth Defects 7:78, 1971.
10. DeMyer W: Holoprosencephaly (cyclopia-arhinencephaly). In: Vinken PJ, Bruyn GW (eds): Handbook of Clinical Neurology. Amsterdam, Elsevier/North Holland Biomedical Press, 1977, Vol 30, pp 431–478.
11. DeMyer W, Zeman W: Alobar holoprosencephaly (arhinencephaly) with median cleft lip and palate: Clinical, electroencephalographic and nosologic considerations. Confin Neurol 23:1, 1963.
12. DeMyer W, Zeman W, Palmer CG: The face predicts the brain: Diagnostic significance of median facial anomalies for holoprosencephaloy (arhinencephaly). Pediatrics 34:256, 1964.
13. Filly RA, Chinn DH, Callen PW: Alobar holoprosencephaly: Ultrasonographic prenatal diagnosis. Radiology 151:455, 1984.
14. Fitz CR: Midline anomalies of the brain and spine. Radiol Clin North Am 29:95, 1982.
15. Fitz CR: Holoprosencephaly and related entities. Neuroradiology 25:225, 1983.
16. Hidalgo H, Bowie J, Rosenberg ER, et al.: In utero sonographic diagnosis of fetal cerebral anomalies. AJR 139:143, 1982.
17. Hill LM, Breckle R, Bonebrake CR: Ultrasonic findings with holoprosencephaly. J Reprod Med 27:172, 1982.
17a. Hoffman-Tretin JC, Horoupian DS, Koenigsberg M, et al.: Lobar holoprosencephaly with hydrocephalus: Antenatal demonstration and differential diagnosis. J Ultrasound Med 5:691, 1986.
18. Kurtz AB, Wapner RJ, Rubin CS, et al.: Ultrasound criteria for in utero diagnosis of microcephaly. JCU 8:11, 1980.
19. Lev-Gur M, Maklad NF, Patel S: Ultrasonic findings in fetal cyclopia. A case report. J Reprod Med 28:554, 1983.
20. Pearce JM, Little DJ, Campbell S: The diagnosis of abnormalities of the fetal central nervous system. In: Sanders RC, James AE (eds): The Principles and Practice of Ultrasonography in Obstetrics and Gynecology, 3d ed. Norwalk, CT, Appleton-Century Crofts, 1985, pp 243–256.
21. Matsunaga E, Shiota K: Holoprosencephaly in human embryos: Epidemiologic studies of 150 cases. Teratology 16:261, 1977.
22. Mayden KL, Tortora M, Berkowitz RL, et al: Orbital diameters: A new parameter for prenatal diagnosis and dating. Am J Obstet Gynecol 144:289, 1982.
23. Pilu G, Romero R, Jeanty P, et al.: Criteria for the antenatal diagnosis of holoprosencephaly. Am J Perinatol 4:41, 1987.
24. Roach E, DeMyer W, Conneally PM, et al.: Holoprosencephaly. Birth data, genetic and demographic analyses of 30 families. Birth Defects 11:294, 1975.

Iniencephaly

Definition
Iniencephaly is a complex developmental abnormality characterized by an exaggerated lordosis of the spine, usually associated with spina bifida and cephalocele.

Epidemiology
It is an extremely rare condition. The reported frequency has varied from 1:896 in England[15] to 1:65,000 in India.[11]

Etiology
Occurrence in siblings has been observed in only 1 patient of 57.[3] Females are more frequently affected than males (M:F ratio = 0.28).[14] Iniencephaly has been reported in association with maternal syphilis[1,10] and with sedative intake.[12] It can be produced in animals by the administration of vinblastine,[5] streptonigrin,[19] and triparanol.[16]

Embryology
Different hypotheses have been postulated. Persistence of the embryonic cervical lordosis at the third week, leading to failure of closure of the neural tube, or abnormal development of the rostral portion of the notocord and somites of the cervicooccipital region are the most widely accepted theories.[14]

Pathology
The criteria for the diagnosis of iniencephaly are (1) imperfect formation of the base of the skull, particularly at the level of the foramen magnum, (2) rachischisis, and (3) exaggerated lordosis of the spine. The spine is short and grossly abnormal, with kyphoscoliosis.

Associated Anomalies
Eighty-four percent of iniencephalic infants have other associated anomalies,[8] including anencephaly, cephaloceles, hydrocephaly, cyclopia, absence of mandible, cleft lip and palate, cardiovascular anomalies, diaphragmatic hernia, single umbilical artery,

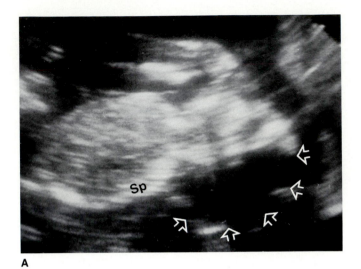
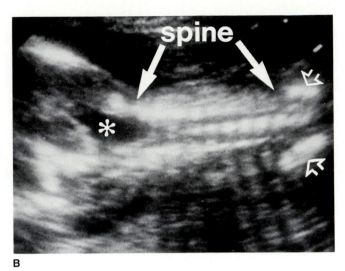

Figure 1–73. A. In this 21-week-old fetus, the diagnosis of iniencephaly was suspected because of the grotesque hyperextension of the head (*arrowheads*). Sp, spine. **B.** In the same fetus, a coronal scan demonstrates the striking shortness of the spine and an occipital cephalocele (X). The arrowheads indicate the iliac wings.

omphalocele, gastroschisis, situs inversus, polycystic kidneys, arthrogryposis, and clubfoot.[3,7,14]

Diagnosis

The two diagnostic clues are extreme dorsal flexion of the head and an abnormally short and deformed spine (Fig. 1–73).[4,9,13,17] The differential diagnosis includes anencephaly, the Klippel-Feil syndrome (shortness of the neck associated with fusion of cervical vertebrae), and a cervical myelomeningocele. Anencephaly can be identified by an absent calvarium. The differential diagnosis with Klippel-Feil syndrome appears to be difficult. As a matter of fact, some authors consider the Klippel-Feil syndrome and iniencephaly as different abnormalities of the same spectrum. However, in the former, gross and devastating abnormalities of the spine are absent. The presence of a cervical myelomeningocele raises the index of suspicion.

Prognosis

This entity is virtually always fatal in the neonatal period.[14] Three long-term survivors have been reported.[18] However, the iniencephalic deformity was very mild in these infants, and it is doubtful that they would have been identified in utero by ultrasound.

Obstetrical Management

The option of pregnancy termination should be offered to the parents before viability. When a definitive diagnosis is made after viability, nonaggressive management is recommended. An important consideration is that iniencephaly could be a cause of obstructed labor because of the hyperextended fetal head associated with hydrocephalus.[2,6] Under these circumstances, a cephalocentesis should be attempted. When this procedure is not enough to accomplish vaginal delivery, an embryotomy may be undertaken to avoid cesarean section.

REFERENCES

1. Abbott ME, Lockhart FAL: Iniencephalus. J Obstet Gynaecol Br Emp 8:236, 1905.
2. Bluett D: Iniencephaly causing obstructed labour. Proc Roy Soc Med 61:1281, 1968.
3. Brodsky I: Four examples of iniencephalus, with a statistical review of the literature. Med J Aust 2:795, 1939.
4. Campbell S, Allan LD, Griffin D, et al.: The early diagnosis of fetal structural abnormalities. In: Lerski RA, Morley P (eds): Ultrasound '82. Oxford, Pergamon Press, 1983, pp 547–563.
5. Cohlan SQ, Kitay D: The teratogenic effect of vincaleukoblastine in the pregnant rat. J Pediatr 66:541, 1965.
6. Cunningham I: Iniencephalus: A cause of dystocia. J Obstet Gynaecol Br Commonw 72:299, 1965.
7. David TJ, Illingworth CA: Diaphragmatic hernia in the southwest of England. J Med Genet 13:253, 1976.
8. David TJ, Nixon A: Congenital malformations associated with anencephaly and iniencephaly. J Med Genet 13:263, 1976
9. Hackeloer BJ, Nitschke S: Fruhdiagnose des Anenzephalus und Inienzephalus durch Ultraschall. Geburtsch Frauenheilk 35:866, 1975.
10. Howkins J, Lawrie RS: Iniencephalus. J Obstet Gynaecol Br Emp 46:25, 1939.
11. Jayant K, Mehta A, Sanghvi LD: A study of congenital malformations in Bombay. J Obstet Gynaecol India 11:280, 1960.
12. Konstantinova B, Kassabov L: Rare congenital malfor-

mations. In: Bertelli A (ed): Teratology: Proceedings of a Symposium Organized by the Italian Society of Experimental Teratology. Como, Italy, 21–22, October 1967. Amsterdam, Excerpta Medica, 1969, pp 223–227.

13. Pearce, JM, Little DJ, Campbell S: The diagnosis of abnormalities of the fetal central nervous system. In: Sanders RC, James AE (eds): The Principles and Practice of Ultrasonography in Obstetrics and Gynecology, 3d ed. Norwalk, CT, Appleton-Century-Crofts, 1985, pp 243–256.

14. Nishimura H, Okamoto N: Iniencephaly. In: Vinken GW, Bruyn PW (eds): Handbook of Clinical Neurology. Amsterdam, Elsevier/North Holland Biomedical Press,

1977, Vol 30, pp 257–268.

15. Paterson SJ: Iniencephalus. J Obstet Gynaecol Br Emp 51:330, 1944.

16. Roux C: Action teratogene du triparanol chez l'animal. Arch Franc Pediatr 21:451, 1964.

17. Santos-Ramos R, Duenhoelter JH: Diagnosis of congenital fetal abnormalities by sonography. Obstet Gynecol 45:279, 1975.

18. Sherk HH, Shut L, Chung S: Iniencephalic deformity of the cervical spine with Klippel-Feil anomalies and congenital elevation of the scapula. J Bone Joint Surg 56-A:1254, 1974.

19. Warkany J, Takacs E: Congenital malformations in rats from streptonigrin. Arch Pathol 79:65, 1965.

Agenesis of the Corpus Callosum

Synonym
Callosal agenesis.

Epidemiology
There is a discrepancy in the reported incidence between autopsy series and those based on pneumoencephalographic studies. In one autopsy study, the frequency was about 1:19 (5.3 percent).[11] On the other hand, one radiologic series based on 6450 pneumoencephalograms found an incidence of 0.7 percent.[14]

Etiology
Agenesis of the corpus callosum (ACC) can occur in chromosomal abnormalities, such as trisomy 13 and trisomy 18 (as part of the holoprosencephalic sequence)[23] and translocations (2 to a chromosome B).[22] Familial occurrence has been documented, suggesting a marked genetic heterogeneity with autosomal dominant, autosomal recessive, and X-linked inheritance.[2,9,11,18,19,21,24] ACC has also been described in the median cleft face syndrome,[8] in the Aicardi syndrome (seizures, chorioretinal lacunae, mental retardation, microcephaly, vertebral anomalies; sex-linked dominant inheritance),[1,24] Andermann syndrome (mental retardation, progressive motor neuropathy; autosomal recessive transmission), F.G. syndrome (mental retardation, macrocephaly, hypotonia), and acrocallosal syndrome (mental retardation, macrocephaly, polydactyly; autosomal recessive transmission).[24] An association with tuberous sclerosis,[10] mucopolysaccharidosis,[17] basal cell nevus syndrome,[5] maternal toxoplasmosis,[4] and maternal rubella[12] has been reported.

Embryology
The corpus callosum is a white matter structure that connects both cerebral hemispheres. Its presence is important in coordinating information and exchanging sensorial stimuli between the two hemispheres. The corpus callosum is derived from the lamina terminalis in the portion of the neural tube cephalic to the rostral neuropore. Until the fourth month of gestation, only the most rostral part of the corpus callosum is formed. The caudal portion develops only after the 5th month.[16,17] The insult responsible for ACC or varying degrees of hypoplasia of the corpus callosum is not known. Logically, an early insult may lead to complete agenesis, whereas a later one will lead to partial agenesis.[11]

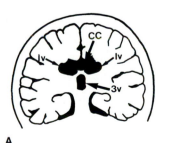
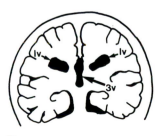

A   B

Figure 1–74. Schematic representation of a normal brain (**A**) and of agenesis of the corpus callosum (**B**). In the absence of the corpus callosum (CC), the lateral ventricles (lv) are set apart, and the third ventricle (3v) is displaced upward.

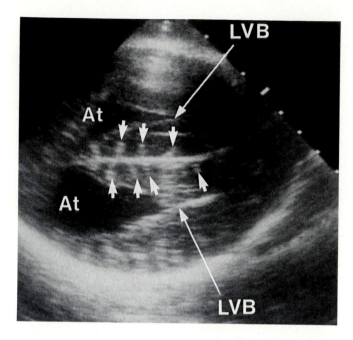

Figure 1–75. Typical ventricular configuration of ACC. The bodies of lateral ventricles (LVB) are of normal size but are markedly separated. The atria (At) are typically enlarged. The arrowheads indicate the abnormal convolutional pattern that is frequently seen in these cases.

Pathology

The defect may be complete or partial.[16,17] In partial ACC, the posterior portion is missing. As a consequence of the absence of the corpus callosum, the two lateral ventricles are set apart, and the third ventricle

may sometimes be displaced upward (Fig. 1–74). In most cases, there is a stable, nonprogressive dilatation of the caudal portion of the lateral ventricles (atria and occipital horns).[11,16,17] The reason for this enlargement is not known. There is no evidence of obstruction along the CSF pathways, since there is neither increased intraventricular pressure or progressive ventriculomegaly.

Associated Anomalies

ACC is frequently associated with other anomalies of the CNS and of other organs, including holoprosencephaly, Dandy-Walker malformation, microcephaly, macrocephaly, median cleft syndrome, and cardiovascular, gastrointestinal, and genitourinary anomalies.[20] ACC may be a part of mendelian syndromes.[24]

Diagnosis

In the newborn, ACC can be diagnosed by both computed tomography[6,15] and sonography[3,13] through the demonstration of (1) increased separation of the lateral ventricles, (2) enlargement of the occipital horns and atria, and (3) upward displacement of the third ventricle.

These findings can also be demonstrated in utero. The increased separation of the normal-sized bodies and the enlargement of the atria and occipital horns of the lateral ventricles result in a typical ultrasound image (Fig. 1–75). Upward displacement of the third ventricle is a very specific sign.[7] However, it was present in only 40 percent of fetuses in

Figure 1–76. A. Axial scan at the level of the bodies of lateral ventricles (LVB) in a 29-week fetus, revealing the typical ventricular configuration of ACC. A cystic structure is seen on the midline (*). At, atrium. **B.** In the mid-coronal scan, the midline cystic lesion (*) can be seen arising from between the thalami (T) and thus is positively identified as an enlarged and upwardly displaced third ventricle.

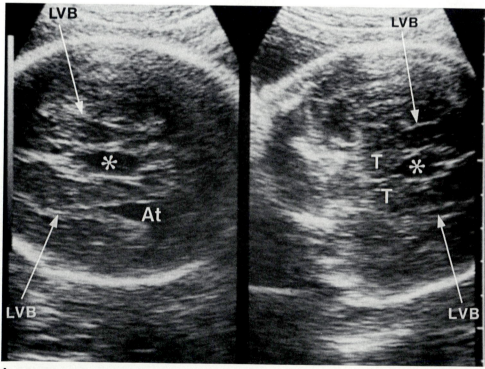

A   B

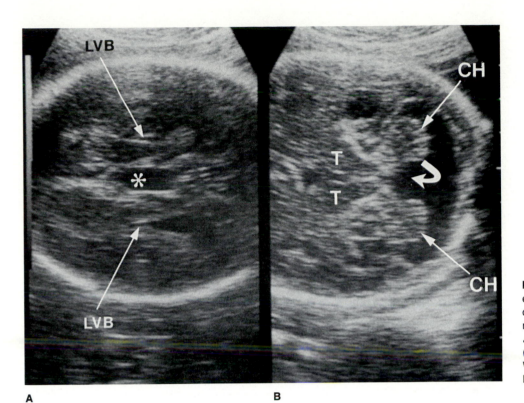

Figure 1–77. In a fetus with ACC, examination of the posterior fossa demonstrates a cystic cisterna magna (*) with lack of fusion (*curved arrow*) of the cerebellar hemispheres (CH). These findings indicate Dandy-Walker malformation. LVB, bodies of lateral ventricles; T, thalami.

our series (Fig. 1–76). When ACC is suspected, orbital measurements should be made, and the fetal face should be examined because of the possible association of this condition with the hypertelorism median cleft syndrome.[8] Investigation of the posterior fossa is also recommended because of the frequent association with Dandy-Walker malformation[11,20] (Fig. 1–77).

Prognosis

The corpus callosum is phylogenetically a recent structure, and its absence is not essential for life functions. Patients with ACC may have neurologic problems, such as seizures, intellectual impairment, and psychosis.[11,16,17] However, these conditions are believed to be caused by associated cerebral anomalies. Isolated ACC may be either a completely asymptomatic finding or revealed during the course of a neurologic examination by subtle deficits, such as inability to match stimuli using both hands (e.g., individuals are unable to discriminate differences in temperature, shape, weight in objects placed in both hands).[9] In our own series of nine cases of ACC identified in utero, severe associated anomalies were found in three (Dandy-Walker malformation, microcephaly, diaphragmatic hernia). Of the remaining six, one infant is affected by moderate paraparesis and five are developing normally.

Obstetrical Significance

The value of an antenatal diagnosis of ACC is twofold. First, it is a condition associated with a broad range of abnormalities of both CNS and other organs. Therefore, identification of this anomaly demands a careful search of fetal anatomy in its entirety. Second, it is important to recognize that the sonographic appearance of ACC may be very similar to that of uncomplicated hydrocephaly. A correct diagnosis could avoid unnecessary intervention. The diagnosis of ACC per se does not require any change in standard obstetrical management.

REFERENCES

1. Aicardi J, Lefebvre J, Lerique-Koechlin A: A new syndrome: Spasm in flexion, callosal agenesis, ocular abnormalities. Electroencephalogr Clin Neurophysiol 19:609, 1965.
2. Andermann E, Andermann F, Joubert M, et al.: Three familial midline malformation syndromes of the central nervous system: Agenesis of the corpus callosum and anterior horn cell disease; agenesis of the cerebellar vermis; and atrophy of the cerebellar vermis. Birth Defects 11:269, 1975
3. Babcock DS: The normal, absent, and abnormal corpus callosum: Sonographic findings. Radiology 151:449, 1984.
4. Bartoleschi B, Cantore GP: Agenesia del corpo calloso in paziente affetto da toxoplasmosi. Riv Neurol 32:79, 1962.

5. Binkley GW, Johnson HH: Epithelioma adenoides cysticum: Basal cell nevi, agenesis of the corpus callosum and dental cysts. Arch Dermatol 63:73, 1951.

6. Byrd SE, Harwood-Nash DC, Fitz CR: Absence of the corpus callosum: Computed tomographic evaluation in infants and children. J Can Assoc Radiol 29:108, 1978.

7. Comstock CH, Culp D, Gonzalez J, et al.: Agenesis of the corpus callosum in the fetus: Its evolution and significance. J Ultrasound Med 4:613, 1985.

8. DeMyer W: The median cleft face syndrome. Differential diagnosis of cranium bifidum occultum, hypertelorism, and median cleft nose, lip and palate. Neurology 17:961, 1967.

9. Dogan K, Dogan S, Louren CI: Agenesis of the corpus callosum in two brothers. Lijec Vjesn 89:377, 1967.

10. Elliot GB, Wollin DW: Defect of the corpus callosum and congenital occlusion of the fourth ventricle with tuberous sclerosis. AJR 85:701, 1961.

11. Ettlinger G: Agenesis of the corpus callosum. In: Vinken GW, Bruyn PW (eds): Handbook of Clinical Neurology. Amsterdam, Elsevier/North Holland Biomedical Press, 1977, Vol 30, pp 285–297.

12. Friedman M, Cohen P: Agenesis of corpus callosum as a possible sequel to maternal rubella during pregnancy. Am J Dis Child 73:178, 1947.

13. Gebarski SS, Gebarski KS, Bowerman RA, et al.: Agenesis of the corpus callosum: Sonographic features. Radiology 151:443, 1984.

14. Grogono JL: Children with agenesis of the corpus callosum. Dev Med Child Neurol 10:613, 1968.

15. Guibert-Trainier F, Piton J, Billerey J, et al.: Agenesis of the corpus callosum. J Neuroradiol 9:135, 1982.

16. Loeser JD, Alvord EC: Clinicopathological correlations in agenesis of the corpus callosum. Neurology 18:745, 1968.

17. Loeser JD, Alvord EC: Agenesis of the corpus callosum. Brain 91:553, 1968.

18. Menkes JH, Philippart M, Clark DB: Hereditary partial agenesis of corpus callosum. Arch Neurol 11:198, 1964.

19. Naiman J, Fraser FC: Agenesis of the corpus callosum. A report of two cases in siblings. Arch Neurol 74:182, 1955.

20. Parrish ML, Roessmann U, Levinsohn MW: Agenesis of the corpus callosum: A study of the frequency of associated malformations. Ann Neurol 6:349, 1979.

21. Shapira Y, Cohen T: Agenesis of the corpus callosum in two sisters. J Med Genet 10:266, 1973.

22. Warkany J: Congenital Malformations. Chicago, Year Book, 1971.

23. Warkany J, Passarge E, Smith LB: Congenital malformations in autosomal trisomy syndromes. Am J Dis Child 112:502, 1966.

24. Young ID, Trounce JQ, Levene MI, et al.: Agenesis of the corpus callosum and macrocephaly in siblings. Clin Genet 28:225, 1985.

Lissencephaly

Synonym
Agyria.

Definition
The term "lissencephaly" indicates the absence of cerebral gyri.

Incidence
Rare.

Etiology
Familial occurrence has been documented. The pattern is suggestive of an autosomal recessive trait.[2,4,5,9,10,13] Lissencephaly has also been found in association with trisomy 18.[8]

Embryology
The gray matter of the cerebral cortex is formed by proliferation of cells that migrate from the primitive neural tube.[14] Lissencephaly is believed to result from failure of migration of these cells. In the absence of these cells, no gyri are formed.[8] This theory is supported by the observation that in lissencephaly, there is abnormal stratification of the cortex.[8]

Pathology
The cerebral gyri are almost completely absent. The surface of the brain is smooth, similar to that found in fetuses before 20 weeks.[3,6,7] Hydrocephalus, agenesis of the corpus callosum, and microcephaly are very often associated with lissencephaly. Thalami are often hypoplastic. Due to the thinness of the white matter, an enlargement of the lateral ventricles, especially in the caudal portion (atria and occipital horns), is frequently found.[6]

Diagnosis
In the newborn, lissencephaly can be diagnosed by demonstrating the absence of cerebral gyri on computed tomography.[5,11] This diagnosis was made recently by ultrasound through the identification of an incomplete opercularization of the insula.[1]

Cerebral gyri can be visualized in the third trimester. Their absence could be used to make a diagnosis. However, prenatal diagnosis based upon this criterion has not been reported. We have made this diagnosis in a patient at risk because of a positive family history by demonstrating the associated ventriculomegaly. Other findings that can be documented with ultrasound include agenesis of the corpus callosum and microcephaly. Failure to visualize the thalamic structures can raise the index of suspicion.

Associated Anomalies

Lissencephaly is commonly associated with other anomalies such as micromelia, club foot, polydactyly, camptodactyly, syndactyly, duodenal atresia, micrognathia, omphalocele, hepatosplenomegaly, and cardiac and renal anomalies. Polyhydramnios is present in 50 percent of cases.[12]

Prognosis

Lissencephaly is invariably fatal by infancy or childhood and it is always associated with severe intellectual impairment (IQ <35). Some infants show neurologic signs of decerebration, seizures, and spastic diplegia.[4,7]

Obstetrical Management

It is unclear if the diagnosis can be made before viability. If ventriculomegaly is identified in a patient at risk because of a previously affected infant, the option of pregnancy termination should be offered to the parents. Lissencephaly is a condition for which pregnancy termination may be offered in the third trimester if a confident diagnosis can be made. This latter requirement has not been met.

REFERENCES

1. Babcock DS: Sonographic demonstration of lissencephaly (agyria). J Ultrasound Med 2:465, 1983.
2. Barth PG, Mullaart R, Stam FC, et al.: Familial lissencephaly with extreme neopallial hypoplasia. Brain Dev 4:145, 1982.
3. Daube JR, Chou SM: Lissencephaly. Two cases. Neurology 16:179, 1966.
4. Dieker H, Edwards RH, Zu Rhein G, et al.: The lissencephaly syndrome. Birth Defects 5:53, 1969.
5. Garcia CA, Dunn D, Trevor R: The lissencephaly (agyria) syndrome in siblings: Computerized tomographic and neuropathologic findings. Arch Neurol 35: 608, 1978.
6. Jellinger K, Rett A: Agyria–pachygyria (lissencephaly syndrome). Neuropaediatrie 7:66, 1976.
7. Larroche JC: Cytoarchitectonic abnormalities (abnormalities of cell migration). In: Vinken GW, Bruyn PW (eds): Handbook of Clinical Neurology. Amsterdam, Elsevier/North Holland Biomedical Press, 1977, Vol 30, pp 479–505.
8. Ludwin SK, Malamud N: Pathology of congenital anomalies of the brain. In: Newton TH, Potts DG (eds): Radiology of the Skull and Brain. Anatomy and Pathology. St. Louis, CV Mosby, 1977, pp 2979–3015.
9. Miller JQ: Lissencephaly in 2 siblings. Neurology 13: 841, 1963.
10. Norman MG, Roberts J, Siroid J, et al.: Lissencephaly. J Can Soc Neurol 3:39, 1976.
11. Ohno K, Enomoto T, Imamoto J, et al.: Lissencephaly (agyria) on computed tomography. J Comput Assist Tomogr 3:92, 1979.
12. Opitz JM: Lissencephaly syndrome. In: Bergsma D (ed): Birth Defects Compendium, 2d ed. New York, Alan R Liss, 1979, p 658.
13. Reznik M, Alberca RS: Hypertelorisme et lissencephalie: Etude d'une forme familiale. (Famille Ma. . .). Acta Neurol Belg 63:970, 1963.
14. Sidman RL, Rakie P: Neuronal migration, with special reference to developing human brain: A review. Brain Res 62:1, 1973.

Intracranial Arachnoid Cysts

Definition

Arachnoid cysts are fluid-filled cavities lined completely or partially by the arachnoid membrane.

Epidemiology

The frequency of this disorder is not known. In most cases, the diagnosis is made at autopsy in an otherwise asymptomatic individual.

Etiology

Arachnoid cysts are classified as primary or secondary. Secondary or acquired cysts result from trauma, meningitis, infarction, or bleeding. Necrotic remnants or hematomas formed after the initial insult are subsequently reabsorbed, and a cyst is formed. In the absence of any obvious cause, the cyst can be considered as primary and regarded to be the consequence

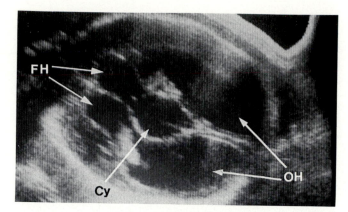

Figure 1–78. Arachnoid cyst at the level of the interhemispheric fissure. Note the echo-spared area (Cy) at the level of the midline and the associated hydrocephalus. FH, frontal horns of the lateral ventricles; OH, occipital horns of the lateral ventricles.

of a developmental abnormality. In practice, it is impossible to be certain that a remote and minor insult is not responsible for the cyst.[10]

Pathology

The meninges are the dura mater, arachnoid, and pia mater. The dura mater (usually referred to as "pachymeninge") is the most external and lines the skull. The arachnoid is the intermediate meninge and is formed by two layers. The pia mater is in direct contact with the surface of the brain. The space between the pia mater and the inner layer of the arachnoid is filled by CSF and called the "subarachnoid space."[10]

Arachnoid cysts are commonly subdivided into subarachnoid and intraarachnoid cysts. The former are lined externally by the inner layer of the arachnoid and internally by the pia mater and represent a localized enlargement of the subarachnoid space. Intraarachnoid cysts are much less frequent and are located between the inner and outer layer of the arachnoid.[10]

Arachnoid cysts have been found anywhere in the CNS, including the spinal canal. The most frequent locations are the surface of the cerebal hemispheres in the sites of the major fissures (sylvian, rolandic, and interhemispheric fissures),[12,13] the region of the sella turcica,[5,8] the anterior fossa, and the middle fossa.[4,11] Less frequently, they are seen in the posterior fossa.[3]

Arachnoid cysts may cause compression of the ventricular system and congenital hydrocephalus.[1,10]

Diagnosis

Arachnoid cysts appear on ultrasound examination as fluid-filled structures inside the intracranial cavity (Fig. 1–78). The differential diagnosis from other cystic lesions may be impossible.[6]

Arachnoid cysts located on the surface of the brain and main fissures should be distinguished from porencephaly and intracranial tumors. However, porencephaly is very often associated with ventriculomegaly and a shift in the midline, both of which are unusual features in arachnoid cysts of the convexities.[10] Furthermore, cystic cavities in porencephaly communicate with the ventricles. Brain tumors are usually located inside the brain substance, whereas arachnoid cysts lie between the skull and brain surface.

Posterior fossa arachnoid cysts must be differentiated from Dandy-Walker syndrome. The main criterion in these cases is the integrity of the cerebellar vermis in arachnoid cysts.[7,9]

In the newborn, the diagnosis can be made by contrast-enhanced computerized tomography. Characteristically, arachnoid cysts do not take up contrast.[2]

Prognosis

Insufficient data are available regarding the prognosis of cases diagnosed either antenatally or in the newborn period. In many cases, arachnoid cysts are asymptomatic, but they may cause epilepsy, mild motor or sensory abnormalities, or hydrocephalus.[10] Depending on the location and extent of the lesion, these cysts can be resectable.[1,10]

Obstetrical Management

If a fluid-filled intracranial lesion suggesting an arachnoid cyst is seen in the second trimester, termination of pregnancy should be discussed with the parents because prognosis is largely unknown and more serious intracranial lesions (e.g., porencephaly or intracranial tumors) cannot be excluded. In the third trimester, when hydrocephalus is not present, there is no reason to modify the mode and time of delivery. In the presence of hydrocephalus with normal skull dimensions, there is no evidence that a cesarean section could improve the outcome, and we believe that a vaginal delivery should be attempted.

REFERENCES

1. Anderson FM, Landing BH: Cerebral arachnoid cysts in infants. J Pediatr 69:88, 1966.
2. Banna M: Arachnoid cysts on computed tomography. AJR 127:979, 1976.
3. DiRocco C, Caldarelli M, DiTrapani G: Infratentorial arachnoid cysts in children. Childs Brain 8:119, 1981.
4. Geissinger JD, Kohler WC, Robinson BW, et al.: Arachnoid cysts of the middle cranial fossa: Surgical considerations. Surg Neurol 10:27, 1978.
5. Harrison MJG: Cerebral arachnoid cysts in children. J Neurol Neurosurg Psychiatry 34:316, 1971.
6. Pilu G, Rizzo N, Orsini LF, et al.: Antenatal detection of cerebral anomalies. Ultrasound Med Biol 12:319, 1986.

7. Pilu G, Romero R, DePalma L, et al.: Antenatal diagnosis and obstetrical management of Dandy-Walker syndrome. J Reprod Med 31:1017, 1986.
8. Ring BA, Waddington M: Primary arachnoid cyst of the sella turcica. AJR 98:611, 1966.
9. Roach ES, Laster DW, Sumner TE, et al.: Posterior fossa arachnoid cyst demonstrated by ultrasound. J Clin Ultrasound 10:88, 1982.
10. Shaw CM, Alvord EC: Congenital arachnoid cysts and their differential diagnosis. In: Vinken PJ, Bruyn GW (eds): Handbook of Clinical Neurology. Amsterdam, Elsevier/North Holland Biomedical Press, 1977, Vol 30, pp 75–135.
11. Smith RA, Smith WA: Arachnoid cysts of the middle cranial fossa. Surg Neurol 5:246, 1976.
12. Starkman SP, Brown TC, Linell EA: Cerebral arachnoid cysts. J Neuropathol Exp Neurol 17:484, 1958.
13. Zingesser L, Schechter M, Gonatas N, et al.: Agenesis of the corpus callosum associated with an interhemispheric arachnoid cyst. Br J Radiol 37:905, 1964.

Intracranial Tumors

Intracranial tumors include epidermoid, dermoid, teratoma, germinoma, medulloblastoma, tuberous sclerosis (Bourneville's disease), neurofibromatosis (Von Recklinghausen's disease), and systemic angiomatosis of the central nervous system and eye (Von Hippel-Lindau's disease).

Incidence
Fetal intracranial tumors are rare. There are obvious difficulties in assessing the incidence of congenital brain neoplasms, because some lesions are asymptomatic or become symptomatic during childhood, adolescence, or even adulthood. Malignancies of the CNS were found to account for 0.04 to 0.18 percent of the total deaths of infants under 1 year of age.[3] It should be stressed that only a very small portion of brain tumors in children seem to arise during fetal life. In a series of 730 neoplasms diagnosed between 1 and 16 years of age, only 56 (7.8 percent) were thought to be congenital.[3]

Etiology
Embryonic tumors are thought to derive from embryologically displaced cells. Brain tumors have been produced in animals by the use of chemical[2] and viral teratogens.[7] The relevance of these experiments to human brain neoplasms is unclear.

Pathology
There are several classifications of congenital brain tumors.[3,5] A commonly used system is shown in Table 1–18. Epidermoid tumors (also known as "cholesteatomas") derive from epithelial cells and frequently appear as cystic lesions, containing a leaf-like material, that originate from the desquamation of the internal epithelial lining. They are most commonly located at the level of the cerebellopontine

TABLE 1–18. CLASSIFICATION OF CONGENITAL INTRACRANIAL TUMORS

Embryonic tumors	Tumors of ependymal origin
Epidermoid	Ependymoma
Dermoid	Subependymal mixed glioma
Teratoma	Choroid plexus papilloma
Germinal tumors	Glioblastoma multiforme
Germinoma	Malignant astrocytoma
Embryonal carcinoma	Tumors associated with genetic diseases
Choriocarcinoma	Tuberous sclerosis (Bourneville's disease)
Endodermal sinus tumor	Neurofibromatosis (Von Recklinghausen's disease)
Teratoma	Systemic angiomatosis of the CNS and eye (Von Hippel–Lindau's disease)
Neuroblastic tumors	Colloid cyst of the third ventricle
Medulloblastoma	Heterotopia and hamartoma
Neuroblastoma	Lipoma
Retinoblastoma	Vascular tumors: hemangioblastoma
Tumors related to embryonal remnant tissues	
Craniopharyngioma	
Chordoma	

Adapted from Mori: Neuroradiology and Neurosurgery. New York, Thieme-Stratton, 1985; Wilson et al. In: Newton, Potts (eds): Radiology of the Skull and Brain. Anatomy and Pathology. St. Louis, CV Mosby, 1977.[11]

angle, suprasellar region, and temporal lobe. Dermoid tumors are characterized by the presence of desquamated epithelium, sebaceous secretions, and hair. They are often connected with the skin surface by a dermal sinus and usually occur in the posterior fossa. Teratomas are tumors derived from the three embryonic layers. They may contain well-differentiated structures, such as hair, bone, or muscle, or undifferentiated structures. In the latter case, they have a tendency toward malignancy. Teratomas usually occur in the pineal region, the suprasellar region, or the fourth ventricle.

Germinomas originate from germ cells and are usually solid lesions occurring in the pineal and suprasellar regions. Tumors originating from differentiated germ cells include choriocarcinoma (trophoblastic cells), endodermal sinus tumor (yolk sac), embryonal carcinoma, and teratoma. Medulloblastoma only arises in the posterior fossa. It is a very malignant lesion that appears as a soft, friable mass often with internal necrosis.

Craniopharyngioma is the most frequent supratentorial tumor in children. It derives from remnants of the craniopharyngeal duct, consists of both cystic and solid components, and occurs in the suprasellar region. Among the tumors that derive from ependymal cells, the one that is most frequently congenital in origin is the choroid plexus papilloma (see p. 34).

Tuberous sclerosis, neurofibromatosis, and systemic angiomatosis of the CNS and eye are autosomal dominant diseases that are characterized by the presence of intracranial tumors. In tuberous sclerosis, multiple neuroglial nodules occur in the cerebral cortex or ventricular system. Neurofibromatosis is associated with brain tumors, such as acoustic neurinoma, multiple meningioma, and glioma. Systemic angiomatosis of the CNS and eye is characterized by the presence of cerebellar hemangioblastoma. The colloid cyst of the third ventricle is thought to derive from the epithelium that forms the roof of the thela choroidea and is located in the anterior portion of the third ventricle.

Intracranial tumors frequently cause obstruction to the normal flow of CSF within the ventricular system and are, therefore, often found in association with obstructive hydrocephalus. Choroid plexus papilloma may cause hydrocephalus by overproduction of cerebrospinal fluid (see p. 34).

Diagnosis

Experience in the prenatal diagnosis of brain neoplasms is limited, because of the rarity of these lesions. Cystic tumors and teratomas are usually characterized by complete loss of the normal intracranial architecture[1,4] (Fig. 1–79). A brain tumor should be suspected when mass-occupying lesions, cystic areas, or solid areas are seen or when there is a change in shape or size of the normal anatomic structures (e.g., a shift in the midline). In some cases, the lesion appears as a low echogenic structure, and it may be difficult to recognize.[8,9] Hydrocephalus is frequently associated with brain tumors and may be the presenting sign. Although ultrasound can detect some fetal intracranial tumors, it does not allow a specific diagnosis of the histologic variety. Identification of brain neoplasm associated with tuberous sclerosis, neurofibromatosis, and systemic angiomatosis of the CNS and eye can be attempted in the patients at risk.

Prognosis

Prognosis depends on a number of factors, including the histologic type and the size and location of the lesion. Congenital intracranial teratomas are usually fatal.[10] The limited experience with the other neoplasms in prenatal diagnosis precludes the formulation of prognostic considerations.

Obstetrical Management

Pregnancy termination can be offered to the parents before viability. Because of the paucity of data, it is impossible to provide strong guidelines for the management of pregnancies complicated by fetal intracranial tumors. The classic teratoma (with impor-

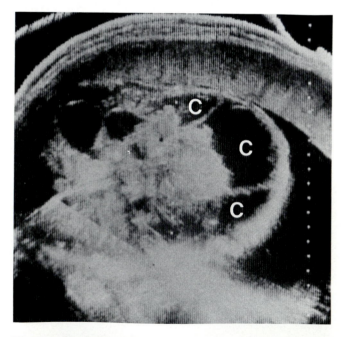

Figure 1–79. Cross-section of the head of a third trimester fetus with intracranial teratoma. Note the complete loss of the normal architecture of the brain, which is replaced by a bizarre pattern of cystic (C) and solid components.

tant distortion of the intracranial anatomy) should be conservatively managed, because it is associated with a very high death rate. Vaginal delivery is recommended. If the tumor is associated with macrocrania, a cephalocentesis to overcome fetopelvic disproportion should be considered.

REFERENCES

1. Crade M: Ultrasonic demonstration in utero of an intracranial teratoma. JAMA 247:1173, 1982.
2. Druckrey H, Ivankovic S, Preussmann R, et al.: Selective induction of malignant tumors of the nervous system by resorptive carcinogens. In: Kirsch WM, Grossi-Paoletti E, Paoletti P (eds): The Experimental Biology of Brain Tumors. Springfield, Charles C Thomas, 1972, pp 85–147.
3. Jellinger K, Sunder-Plassmann M: Connatal intracranial tumours. Neuropadiatrie 4:46, 1973.
4. Kirkinen P, Suramo I, Jouppila P, et al.: Combined use of ultrasound and computed tomography in the evaluation of fetal intracranial abnormality. J Perinat Med 10:257, 1982.
5. Koos W, Miller MH: Intracranial Tumors of Infants and Children. Stuttgart, G Thieme, 1971.
6. Mori K: Anomalies of the Central Nervous System. Neuroradiology and neurosurgery. New York, Thieme-Stratton, 1985.
7. Rapp F, Pauluzzi S, Waltz TA, et al.: Induction of brain tumors in newborn hamsters by simian adenovirus SA7. Cancer Res 29:1173, 1969.
8. Sauerbrei EE, Cooperberg PL: Cystic tumors of the fetal and neonatal cerebrum: Ultrasound and computed tomographic evaluation. Radiology 147:689, 1983.
9. Strassburg HM, Sauer M, Weber S, et al.: Ultrasonographic diagnosis of brain tumors in infancy. Pediatr Radiol 14:284, 1984.
10. Whittle IR, Simpson DA: Surgical treatment of neonatal intracranial teratoma. Surg Neurol 15:268, 1981.
11. Wilson CB, Moossy J, Boldrey EB, et al.: Pathology of intracranial tumors. In: Newton TH, Potts DG (eds): Radiology of the Skull and Brain. Anatomy and Pathology. St Louis, CV Mosby, 1977, pp 3016–3048.

Acrania

Definition

Acrania is a developmental abnormality characterized by a partial or complete absence of the calvarium, with complete but abnormal development of brain tissue.[2]

Incidence

Unknown. Very few cases have been reported in the world literature.[1,2]

Embryology

After the closure of the anterior neuropore, which occurs at the fourth week, migration of the mesenchymal tissue under the ectoderm overlying the future cerebral hemispheres takes place. The ectoderm will give rise to the skin of the scalp, and the mesenchymal tissue will form the muscle and bone. Acrania results from a failure of mesenchymal migration.[2]

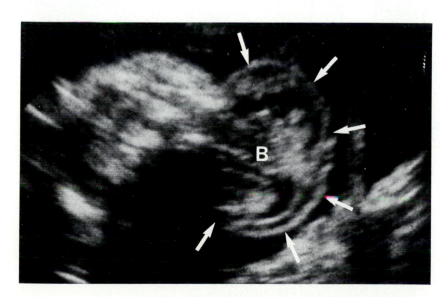

Figure 1–80. Longitudinal scan of the cephalic pole of a fetus with acrania. The calvarium is absent. The brain tissue (B) is covered by a thin membrane (*arrows*).

Etiology
Unknown. Only sporadic cases have been reported.[1,2] We have seen pathologic findings very similar to those pathognomonic of acrania in three fetuses with amniotic band syndrome.

Pathology
The calvarian dermal bones of the skull, the related musculature, and dura mater are absent. The hemispheres are present but grossly abnormal and are covered by a thin membrane. Cerebellum, brain stem, and cranial nerves are normal.

Associated Anomalies
Cleft lip and palate, and talipes.[2]

Diagnosis
The condition is identified by the absence of the calvarium. The cerebral hemispheres are surrounded by a thin membrane[2] (Fig. 1–80). Differential diagnosis includes anencephaly and large encephaloceles. In the former case, cerebral tissue is completely absent. In the latter case, some remnant of the cranial vault can always be detected. A distinction should also be made between acrania and conditions characterized by lack of mineralization of the skull bones (hypophosphatasia, osteogenesis imperfecta). In these skeletal dysplasias, the intracranial anatomy is normal, and the brain is surrounded by a thick layer of tissue representing soft tissues and unossified bone. Bowing or shortening of long bones is generally found.

Prognosis
Acrania is uniformly lethal.

Obstetrical Management
Pregnancy termination can be offered to the parents any time the condition is diagnosed.

REFERENCES

1. Kristoffersen K, Pedersen BN, Secher NJ, et al.: Akrani og spina bifida diagnosticeret ved bestemmelse af alfa fotoprotein i 16. graviditetsuge. Ugeskr Laeger 137:1719, 1975.
2. Mannes EJ, Crelin ES, Hobbins JC, et al.: Sonographic demonstration of fetal acrania. AJR 139:181, 1982.

Choroid Plexus Cyst

Incidence
Cysts of the choroid plexus are found in 50 percent of brains serially autopsied.[11]

Etiopathogenesis
These cysts are thought to arise from neuroepithelial folds within the choroid plexus that become fil-

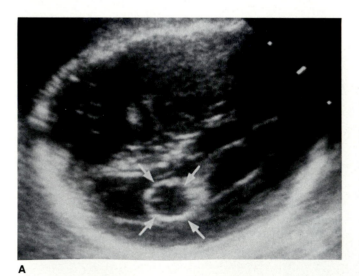
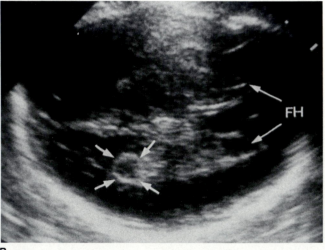

A

B

Figure 1–81. A. Axial scan of the head of a 21-week fetus. The arrows point to a cyst inside the choroid plexus. **B.** Three weeks later, the cyst has considerably diminished in size. Note the normal size of the ventricles. A further scan performed 2 weeks later failed to reveal any anomaly of the choroid plexus. The infant was normal at birth. FH, frontal horns.

led with fluid and cellular debris.[11,12] In autopsy specimens, they are usually less than 1 cm in diameter.[11,12]

Pathology
Cysts are lined by the ependyma and deeply enfolded within the choroid plexus. They may be bilateral. Generally, they are asymptomatic unless they obstruct the flow of CSF, causing hydrocephaly.[1,2,4,5,8,9]

Diagnosis
A round hypoechogenic area can be seen within the texture of the choroid plexus, most frequently at the level of the atrium of the lateral ventricle[3,6,7] (Fig. 1–81). This condition should be differentiated from choroid plexus papilloma, which generally produces an echogenic image and subependymal hemorrhages, which are rare in the fetus and are located below the choroid plexus.

Prognosis
Ten cases of fetal choroid plexus cysts have been reported.[3,7,10] In six cases this was the only anomaly identified. In four, the choroid plexus cyst was bilateral and associated with severe anomalies, such as trisomy 18 (three cases), omphalocele, obstructive uropathy, and ventricular septal defect.[10] In the cases of isolated choroid plexus cysts, the lesion spontaneously disappeared before the 28th week (in five cases before the 24th week). The infants were neurologically normal at birth. Hydrocephalus has been reported occasionally in infants and adults with choroid plexus cysts.[1,2,4,5,8,9]

Obstetrical Management
The limited experience available with these lesions suggests that they are clinically benign. Serial scans to monitor their status and exclude the development of hydrocephalus are indicated. There is no reason to modify standard obstetrical management.[3] However, the occurrence of hydrocephalus, chromosomal abnormalities, and other associated anomalies has been reported, and, therefore, a careful survey of the fetal anatomy and a fetal karyotype seem indicated.[10a]

REFERENCES

1. Andreussi L, Cama A, Cozzutto C, et al.: Cyst of the choroid plexus of the left lateral ventricle. Surg Neurol 12:53, 1979.
2. Baker GS, Gottlieb CM: Cyst of the choroid plexus of the lateral ventricle causing disabling headache and unconsciousness: Report of case. Mayo Clin Proc 31:95, 1956.
3. Chudleigh P, Pearce JM, Campbell S: Short communications. The prenatal diagnosis of transient cysts of the fetal choroid plexus. Prenatal Diagn 4:135, 1984.
4. DeLaTorre E, Alexander E, Courtland HD, et al.: Tumors of the lateral ventricles of the brain: Report of eight cases, with suggestions for clinical management. J Neurosurg 20:461, 1963.
5. Dempsey RJ, Chandler WF: Choroid plexus cyst in the lateral ventricle causing obstructive symptoms in an adult. Surg Neurol 15:116, 1981.
6. Fakhry J, Schechter A, Tenner MS, et al.: Cysts of the choroid plexus in neonates: Documentation and review of the literature. J Ultrasound Med 4:561, 1985.
7. Friday RO, Schwartz DB, Tuffli GA: Spontaneous intrauterine resolution of intraventricular cystic masses. J Ultrasound Med 4:385, 1985.
8. Giorgi C: Symptomatic cyst of the choroid plexus of the lateral ventricle. Neurosurgery 5:53, 1979.
9. Neblett CR, Robertson JW: Symptomatic cysts of the telencephalic choroid plexus. J Neurol Neurosurg Psychiatry 34:324, 1971.
10. Nicolaides KH, Rodeck CH, Gosden CM: Rapid karyotyping in non-lethal fetal malformations. Lancet 1:283, 1986.
10a. Ostlere SJ, Irving HC, Lilford RJ: Choroid plexus cysts in the fetus. Lancet 1:1491, 1987.
11. Shuangshoti S, Netsky MG: Neuroepithelial (colloid) cysts of the nervous system: Further observations on pathogenesis, location, incidence and histochemistry. Neurology 16:887, 1966.
12. Shuangshoti S, Netsky MG: Histogenesis of choroid plexus in man. Am J Anat 118:283, 1966.

Aneurysm of the Vein of Galen

Synonym
Varix of the vein of Galen.

Definition
Aneurysm of the vein of Galen (AVG) is a complex arteriovenous malformation ranging in appearance from a gigantic aneurysmal enlargement of the vein of Galen to multiple communications between the system of the vein of Galen and the cerebral arteries (carotid or vertebrobasilar systems).

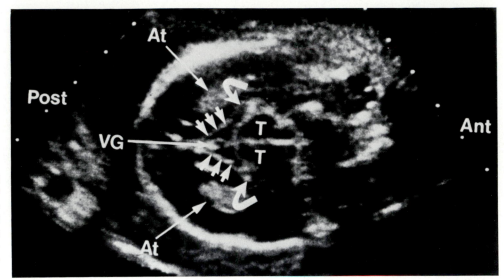

Figure 1–82. Axial scan of the fetal head, showing the normal anatomy of the vein of Galen (VG). Straight arrows point to the medial contour of the occipital lobes. Curved arrows point to the ambient cisterns. T, Thalami; At, atria of ventriculi; Ant, anterior; Post, posterior.

Incidence

Unknown. Less than 200 cases had been reported in the literature up to 1984.[9] It is more common in males than females (M:F ratio = 2:1).[7]

Embryology

The cerebral vessels derive from a primitive plexus that differentiate in both arteries and veins. There is controversy about the chronology of the derangement giving rise to cerebral arteriovenous malformations (AVM). According to some authors, the primary

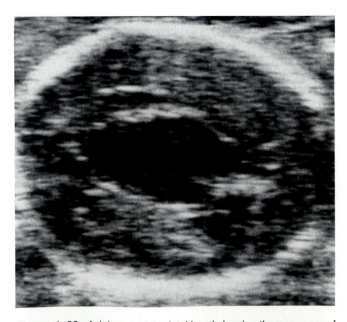

Figure 1–83. Axial scan of the fetal head showing the aneurysm of the vein of Galen as a large interhemispheric cystic mass.

defect occurs early, during the phase of differentiation of the angioblasts to form primitive capillaries, arteries, and veins.[6] Others believe that AVM arises during the late histologic differentiation of the primitive vessels into adult vessels.[5]

Pathology and Clinical Presentation

The vein of Galen is the major cerebral vein. It runs superoposteriorly to the thalami within a subarachnoid space known as the "vein of Galen cystern." It joins the inferior sagittal sinus, which runs along the lower edge of the cerebral falx to form the straight sinus (Fig. 1–82). In cases of AVG, an aneurysmal dilatation of the vein of Galen is usually found in association with varying patterns of arteriovenous communication.[3]

The clinical presentation of AVG depends on the type of lesion. Large arteriovenous communications result in significant intracranial shunt and usually appear in the neonatal period with high output congestive heart failure. In some patients, up to 80 percent of the cardiac output is diverted to the cerebral circulation.[5] Diversion of blood from the cerebral circulation may lead to infarction of the brain and porencephaly. High output heart failure may also result in reduction of coronary blood flow, myocardial ischemia, and infarction.[3] Hydrocephalus is frequently found, and it is thought to result from either compression of the aqueduct of Sylvius by the dilated vessel or from increased intracranial venous pressure. In other cases characterized by milder arteriovenous communication, AVG may occur during the first year of age with macrocrania, subarachnoidal hemorrhages, and seizures. In a third group of patients, the condition becomes symptomatic later in life, with headache, syncope, seizures, and subarachnoid hemorrhages.[1,3]

Associated Anomalies
Hydrocephalus, porencephaly, and nonimmune hydrops.

Diagnosis
Prenatal diagnosis or visualization of this condition has been reported.[2,4,9] The aneurysm appeared as a median, tubular, fluid-filled area extending posteriorly from above the thalami to the straight sinus or to the torcular Herophili. In our own case, a gigantic cystic structure was seen extending superiorly between the hemispheres (Fig. 1–83). A differential diagnosis with other cystic intracranial lesions may be impossible on purely morphologic ground. The use of Doppler ultrasound has proved useful in the newborn,[8] as well as in utero,[2] by demonstrating the presence of blood flow within the lesion.

Prognosis
It is likely that only the severe forms of AVG will be detectable in utero. In these cases, a careful evaluation of the fetal anatomy in search of signs of nonimmune hydrops and destructive lesions of the cerebral parenchyma is recommended, because these conditions have a major impact on the prognosis. Early treatment is mandatory in the forms occurring in the neonatal period to prevent both cerebral and myocardial infarction. Total excision of the lesion may not be possible because of the presence of a huge fistulous tract. In these cases, embolism or surgical ligation of the feeding arteries is commonly performed.[3]

Newborn infants with congenital heart failure have a very poor outcome. In a group of nine treated neonates, eight died, and the only survivor developed severe neurologic deficit.[3] A similar mortality rate was found in untreated neonates. In older infants, the prognosis is much better. The mortality rate after treatment was 20 percent, and all survivors were normal.[3]

Obstetrical Management
The option of pregnancy termination should be offered before viability. After this point, management depends on the presence or absence of ultrasonically detectable cerebral damage or hydrops. If severe porencephaly is found, we feel that a nonaggressive management should be offered to the parents. Because the mortality rate of AVG associated with hydrops is very high despite treatment, the options should be discussed with the parents. Alternatives include either an elective cesarean section as soon as pulmonic maturity is reached or nonaggressive management. No data are available indicating the optimal mode of delivery of fetuses with AVG.

REFERENCES

1. Diebler C, Dulac O, Renier D, et al.: Aneurysms of the vein of Galen in infants aged 2 to 15 months. Diagnosis and natural evolution. Neuroradiology 21:185, 1981.
2. Hirsch JH, Cyr D, Eberhardt H, et al.: Ultrasonographic diagnosis of an aneurysm of the vein of Galen in utero by duplex scanning. J Ultrasound Med 2:231, 1983.
3. Hoffman HJ, Chuang S, Hendrick EB, et al.: Aneurysms of the vein of Galen. Experience at the Hospital for Sick Children, Toronto. J Neurosurg 57:316, 1982.
4. Mao K, Adams J: Antenatal diagnosis of intracranial arteriovenous fistula by ultrasonography. Case report. Br J Obstet Gynaecol 90:872, 1983.
5. Mori K: Vascular malformations. In: Anomalies of the Central Nervous System. Neuradiology and Neurosurgery. New York, Thieme-Stratton, 1985, pp 169–186.
6. Olivecrona H, Ladenheim J: Congenital Arteriovenous Aneurysms of the Carotid and Vertebral Arterial Systems. Berlin, Springer, 1957.
7. Rosenberg AW: A vascular malformation drained by the great vein of Galen. Report of a case. Bull Los Angeles Neurol Soc 20:196, 1955.
8. Sivakoff M, Nouri S: Diagnosis of vein of Galen arteriovenous malformation by two-dimensional ultrasound and pulsed Doppler method. Pediatrics 69:84, 1982.
9. Vintzileos AM, Eisenfeld LI, Campbell WA, et al.: Prenatal ultrasonic diagnosis of arteriovenous malformation of the vein of Galen. Am J Perinatol 3:209, 1986.

The Face

Normal Anatomy of the Face

The fetal face can be studied with ultrasound very early in gestation. Several elements of the normal anatomy (orbits, forehead) can be identified as early as the 12th week of gestation. Before 14 weeks, the soft tissues of the face are too thin to be reliably imaged with current ultrasound equipment. After this time, forehead, orbits, nose, lips, and ears can be consistently identified[1,4] and studied in detail. A systematic approach to the examination of the fetal face should include sagittal, axial, and coronal planes.

SAGITTAL PLANES

Sagittal planes of the fetal face are useful in the assessment of the normality of the profile: forehead, nose, and jaw (Fig. 2–1). Ears are well visualized in parasagittal scans tangential to the calvarium. In late gestation, significant details of the anatomy of the external ear can be seen. The helix, scaphoid fossa, triangular fossa, concha, antihelix, tragus, antitragus, intertragic incisure, and lobule can be identified (Fig. 2–2).

AXIAL PLANES

An axial scan slightly caudad to the one commonly used for the determination of the biparietal diameter easily reveals both orbits. This view (Fig. 2–3) can be used for determination of the ocular biometry.[2,3] Nomograms for binocular distance, interocular distance, and ocular diameter (Fig. 2–4, Table 2–1) are available. One type of nomogram is utilized for the evaluation of ocular biometry when the gestational age is known (Figs. 2–5, 2–6, 2–7). If the gestational age is uncertain, nomograms constructed with the biparietal diameter as the independent variable can be utilized (Figs. 2–8, 2–9, 2–10). By moving the transducer caudally, the anterior palate can be visualized, and a slight angulation will allow visualization of the tongue within the oral cavity (Fig. 2–11).

CORONAL PLANES

The coronal planes are the most important ones in the evaluation of the integrity of facial anatomy. Figure 2–12 illustrates a sequence of scans tangential to the

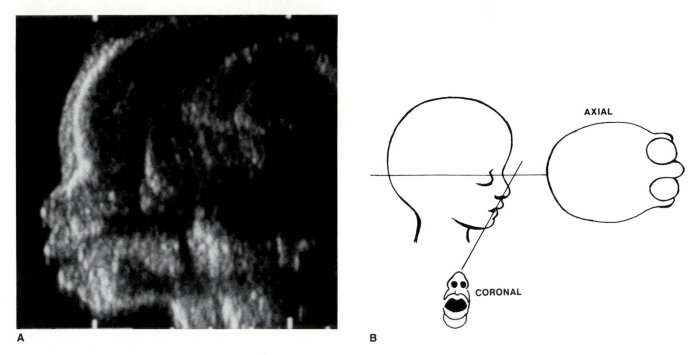

A

B

Figure 2–1. A. Fetal profile at 25 weeks. **B.** Schematic representation of the scanning planes to be used for obtaining axial and coronal views of the fetal face. *(Figure A reproduced with permission from Pilu et al.: Am J Obstet Gynecol 155:45, 1986.)*

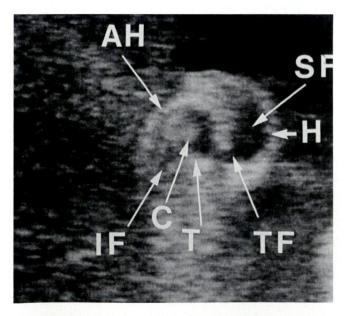

Figure 2–2. The helix (H), scaphoid fossa (SF), triangular fossa (TF), concha (C), antihelix (AH), tragus (T), and intertragic incisure (IF) can be seen in this view of the fetal ear.

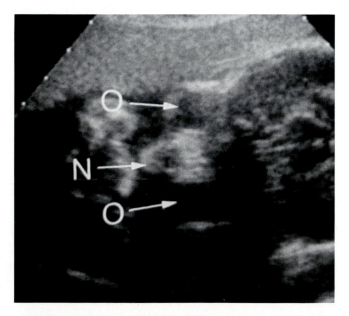

Figure 2–3. Axial scan passing through the orbits (O) of a normal third trimester fetus. N, nasal process. (*Reproduced with permission from Pilu et al.: Am J Obstet Gynecol 155:45, 1986.*)

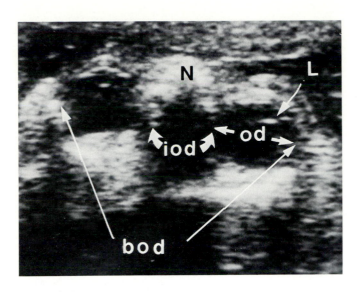

Figure 2–4. The ocular diameter (od), interocular distance (iod), and binocular distance (bod) are demonstrated in this scan. The lens (L) is visible in the eye. N, nasal process.

forehead. Orbits, eyelids, nose, and lips are well visualized. The tip of the nose, the alae nasi, and the columna are seen above the upper lip. The nostrils typically appear as two little anechoic areas (Fig. 2–13). In this scanning plane, it is possible to evaluate movements of the mouth, including protrusion of the tongue, "chewing" movements, and wide opening of the mouth (Fig. 2–14). By tilting the transducer, it is sometimes possible to visualize the intranasal portion of the upper airways (Fig. 2–15).

The lens, iris, pupil, cornea, and extraocular structures such as muscles, retro-orbital fat, and optic nerve may be visualized. Movements of both eyes are not synchronous and conjugated, limiting the possibility of the prenatal diagnosis of strabismus.[1a]

This chapter focuses on the anomalies more frequently found during the course of prenatal diagnosis. It is divided into anomalies of the orbits, nose, lip, palate and mandible. Besides these dysmorphic

TABLE 2–1. GROWTH OF THE OCULAR PARAMETERS

Age (weeks)	Binocular Distance (mm)			Interocular Distance (mm)			Ocular Diameter (mm)		
	5th	50th	95th	5th	50th	95th	5th	50th	95th
11	5	13	20	—	—	—	—	—	—
12	8	15	23	4	9	13	1	3	6
13	10	18	25	5	9	14	2	4	7
14	13	20	28	5	10	14	3	5	8
15	15	22	30	6	10	14	4	6	9
16	17	25	32	6	10	15	5	7	9
17	19	27	34	6	11	15	5	8	10
18	22	29	37	7	11	16	6	9	11
19	24	31	39	7	12	16	7	9	12
20	26	33	41	8	12	17	8	10	13
21	28	35	43	8	13	17	8	11	13
22	30	37	44	9	13	18	9	12	14
23	31	39	46	9	14	18	10	12	15
24	33	41	48	10	14	19	10	13	15
25	35	42	50	10	15	19	11	13	16
26	36	44	51	11	15	20	12	14	16
27	38	45	53	11	16	20	12	14	17
28	39	47	54	12	16	21	13	15	17
29	41	48	56	12	17	21	13	15	18
30	42	50	57	13	17	22	14	16	18
31	43	51	58	13	18	22	14	16	19
32	45	52	60	14	18	23	14	17	19
33	46	53	61	14	19	23	15	17	19
34	47	54	62	15	19	24	15	17	20
35	48	55	63	15	20	24	15	18	20
36	49	56	64	16	20	25	16	18	20
37	50	57	65	16	21	25	16	18	21
38	50	58	65	17	21	26	16	18	21
39	51	59	66	17	22	26	16	19	21
40	52	59	67	18	22	26	16	19	21

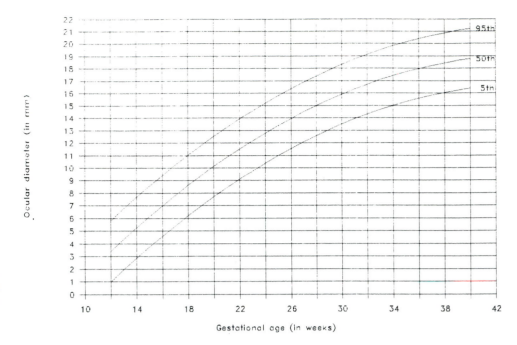

Figure 2–5. Ocular diameter versus gestational age. This nomogram and the one displayed in Figure 2–8 are utilized for the diagnosis of micro-phthalmia.

anomalies, ultrasound examination of the face can identify less common and more benign anomalies such as lacrimal duct cysts and hemangiomas.[1b] Congenital obstruction of the nasolacrimal duct results in cystic dilatation of the proximal part of the duct (dacrocystocele). It has been identified prenatally as a hypoechogenic mass inferior to the globe. The differential diagnosis includes an anterior cephalocele, hemangiomas, and dermoid cyst. Hemangiomas generally have a solid appearance or multiple septae. Dermoid cysts usually have a superolateral location. Anterior cephaloceles may be difficult to differentiate

from these lesions. The presence of hydrocephaly should raise the index of suspicion for a cephalocele. Dacrocystoceles resolve spontaneously in 78 percent of cases by 3 months and in 91 percent of cases by 6 months. Hemangiomas of the fetal face have been recognized prenatally. They appear as exophytic lesions with echogenicity similar to the placenta. Pulsation may be identified. The differential diagnosis includes cephaloceles and teratomas of the face. The cavernous variety of hemangiomas generally disappears spontaneously. A giant hemangioma may be associated with thrombocytopenia (Kasabach-Merritt

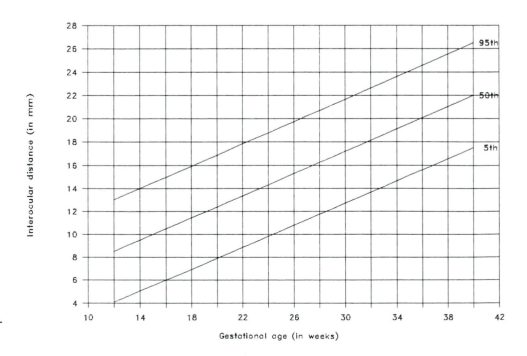

Figure 2–6. Interocular distance versus gestational age.

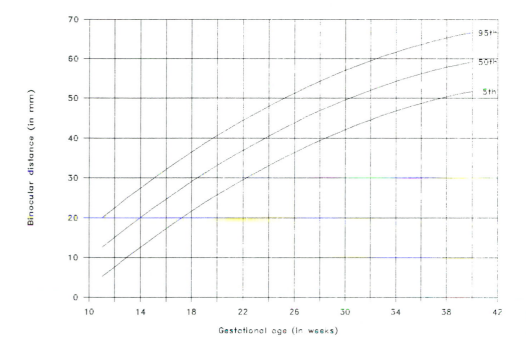

Figure 2–7. Binocular distance versus gestational age.

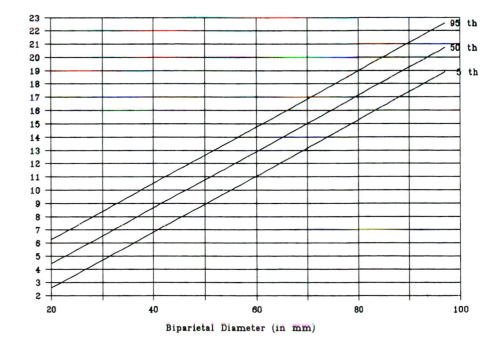

Figure 2–8. Ocular diameter versus biparietal diameter.

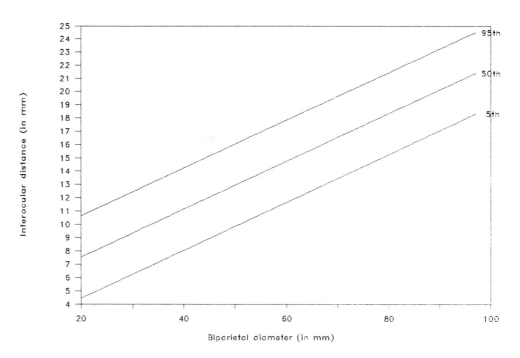

Figure 2–9. Interocular distance versus biparietal diameter.

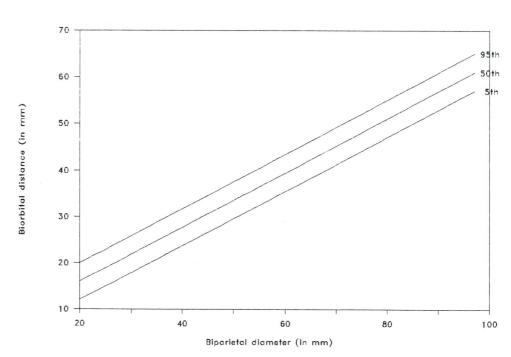

Figure 2–10. Binocular distance versus biparietal diameter.

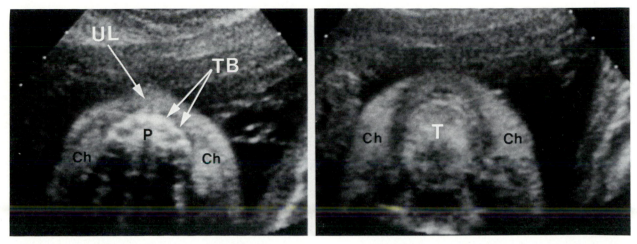

Figure 2–11. Axial scan of the lower fetal face demonstrating the upper lip (UL) and the anterior palate (P). The teethbuds (TB) and cheeks (Ch) can be seen. At a slightly lower level, the tongue (T) is seen filling the oral cavity. *(Reproduced with permission from Pilu et al.: Am J Obstet Gynecol 155:45, 1986.)*

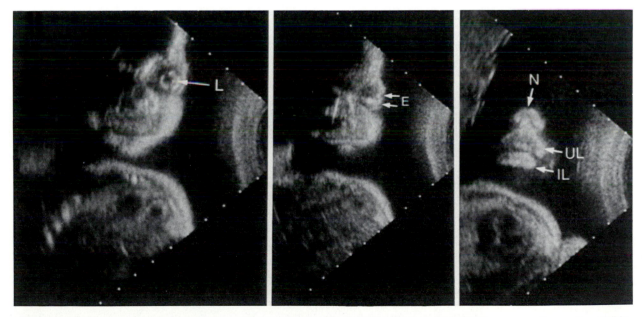

Figure 2–12. Cross sectional sweep from posterior to anterior, demonstrating the lens (L) inside the corpus vitreum, the eyelids (E), the upper and inferior lip (UL and IL), and the nose (N). *(Reproduced with permission from Pilu et al.: Am J Obstet Gynecol 155:45, 1986.)*

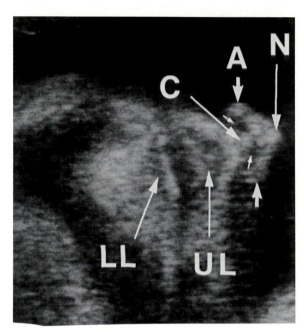

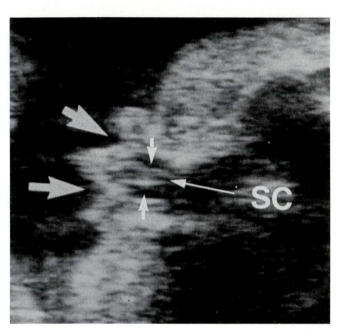

Figure 2–13. The tip (N) of the nose, the alae nasi (A), and the columna (C) are seen above the upper lip (UL). The nostril typically appears as two little anechoic areas (*tiny arrows*). LL, lower lip.

Figure 2–15. Transverse sections reveal the intranasal portion of the upper airways (*small arrows*) between the concha and the septal cartilage (SC). Large arrows, nostrils.

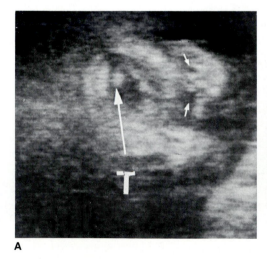

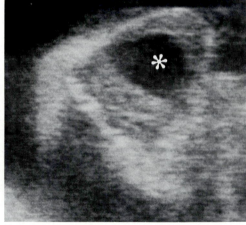

Figure 2–14. A. Coronal scan permits the visualization of the tongue (T) protruding. *Small arrows,* nostrils. **B**. Wide opening of the mouth (*) in the same fetus.

A

B

syndrome). Complications of hemangiomas include ulceration, bleeding, infection and scar formation.[3a]

REFERENCES

1. Benacerraf BR, Frigoletto FD, Bieber FR: The fetal face: Ultrasound examination. Radiology 153:495, 1984.
1a. Birnholz JC: Ultrasonic fetal ophthalmology. Early Hum Dev 12:199, 1985.
1b. Davis WK, Mahony BS, Carroll BA, Bowie JD: Antenatal sonographic detection of benign dacrocystoceles (lacrimal duct cysts). J Ultrasound Med 6:461, 1987.
2. Jeanty P, Dramaix-Wilmet M, Van Gansbeke D, et al.: Fetal ocular biometry by ultrasound. Radiology 143:513, 1982.
3. Mayden KL, Tortora M, Berkowitz RL, et al.: Orbital diameters: A new parameter for prenatal diagnosis and dating. Am J Obstet Gynecol 144:289, 1982.
3a. Pennell RG, Baltarowich OH: Prenatal sonographic diagnosis of a fetal facial hemangioma. J Ultrasound Med 5:525, 1986.
4. Pilu G, Reece EA, Romero R, et al.: Prenatal diagnosis of craniofacial malformations with ultrasonography. Am J Obstet Gynecol 155:45, 1986.

ANOMALIES OF THE ORBITS

Hypertelorism

Synonym
Euryopia.

Definition
Hypertelorism is an increased interocular distance.

Incidence
Rare.

Embryology and Pathogenesis
In early developmental stages of the human embryo, the eyes are placed laterally in the primitive face in a fashion similar to that of lower animals with panoramic vision. As gestation progresses, they migrate toward the midline, creating favorable conditions for the development of stereoscopic vision (Fig. 2–16). Three different mechanisms have been postulated to be responsible for hypertelorism[23]: (1) primary arrest in the forward migration of the eyes, (2) secondary arrest due to the presence of a midline tumor, such as a frontal meningoencephalocele, or (3) abnormal growth vectors of the skull bones manifested through an enlargement of the lesser wings of the sphenoid.[42] Another hypothesis is that hypertelorism is due to abnormal growth of the splachnocranium associated with maldevelopment of the bones derived from the first branchial arches.[41]

Pathology
Three parameters have been used to quantitate ocular spacing in infants and adults: interpupillary distance,[30,55,58,61,88] canthal distance, and interorbital distance. Canthal measurements include the distance between the two medial canthi (intercanthal) and the distance between the two external canthi (outer canthal). These measurements are obtained from frontal view photographs.[12,30,45,55,61,69,93,94] Another commonly used parameter is the canthal index, which is the ratio between the inner and outer

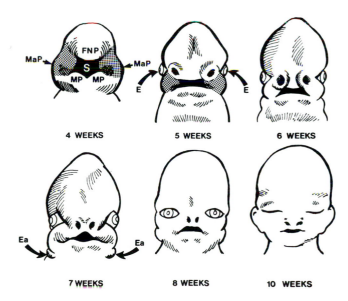

Figure 2–16. Schematic representation of the development of the facial structures from the 4th to 10th week of gestation. In the earliest stages, the primitive eyes (E) are positioned on both sides of the cephalic pole. As gestation progresses, they migrate toward the midline. FNP, frontonasal prominence; MaP, maxillary prominence; MP, mandibular prominence; Ea, ears; S, stomodeum.

TABLE 2–2. MALFORMATIONS AND SYNDROMES ASSOCIATED WITH HYPERTELORISM

Hypertelorism with other median plane facial malformations
Median cleft face syndrome: V-shaped frontal hairline (widow's peak), cranium bifidum occultum, median cleft nose (bifid nose, Doggennase), median cleft lip and palate[14,20,84,95]
Frontal, ethmoidal, or sphenoidal meningoencephalocele
Frontal, ethmoidal, or sphenoidal dermoid–lipoma–teratoma
Nasal glioma
Nasofrontal mucoceles, segmental vitiligo, and porencephaly[106]

Hypertelorism with miscellaneous facial defects
Proboscis lateralis[20]
Facial clefts other than median[20]
Facial hemangioma[66]
Extra nares[28]

Hypertelorism with other prominent skull dysplasias
Craniosynostosis with or without syndactyly[83]
  Apert[14]
  Crouzon syndrome
  Pfeiffer syndrome
  Carpenter syndrome
  Kleeblattschaedel
Thickened skull
  Albers-Schonberg disease
  Craniometaphyseal dysplasia of Pyle
Metopism[105]

Hypertelorism with teeth defects[(36)]
Rieger syndrome with teeth hypoplasia[62]

Hypertelorism with prominent neurologic and brain defects
Hydrocephalus, any prenatal type including myelomeningocele (Chiari malformation, Arnold-Chiari malformation)
Megalencephaly with generalized skull enlargement[21]
  Anatomic megalencephaly: simple autosomal dominant[21]
  Metabolic megalencephaly, particularly mucopolysaccharidosis
Familial neurovisceral lipidosis syndrome
Lissencephaly[90]
Agenesis of the septum pellucidum[82]
Agenesis of the corpus callosum[34]
  With microcephaly and mild extremity malformation[47,75]
  Arhinencephaly; hypertelorism with arhinecephaly very rare; hypotelorism very common[22,24]
  Possibly patients with Meckel-Gruber dysencephalia splanchnocystica syndrome[22]
Peripheral neuritis, ulnar[104]
G syndrome of dysphagia–dysphonia, ear anomalies, and hypospadias[80]
Essential tremor and nyctalopia[64]
Bilateral deafness–microtia S (Mengel-Konigsmark-Berlin-McKusick syndrome)[64]
Pinsky-DiGeorge-Harley-Baird oculocerebral syndrome of microphthalmus, iris dysplasia, severe retardation, and spastic tetraplegia[86]
Cerebrohepatorenal syndrome of high forehead, hepatomegaly, hypotonia, mild skeletal malformation; patients may have only canthal rather than orbital hypertelorism[47]
Cerebral gigantism[99,108]
Familial mild mental retardation[29]

Hypertelorism with other prominent ocular defects
Waardenburg syndrome of dystopia canthorum, white forelock, and deafness[107]
Rieger syndrome of iris dysplasia, hypodontia, and questionable myotonic dystrophy[19,62]
With heterotopia of the macula and pseudoexotropia
Fraser syndrome of cryptophthalmia, ear and genital malformations
Iris dysplasia and mental retardation[19]
Stickler syndrome of arthroophthalmopathy: myopia, retinal detachment, micrognathia, cleft palate, and marfanoid habitus, with hyperextensible joints[81]
Wildervanck I–Waardenburg–Franceschetti–Klein syndrome, cervicooculoacoustic syndrome of congenital deafness, abducens paralysis, frequently other face and tooth deformities and heterochromia of the irises[64]
Wildervanck II syndrome of microphthalmia and blepharophimosis with facial dysmorphia, dysostosis zygomatica–maxillomandibulofacialis[64]
Mohr syndrome of conduction deafness, short stature, and multiple minor facial and skeletal malformations; autosomal recessive; patients probably have only dystopia canthorum and not true hypertelorism
Freeman-Sheldon whistling face syndrome of short stature, whistling, pursed appearance of lips, blepharophimosis, ptosis, strabismus, subcutaneous ridge across lower forehead, and scoliosis[98]
Familial telecanthus–hypospadias–multiple minor malformations syndrome—see under hypertelorism with sex organ malformations
Nyctalopia and tremor[63]
Miscellaneous ocular defects[8]
Corneal ulceration, pseudoexophthalmos, bifid tongue, and extremity and digital malformations[48]
Microphthalmus, iris dysplasia, corneal opacity, severe retardation, and spastic cerebral tetraplegia[86]

Hypertelorism with cleft lip/palate
Ordinary cleft lip and palate[3,32,74]
Robert syndrome of cleft lip and palate with tetraphocomelia and genital enlargement[39,47]
Cleft lip, iridochoroidal coloboma, and deafness[50]
Juberg-Hayward syndrome of oral–cranial–digital anomalies[56]
Orofaciodigital syndrome I and II[39]
Meckel-Gruber syndrome[22]
Median cleft face syndrome[14,20,95]
Cleft lip/palate, tetraperomelia, deformed pinna, scarcity of hair, and hypoplastic nipples[39]
Oral duplication (two hard palates and dental arches)[39]
Hypertelorism, microtia, and facial clefting (HMC syndrome)[9]
Cleft lip with cutis gyrata and acanthosis nigricans[7]

Hypertelorism with prominent skin manifestations and frequent mental retardation
Riley-Day syndrome[47]; true hypertelorism doubtful
Albinism syndrome[64]
Segmental vitiligo, porencephaly, and nasofrontal mucoceles[106]
Leopard syndrome of multiple lentigines, pulmonary stenosis, and cardiac conduction defects with dysrhythmia[38]
Basal cell nevus syndrome[47]
Hypohidrotic ectodermal dysplasia syndrome
Sjogren-Larsen syndrome
G-syndrome of dyschondroplasia, cutis laxa, trigonocephaly (?), polysyndactyly, and kewpie doll facies[80]

TABLE 2–2. (*Continued*)

With elastic tissue deficiency[47]

Bonham-Carter syndrome of mottled skin and congenital heart disease

Ehlers-Danlos syndrome

Acanthosis nigricans, cutis gyrata, and cleft palate[7]

Dubowitz syndrome of dwarfism, eczematous skin, hypospadias, large ears, micrognathia, aplasia of lateral half of eyebrows, and photosensitivity[27]

Short stature, prominent forehead, cutis laxa, pseudoathetosis[17]

Anhidrosis and abnormal nails[109]

Facial hemangioma[66]

Ichthyosis and polysyndactyly[60]

Hypertelorism with prominent skeletal malformations

Otopalatodigital syndrome

Arthrogryposis multiplex congenita, Guerin-Stern syndrome[64]

Larsen syndrome of flattened facies, cleft palate, and multiple congenital joint dislocations

Pterygium syndrome[40]

Roberts tetraphocomelia syndrome with cleft palate and genital enlargement[47,91]

With cardiac and digital malformations[25]

Seckel dwarf; hypertelorism doubtful

Mohr syndrome of polysyndactyly, cleft tongue, micrognathia, and epilepsy

Papillon-League syndrome of orodigitofacial dysostosis[64]

Sprengel deformity[57,60,66,89,102]

With poor frontal development of the skull[53]

DeLange typus degenerativus Amstelodamensis[64]; hypertelorism doubtful

Cleft lip and multiple vertebral malformations[43]; Fara–Chlupackova–Hrivnalsova syndrome; dysmorphia otofaciocervicalis familiaris

Cleidocranial dysostosis[64]

Chondrodystrophia calcificans congenita[64]

Achondroplastic dwarfism

Russell-Silver dwarf[64]

Craniodiaphyseal dysplasia

Robinow–Silverman–Smith syndrome of dyschondroplasia[92]

Craniometaphyseal dysplasia of Pyle[100]

Coffin syndrome: short stature, midface hypoplasia, pectus carinatum, multiple exostoses[13]

Short stature–webbed neck Turner–Noonan–Boonevie–Ulrich phenotype

Noonan syndrome: Turner phenotype in male with normal karyotype[15,52,64,78,87]

Nielsen syndrome: Combination of Klippel-Feil syndrome and Bonnevie-Ulrich syndrome[64]

Melnick-Needles osteodysplasia syndrome[64]

Bonnevie-Ulrich syndrome of Turnerlike phenotype with normal karyotype[87]

F syndrome of acropectorovertebral dysplasia[43,44]

Short thumbs; see Chromosomal anomalies, Ring D-13

Fanconi–v. Albestini-Zellweger syndrome of osteopathia acidotica pseudorachitica

Aminopterin embryopathy syndrome of craniosynostosis, extremity malformations, frequently severe cerebral

malformations with anencephaly, hydrocephalus, and meningomyelocele[47]

Intermittent muscular weakness with small stature, hypodontia, extrasystoles, and multiple minor developmental anomalies[4]

Polydactyly and undescended testes[10]

Brevicollis[20]

Klippel-Feil syndrome[20]

Polysyndactyly and ichthyosis[60]

Mutilating acropathy[49]

Broad thumbs[89]

Dubowitz syndrome of dwarfism, eczematous skin, hypospadias, large ears, micrognathia, aplasia of lateral half of eyebrows, and photosensitivity[27]

Campomelic syndrome of bowed legs, macrocephaly, micrognathia, and cleft palate[101]

Extremity and digital malformations with bifid tongue and pseudoexophthalmus[48]

Syndactyly, short neck, microstomia, cutis laxa, and agenesis of the small intestine

Hypertelorism with sexual organ malformations

Familial telecanthus-hypospadias–multiple minor malformations syndrome[12,70,72,79,80]

Aarskog syndrome of short stature, ptosis, short stubby nose, broad upper lip, and genital malformations[1,35]

Dubowitz syndrome with hypospadias

Cryptorchidism and polydactyly[10]

Hypertelorism with chromosomal anomalies

Wolf syndrome of 4p−[71,72,96]

5p− cri du chat[72]

Translocation t (lp−; 17q+)[31]

Translocation t (2; 13) (q32; q33): broad cranium, short nose, elongated lip, and micrognathia[33]

Trisomy for short arm of 10[51]

Ring D[65,76]

18p, 18q− syndromes[47]

Turner XO syndrome

48 XXXX

49 XXXXY[5,85]

49 XXXXX[64]

47 XX + G cat's eye syndrome

Trisomy 14 (D-2)[103]

Partial trisomy 7: coloboma, urinary malformation, small stature, and mental retardation[77]

Trisomy 9: microbrachycephaly, antimongoloid palpebral fissures, phalangeal hypoplasia, and mental retardation[6]

Deletion of short arm of 13–15 chromosome[18]

Extra fragment macrobrachycephaly, thoracic and cardiac malformations[66]

Mosaic (46, XY − D, + Dr) and (45, XY − D)[65]

Hypertelorism with miscellaneous conditions

Hypercalcemia with supravalvular aortic stenosis (Fanconi-Schlesinger syndrome, Williams-Bensen syndrome)

Potter syndrome of renofacial dysplasia

Hypertelorism with inguinal hernia[2,29]

Lymphedema and yellow nails[59]

AIDS dysmorphism[66a]

Adapted from DeMyer. In: Vinken, Bruyn (eds): *Handbook of Clinical Neurology.* Amsterdam, Elsevier/North Holland Biomedical Press, 1977, Vol 30, pp 235–255.

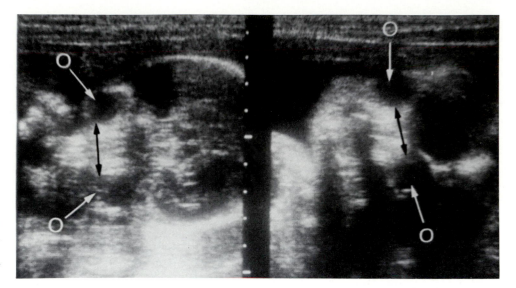

Figure 2–17. Axial and coronal scans passing through the orbits (O) of a 26-week fetus with hypertelorism. The interorbital distance (*black arrows*) is increased.

canthal distance.[84] Interorbital distance is measured on posteroanterior radiograms.[12,16,37,46,74,97]

Analysis of the literature is somewhat confusing, and many authors have used intercanthal distance to define hypertelorism. However, there are anomalies of the soft tissues of the face that can lead to changes in intercanthal distances without affecting interorbital distance (epicanthal folds, dystopia canthorum, cryptophthalmus). It is now well established that the definition of hypertelorism is based on radiographic interorbital measurements.[23]

In the overwhelming number of cases, hypertelorism is bilateral, although some unilateral cases have been reported in such conditions as plagiocephaly and proboscis lateralis.[23,26]

Hypertelorism can be either an isolated finding or associated with other clinical syndromes or malformations. Table 2–2 is an exhaustive classification, provided by DeMyer, of hypertelorism according to associated abnormalities.[23]

A few entities deserve to be considered in more detail. The most common syndromes with hypertelorism are the median cleft syndrome and craniosynostoses. The median cleft face syndrome, or frontonasal dysplasia, is characterized in its most severe expression by hypertelorism, median cleft lip with or without a median cleft of the hard palate and nose, and cranium bifidum occultum. At the other end of the spectrum is the infant with only mild hypertelorism and broad nasal root.[14,20,23] Agenesis of the corpus callosum has been described in these infants.[20,34] The median cleft face syndrome is usually a sporadic disease, although a few familial cases consistent with an autosomal dominant form of inheritance have been reported.[14] Among the craniosynostoses, hypertelorism can be consistently found in Apert, Crouzon, and Carpenter syndromes. For a more detailed discussion of the subject the reader is referred to the section on craniosynostoses, page 369.

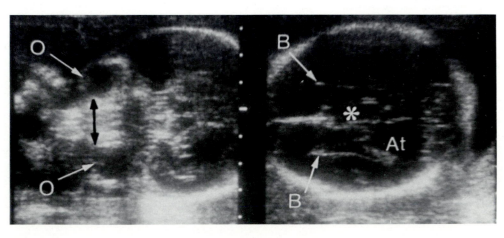

Figure 2–18. In the same fetus as in Figure 2–17, an axial scan passing through the lateral ventricles demonstrates the typical enlargement of the atria (At), widely separated bodies (B), and upward displacement of the third ventricle (*) pathognomonic of agenesis of the corpus callosum. O, orbits.

Diagnosis

Nomograms indicating the normal values of the ultra-sound measurements of the interorbital distance in the fetus are now available.[54,68] By using these nomograms, the prenatal diagnosis of hypertelorism in a case of median cleft face syndrome has been reported.[11] We have been able to identify hypertelorism in one fetus with agenesis of the corpus callosum, Dandy-Walker malformation, double outlet right ventricle, bilateral clubfeet, and normal chromosomes (Figs. 2–17, 2–18). However, the accuracy of sonography in the diagnosis of hypertelorism has not been established in a large series of cases.

Prognosis and Obstetrical Management

Hypertelorism per se results only in cosmetic problems and possible impairment of stereoscopic binocular vision. For severe cases, a number of operative procedures, such as canthoplasty, orbitoplasty, surgical positioning of the eyebrows, and rhinoplasty, have been proposed. It should be stressed that "hypertelorism by itself has little or no status as an entity, does not serve to identify a unitary group of syndromes, and by itself it does not constitute a diagnosis."[23] Therefore, a careful survey for associated anatomic anomalies and a karyotype is mandatory. The obstetrical management depends on the precise diagnosis. Hypertelorism per se does not require a change in standard obstetrical care. The median cleft face syndrome is usually associated with normal intelligence and life span. However, there is a high likelihood of mental retardation when either extracephalic anomalies or an extreme degree of hypertelorism is found.[23] The severity of the cosmetic disturbance should not be underestimated, because this syndrome may be associated with extremely grotesque features.

REFERENCES

1. Aarskog D: A familial syndrome of short stature associated with facial dysplasia and genital anomalies. J Pediatr 77:856, 1970.
2. Abernethy DA: Hypertelorism in several generations. Arch Dis Child 2:361, 1927.
3. Aduss H, Pruzansky S, Miller M: Interorbital distance in cleft lip and palate. Teratology 4:171, 1971.
4. Andersen ED, Krasilnikoff PA, Overvad H: Intermittent muscular weakness, extrasystoles, and multiple developmental anomalies. Acta Paediatr Scand 60:559, 1971.
5. Atkins L, Connelly JP: XXXXY sex-chromosome abnormality. Am J Dis Child 106:514, 1963.
6. Baccichetti C, Tenconi R: A new case of trisomy for the short arm of No. 9 chromosome. J Med Genet 10:296, 1973.
7. Beare JM, Dodge JA, Nevin NC: Cutis gyratum, acanthosis nigricans and other congenital anomalies. A new syndrome. Br J Dermatol 81:241, 1969.
8. Berliner ML, Gartner S: Hypertelorism. Arch Ophthalmol 24:691, 1940.
9. Bixler D, Christian JC, Gorlin RJ: Hypertelorism, microtia, and facial clefting: A new inherited syndrome. Birth Defects 5:77, 1969.
10. Bunge RG, Bradbury JT: Two unilaterally cryptorchid boys with spermatogenic precocity in the descended testis, hypertelorism and polydactyly. J Clin Endocrinol 19:1103, 1959.
11. Chervenak FA, Tortora M, Mayden K, et al.: Antenatal diagnosis of median cleft face syndrome: Sonographic demonstration of cleft lip and hypertelorism. Am J Obstet Gynecol 149:94, 1984.
12. Christian JC, Bixler D, Blythe SC, et al.: Familial telecanthus with associated congenital anomalies. Birth Defects 5:82, 1969.
13. Coffin GS, Siris E, Wegienka LC: Mental retardation with osteocartilaginous anomalies. Am J Dis Child 112:205, 1966.
14. Cohen MM, Sedano HO, Gorlin RJ, et al.: Frontonasal dysplasia (median cleft face syndrome): Comments on etiology and pathogenesis. Birth Defects 7:117, 1971.
15. Collins E, Turner G: The Noonan syndrome—A review of the clinical and genetic features of 27 cases. J Pediatr 83:941, 1973.
16. Currarino G, Silverman FN: Orbital hypotelorism, arhinencephaly, and trigonocephaly. Radiology 74:206, 1960.
17. De Barsy AM, Moens E, Dierckx L: Dwarfism, oligophrenia, and elastic tissue hypoplasia: A new syndrome? Lancet 2:47, 1967. Helv Paediatr Acta 23:305, 1968.
18. De Grouchy J, Salmon C, Salmon D, et al.: Deletion du bras court d'un chromosome 13-15, hypertelorisme et phenotype haptoglobine HPO dans une même famille. Ann Genet 9:80, 1966.
19. De Hauwere RC, Leroy JG, Adriaenssens K, et al.: Iris dysplasia, orbital hypertelorism, and psychomotor retardation: A dominantly inherited developmental syndrome. J Pediatr 82:679, 1973.
20. DeMyer W: The median cleft face syndrome. Differential diagnosis of cranium bifidum occultum, hypertelorism, and median cleft nose, lip and palate. Neurology 17:961, 1967.
21. DeMyer W: Megalencephaly in children. Clinical syndromes, genetic patterns, and differential diagnosis from other causes of megalocephaly. Neurology 22:634, 1972.
22. DeMyer W: Holoprosencephaly (cyclopia-arhinencephaly). In: Vinken PJ, Bruyn GW (eds): Handbook of Clinical Neurology. Amsterdam, Elsevier/North Holland Biomedical Press, 1977, Vol 30, pp 431–478.
23. DeMyer W: Orbital hypertelorism. In: Vinken PJ, Bruyn GW (eds): Handbook of Clinical Neurology. Amsterdam, Elsevier/North Holland Biomedical Press, 1977, Vol 30, pp 235–255.
24. DeMyer W, Zeman W: Alobar holoprosencephaly (arhinencephaly) with median cleft lip and palate:

Clinical, electroencephalographic and nosologic considerations. Confin Neurol 23:1, 1963.

25. Desvignes P, Blanck C: Un hypertelorisme avec malformations generales associees. Arch Ophthalmol 26:769, 1966.

26. Divry D, Evrard E: Plagiocephalie et hypertelorisme unilateral chez un epileptique. J Belg Neurol Psychiatry 35:75, 1935.

27. Dubowitz V: Familial low birthweight dwarfism with an unusual facies and a skin eruption. J Med Genet 2:12, 1965.

28. Erich JB: Nasal duplication. Report of case of patient with two noses. Plast Reconstruct Surg 29:159, 1962.

29. Falchi G, Gerlini F: Ipertelorismo di Greig. Lattante 30:202, 1959.

30. Feingold M, Bossert WH: Normal values for selected physical parameters: An aid to syndrome delineation. Birth Defects 10:1, 1974.

31. Ferrari I, Hering SE: Case report: Reciprocal translocation, t(1p−;17q+), in a patient with multiple anomalies. Birth Defects 5:132, 1969.

32. Figalova P, Hajnis K, Smahel Z: The interocular distance in children with clefts before the operation. Acta Chir Plast 16:65, 1974.

33. Forabosco A, Dutrillaux B, Toni G, et al.: Translocation equilibree t (2;13) (q32; q33) familiale et trisomie 2q partielle. Ann Genet 16:255, 1973.

34. Francois J, Eggermont E, Evens L, et al.: Agenesis of the corpus callosum in the median facial cleft syndrome and associated ocular malformations. Am J Ophthalmol 76:241, 1973.

35. Furukawa CT, Hall BD, Smith DW: The Aarskog syndrome. J Pediatr 81:1117, 1972.

36. Gaard RA: Ocular hypertelorism of Grieg: A congenital craniofacial deformity. Am J Orthodont 47:205, 1961.

37. Gerald BE, Silverman FN: Normal and abnormal interorbital distances, with special reference to mongolism. AJR 95:154, 1965.

38. Gorlin RJ, Anderson RC, Blaw M: Multiple lentigenes syndrome. Complex comprising multiple lentigenes, electrocardiographic conduction abnormalities, ocular hypertelorism, pulmonary stenosis, abnormalities of genitalia, retardation of growth, sensorineural deafness, and autosomal dominant hereditary pattern. Am J Dis Child 117:652, 1969.

39. Gorlin RJ, Cervenka J, Pruzansky S: Facial clefting and its syndromes. Birth Defects 7:3, 1971.

40. Gorlin RJ, Heddie MS, Sedano O, et al.: Popliteal pterygium syndrome. A syndrome comprising cleft lip–palate, popliteal and intercrural pterygia, digital and genital anomalies. Pediatrics 41:503, 1968.

41. Walker DG: Malformations of the Face. Edinburgh, Livingstone, 1961.

42. Grieg, D: Hypertelorism. A hitherto undifferentiated congenital cranio-facial deformity. Edinb Med J 31: 560, 1924.

43. Gros C, Sacrez R, Levy JM, et al.: Hypertelorisme avec malformations cranio-faciales encephaliques et vertebrales multiples. J Radiol 44:635, 1963.

44. Grosse FR, Hermann J, Opitz JM: The F-form of acropectoro-vertebral dysplasia: The F-syndrome. Birth Defects 5:48, 1969.

45. Gunther H: Konstitutionelle Anomalien des Augenabstandes und der Interorbitalbreite. Virchows Arch [Pathol Anat] 290:373, 1933.

46. Hansman CF: Growth of interorbital distance and skull thickness as observed in roentgenographic measurements. Radiology 86:87, 1966.

47. Holmes LB, Moser H, Halldorsson S, et al.: Mental Retardation. An Atlas of Diseases with Associated Physical Abnormalities. New York, Macmillan, 1972.

48. Hornblass A, Dolan R: Oculofacial anomalies and corneal ulceration. Ann Ophthalmol 6:575, 1974.

49. Hozay J: Sur une dystrophie familiale particuliere. (Inhibition précoce de la croissance et osteolyse non mutilante acrales avec dysmorphic faciale). Rev Neurol 89:245, 1953.

50. Hussels IE: L-Midface syndrome with iridochoroidal coloboma and deafness in a mother: Microphthalmia in her son. Birth Defects 7:269, 1971.

51. Hustinx W, Ter-Haar BGA, Scheres JMJ, et al.: Trisomy for the short arm of chromosome No. 10. Clin Genet 6:408, 1974.

52. Jackson LG, Lefrak S: Familial occurrence of the Noonan syndrome. Birth Defects 5:36, 1969.

53. James FE: Hypertelorism associated with poor frontal development of skull and bilateral Sprengel's shoulders. Br Med J 1:1019, 1959.

54. Jeanty P, Romero R: Fetal ocular biometry. In: Obstetrical Ultrasound. New York, McGraw-Hill, 1984, pp 93–98.

55. Johr P: Tableaux de mensurations des distances oculaires et craniennes. J Genet Hum 2:147, 1953.

56. Juberg RC, Hayward JR: A new familial syndrome of oral, cranial, and digital anomalies. J Pediatr 74:755, 1969.

57. Keats TE: Ocular hypertelorism (Greig's syndrome) associated with Sprengel's deformity. AJR 110:119, 1970.

58. Kerwood LA, Lang-Brown H, Penrose LS: The interpupillary distance in mentally defective patients. Hum Biol 26:313, 1954.

59. Kleinman PK: Congenital lymphedema and yellow nails. J Pediatr 83:454, 1973.

60. Korting G, Ruther H: Ichthyosis vulgaris and akrofaciale dysostose. Arch Belg Derm Syph 197:91, 1954.

61. Laestadius ND, Aase JM, Smith DW: Normal inner canthal and outer orbital dimensions. J Pediatr 74:465, 1969.

62. Langdon JD: Rieger's syndrome. Oral Surg 30:788, 1970.

63. Laubichler W, Stenzel A: Ein Greig-Syndrom mit essentiellem Tremor. Nervenarzt 35:310, 1964.

64. Leiber B, Olbrich G: Die klinischen Syndrome. Munich, Urban & Schwarzenberg, 1972.

65. Lejeune J, Lafourcade J, Berger R, et al.: Le phenotype [Dr;] Etude de trois cas de chromosomes D en anneau. Ann Genet 11:79, 1968.

66. MacGillivray RC: Hypertelorism with unusual associated anomalies. Am J Ment Defic 62:288, 1957.

66a. Marion RW, Wiznia AA, Hutcheon RG, Rubinstein A: Fetal AIDS syndrome score: Correlation between severity of dysmorphism and age at diagnosis of immunodeficiency. JAMA 141:429, 1987.

67. Massimo L, Vianello MG: Syndrome de malformations multiples avec un chromosome supplementaire chez une petite fille. Ann Paediatr 204:244, 1965.

68. Mayden KL, Tortora M, Berkowitz RL, et al.: Orbital diameters: A new parameter for prenatal diagnosis and dating. Am J Obstet Gynecol 144:289, 1982.

69. Mehes K, Kitzveger E: Inner canthal and intermamillary indices in the newborn infant. J Pediatr 85:90, 1974.

70. Michaelis E, Mortier W: Association of hypertelorism and hypospadias—The BBB-syndrome. Helv Paediatr Acta 27:575, 1972.

71. Miller JQ: Microcephaly mental retardation and hypertelorism in chromosome deletion studies. Neurology 23:1141, 1973.

72. Miller OJ, Warburton D, Breg WR: Deletions of group B chromosomes. Birth Defects 5:100, 1969.

73. Morin JD, Hill JC, Anderson JE, et al.: A study of growth in the interorbital region. Am J Ophthalmol 56:895, 1963.

74. Moss ML: Hypertelorism and cleft palate deformity. Acta Anat 61:547, 1965.

75. Neu RL, Kajii T, Gardner LI, et al.: A lethal syndrome of microcephaly with multiple congenital anomalies in three siblings. Pediatrics 47:610, 1971.

76. Niebuhr E, Ottosen J: Ring chromosome D(13) associated with multiple congenital malformations. Ann Genet 16:157, 1973.

77. Noel B, Mottett J, Nantois Y, et al.: Contribution à l'identification du petit chromosome submetacentrique surnumeraire dans le syndrome des yeux de chat. J Genet Hum 21:23, 1973.

78. Noonan JA: Hypertelorism with Turner phenotype. A new syndrome with associated congenital heart disease. Am J Dis Child 116:373, 1968.

79. Opitz JM, Summitt RL, Smith DW: The BBB syndrome. Familial telecanthus with associated congenital anomalies. Birth Defects 5:86, 1969.

80. Opitz JM, Frias JL, Gutenberger JE, et al.: The G syndrome of multiple congenital anomalies. Birth Defects 5:95, 1969.

81. Opitz J, France T, Herrmann J, et al.: The Stickler syndrome. N Engl J Med 286:546, 1972.

82. Pelc S, Bollaert A: Contribution a l'etude des dysostoses craniofaciales (hypertelorisme) coexisant avec des malformations cerebrales (commissurales). J Belg Radiol 51:103, 1968.

83. Pendl G, Zimprich H: Ein Beitrag zum Syndrom des Hypertelorismus Greig. Helv Paediatr Acta 26:319, 1971.

84. Peterson MQ, Cohen MM, Sedana HO, et al.: Comments on frontonasal dysplasia, ocular hypertelorism and dystopia canthorum. Birth Defects 7:120, 1971.

85. Pfeiffer RA: Beitrag zum Erscheinungsbild der XXXXY-konstitution. Z Kinderheilk 87:356, 1962.

86. Pinsky L, DiGeorge AM, Harley RD, et al.: Microphthalmos, corneal opacity, mental retardation, and spastic cerebral palsy. An oculocerebral syndrome. J Pediatr 67:387, 1965.

87. Polani PE: Turner phenotype with normal sex chromosomes. Birth Defects 5:24, 1969.

88. Pryor HB: Objective measurement of interpupillary distance. Pediatrics 44:973, 1969.

89. Reilly W: Hypertelorism. Report of 4 cases. JAMA 96:1929, 1931.

90. Reznik M, Alberca-Serrano R: Familial form of hypertelorism associated with lissencephalia with the clinical picture of a form of mental retardation associated with epilepsy and spastic paraplegia. J Neurol Sci 1:40, 1964.

91. Roberts JB: A child with double cleft of lip and palate, protrusion of the intermaxillary portion of the upper jaw and imperfect development of the bones of the four extremities. Ann Surg 70:252, 1919.

92. Robinow M, Silverman FN, Smith HD: A newly recognized dwarfing syndrome. Am J Dis Child 117:645, 1969.

93. Romanus T: Interocular–biorbital index. A gauge of hypertelorism. Acta Genet 4:117, 1953.

94. Schroll K: Hypertelorismus and interkanthale Distanz. Klin Monatsbl Augenheilkd 163:56, 1973.

95. Sedano HO, Cohen MM, Jirasek J, et al.: Frontonasal dysplasia. J Pediatr 76:906, 1970.

96. Sedano HO, Look RA, Carter C, et al.: B group short-arm deletion syndromes. Birth Defects 7:89, 1971.

97. Siedband GN: Roentgen-study of the development of the frontal sinus and the interorbital distance in the half-axial view during infancy and childhood. Ann Paediatr 206:175, 1966.

98. Smith D, Jones KL: Recognizable Patterns of Human Malformation; genetic, embryologic and clinical aspects. Philadelphia, Saunders, 1982.

99. Sotos JF, Dodge PR, Muirhead D, et al.: Cerebral gigantism in childhood. A syndrome of excessively rapid growth with acromegalic features and a nonprogressive neurologic disorder. N Engl J Med 271:109, 1964.

100. Spranger J, Paulsen K, Lehmann W: Die kraniometaphysare Dysplasie (Pyle). Z Kinderheilk 93:64, 1965.

101. Storer J, Grossman H: The campomelic syndrome. Congenital bowing of limbs and other skeletal and extraskeletal anomalies. Radiology 111:673, 1974.

102. Stracker O: Hypertelorismus. Wien Med Wochenschr 101:469, 1951.

103. Murken JD, Bauchinger M, Palitzsch D, et al.: Trisomie D-2 bei einem 2-1/2 jahrigen Madchen (47, XX, 14+). Hum Genet 10:254, 1970.

104. Symonds CP: Bilateral ulnar neuritis in association with skeletal deformities: Hypertelorism. Proc R Soc Med 20:1241, 1927.

105. Tan K: The metopic fontanelle. Am J Dis Child 124:211, 1972.

106. Tay C: Porencephaly, nasofrontal mucoceles, hypertelorism and segmental vitiligo. Report of a new neurocutaneous disorder. Singapore Med J 11:253, 1970.

107. Ulivelli A, Silenzi M: Hypertelorism and Waardenburg's syndrome. Helv Paediatr Acta 24:123, 1969.

108. Villaverde M, DaSilva J: Soto's syndrome—Hypertelorism, antimongoloid slant of eye, and high arched palate complex. J Med Soc NJ 68:805, 1971.

109. Whitwell GPB: A case of ectodermal defect associated with hypertelorism. Br J Dermatol 43:648, 1931.

Hypotelorism

Synonym
Stenopia.

Definition
Hypotelorism is a decreased interorbital distance.

Incidence
Very rare.

Etiology
With exceedingly rare exceptions,[1,7] hypotelorism has always been found in association with other severe anomalies (Table 2–3). The main association is with the holoprosencephalic malformation sequence.

Embryology and Pathogenesis
The craniofacial skeleton originates from a mesenchymal mass that has a dual origin: the mesoderm and the neural crest that migrate into the region. There is a close correlation between the development of the midline facial structures (forehead, nose, interorbital structures, and upper lip) and the differentiation process of the forebrain. Both events are probably induced by the prechordal mesenchyma, the tissue interposed between the prosencephalon and the roof of the primitive mouth (stomodeum). Therefore, midline defects of the face, such as hypotelorism, are frequently associated with cerebral anomalies, mainly holoprosencephaly.[6,8,9]

Although there is some controversy about the precise nature of the process,[6,8] an interference with the activity of the prechordal mesenchyma would lead to defects in both areas, brain and face. The facial anomalies encompass a broad range of defects that are due to aplasia or varying degrees of hypoplasia of the median facial structures. Underdevelopment of the skeleton of the face would result in medial displacement of the orbits. The cerebral anomalies are mainly due to varying degrees of failure of cleavage of the prosencephalon, with incomplete division of the cerebral hemispheres and underlying structures (see pp. 59–65).

Hypotelorism can also be found in association with trigonocephaly,[8] microcephaly,[8] Meckel syndrome,[5] and chromosomal aberrations.[2,10,12,16] It is unclear from some of the reports of hypotelorism whether it occurred as an isolated finding or as a part of a holoprosencephalic malformation sequence.

Pathology and Associated Anomalies
The interorbital distance is reduced, and severe associated anomalies are almost always present.[7] Other facial anomalies can occur as a part of the holoprosencephalic sequence. The classification suggested by DeMyer[9] is shown in Table 1–17.

Diagnosis
The diagnosis is based on demonstration of a reduced interocular distance (Table 2–1, Figs. 2–6, 2–9, 2–19). The prenatal diagnosis of hypotelorism, always in association with holoprosencephaly, has been reported in the literature several times.[3,4,13,14,15]

Prognosis and Obstetrical Management
Prognosis and management depend entirely on the associated malformations. A careful survey of the fetal anatomy and karyotyping must be performed.

TABLE 2–3. ANOMALIES ASSOCIATED WITH HYPOTELORISM

Holoprosencephaly[5, 6, 8, 9]
Trigonocephaly[8]
Oculodentodigital dysplasia[11]
Microcephaly[8]
Meckel syndrome[5]
Maternal phenylketonuria[16]
Chromosomal aberrations
  Trisomy 13[16]
  Trisomy 21[10]
  18 p−[16]
  5p−[2]
  14 q+[12]

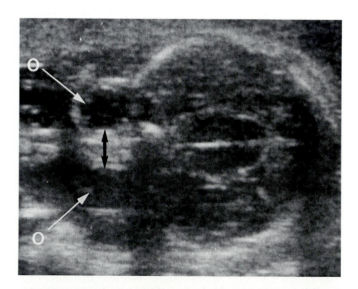

Figure 2–19. Axial scan passing through the orbits (O) in a 22-week fetus with alobar holoprosencephaly. The interorbital distance (*black arrows*) is obviously decreased. (*Reproduced with permission from Pilu et al.: Am J Obstet Gynecol 155:45, 1986.*)

REFERENCES

1. Ben-Hur N, Ashur H, Musseri M: An unusual case of median cleft lip with orbital hypotelorism—A missing link in the classification. Cleft Palate J 15:365, 1978.
2. Breg WR: Chromosome 5p− syndrome. In: Bergsma D (ed): Birth Defects Compendium, 2d ed. New York, Alan R. Liss, 1979, pp 205–206.
3. Chervenak FA, Berkowitz RL, Romero R, et al.: The diagnosis of fetal hydrocephalus. Am J Obstet Gynecol 147:703, 1983.
4. Chervenak FA, Isaacson G, Mahoney MJ, et al.: The obstetric significance of holoprosencephaly. Obstet Gynecol 63:115, 1984.
5. Cohen MM: An update on the holoprosencephalic disorders. J Pediatr 101:865, 1982.
6. Cohen MM, Jirasek JE, Guzman RT: Holoprosencephaly and facial dysmorphia: Nosology, etiology and pathogenesis. Birth Defects 7:125, 1971.
7. Converse JM, McCarthy JG, Wood-Smith D: Orbital hypotelorism. Pathogenesis, associated facio-cerebral anomalies, surgical correction. Plast Reconstr Surg 56:389, 1975.
8. DeMyer W: Holoprosencephaly. (Cyclopia-arhinencephaly). In: Vinken PJ, Bruyn GW (eds): Handbook of Clinical Neurology. Amsterdam, Elsevier/North Holland Biomedical Press, 1977, Vol 30, p 431.
9. DeMyer W, Zeman W, Palmer CG: The face predicts the brain: Diagnostic significance of median facial anomalies for holoprosencephaly (arhinencephaly). Pediatrics 34:256, 1964.
10. Gerald BE, Silverman FN: Normal and abnormal interorbital distances with special reference to mongolism. AJR 95:154, 1965.
11. Gorlin RJ, Meskin LH, St Geme JW: Oculodentodigital dysplasia. J Pediatr 63:69, 1963.
12. Hecht F, Wyandt HE: Chromosome 14q proximal partial trisomy syndrome. In: Bergsma D (ed): Birth Defects Compendium, 2d ed. New York, Alan R. Liss, 1979, pp 209–210.
13. Mayden KL, Tortora M, Berkowitz RL, et al.: Orbital diameters: A new parameter for prenatal diagnosis and dating. Am J Obstet Gynecol 144:289, 1982.
14. Pilu G, Reece EA, Romero R, et al.: Prenatal diagnosis of cranio facial malformations with ultrasonography. Am J Obstet Gynecol (155:45, 1986.)
15. Pilu G, Romero R, Jeanty P, et al.: Criteria for the antenatal diagnosis of holoprosencephaly. Am J Perinatol 4:41, 1987.
16. Smith DW, Jones KL: Recognizable Patterns of Human Malformation: Genetic, Embryologic, and Clinical Aspects, 3d ed: Philadelphia, Saunders, 1982.

Microphthalmia

Definition
Decreased size of the eyeball. The term "anophthalmia" refers to absence of the eye. However, it should be reserved for the pathologist, who must demonstrate not only absence of the eye but also of optic nerves, chiasma, and tracts.

Incidence
The incidence is difficult to define. Microphthalmia/anophthalmia is responsible for 4 percent of cases of congenital inheritable blindness.[5]

Etiology/Pathology
Microphthalmia is generally associated with other anomalies. On rare occasions it occurs in the absence of other ocular and systemic malformations and the term "nanophthalmous" is used. Microphthalmia can occur as a sporadic disorder or as a condition inherited with an autosomal dominant, recessive, or X-linked pattern.[4] Microphthalmia can be unilateral or bilateral. The term "cryptophthalmia" refers to a condition in which there is fusion of the eyelids, and it is frequently associated with microphthalmia.

Diagnosis
The diagnosis can be suspected by demonstrating an orbital diameter below the 5th percentile for gestational age (Table 2–1, Fig. 2–5). It should be stressed that this is a statistical definition of microphthalmia. Some normal infants will fall within this range. A careful examination of the intraorbital anatomy is indicated to identify lens, pupil, and optic nerve.[1] The diagnosis of this condition has been reported twice. One fetus had Fraser syndrome, and the other hemifacial microsomia (Goldenhar-Gorlin syndrome). In the former case, the diagnosis was made in a patient at risk for this autosomal recessive condition.[2] In the latter case, the diagnosis was possible by detecting unilateral microphthalmia and a deformed ipsilateral ear.[3] Table 2–4 illustrates conditions associated with microphthalmia that can be diagnosed in utero. Once the diagnosis is suspected, a search for associated anomalies is indicated. The sonographer should concentrate on the identification of microtia, micrognathia, syndactyly, camptodactyly, median cleft, feet abnormalities (rockerbottom and talipes), hemivertebrae, and congenital heart defects. Karyotyping is indicated, because several

TABLE 2–4. CONDITIONS ASSOCIATED WITH MICROPHTHALMIA

1. Chromosomal
  Partial trisomy 10q
  Triploidy
  Trisomy 13
  4p−
  13q−
  Trisomy 4p
  Trisomy 9 mosaic
  Trisomy 18
  18q−

2. Environmental
  Fetal toxoplasmosis
  Fetal rubella
  Fetal alcohol syndrome
  Fetal varicella
  Maternal phenylketonuria

3. Syndrome
  CHARGE association (sporadic)
    Coloboma sequence (ranging from coloboma to
      microphthalmia)
    Heart defects (tetralogy of Fallot, double outlet right ventricle
      with atrioventricular canal, atrial and ventricular septal
      defects)
    Atresia of choanae
    Growth retardation (postnatal)
    Genital abnormalities 75% (males with testicular hypoplasia)
    Ear anomalies 88% (microtia, deafness)
    Micrognathia (rare)
  Frontonasal dysplasia (median cleft face syndrome) (sporadic)
    Ocular hypertelorism (only rarely microphthalmia)
    Median cleft
    Bifid nose
  Fraser syndrome (autosomal recessive)
    Cryptophtalmos
    Hypoplastic notched nares
    Incomplete development of genitalia
  Goldenhar-Gorlin syndrome (sporadic)
    Ipsilateral ear anomalies
    Vertebral anomalies

3. Syndrome (cont.)
  Lenz syndrome (X-linked)
    Coloboma
    Cataracts
    Unilateral or bilateral renal agenesis
    Hydroureter
  Goltz syndrome (poikiloderma with focal dermal hypoplasia)
    (sporadic)
    Syndactyly
    Cutaneous abnormalities
    Dental abnormalities
  Hallerman-Streiff syndrome (dominant)
    Frontal bossing
    Micrognathia
    Small nose
  Oculodentodigital syndrome (oculodentodigital dysplasia)
    (autosomal dominant)
    Syndactyly
    Camptodactyly of fifth finger
    Enamel hypoplasia
    Thin hypoplastic nose
  Pena-Shokeir II syndrome (autosomal recessive)
    Microcephaly (?)
    Cataracts
    Camptodactyly
    Flexion contraction of elbows and knees
    Rocker-bottom foot
  Facioauriculovertebral spectrum (first and second branchial arch)
    (sporadic)
    Unilateral involvement in 70% of cases
    Micrognathia
    Malar hypoplasia
    Hypoplasia of the maxilla
    Microtia
    Hemivertebrae or hypoplasia of vertebrae
  Fanconi syndrome (autosomal recessive)
    Pancytopenia
    Enhanced chromosomal breakage
    Splenic hypoplasia

chromosomal disorders can be associated with microphthalmia. (Fig 1–71 shows a case of anophthalmia.)

Prognosis and Obstetrical Management
Management depends on the specific syndrome responsible for microphthalmia.

REFERENCES

1. Birnholz JC: Ultrasonic fetal ophthalmology. Early Hum Devel 12:199, 1985.
2. Feldman E, Shalev E, Weiner E, et al.: Microphthalmia—Prenatal ultrasonic diagnosis: A case report. Prenatal Diagn 5:205, 1985.
3. Tamas DE, Mahony BS, Bowie JD, et al.: Prenatal sonographic diagnosis of hemifacial microsomia (Goldenhar-Gorlin syndrome). J. Ultrasound Med 5:461, 1986.
4. Warburg M: The heterogeneity of microphthalmos. International Ophthalmology 4:45, 1981.
5. Warburg M: Congenital blindness. In: Emery AEH, Rimoin DL (eds): Principles and Practice of Medical Genetics. Edinburgh, Churchill Livingston, 1983, pp 474–479.

ANOMALIES OF THE NOSE

Arhinia

Definition
Absence of the nose.

Incidence
Unknown. It is an extremely rare condition.

Etiology and Associated Anomalies
Unknown in most cases. It may occur as an isolated malformation or be part of a malformation complex, such as holoprosencephaly[2] or mandibulofacial dysostosis (Treacher Collins syndrome).[1]

Embryology
The nasal cavity originates from the nasal sacs which are paired invaginations of the ectoderm. The nasal sacs are originally separated from the oral cavity by the oronasal membrane, which subsequently undergoes reabsorption. At about 6 weeks of gestation, the primitive nasal and oral cavities communicate freely through an opening that is then progressively closed by the developing palate. At about 12 weeks gestation, when the lateral palatine processes fuse medially with the nasal septum, the oral and the two nasal cavities are formed and separated. The external nose derives from the lower portion of the frontonasal prominence, which merges on both sides with the maxillary processes (Fig. 2–16).

Failure of development of the frontonasal prominence results in complete or partial nasal aplasia. In the holoprosencephalic sequence, this defect is part of a complex spectrum of midfacial anomalies that are thought to arise from a primitive defect of the pre-chordal mesenchyma, the tissue responsible for the induction of both facial and cerebral structures (see p. 60).

Pathology
In arhinia, a concavity extending from the forehead to the upper lip is usually seen in the position normally occupied by the nose. In unilateral aplasia, a small pit is often seen in the area of the nostril.

Diagnosis
The diagnosis can be easily made by using both axial and longitudinal scans of the fetal face.[3] A careful survey for associated anomalies is mandatory. (see Fig. 2–25).

Prognosis and Obstetrical Management
These depend on the associated anomalies. Isolated arhinia is compatible with life and does not require alteration in obstetrical care.

REFERENCES
1. Berndorfer A: Uber die seitliche Nasenspalte. Acta Otolaryngol 55:163, 1962.
2. DeMyer W: Holoprosencephaly (cyclopia-arhinencephaly). In: Vinken PJ, Bruyn GW (eds): Handbook of Clinical Neurology. Amsterdam, Elsevier/North Holland Biomedical Press, 1977, Vol 30, pp 431–478.
3. Pilu G, Romero R, Jeanty P, et al.: Criteria for the diagnosis of holoprosencephaly. Am J Perinatol 4:41, 1987.

Proboscis

Definition
A proboscis is a trunklike appendage with either one or two internal openings, usually associated with absence of the nose.

Incidence
Unknown. Cyclopia and cebocephaly, two of the main conditions in which a proboscis is present, have been reported to occur in 1:40,000 and 1:16,000 births, respectively.[3,7]

Embryology
Normal development of the nose is discussed above. The presence of a proboscis is almost always found in association with holoprosencephaly. It has been suggested that in these cases, a primary disorder of the

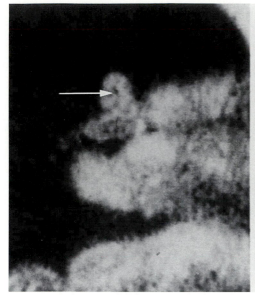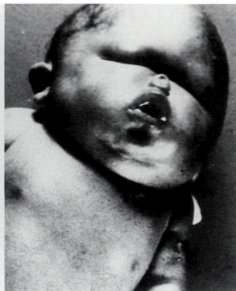

Figure 2–20. Anterior coronal scan of the face of a fetus with cebocephaly. The presence of a proboscis is inferred by the tubular appearance of the nasal appendage and by the presence of a single median nostril (*arrow*). An image of the stillborn infant is provided for comparison. *(Reproduced with permission from Pilu et al.: Am J Obstet Gynecol 155:45, 1986.)*

prechordal mesenchyma results in an abnormal induction of the midfacial structures. Abnormal development of the nasal prominences may lead to a fusion of the olfactory placodes and formation of a proboscis. Derangement in the morphogenesis of the medial facial structures may lead to different positions of the proboscis with regard to the eye(s).[2–4]

Pathology and Associated Anomalies

The proboscis usually has a single central opening. According to the classification of holoprosencephalic facies suggested by DeMyer (Table 1–17), the proboscis may be inserted either above the orbit(s) (cyclopia, ethmocephaly) or in a normal position between the orbits (cebocephaly). The openings of the proboscis have no connection with the choanae. The ethmoid, the nasal conchae, and the nasal and lacrimal bones are absent. Typically, in cyclopia, ethmocephaly, and cebocephaly, there is no cleft of the lip and palate. The presence of a proboscis has rarely been reported in the absence of holoprosencephaly.[8] In these cases, there is usually unilateral nasal aplasia, and the proboscis is found in the position normally occupied by the missing nasal structures. In rare cases, a bilateral proboscis has been found.[8]

Diagnosis

The diagnosis relies on the demonstration of a trunk-like structure, usually with a single central opening either occupying the normal position of the nose[6] or hanging above the orbits[1,5] (Fig. 2–20).

Prognosis and Obstetrical Management

Most cases will be associated with holoprosencephaly, which was discussed in the previous chapter (see pp. 59–64). A karyotype should be performed.

REFERENCES

1. Benacerraf BR, Frigoletto FD, Bieber FR: The fetal face: Ultrasound examination. Radiology 153:495, 1984.
2. Cohen MM, Jirasek JE, Guzman RT, et al.: Holoprosencephaly and facial dysmorphia: nosology, etiology and pathogenesis. Birth Defects 7(7):125, 1971.
3. DeMyer W: Holoprosencephaly (cyclopia-arhinencephaly). In: Vinken PJ, Bruyn GW (eds): Handbook of Clinical Neurology. Amsterdam, Elsevier/North Holland Biomedical Press, 1977, Vol 30, pp 431–478.
4. DeMyer W, Zeman W: Alobar holoprosencephaly (arhinencephaly) with median cleft lip and palate: Clinical, electroencephalographic and nosologic considerations. Confin Neurol 23:1, 1963.
5. Filly RA, Chinn DH, Callen PW: Alobar holoprosencephaly: Ultrasonographic prenatal diagnosis. Radiology 151:455, 1984.
6. Pilu G, Reece E A, Romero R, et al.: Prenatal diagnosis of craniofacial malformations with ultrasonography. Am J Obstet Gynecol 155:45, 1986.
7. Roach E, DeMyer W, Conneally PM, et al.: Holoprosencephaly. Birth data, genetic and demographic analyses of 30 families. Birth Defects 11:294, 1975.
8. Warkany J: Malformation of the respiratory tract. In: Congenital Malformations. Chicago, Year Book, 1971, pp 587–615.

ANOMALIES OF THE LIP AND PALATE

Facial Clefting

Synonyms
Cleft lip and cleft palate.

Definition
This term refers to a wide spectrum of lateral clefting defects usually involving the upper lip, the palate, or both. Median cleft lip and palate is a different entity and will be discussed separately (see p. 105).

Incidence
Facial clefting is the second most common congenital malformation, accounting for 13 percent of all anomalies.[8] Its incidence in the United States has been estimated to be 1:700 live births.[8] In 50 percent of patients, both lip and palate are defective, whereas either the lip or the palate alone is involved in 25 percent of patients each.[2]

Etiology
In the vast majority of patients, cleft lip (CL) and cleft palate (CP) have a multifactorial etiology, with both genetic and environmental factors accounting for the defect.[7] The empiric risks of recurrence for these cases are reported in Table 2–5. CL with or without CP and isolated CP are two different anomalies. With exceedingly rare exceptions, recurrences are type specific. If the index case has CL–CP, there is no increased risk for isolated CP, and vice versa. In some cases, facial clefts are a part of well-established mendelian, chromosomal, and nongenetic syndromes. Gorlin et al.[8] list 72 possible associations (Table 2–6).

CL–CP and isolated CP can occur as a component of a well-defined syndrome in 3 percent of the cases (syndromic) and in 97 percent of cases is nonsyndromic. Of nonsyndromic defects, CL–CP represents 75 percent of all clefting malformations (25 percent isolated CL and 50 percent CL+CP), and isolated cleft palate represents 25 percent. CL–CP can occur as a result of a multifactorial defect or the combination of an autosomal dominant with incomplete expressivity and penetrance (25 percent) or a sporadic disorder (75 percent). The male:female ratio is 2:1, and the left side is involved twice as often as the right.

The genetic basis of isolated CP is less well established but is thought to be similar to CL–CP. The female:male ratio is 2:1. If the parent affected is the mother, the recurrence risk is decreased, and if it is the father, the recurrence risk is increased.[6] The opposite is true for CL–CP. The claimed risk associated with diazepam and steroidal agents intake has not been confirmed in carefully controlled studies. Chromosomal abnormalities are present in less than 1 percent of clefting abnormalities.[13]

Embryology
Shortly after the third week of gestation, outgrowths of mesenchyma result in the formation of ectodermal elevations that surround the primitive oral cavity or stomodeum. These structures (frontonasal prominence, maxillary prominence, and mandibular prominence) are separated by grooves (Fig. 2–16). Progressive growth of the prominences obliterates the grooves. Cleft lip results from the persistence of the grooves. Collapse of the mesenchymal tissue under the groove leads to the formation of the cleft (Fig. 2–21).[12]

The palate originates from the fusion of three palatine processes. The median originates from the medial nasal prominences, and the two lateral ones originate from the maxillary processes. The palatine processes fuse also with the nasal septum, which divides the nasal cavities (Fig. 2–22). Cleft palate is the consequence of lack of fusion of these structures.[12]

TABLE 2–5. INCIDENCE OF CLEFT LIP/PALATE AND ISOLATED CLEFT PALATE IN RELATIVES OF SIMILARLY AFFECTED PERSONS

Affected Parents	Affected Siblings	Affected Relatives	Cleft Lip/ Palate	Isolated Cleft Palate
None	None	None	0.1	0.04
None	1	None	4	2
None	1	1	4	7
None	2	None	9	1*
1	None	None	4	6
1	1	None	17	15

Percent Risk for Each Subsequent Child

* The authors have no explanation for this puzzling observation.
Adapted from Curtis et al.: Am J Dis Child 102:853, 1961.

TABLE 2–6. MALFORMATION AND SYNDROMES ASSOCIATED WITH FACIAL CLEFTING

Autosomal dominant cleft syndromes

1. Cleft lip or palate or both and lip pits (Van der Woude syndrome)
2. Cleft lip or palate or both and ankyloblepharon filiforme adnatum
3. Cleft lip/palate, lobster claw deformity, dacrocystitis, and hypodontia (most sporadic cases)
4. Cleft lip or palate or both and enlarged parietal foramina (uncertain)
5. Cleft lip or palate or both and congenital neuroblastoma
6. Cleft lip or palate or both and popliteal pterygia
7. Cleft palate and hereditary arthroophthalmopathy
8. Cleft palate, retinal detachment and myopia
9. Cleft palate, retinal detachment and joint hypermobility
10. Cleft lip or palate or both and multiple nevoid basal cell carcinoma
11. Cleft palate and the Apert syndrome
12. Cleft palate and the Marfan syndrome
13. Cleft lip or palate or both and the Waardenburg syndrome
14. Cleft palate and mandibulofacial dysostosis
15. Cleft palate and congenital spondyloepiphyseal dysplasia
16. Cleft lip/palate, hypohidrosis, thin wiry hair and dystrophic nails
17. Cleft palate, camptodactyly, and clubfoot

Autosomal recessive cleft syndromes

1. Cleft lip/palate, tetraphocomelia, and penile or clitoral enlargement
2. Cleft lip/palate and pseudothalidomide syndrome
3. Cleft palate and Klippel-Feil syndrome (genetic pattern uncertain)
4. Cleft palate and chondrodysplasia punctata
5. Cleft palate and multiple congenital dislocations (Larsen syndrome)
6. Cleft palate and diastrophic dwarfism
7. Cleft palate and the Smith–Lemli–Opitz syndrome
8. Cleft palate and the Meckel syndrome
9. Cleft palate and the multiple pterygium syndrome
10. Cleft lip or palate or both and cryptophthalmia syndrome
11. Cleft lip/palate, ocular hypertelorism, and microtia
12. Cleft lip/palate, microcephaly, and hypoplasia of radii and thumbs
13. Cleft lip/palate, tetraperomelia, deformed pinna, and ectodermal dysplasia
14. Cleft palate, stapes fixation and oligodontia
15. Cleft palate and cerebrocosto mandibular syndrome
16. Cleft palate and orofaciodigital syndrome II
17. Cleft palate and new chondrodysplasia
18. Cleft palate, median cleft lip, and unknown lethal chondrodysplasia

X-Linked cleft syndromes

1. Otopalatodigital syndrome (probably XLR)
2. Orofaciodigital syndrome I (XLD, lethal in male)
3. Cleft uvula, familial nephrons, deafness, congenital urinary tract, and digital anomalies (XLR, ?)
4. Cleft palate, micrognathia, talipes equinovarus, atrial septal defect, and persistence of left superior vena cava (XLR)

Nongenetic cleft syndromes

1. Robin syndrome (rare familial occurrence)
2. Cleft lip/palate and cleft larynx
3. Cleft lip/palate and laryngeal web
4. Cleft lip or palate or both and thoracopagous twins
5. Facial clefts and amniotic band syndrome
6. Cleft lip or palate or both and forearm bone aplasia
7. Cleft lip or palate or both and congenital heart disease
8. Cleft lip or palate or both and anencephaly
9. Cleft palate and Brachmann-DeLange syndrome
10. Cleft palate and glossopalatine ankylosis
11. Cleft lip/palate and lateral proboscis
12. Premaxillary agenesis (may also occur with trisomy 13 and 18p−)
13. Cleft lip or palate or both and encephalomeningocele
14. Cleft lip or palate or both and median cleft face syndrome
15. Cleft palate and congenital oral teratoma
16. Cleft palate and buccopharyngeal membrane persistence
17. Cleft palate and oral duplication
18. Cleft palate and bilateral femoral dysplasia

Gross chromosomal cleft syndromes

1. 4p−
2. 5p−
3. Trisomy C mosaicism
4. Trisomy 13
5. Dp−
6. 14q−
7. Trisomy 18
8. 18p−
9. 18q−
10. Trisomy 21
11. XXXXY syndrome
12. Various translocations
13. Supernumerary G-sized fragment
14. Monosomy G
15. Triploidy

XLR, X-linked recessive; XLD, X-linked dominant.
Adapted from Gorlin et al.: Birth Defects 7 (7): 3, 1971.

Pathology

Facial clefts encompass a broad spectrum of severity, ranging from minimal defects, such as a bifid uvula, linear indentation of the lip, or submucous cleft of the soft palate, to large deep defects of the facial bones and soft tissues (Fig. 2–23). The typical CL will appear as a linear defect extending from one side of the lip into the nostril. CP associated with CL may extend through the alveolar ridge and hard palate, reaching the floor of the nasal cavity or even the floor of the orbit. Isolated cleft palate may include defects of the hard palate, the soft palate, or both or the submuco-

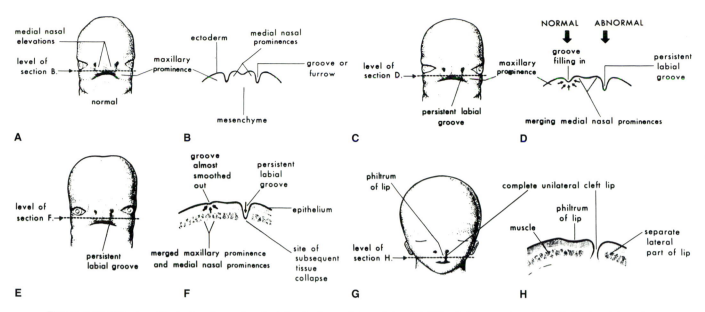

Figure 2–21. Drawings illustrating the embryologic basis of complete unilateral cleft lip. **A.** Five-week embryo. **B.** Horizontal section through the head, illustrating the grooves between the maxillary prominences and the medial nasal prominences. **C.** Six-week embryo, showing a persistent labial groove on the left side. **D.** Horizontal section through the head, showing the disappearance of the groove on the right side because of proliferation of the mesenchyma (*arrows*). **E.** Seven-week embryo. **F.** Horizontal section through the head, showing that the epithelium on the right has almost been pushed out of the groove between the maxillary prominence and medial nasal prominence. **G.** Ten-week fetus with a complete unilateral cleft lip. **H.** Horizontal section through the head following stretching of the epithelium and breakdown of the tissues in the floor of the persistent labial groove on the left side.[12] *(Reproduced with permission from Moore: The Developing Human: Clinically Oriented Embryology, 2d ed. Philadelphia, Saunders, 1977.)*

sal tissue. CL is bilateral in 20 percent of patients, whereas CL–CP is bilateral in 25 percent of cases.[11]

Associated Anomalies

Associated anomalies are found in 50 percent of patients with isolated CP and in only 13 percent of those with CL–CP.[9] An incidence of 60 percent has been found in embryos and fetuses with facial clefting.[10] In the majority of patients, the associated anomalies do not conform to an established syndrome. In cases of either isolated CL or CP, the most frequent anomaly is clubfoot, whereas in cases of CL–CP, it is polydactyly.[8] Of particular importance is the association with congenital heart disease.[3] No specific pattern could be identified.[18] Specific associations with well-described syndromes are shown in Table 2–6.

Diagnosis

The sonographic diagnosis of CL–CP in the fetus depends on demonstration of a groove extending from one of the nostrils inside the lip and possibly the alveolar ridge. Both axial and coronal planes can be used. In our experience, coronal scans have proved to be the most informative (Fig. 2–24). Several cases of prenatal diagnosis of CL–CP have been reported in the literature.[1,4,5,14,15,17] However, it must be stressed that in all these cases, the facial lesions were quite

large. The accuracy of ultrasound in detecting small lesions has not been established. At present the ultrasound diagnosis of isolated CP appears difficult.[14] In cases at risk for mendelian syndromes associated with isolated CP, fetoscopy could be diagnostic.[16] We have seen several cases of both CL and CP associated with polyhydramnios, and, therefore,

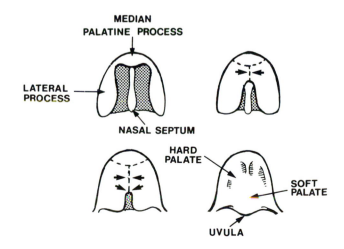

Figure 2–22. The palate derives from the fusion of the median and lateral palatine processes. Merging with the outgrowing nasal septum results in the separation of the oral and nasal cavities.

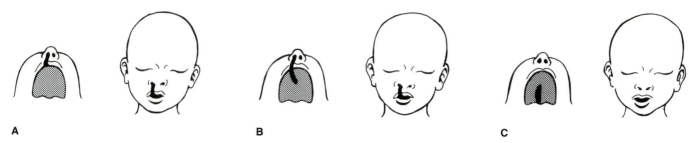

A   **B**   **C**

Figure 2–23. Schematic representation of various types of cleft lip and cleft palate. **A.** Unilateral cleft lip. **B.** Unilateral cleft lip and palate. **C.** Unilateral cleft palate.

we believe that an increased amount of amniotic fluid is an indication for careful examination of the fetal face.

Prognosis

Minimal defects, such as linear indentations of the lips or submucosal cleft of the soft palate, may not require surgical correction. Larger defects cause cos-

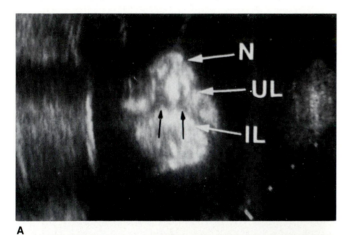

A

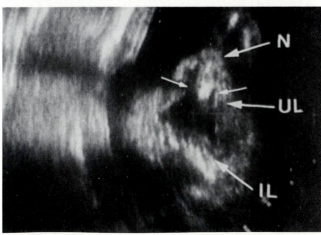

B

Figure 2–24. A. Coronal scan of the face of a 26-week fetus with bilateral cleft lip and palate. Two grooves (*black arrows*) are seen extending from both sides of the upper lip (UL) into the nostrils. N, nose; IL, inferior lip. **B.** A slight posterior angulation of the transducer allows visualization of the defects extending into the hard palate (*thin arrows*).

metic, swallowing, and respiratory problems. Recent advances in surgical technique have produced good cosmetic and functional results. However, prognosis depends primarily on the presence and type of associated anomalies.[13]

Obstetrical Management

A careful survey for associated anatomic defects is indicated. The advisability of karyotype is controversial in view of the low incidence of chromosomal anomalies in clefting defects. In the absence of other anomalies, fetal CL–CP does not require a change in standard obstetrical care. Infants should be delivered in a tertiary center because of the possibility of respiratory and feeding problems.

REFERENCES

1. Benacerraf BR, Frigoletto FD, Bieber FR: The fetal face. Ultrasound examination. Radiology 153:495, 1984.
2. Biggerstaff RH: Classification and frequency of cleft lip and/or palate. Cleft Palate J 6:40, 1969.
3. Boeson I, Melchior JC, Terslev E, et al.: Extracardiac congenital malformations in children with congenital heart diseases. Acta Paediatr (Suppl.) 146:28, 1963.
4. Chervenak FA, Tortora M, Mayden K, et al.: Antenatal diagnosis of median cleft face syndrome: Sonographic demonstration of cleft lip and hypertelorism. Am J Obstet Gynecol 149:94, 1984.
5. Christ JE, Meininger MG: Ultrasound diagnosis of cleft lip and cleft palate before birth. Plast Reconstr Surg 68:854, 1981.
6. Curtis EJ, Fraser FC, Warburton D: Congenital cleft lip and palate. Am J Dis Child 102:853, 1961.
7. Fraser FC: The genetics of cleft lip and cleft palate. Am J Hum Genet 22:336, 1970.
8. Gorlin RJ, Cervenka J, Pruzansky S: Facial clefting and its syndromes. Birth Defects 7(7):3, 1971.
9. Ingalls TH, Taube IE, Klingberg MA: Cleft lip and cleft palate: Epidemiologic considerations. Plast Reconstr Surg 34:1, 1964.
10. Kraus BS, Kitamura H, Ooe T: Malformations associated with cleft lip and palate in human embryos and fetuses. Am J Obstet Gynecol 86:321, 1963.
11. Meskin LH, Pruzansky S, Gullen WH: An epidemiologic investigation of factors related to the extent of

facial clefts. 1. Sex of the patient. Cleft Palate J 5:23, 1968.
12. Moore KL: The Developing Human: Clinically Oriented Embryology, 2d ed. Philadelphia, Saunders, 1977.
13. Pashayan HM: What else to look for in a child born with a cleft of the lip and palate. Cleft Palate J 20(1):54–82, 1983.
14. Pilu G, Reece EA, Romero R, et al.: Prenatal diagnosis of craniofacial malformations with ultrasonography. Am J Obstet Gynecol 155:45, 1986.
15. Pilu G, Romero R, Rizzo N, et al.: Criteria for the antenatal diagnosis of holoprosencephaly. Am J Perinatol 4:41, 1987.
16. Rodeck CH, Nicolaides KH: The use of fetoscopy for prenatal diagnosis and treatment. Semin Perinatol 7:118, 1983.
17. Savoldelli G, Schmid W, Schinzel A: Prenatal diagnosis of cleft lip and palate by ultrasound. Prenat Diagn 2:313, 1982.
18. Shah CV, Pruzansky S, Harris WS: Cardiac malformations with facial clefts: With observations on the Pierre Robin syndrome. Am J Dis Child 119:238, 1970.

Median Cleft Lip

Synonyms
Complete median cleft lip, pseudomedian cleft lip, and premaxillary agenesis.

Definition
A quadrangular or triangular median defect of the upper lip, possibly extending posteriorly to the nose.

Incidence
Median cleft lip (MCL) accounts for 0.2 to 0.7 percent of all cases of cleft lip.[1,4]

Embryology
The median portion of the upper lip and maxilla derives from the frontonasal prominence, which joins the maxillary prominences (Fig. 2–16). In cases of median cleft lip, there is absence or underdevelopment of this portion.

There is a close correlation between the development of the midline facial structures and the differentiation process of the forebrain. Both events are probably induced by the prechordal mesenchyma, the tissue interposed between the prosencephalon, and the roof of the primitive mouth (stomodeum). Therefore, midline defects of the face, such as MCL,

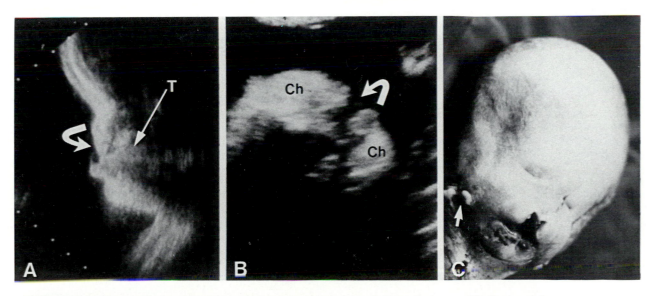

Figure 2–25. Median cleft lip in a third trimester holoprosencephalic fetus. **A.** Midsagittal scan of the face reveals an unusually high position of the tongue (T) inside the oral cavity, as well as absence of the nose (*curved arrow*). **B.** Axial scan of the palate demonstrating a large quadrangular median cleft (*curved arrow*). Ch, cheeks. **C.** Postnatal appearance of the stillborn infant. Note the median cleft lip and palate, absence of the nose, anophthalmia, and low set ears (*arrow*). (*Reproduced with permission from Pilu et al.: Am J Obstet Gynecol 155:45, 1986.*)

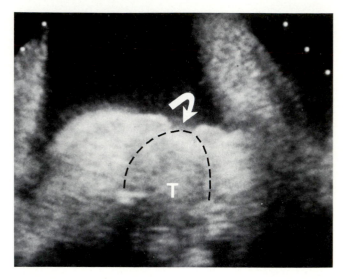

Figure 2–26. Axial scan at midfacial level in a third trimester fetus with holoprosencephaly and a large cleft of the palate. The seemingly intact appearance of the palate is due to the tongue (T) filling the defect. A correct diagnosis could be made by observing the midline cleft of the upper lip (*curved arrow*), as well as the active movement of the tongue.

are frequently associated with cerebral anomalies, such as holoprosencephaly (see Fig. 1–64, Table 1–17).[3]

Etiology and Pathology

MCL has been described only as part of two distinct syndromes: MCL with orbital hypotelorism,[3] which is a synonym for holoprosencephaly, and MCL with orbital hypertelorism.[2] In the former case, there is absence of the premaxillary bone, nasal septum, nasal bones, and crista galli. The ethmoid bone that sets the interorbital distance is hypoplastic. The secondary palate may or may not be involved. For a detailed description of the other facial and cerebral findings, see the section on hypotelorism in this chapter and the section on holoprosencephaly in Chapter 1. MCL with hypertelorism (also known as "median cleft face syndrome" or "frontonasal dysplasia") is characterized by the presence of a bifid nose and cranium bifidum occultum. The premaxilla is usually present. The brain is normal in most cases.

Diagnosis

The diagnosis relies on the demonstration of a wide central defect involving both the upper lip and the palate.[5,6] In our experience, the defect is better demonstrated in axial scans of the palate (Fig. 2–25). A useful hint for the diagnosis is the visualization of the tongue in a higher than normal position within the oral cavity. The sonographer should be alerted to a possible pitfall in the diagnosis of MCL. On occasion, the defect may be filled by the tongue, giving a false impression of an intact palate (Fig. 2–26). Recognition of MCL should immediately prompt a careful ultrasound investigation of the entire fetal anatomy, with special attention to the intracranial contents. Orbital measurements will identify hypotelorism or hypertelorism.

Prognosis and Obstetrical Management

Prognosis depends entirely on the association with other anomalies. MCL syndrome is associated in 80 percent of cases with normal intelligence.[2] Radical cosmetic surgery may be required. Alobar holoprosencephaly is uniformly lethal.

REFERENCES

1. Davis WB: Congenital deformities of the face: Types found in a series of one thousand cases. Surg Gynecol Obstet 61:201, 1935.
2. DeMyer W: The median cleft face syndrome. Neurology 17:961, 1967.
3. DeMyer W, Zeman W: Alobar holoprosencephaly (arhinencephaly) with median cleft lip and palate: Clinical, electroencephalographic and nosologic considerations. Confin Neurol 23:1, 1963.
4. Fogh-Andersen P: Rare clefts of the face. Acta Chir Scand 129:275, 1965.
5. Pilu G, Reece EA, Romero R: Prenatal diagnosis of craniofacial malformations with ultrasonography. Am J Obstet Gynecol 155:45, 1986.
6. Pilu G, Romero R, Jeanty P, et al.: Criteria for the antenatal diagnosis of holoprosencephaly. Am J Perinatol 4:41, 1987.

Epignathus

Definition

A teratoma that arises from the oral cavity or pharynx.

Incidence

Two percent of all pediatric teratomas occur in the nasopharyngeal area (including oral, tonsillar, and

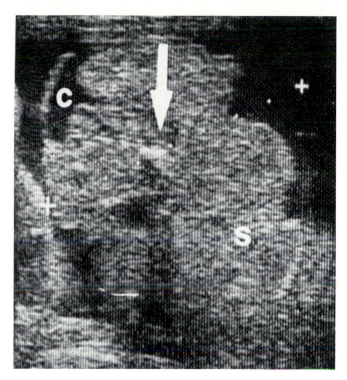

Figure 2–27. Sonogram of a 32-week fetus, demonstrating a complex mass with solid (S) and cystic (C) components. The arrow points to areas of calcification with acoustic shadowing. *(Reproduced with permission from Chervenak et al.: J Ultrasound Med 3:235, 1984.)*

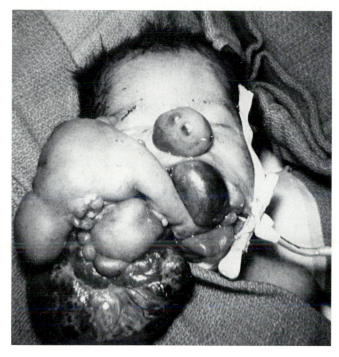

Figure 2–29. Mass arising from the palate, obstructing the mouth opening and nostril of the neonate. *(Reproduced with permission from Chervenak et al.: J Ultrasound Med 3:235, 1984.)*

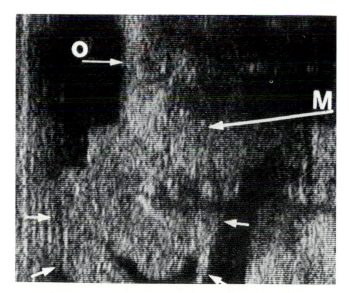

Figure 2–28. Coronal scan of the same fetus as in Figure 2–27, with arrows outlining the mass. O, orbit; M, mouth area; mouth not visualized. *(Reproduced with permission from Chervenak et al.: J Ultrasound Med 3:235, 1984.)*

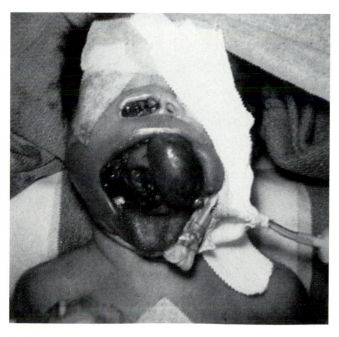

Figure 2–30. Appearance of mass after resection. *(Reproduced with permission from Chervenak et al.: J Ultrasound Med 3:235, 1984.)*

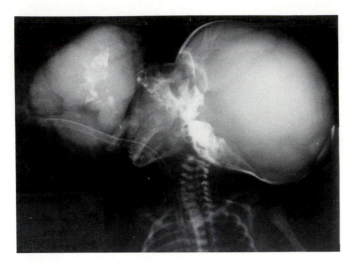

Figure 2–31. Radiograph showing the relation of the mass to the skull and calcifications in the mass. *(Reproduced with permission from Chervenak et al.: J Ultrasound Med 3:235, 1984.)*

basicranial areas).[5] Most of approximately 100 cases have been reported in newborns.[6,8]

Pathology
Most tumors arise from the sphenoid bone. Some arise from the hard and soft palate, the pharynx, the tongue, and jaw. From their sites of origin, the tumors grow into the oral or nasal cavity or intracranially. Most tumors are benign. Histologically, they consist of tissues derived from any of the three germinal layers. Most often they contain adipose tissue, cartilage, bone, and nervous tissue. These tumors can fill the mouth and airways and lead to acute asphyxia immediately after birth. Obstruction of the mouth is responsible for polyhydramnios.

Associated Anomalies
Six percent of these tumors have associated anomalies.[5] They include cleft palate, multiple facial hemangiomas, branchial cysts, hypertelorism, umbilical hernia, and congenital heart defects. Facial anomalies have been attributed to the mechanical effects of the tumor on developing structures.[1,2,4,9]

Diagnosis
Antenatal sonographic findings have been reported in two fetuses.[3,7] A solid tumor emanating from the fetal oral cavity is suggestive of this condition (Figs. 2–27 through 2–31). Calcifications and cystic components may be visualized. Differential diagnosis include neck teratomas, cephaloceles, conjoined twins,

and other tumors of the facial structures. Polyhydramnios is usually present.[8] A careful examination of the CNS anatomy is important because the tumor may grow intracranially.

Prognosis
The outlook depends on the size of the lesion and the involvement of vital structures. Lesions detected antenatally have been very large. Polyhydramnios has been associated with poor prognosis.[8] Soft tissue dystocia can occur. The major cause of neonatal death is asphyxia because of airway obstruction. Surgical resection and normal postoperative course are possible and have been documented.[8] There are no reported cases of malignancies. Two cases of epignathus have been diagnosed in our institution, and both infants died. One died immediately after birth and the other after progressive respiratory failure.

Obstetrical Management
Management in the third trimester depends on the size of the lesion. Infants with large tumors are best delivered by cesarean section. An expert pediatric team must be available for intubation of the infant.

REFERENCES

1. Amarjit S, Singh A, Singh R: Nasopharyngeal teratoma. Indian J Cancer 14:367, 1977.
2. Carney JA, Thompson DP, Johnson CL, et al.: Teratomas in children: Clinical and pathologic aspects. J Pediatr Surg 7:271, 1972.
3. Chervenak FA, Tortora M, Moya FR, et al.: Antenatal sonographic diagnosis of epignathus. J Ultrasound Med 3:235, 1984.
4. Fraumeni JF Jr, Li FP, Dalager N: Teratomas in children: Epidemiologic features. J Natl Cancer Inst 51:1425, 1973.
5. Gilman PA: Epidemiology of human teratomas. In: Damjanov I, Knowles BB, Solter D (eds): The Human Teratomas. Experimental and Clinical Biology. Clifton, New Jersey, Humana Press, 1983, p 94.
6. Hawkins DB, Park R: Teratoma of the pharynx and neck. Ann Otol Rhinol Laryngol 81:848, 1972.
7. Kang KW, Hissong SL, Langer A: Prenatal ultrasonic diagnosis of epignathus. J Clin Ultrasound 6:330, 1978.
8. Shah BL, Vasan U, Raye JR: Teratoma of the tonsil in a premature infant. Case report and review of the literature. Am J Dis Child 133:79, 1979.
9. Wilson JW, Gehweiler JA: Teratoma of the face associated with a patent canal extending into the cranial cavity (Rathke's pouch) in a three-week-old child. J Pediatr Surg 5:349, 1970.

ABNORMALITIES OF THE MANDIBLE

Robin Anomalad

Synonyms

Cleft palate, micrognathia and glossoptosis, and Pierre Robin syndrome.

Definition

This anomalad is characterized by the association of micrognathia and glossoptosis. Frequently, a posterior cleft palate or a high arched palate is present.[3]

Incidence

The frequency is 1:30,000.[2]

Etiology

In 40 percent of cases, the anomaly is isolated and is mostly sporadic, although familial cases suggesting both autosomal recessive[8] and autosomal dominant[1] patterns of transmission have been reported. This anomalad is most frequently seen in association with other anomalies or with recognized genetic and nongenetic syndromes (Table 2–7).

Embryology

The mandible arises from the merging of the two mandibular prominences that inferiorly delimit the stomodeum. The palate originates from the fusion of the three palatine processes. The median derives from the frontonasal prominence and the two lateral ones originate from the maxillary processes.

It has been suggested that the three components of the anomalad are related. The primary disorder is probably an early hypoplasia of the mandible. This would lead to posterior displacement of the tongue, thus preventing the normal closure of the posterior palatine processes.[4]

Pathology

The hypoplasia of the mandible leads to foreshortening of the floor of the mouth and reduction of the size of the oral cavity. As a consequence, there is a tendency to glossoptosis, which may alter the development of the palate and lead to a posterior cleft or a high arched deformity.[1]

Associated Anomalies

The Robin anomalad is found as an isolated lesion in 39 percent of all patients. In 36 percent, one or more associated anomalies are found, but these do not conform to a well-established syndrome. In 25 percent of patients, a known syndrome is found.[2]

Diagnosis

Only one case of Robin anomalad has been identified in utero thus far.[6] The diagnosis relied upon the demonstration of micrognathia in a midsagittal scan of the face (Fig. 2–32). The hypoplasia of the mandible could not be detected in the second trimester. This suggests the possibility of a progressive course, which may preclude an early diagnosis.[6]

Polyhydramnios was seen in the reported case. It is likely to result from failure to swallow as a consequence of the glossoptosis.[6] Sonographers should suspect Robin anomalad when polyhydramnios is associated with micrognathia. A posterior cleft palate is frequently present, but it may be difficult to detect with ultrasound. The difficulties in imaging this part of the fetal anatomy make this diagnosis unlikely.

A careful survey of fetal anatomy is indicated. Because congenital heart disease occurs in 10 percent

TABLE 2–7. SYNDROMES ASSOCIATED WITH THE ROBIN ANOMALAD

Genetic syndromes
  Monogenic syndromes
    Diastrophic dysplasia
    Stickler syndrome (congenital myopia associated with irregular articular surfaces)
    Spondyloepiphyseal dysplasia
    Beckwith-Wiedemann (omphalocele, visceromegaly, macroglossia, neonatal hypoglycemia)
    Myotonic dystrophy (weakness of facial, neck, and distal limb muscles)
    Campomelic syndrome
  Chromosomal
    Trisomy 11q+
Nongenetic syndromes
  Fetal alcohol syndrome
  Fetal hydantoin syndrome
  Fetal trimethadione syndrome

Adapted from Cohen: J Oral Surg 34:587, 1976.

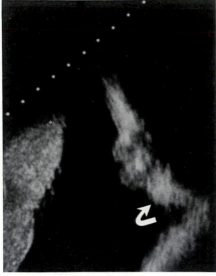
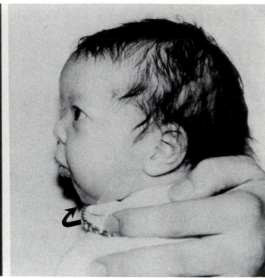

A   **B**

Figure 2–32. A. Midsagittal scan of the face of a 35-week fetus with Robin anomalad. Micrognathia is evident (*curved arrow*). **B.** A side view of the infant is provided for comparison. *(Reproduced with permission from Pilu et al.: Am J Obstet Gynecol 154:630, 1986.)*

of affected neonates,[3] fetal echocardiography is recommended.

Prognosis

The Robin anomalad is in many cases a neonatal emergency. Glossoptosis may lead to obstruction of the airways and suffocation. Many cases of sudden death have been described. Infants have difficulties feeding because of the ball valve effect of the tongue in the oropharynx and because of vomiting.[3,5,7] This leads to failure to thrive. However, with proper assistance, these infants may overcome these difficulties. With time there is some growth of the mandible.

Obstetrical Management

If a prenatal diagnosis is made, the sonographer should look for associated anomalies. It is mandatory that a pediatrician be present in the delivery room and be prepared to intubate the infant. This procedure may be lifesaving. Karyotype should be considered.

REFERENCES

1. Bixler D, Christian JC: Pierre Robin syndrome occurring in two related sibships. Birth Defects 7(7):67, 1971.
2. Cohen MM: The Robin anomalad—its nonspecificity and associated syndromes. J Oral Surg 34:587, 1976.
3. Dennison WM: The Pierre Robin syndrome. Pediatrics 36:336, 1965.
4. Hanson JW, Smith DW: U-shaped palatal defect in the Robin anomalad: Developmental and clinical relevance. J Pediatr 87:30, 1975.
5. Lewis MB, Pashayan HM: Management of infants with Robin Anomaly. Clin Pediatr 19:519, 1980.
6. Pilu G, Romero R, Reece EA, et al.: The prenatal diagnosis of Robin anomalad. Am J Obstet Gynecol 154:630, 1986.
7. Poole AE, Greene I, Greenstein RM: Feeding problems in Robin anomalad: A report of 4 cases. Birth Defects 18(1):151, 1982.
8. Smith JL, Stowe FR: The Pierre Robin syndrome (glossoptosis, micrognathia, and cleft palate): A review of 39 cases with emphasis on associated ocular lesions. Pediatrics 27:128, 1961.

Otocephaly

Synonyms

Synotia and melotia.

Definition

Otocephaly is a grotesque anomaly characterized by absence or hypoplasia of the mandible, proximity of the temporal bones, and abnormal horizontal position of the ears.

Incidence

Unknown. It seems to be an extremely rare disorder.

Embryology

The mandible arises from the fusion of the two mandibular prominences that inferiorly delimit the stomodeum. The primitive external ears are located laterally and inferiorly to the mandibular prominences, and they migrate (Fig. 2–16). Otocephaly is thought to result from failure of development of the mandible, possibly secondary to a defect in neural crest cell migration.[3] Absence or extreme hypoplasia of the mandible leads to an abnormal position of the ears, which are horizontal, with the lobules located close to the midline. A spectrum of anatomic lesions ranging from ears closely apposed to the midline (synotia), agnathia, absence of the mouth to varying degrees of micrognathia and low set ears (melotia) is possible.

Etiology

Unknown. Otocephaly may be part of very severe malformation complexes, such as conjoined twins and holoprosencephaly.[4] This malformation has been produced experimentally by X-irradiation and administration of streptonigrin in mice.[2,4]

Associated Anomalies

Holoprosencephaly, neural tube defects, cephaloceles, midline proboscis, hypoplastic tongue, tracheoesophageal fistula, cardiac anomalies, and adrenal hypoplasia.

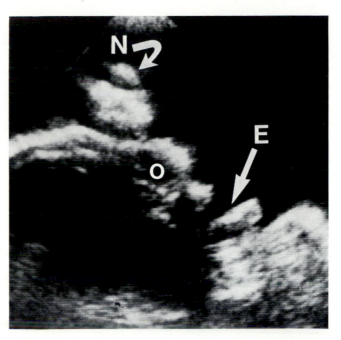

Figure 2–33. A. Midsagittal scan of the face of a fetus with otocephaly and holoprosencephaly. The nasal appendage (N) can be seen arising from the forehead superiorly to the orbits (O). A well-defined ear (E) is seen implanting in the lower face. *(Courtesy of Prof. A. Ianniruberto.)*

Diagnosis

This condition should be suspected when it is impossible to visualize the jaw and the ears are seen in a very low position (Fig. 2–33). It is likely that this

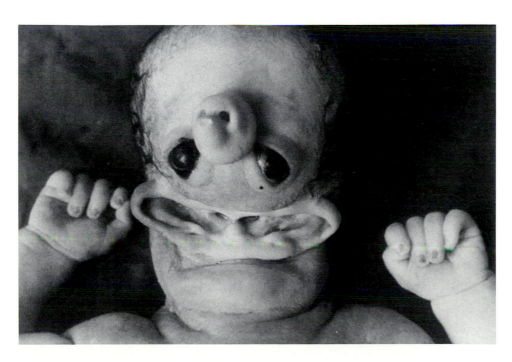

Figure 2–33. B. Frontal view of the stillborn infant. Note synotia, hypotelorism, towering skull, and a proboscis. *(Courtesy of Prof. A. Ianniruberto.)*

condition will be identified in fetuses with very severe associated anomalies, such as anencephaly, holoprosencephaly, and cephaloceles.[1] Milder expressions of otocephaly may be difficult to distinguish on prenatal ultrasound studies from other conditions characterized by very low set ears, such as Treacher-Collins syndrome.[1]

We have recently diagnosed this condition in a fetus with polyhydramnios and an absent stomach. It must be considered, therefore, in the differential diagnosis of esophageal atresia.

Prognosis and Obstetrical Management
This condition is incompatible with life. Pregnancy termination could be offered any time in a pregnancy when a confident diagnosis is made.

REFERENCES

1. Cayea PD, Bieber FR, Ross MJ, et al.: Sonographic findings in otocephaly (synotia). J Ultrasound Med 4:377, 1985.
2. Giroud A, Martinet M, Deluchat C: Otocephalie. Compt. Rend. Xod. Franc, Oto-rhino-laryngect. Cong. (Paris), 1965.
3. Johnston MC, Sulik KK: Some abnormal patterns of development in the craniofacial region. Birth Defects 15:23, 1979.
4. Warkany J: Congenital Malformations. Chicago, Year Book, 1971, p 1309.

3

The Neck

Normal Anatomy of the Neck

Current ultrasound equipment allows the visualization of the main anatomic structures of the neck: upper airways and esophagus,[1,2] vessels,[2] and spine.

A detailed investigation of the cervical structures is usually possible as early as the 18th week of gestation. However, flexion of the head and an unfavorable position of the fetus, can make the examination difficult. A midsagittal scan of the fetal neck at 25 weeks of gestation is provided in Figure 3–1. Most anatomic components of this area are demonstrated in this view. The tongue is seen filling the oral cavity. Shadowing from the facial bones

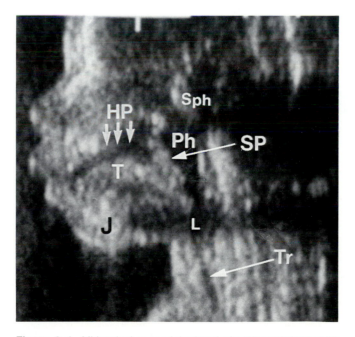

Figure 3–1. Midsagittal scan of the head of a 25-week fetus. The tongue (T) is seen filling the oral cavity. The pharynx (Ph) is delimited anteriorly and superiorly by the soft palate (SP) and the sphenoid (Sph), respectively, and it can be traced inferiorly to the larynx (L), which is partly obscured by acoustic shadowing arising from the jaw (J). The trachea (Tr) is seen in the midportion of the neck. HP, hard palate.

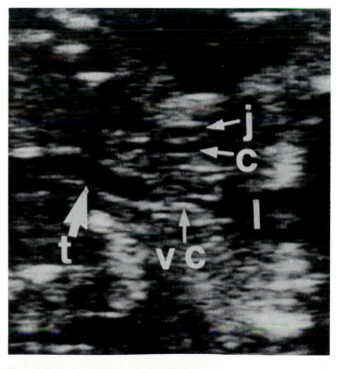

Figure 3–2. A slightly angled sagittal scan of the fetal neck, revealing the continuity between the larynx (l) and trachea (t). The common carotid artery (c) and jugular vein (j) are also demonstrated. At the level of the larynx, the vocal cords (vc) are presumably seen.

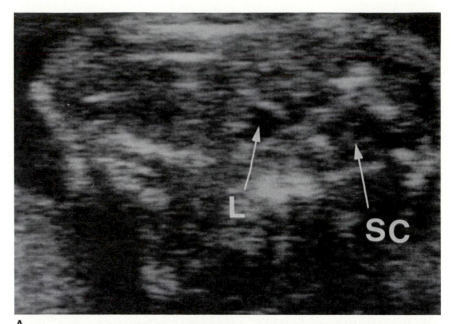

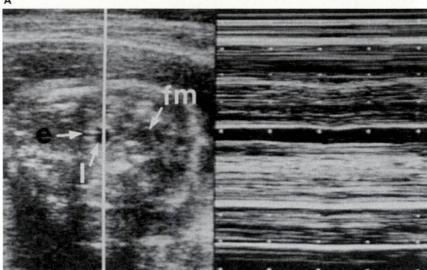

Figure 3–3. A. In this axial scan slightly caudal to the skull base, the larynx (L) is seen in the midportion of the neck, anterior to the cervical spine. SC, spinal cord. **B.** Simultaneous real-time, M-mode representation of a contraction movement of the vestibulum of the larynx (l). The epiglottis (e) is seen anteriorly to the larynx. fm, foramen magnum.

obscures the hard palate, but its position can be inferred by the curvature of the tongue and by the soft palate. Real-time examination greatly enhances the understanding of these structures, since movement of both the tongue and the soft palate is frequently seen. Behind the soft palate and below a high-level echo complex presumably arising from the sphenoid, the fluid-filled pharyngeal cavity is seen and can be followed until it bifurcates into the larynx and hypopharynx. The esophagus is not usually seen.

With slight angulation of the transducer, the main neck vessels, the common carotid artery, and the jugular veins are readily demonstrated. At closer inspection, minute details, such the vocal cords, may be appreciated (Fig. 3–2).

Sagittal scans directed from posterior to anterior allow one to evaluate the soft tissues overlying the spine (see Fig. 1–23).

In axial planes, the previously described structures can be recognized as well. On real-time ultrasound examination, it is frequently possible to demonstrate the contractions of the vestibulum of the larynx (Fig. 3–3).

REFERENCES

1. Cooper C, Mahony BS, Bowie JD, et al.: Ultrasound evaluation of the normal fetal upper airway and esophagus. J Ultrasound Med 4:343, 1985.
2. Jeanty P, Romero R: Obstetrical Ultrasound. New York, McGraw-Hill, 1984.

Cystic Hygroma

Synonyms
Lymphangioma and jugular lymphatic obstructive sequence.

Definition
The term "hygroma" means moist tumor. Cystic hygromas are anomalies of the lymphatic system characterized by single or multiple cysts within the soft tissues, usually involving the neck.

Incidence
Cystic hygromas were found in 1 in 200 spontaneously aborted fetuses with crown–rump length greater than 3 cm.[2]

Etiopathogenesis
Cystic hygromas are frequently found in association with chromosomal aberrations (mainly Turner's syndrome). Table 3–1 shows other syndromes or conditions reported in association with cystic hygromas. When isolated, this anomaly can be inherited as an autosomal recessive trait.[5] Webbed necks or redundant skin are found in genetic and nongenetic syndromes, such as Noonan's syndrome, familial pterygium colli, and fetal alcohol syndrome.

In the embryo, the lymphatic system drains into the jugular lymphatic sac. A communication between this primitive structure and the jugular vein is formed at 40 days of gestation (conceptional age). Failure of development of this communication results in lymphatic stasis. Dilatation of the lymphatic channels leads to the clinical manifestations of the jugular lymphatic obstructive sequence[17] (Figs. 3–4, 3–5).

Dilatation of the jugular lymphatic sac leads to the formation of cystic structures in the cervical region. If a connection between the lymphatic and the venous system does not occur at this point, a progressive peripheral lymphedema and nonimmune hydrops will develop, leading to early intrauterine death (Figs. 3–6, 3–7).[3] If the connection is formed, the sequence is interrupted, and the fluid collections are resorbed. The redundant skin will give rise to webbed neck (pterygium colli), which is a typical manifestation of Turner's syndrome and of many other genetic and nongenetic conditions. Uplifting and anterior rotation of the ears and an abnormal hair pattern are other consequences of overdistention of the jugular lymphatic sac. Distention of the tributary lymphatics may result in peripheral lymphedema, which in turn may give rise to redundancy of the skin of the face and puffy hands and feet, with deep-set narrow nails (Fig. 3–5). It has also been suggested that transitory ascites may result in laxity of the anterior abdominal wall and prune-belly syndrome.[17]

Pathology
Overdistention of the jugular lymphatic sacs that are located in both sides of the neck results in the formation of a cystic structure that is usually partitioned by a thick fibrous band corresponding to the nuchal ligament. Within the cystic structure, thinner septa are seen and are thought to derive from either fibrous structures of the neck or deposits of fibrin.[4] The size of the lesions may vary greatly from small collections of fluid to enormous cysts that may be larger than the fetus. In cases of generalized hydrops, pleural effusions, ascites, and severe skin edema are present.

Associated Anomalies
Cystic hygromas are very frequently associated with chromosomal aberrations (Table 3–1) and, consequently, with a wide variety of anatomic defects.

Diagnosis
The diagnosis of cystic hygroma relies on the demonstration of cystic structures usually located in the occipitocervical region.[1,3,4,7–15] These lesions have a typical honeycomb appearance due to the presence of multiple septa. Large lesions are usually characterized by a thick septum dividing the cyst along the

TABLE 3–1. KARYOTYPE IN 60 CASES OF FETAL CYSTIC HYGROMA

Karyotype	No. of Cases (%)
Abnormal karyotype	
Turner's syndrome	
45 XO	30 (50)
Mosaic	1 (1.6)
Trisomy 21	4 (6.6)
Trisomy 18	3 (5)
Trisomy 13	2 (3.3)
47 XXY	1 (1.6)
Total	41 (68)
Normal karyotype	11 (18)
Karyotype not available	8 (13)

Data derived from Bluth et al.: South Med J 77:1335, 1984; Chervenak et al.: N Engl J Med 309:822, 1983; Garden et al.: Am J Obstet Gynecol 154:221, 1986; Greenberg et al.: Clin Genet 24:389, 1983; Pearce et al.: Prenat Diagn 4:371, 1984; Redford et al.: Prenat Diagn 4:327, 1984; and from cases collected by the authors.

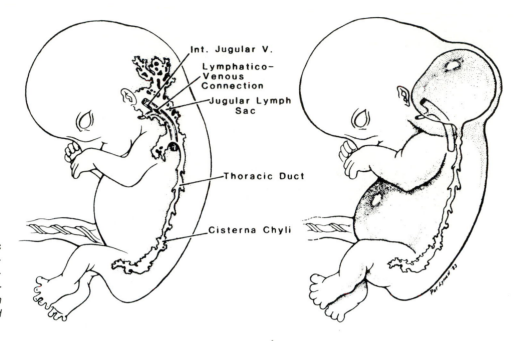

Figure 3–4. Left. Normal lymphatic system in the fetus. Right. Cystic hygroma has developed as a consequence of lymphatic obstruction. *(Reproduced with permission from Chervenak et al.: N Engl J Med 309:822, 1983.)*

anteroposterior axis, the sonographic counterpart of the nuchal ligament[4] (Figs. 3–8, 3–9).

A careful evaluation of the fetal anatomy is indicated for identification of other anatomic abnormalities, as well as signs of nonimmune hydrops. Most patients have decreased amounts of amniotic fluid, and a few have either normal fluid or polyhydramnios.

The diagnosis of cystic hygroma has been made in the first trimester.[9] The differential diagnosis includes cervical meningocele (Fig. 3–10), cephaloceles, neck tumors, and subcutaneous edema. The distinction is often difficult.[7,11] A useful diagnostic hint is the typical multiseptate appearance of cystic hygromas. With a cephalocele, it is usually possible to demonstrate a bony defect in the skull.[13] The presence of hydrocephalus increases the index of suspicion for a cephalocele. Hydrops and generalized edema are more frequently associated with cystic hygromas. Amniotic fluid alpha-fetoprotein may be either elevated or normal in both conditions.[13] Neck tumors usually have a complex appearance.

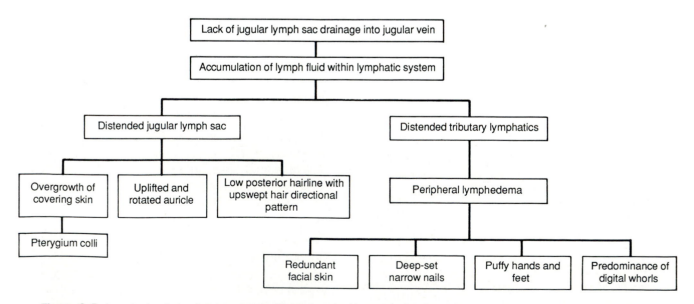

Figure 3–5. Lymphatic obstructive sequence. *(Reproduced with permission from Smith: Recognizable Patterns of Human Malformation: Genetic Embryologic and Clinical Aspects, 3rd ed. Philadelphia, Saunders, 1982, p 472.)*

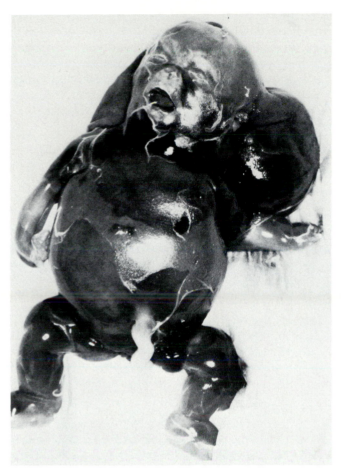

Figure 3–6. Midtrimester fetus with jugular lymphatic obstructive sequence. Note the presence of ascites, skin edema, and cystic hygromas.

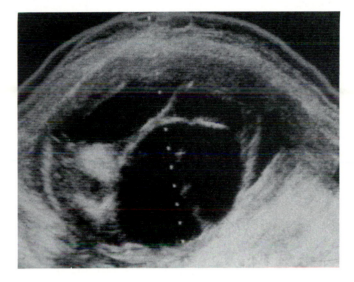

Figure 3–8. Cystic hygroma. Transverse section of the fetal neck. Typical multiseptate appearance.

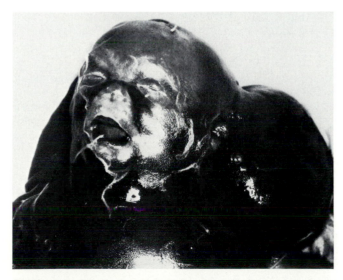

Figure 3–7. Closer view of the fetus shown in Figure 3–6. Cystic hygromas are seen as massive paracervical bilateral masses.

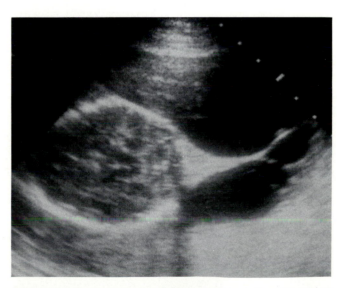

Figure 3–9. Cystic hygroma. Note the presence of septae and an intact skull. This section is an axial scan at the level of the BPD.

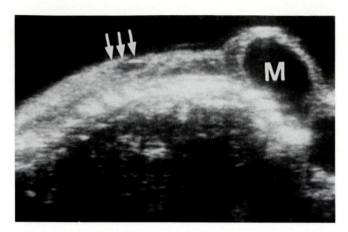

Figure 3–10. Cervical meningocele (M) may mimic a cystic hygroma. A spinal defect extending to the thoracic area is visible (*arrows*). Note the absence of septae in the cystic mass.

Prognosis

The prognosis is different depending on the presence or absence of associated hydrops. In our experience, the mortality rate of cystic hygromas with hydrops is 100 percent. In many cases, intrauterine demise occurs within the first two trimesters of pregnancy. In a review of 40 cases reported in three series in the literature,[3,7,10] most had hydrops. Thirteen (33 percent) died in utero usually within a few weeks of the diagnosis, two (5 percent) died in the early neonatal period, and the rest were electively aborted.

Prognostic data about fetal cystic hygromas without associated hydrops are scanty. Of a total of 41 infants with cystic hygromas of the head and neck reported in two different series,[6,16] 37 (90 percent) required operations. Sixteen (31 percent) developed symptoms of airway obstruction or swallowing difficulties. Facial nerve palsy as a consequence of the operation occurred in 10 (24 percent). In some infants with cystic hygromas, mandibular maldevelopment, problems of malocclusion, and tooth eruption occurred. An early partial glossectomy may be required to allow normal speech development.

The natural history of fetal cystic hygromas has not been clearly established. Some infants diagnosed in the second trimester with isolated hygromas may develop nonimmune hydrops as gestation progresses. Others may undergo canalization of the lymphatic channels and resolution of the hygromas. Regression results in redundant skin in the cervical region and webbed neck.

Obstetrical Management

Determination of fetal karyotype is recommended in all cases. This information is of diagnostic value for the index pregnancy and useful in the counseling of future pregnancies. The option of pregnancy termination should be offered before viability. After viability, fetuses with associated hydrops should probably be managed nonaggressively because of the extremely poor prognosis. In the presence of isolated cystic hygromas, no modification of standard obstetrical management is required. On some occasions, cystic hygromas have been associated with prolongation of the second stage of labor.[6] A cesarean section may be indicated if there are gigantic lesions. Infants must be delivered in a tertiary care center, because there is a high frequency of airway obstruction.[16]

REFERENCES

1. Bluth EI, Maragos VA, Merritt CRB: Antenatal diagnosis of Turner's syndrome. South Med J 77:1335, 1984.
2. Byrne J, Blanc WA, Warburton D, et al.: The significance of cystic hygroma in fetuses. Hum Pathol 15:61, 1984.
3. Chervenak FA, Isaacson G, Blakemore KJ, et al.: Fetal cystic hygroma. Cause and natural history. N Engl J Med 309:822, 1983.
4. Chervenak FA, Isaacson G, Tortora M: A sonographic study of fetal cystic hygromas. J Clin Ultrasound 13:311, 1985.
5. Dallapiccola B, Zelante L, Perla G, et al.: Prenatal diagnosis of recurrence of cystic hygroma with normal chromosomes. Prenat Diagn 4:383, 1984.
6. Emery PJ, Bailey CM, Evans JNG: Cystic hygroma of the head and neck. A review of 37 cases. J Laryngol Otol 98:613, 1984.
7. Garden AS, Benzie RJ, Miskin M, Gardner HA: Fetal cystic hygroma colli: Antenatal diagnosis, significance, and management. Am J Obstet Gynecol 154:221, 1986.
8. Greenberg F, Carpenter RJ, Ledbetter DH: Cystic hygroma and hydrops fetalis in a fetus with trisomy 13. Clin Genet 24:389, 1983.
9. Gustavii B, Edvall H: First-trimester diagnosis of cystic nuchal hygroma. Acta Obstet Gynecol Scand 63:377, 1984.
10. Newman DE, Cooperberg PL: Genetics of sonographically detected intrauterine fetal cystic hygromas. J Can Assoc Radiol 35:77, 1984.
11. Nicolini U, Ferrazzi E, Massa E, et al.: Prenatal diagnosis of cranial masses by ultrasound: Report of five cases. J Clin Ultrasound 11:170, 1983.
12. Pearce JM, Griffin D, Campbell S: Cystic hygroma in trisomy 18 and 21. Prenat Diagn 4:371, 1984.
13. Pearce JM, Griffin D, Campbell S: The differential prenatal diagnosis of cystic hygromata and encephalocele by ultrasound examination. J Clin Ultrasound 13:317, 1985.
14. Phillips HE, McGahan JP: Intrauterine fetal cystic hygromas: Sonographic detection. AJR 136:799, 1981.
15. Redford DHA, McNay MB, Ferguson-Smith ME, et al.: Aneuploidy and cystic hygroma detectable by ultrasound. Prenat Diagn 4:377, 1984.
16. Seashore JH, Gardiner LJ, Ariyan S: Management of giant cystic hygromas in infants. Am J Surg 149:459, 1985.
17. Smith DW, Jones, KL: Recognizable Patterns of Human Malformation: Genetic Embryologic and Clinical Aspects, 3d ed. Philadelphia, Saunders, 1982, p 472.

Goiter

Synonym
Thyromegaly.

Definition
Goiter is an enlargement of the thyroid gland.

Incidence
Rare.

Etiology
Goiter can be associated with hyperthyroidism, hypothyroidism, or a euthyroid state. In the newborn period, goiter is most commonly associated with hypothyroidism.

Maternal Grave's disease may result in neonatal thyrotoxicosis and goiter. Two varieties of this condition are recognized. The self-limited type is thought to result from transplacental passage of a thyroid-stimulating substance, such as long-acting thyroid stimulant (LATS). The second variety appears to be transmitted with an autosomal dominant pattern, and has a predilection for females and a protracted clinical course.[6]

Goiters associated with hypothyroidism can be the result of iodine intoxication, iodine deficiency, or congenital metabolic disorders of thyroid synthesis. Congenital hypothyroidism occurs in 1 in 3600 to 4000 live births.[5] Seventy-four percent of hypothyroid infants have primary thyroid dysgenesis (absent or hypoplastic thyroid gland), 13 percent have thyroid dyshormonogenesis, 3 to 4 percent have secondary (pituitary) or tertiary (hypothalamic) hypothyroidism, and 10 percent have hypothyroidism secondary to intrauterine exposure to antithyroid medications. Of these causes, only thyroid dyshormonogenesis and drug-induced hypothyroidism are associated with goiter in the newborn period. The two drugs primarily responsible for the latter are iodide preparations and propylthiouracil (PTU). Iodide preparations are administered as expectorant medications and radiopaque dyes are used in amniography.[9] Maternal ingestion of as little as 12 mg/day may result in congenital hypothyroidism.[3] The ratio of mothers exposed to PTU to hypothyroid infants is 100:1.[2] These drugs cross the placenta readily and block thyroid synthesis in the fetal gland. Goiter is a rare finding in drug-induced fetal hypothyroidism.

Iodine deficiency is a cause of endemic hypothyroidism in certain parts of the world. Newborns frequently have goiters. An enzymatic deficiency impairing the synthesis of T4 or T3 can result in hypothyroidism with goiter, goiter with euthyroidism, or hypothyroidism without goiter. Six different enzymatic defects have been recognized. They are transmitted as an autosomal recessive trait and, therefore, have a 25 percent recurrence rate. The reader is referred to specialized texts for a full description of these defects.[4] Although some of these enzymatic defects can occur with congenital goiter, in most cases, enlargement of the thyroid gland appears later in life.

Diagnosis
The diagnosis is based on identification of a neck mass that is solid, anterior, and symmetrical and may result in hyperextension of the fetal head.[1,10] Obstruction of the esophagus may lead to polyhydramnios. The differential diagnosis includes cystic hygroma, branchial cleft cysts, cervical meningocele, and hemangiomas of the neck. Cystic hygromas are purely cystic lesions with a typical honeycomb appearance. Branchial cleft cysts are purely cystic masses located on the anterior border of the sternomastoid muscle. Hemangiomas can appear as cystic or solid masses. Teratomas are generally large tumors that have both solid and cystic elements. A prenatal diagnosis of hypothyroidism was reported recently when a high thyroid-stimulating hormone (TSH) concentration in amniotic fluid was determined in a fetus with a goiter[7,8] (Fig. 3–11). This technique requires concentration of amniotic fluid. A concentration of TSH above 0.8 μU/ml in the second trimester or 0.4 μU/ml in the third trimester are suggestive of hypothyroidism.[8]

Prognosis
Goiter may cause dystocia by extending the fetal head during the normal course of labor. It can also lead to acute respiratory failure if the enlarged gland obstructs the airways. The prognosis depends on the basic cause of the goiter. Neonatal hyperthyroidism is transient in most cases, but hypothyroidism requires treatment. In both instances, the goiter generally resolves. Sixty percent of neonates with Grave's disease have a benign course, 20 percent have symptoms after 6 months, and the remaining 20 percent have neonatal hyperthyroidism leading to death. In most cases, the disease subsides spontaneously within 1 to 3 months. Therapy of hypothyroid infants is extremely important, since untreated infants develop serious mental retardation.

Obstetrical Management
The most serious complication of congenital goiter is respiratory distress due to obstruction of the airway. Therefore, these infants should be delivered in a

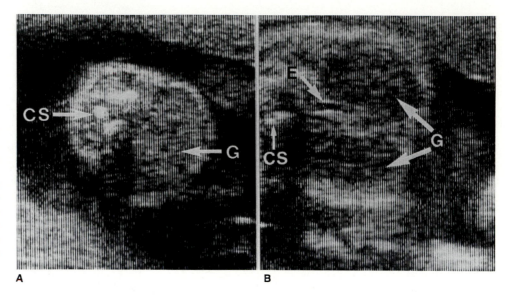

Figure 3–11. **A.** Fetal goiter at 27 weeks. The back of the neck and cervical spine (CS) are on the left. Echolucent areas are evident within the substance of the goiter (G). **B.** Fetal goiter at 36 weeks. The cervical spine is again on the left. Swallowed amniotic fluid is visible within the esophagus (E). The goiter is clearly bilobed in this view. *(Reproduced with permission from Kourides et al.: J Clin Endocrinol Metab 59:1016, 1984)*

center where resuscitation can be performed immediately after birth. A prenatal diagnosis of the functional state of the thyroid gland (hypothyroidism versus hyperthyroidism) can be attempted by assessing levels of TSH in the amniotic fluid.[7,8] Fetal goiter is not an indication to alter standard obstetrical management.

REFERENCES

1. Barone CM, Van Natta FC, Kourides IA, et al.: Sonographic detection of fetal goiter, an unusual cause of hydramnios. J Ultrasound Med 4:625, 1985.
2. Burrow GN, Ferris TF: Thyroid disease. In: Medical Complications During Pregnancy, 2d ed. Philadelphia, Saunders, 1982, p 200.
3. Carswell F, Kerr MM, Hutchinson JH: Congenital goiter and hypothyroidism produced by maternal ingestion of iodides. Lancet 1:1241, 1970.
4. DeGroot LJ, Stanbury JB: The Thyroid and Its Diseases, 4th ed. New York, Wiley, 1975.
5. Fisher DA, Dussault JH, Foley TP Jr, et al.: Screening for congenital hypothyroidism. Results of screening 1 million North American infants. J Pediatr 94:700, 1979.
6. Hollingsworth DR, Mabry CC: Congenital Grave's disease. Am J Dis Child 130:148, 1976.
7. Kourides IA, Berkowitz RL, Pang S, et al.: Antepartum diagnosis of goitrous hypothyroidism by fetal ultrasonography and amniotic fluid thyrotropin concentration. J Clin Endocrinol Metab 59:1016, 1984.
8. Kourides IA, Heath CV, Ginsberg-Fellner F: Measurement of thyroid-stimulating hormone in human amniotic fluid. J Clin Endocrinol Metab 54:635, 1982.
9. Rodesch F, Casmus M, Ermans AM, et al.: Adverse effect of amniofetography on fetal thyroid function. Am J Obstet Gynecol 126:723, 1976.
10. Weiner S, Scharf JI, Bolognese RJ, et al.: Antenatal diagnosis and treatment of a fetal goiter. J Reprod Med 24:39, 1980.

Teratoma of the Neck

Synonyms
Cervical teratoma and thyroid teratoma.

Definition
Germ cell tumor located in the neck.

Incidence
One hundred thirty cases have been reported as of 1983.[3] There is no sexual predilection.

Etiology
The anomaly is sporadic, and the causes are unknown. One familial case has been reported in the literature.[5]

Pathology
Ninety percent of all teratomas are recognized at birth or soon thereafter.[7] Tumors are generally unilateral and encapsulated. They vary in size and generally consist of a mixture of cystic and solid components.

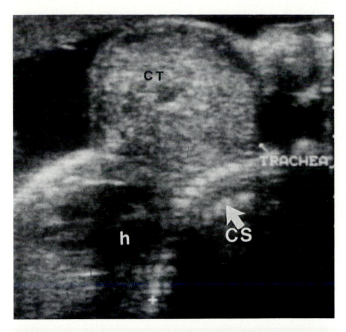

Figure 3–12. Cervical teratoma (CT). A solid mass is seen in the anterior aspect of the fetal neck. CS, cervical spine; h, heart.

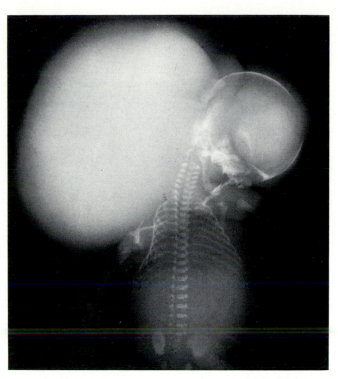

Figure 3–14. Postnatal radiograph showing cervical teratoma.

Malignant transformation is extremely rare, and there are no reports of recurrence after complete surgical excision in the neonatal period.[8] Calcification can be detected in 50 percent of cases.[3] Neural tissue is the predominant histologic component. Obstruction of the airway by the tumor may lead to acute respiratory failure during the newborn period.[3] Polyhydramnios has been reported as a complication in 30 percent of patients and is thought to result from esophageal obstruction.[8] A correlation between the size of the mass and polyhydramnios has been reported. Masses larger than 10 cm are more likely to be associated with this complication than are smaller tumors.[4]

Associated Anomalies

These are very uncommon. Isolated patients have had pulmonary hypoplasia, imperforate anus,[9] trisomy 13,[1] and chondrodystrophia fetalis[9] in association with these tumors.

Diagnosis

The diagnosis relies on demonstration of a complex mass in the cervical region (Figs. 3–12 to 3–14).[10] The differential diagnosis includes cystic hygroma, goiter, branchial cysts, cervical meningocele, neuroblastoma of the neck, and hemangiomas of the neck. Cystic hygromas are purely cystic lesions with a typical honeycomb appearance. Cervical meningoceles appear as masses of the neck, and a spinal defect can be demonstrated. Cervical myelomeningoceles can give a mixed pattern, but their location and the presence of an associated spinal defect should be diagnostic.[6] Goiters are solid, generally devoid of cystic compo-

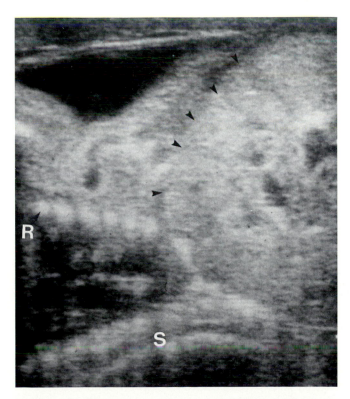

Figure 3–13. Cervical teratoma is seen as a complex mass above the apex of the chest. Arrows point to the margins of the tumor. The complex nature of the mass is apparent. S, spine; R, ribs.

nents, symmetrical, anterior, and generally do not reach the size achieved by some teratomas. Branchial cleft cysts are purely cystic masses located in the anterior border of the sternomastoid muscle. Hemangiomas can appear as cystic or solid masses. A differentiation between mesenchymal tumors and teratomas may not be possible because the former are generally solid tumors. Neuroblastomas of the neck can produce masses of mixed consistency.[2] Polyhydramnios is a frequent finding. Calcifications are present in 40 to 45 percent of the cases.[8]

Prognosis

A stillbirth rate of 17 percent has been reported.[4,7] The mortality rate of untreated infants has varied from 80 to 100 percent.[3,8] Upper airway obstruction is the major cause of death. Operative mortality is 9 to 15 percent.[3,8] Most tumors are benign, and no recurrences have been reported after total excision in the neonatal period.

Obstetrical Management

Large tumors may cause dystocia, and a cesarean section is indicated in these instances. In the presence of small tumors, standard obstetrical care should not be altered. Serial scans are indicated to monitor tumor growth and amniotic fluid volume. Delivery in a tertiary care center is mandatory, and a pediatric team must be prepared to intubate the infant immediately after birth if necessary. An amniogram may be considered in patients with severe polyhydramnios

as an indirect mean to assess the degree of tracheoesophageal obstruction.

REFERENCES

1. Dische MR, Gardner HA: Mixed teratoid tumors of the liver and neck in trisomy 13. Am J Clin Pathol 69:631, 1978.
2. Gadwood KA, Reynes CJ: Prenatal sonography of metastatic neuroblastoma of the neck. J Clin Ultrasound 11:512, 1983.
3. Gundry SR, Wesley JR, Klein MD, et al.: Cervical teratomas in the newborn. J Pediatr Surg 18:382, 1983.
4. Hajdu SI, Faruque AA, Hajdu EO, et al.: Teratoma of the neck in infants. Am J Dis Child 111:412, 1966.
5. Hurlbut HJ, Webb HW, Moseley T: Cervical teratoma in infant siblings. J Pediatr Surg 2:424, 1967.
6. Kagan AR, Steckel RJ: Cervical mass in a fetus associated with maternal hydramnios. AJR 140:507, 1983.
7. Newstedt JR, Shirkey HC: Teratoma of the thyroid region. Am J Dis Child 107:88, 1964.
8. Rosenfeld CR, Coln CD, Duenhoelter JH: Fetal cervical teratoma as a cause of polyhydramnios. Pediatrics 64:176, 1979.
9. Silberman R, Mendelson IR: Teratoma of the neck. Report of two cases and review of the literature. Arch Dis Child 35:159, 1960.
10. Trecet JC, Claramunt V, Larraz J, et al.: Prenatal U/S diagnosis of fetal teratoma of the neck. J Clin Ultrasound 12:509, 1984.

Fetal Nuchal Skin Thickening

Definition

Increased soft tissue thickening in the posterior aspect of the neck.

Diagnosis

Diagnosis is made by the detection of soft tissue nuchal thickness above 5 mm in a fetus between 15 and 20 weeks of gestation. The measurement is generally taken in an axial plane at the level of the thalami, but it can also be taken in sagittal sections of the fetal neck (Figs. 3–15, 3–16)[1,2]

Significance

Increased soft tissue thickening in the nuchal region is one of the eight major criteria for the diagnosis of trisomy 21 in newborn infants.[5,9,12] It is present in 80 percent of newborns with trisomy 21[5,9] and in 45 percent of midtrimester fetuses with trisomy 21 and

in only 0.06 percent of normal fetuses. These data are based on a series of 1704 consecutive midtrimester amniocenteses, of which there were 11 fetuses with trisomy 21.[1,2] If these data are confirmed, fetal nuchal thickening can be used as a means of identifying fetuses at risk for trisomy 21 in a low-risk population (maternal age below 35 years). The value of this approach though, has been challenged recently.[13]

Other conditions associated with redundancy of the skin at the level of the neck in the newborn period and, therefore, skin thickening include:

Chromosomal Syndromes[10]

1. 13q syndrome
2. XXXX syndrome
3. XXXXY syndrome
4. Trisomy 18
5. 18p− syndrome

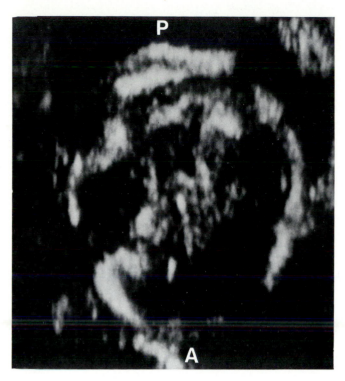

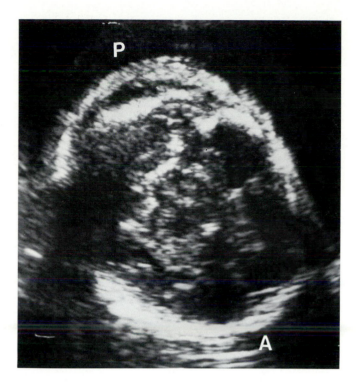

Figure 3–15. Axial scan of a normal fetal head close to the base of the skull. Note the occipital region devoid of soft tissue. P, posterior; A, anterior.

Figure 3–16. Down syndrome fetus. The head is scanned at the same level as in Figure 3–15. Note the nuchal skin thickening. P, posterior; A, anterior. *(Courtesy of Dr. B. Benacerraf.)*

Nonchromosomal Disorders

1. Multiple pterygium syndrome (Escobar syndrome): Characterized by pterygia of the neck, axillae, elbows, and knees, micrognathia, campodactyly, syndactyly, and rocker-bottom feet (autosomal recessive)[4]
2. Klippel-Feil sequence: consists of fusion of the cervical vertebrae; other associated anomalies include congential heart defects (ventricular septal defect is the most common),[6] deafness (30 percent),[8] and cleft palate (sporadic in most cases, autosomal dominant with variable expression)[6,8]
3. Zellweger syndrome (cerebrohepatorenal syndrome): large forehead with shallow supraorbital ridges, flat facies (have been confused with infants with Down syndrome), mild micrognathia, macrogyria, polymicrogyria, hepatomegaly, cystic kidney disease, contractures in extremities, equinovarus, simian crease, elevated serum iron (autosomal recessive)[3,7,11]

REFERENCES

1. Benacerraf BR, Barss VA, Laboda LA: A sonographic sign for the detection in the second trimester of the fetus with Down's syndrome. Am J Obstet Gynecol 151:1078, 1985.
2. Benacerraf BR, Frigoletto FD, Laboda LA: Sonographic diagnosis of Down syndrome in the second trimester. Am J Obstet Gynecol 153:49, 1985.
3. Bowen P, Lee CSN, Zellweger H, et al.: A familial syndrome of multiple congenital defects. Bull Hopkins Hosp 114:402, 1964.
4. Escobar V, Bixler D, Gleiser S, et al.: Multiple pterygium syndrome. Am J Dis Child 132:609, 1978.
5. Hall B: Mongolism in newborn infants. An examination of the criteria for recognition and some speculations on the pathogenic activity of the chromosomal abnormality. Clin Pediatr 5:4, 1966.
6. Morrison SG, Perry LW, Scott LP: Congenital brevicollis (Klippel-Feil syndrome) and cardiovascular anomalies. Am J Dis Child 115:614, 1968.
7. Opitz JM, ZuRhein GM, Vitale L, et al.: The Zellweger syndrome. Birth Defects 5:144, 1969.
8. Palant DJ, Carter BL: Klippel-Feil syndrome and deafness. Am J Dis Child 123:218, 1972.
9. Rex AP, Preus M: A diagnostic index for Down syndrome. J Pediatr 100:903, 1982.
10. Smith D, Jones KL: Recognizable Patterns of Human Malformation, 3d ed. Vol VII in Series Major Problems in Clinical Pediatrics. Philadelphia, Saunders, 1982.
11. Smith DW, Optiz JM, Inhorn SL: A syndrome of multiple developmental defects including polycystic kidneys and intrahepatic biliary dysgenesis in two siblings. J Pediatr 67:617, 1965.
12. Stephens TD, Shepard TH: The Down syndrome in the fetus. Teratology 22:37, 1980.
13. Toi A, Simpson GF, Filly RA: Ultrasonically evident fetal nuchal skin thickening: Is it specific for Down syndrome? Am J Obstet Gynecol 156:150, 1987.

4

The Heart

Approach to the Examination of the Fetal Heart

The first technique used for the sonographic evaluation of the fetal heart was M-mode ultrasound. Using this method, Winsberg reported quantitative evaluation of the fetal cardiac chambers in 1972.[26] However, the use of M-mode echocardiography in the fetus was limited because of the difficulties inherent in examining a moving fetus with a single, pencil-like sound beam. The next step was the use of real-time-directed M-mode that allowed the orientation of the single beam on the bidimensional image. Using this technique, Ianniruberto et al.,[10] DeLuca et al.,[6] and Wladimiroff and McGhie[27] described the quantitative and qualitative anatomy of the fetal heart.

The feasibility of the prenatal diagnosis of congenital heart disease was first established by Kleinman et al.[13] A major breakthrough toward the reproducibility of fetal echocardiography was the introduction of high-resolution real-time equipment. This equipment allowed detailed investigation of the anatomy of the fetal heart beginning in early pregnancy. In 1980, Allan et al.[3] described a systematic approach to the bidimensional examination of the fetal heart. In recent years, the experience collected in several laboratories has demonstrated the reliability of prenatal diagnosis of cardiac structural and functional abnormalities.[1,4,11–14,17,21–23]

ULTRASOUND BIDIMENSIONAL INVESTIGATION OF THE FETAL HEART: A SEQUENTIAL APPROACH

The main objective of fetal echocardiography is the prenatal diagnosis of congenital heart disease. Cardiac abnormalities encompass a broad spectrum of structural disorders, ranging from a simple communication between two cardiac chambers to an almost complete rearrangement of the connections between the different cardiac segments. This demands a systematic approach to the investigation of the fetal heart. In our laboratory, we use a "sequential approach" that depends on the recognition of the morphology and connections of the three segments of the fetal heart: atria, ventricles, and great vessels.

Sequential analysis for the diagnosis of congenital

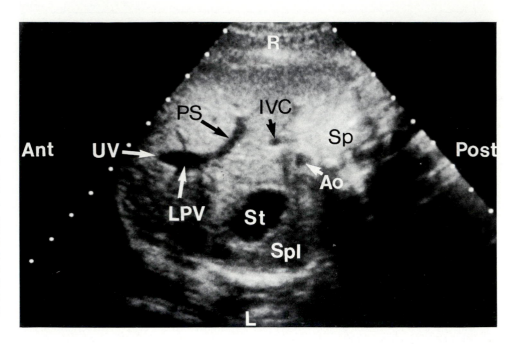

Figure 4–1. Transverse cross-section of the upper fetal abdomen. Study of the intraabdominal organs permits definition of the visceral situs. With situs solitus, the stomach (St) and the spleen (Spl) are on the left. The position of the hilum of the liver, normally on the right, can be inferred by following the umbilical vein (UV) into the left portal vein (LPV), which bends into the portal sinus (PS). The abdominal aorta (Ao) and inferior vena cava (IVC) can be seen on both sides of the spine (Sp). Ant, anterior; Post, posterior; L, left, R, right.

heart disease was first introduced by Van Praagh[24] and subsequently modified by Shinebourne et al.[19] In recent years, this type of approach, conceived for the pathologic and angiographic examination of the heart, has been applied to echocardiography in the postnatal period.[9] Such methodology appears extremely suitable for fetal cardiac studies. In this section, we adhere to the elegant approach to diagnosis and classification of congenital heart disease advocated by Becker and Anderson.[5]

The main steps of sequential analysis are:

1. Position of the heart within the body
2. Identification of the cardiac chambers
3. Study of the atrioventricular connections
4. Study of the ventriculoarterial connections

An ideal echocardiographic examination should begin with determination of the position of the head and the spine, establishing the right and left sides of the fetus. The next step, identification of the visceral situs, is important for two reasons: (1) the arrangement of the abdominal organs predicts the relative position of the right and left atria with a high degree of accuracy (this information is extremely valuable because, in many cases, fetal echocardiography does not distinguish the morphologic left from the right atrium) and (2) anomalies of the visceral situs are very frequently associated with cardiac abnormalities (e.g., cardiosplenic syndromes). Three conditions are possible: situs solitus (normal), situs inversus (mirror image of situs solitus), and situs ambiguous, also known as isomeric situs. This term refers to a condition in which there is an abnormal arrangement of the thoracic and abdominal organs (see sections on asplenia and polysplenia syndromes).

The visceral situs can be easily identified in the fetus by using ultrasound in a transverse cross-section of the upper abdomen. In this view, the stomach and spleen are normally positioned on the left. The portal sinus, which topographically corresponds to the hilum of the liver, can be seen to the right. Anterior to the spine, the abdominal aorta and inferior vena cava are seen on both sides of the spine. The abdominal aorta is to the left and appears as a round structure, and the inferior vena cava is to the right and is flattened and more anterior (Fig. 4–1). Recognition of the relative positions of the aorta and inferior vena cava is of special importance in identifying the atrial chambers, since the morphologic right atrium is almost invariably on the same side of the inferior vena cava.[5]

Since the fetal heart is almost horizontal, a transverse cross-section of the thorax above the level of the diaphragm will demonstrate a four chamber view.[3] In this plane of section, it is easy to recognize the apex and base of the heart and to assess the position of the heart inside the chest. Normally, the heart is in the left side of the chest with the apex pointing toward the left, the right ventricle and atrium being anterior to the left ventricle and atrium (levocardia) (Fig. 4–2). In dextrocardia, the heart is in the right side of the chest, and the apex points toward the right. In mesocardia, the heart occupies a central position inside the chest and the apex points anteriorly. Dextrocardia and mesocardia should be differentiated from those conditions in which the position of the heart is altered due to external compression (e.g., diaphragmatic hernia, lung tumors). In these cases, the term "dextroposition of the heart" is more appropriate.

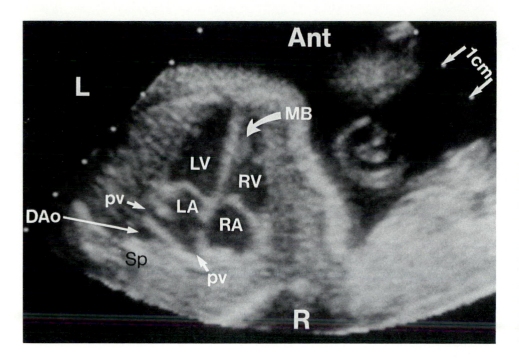

Figure 4–2. Apical four chamber view of the fetal heart. Note the moderator band (MB) and the more apical insertion of the leaflets of the tricuspid valve (unlabeled) on the ventricular septum, distinguishing the morphologic right ventricle from the left. The interatrial septum is interrupted in its central portion by the foramen ovale. The pulmonary veins (pv) can be seen entering the left atrium (LA). RA, right atrium; LV, left ventricle; RV, right ventricle; Sp, spine; DAo, descending aorta; R, right; L, left; Ant, anterior.

The four chamber view of the fetal heart provides important anatomic information. The interatrial septum separating the two atrial chambers can be seen. Normally, the pulmonary veins are connected to the left atrium, and the two atrial chambers communicate through the foramen ovale, an orifice in the center of the interatrial septum that separates the superior septum secundum and the inferior septum primum (Fig. 4–3). The foramen ovale is guarded by a valve that opens toward the left atrium.

The two atrial chambers are connected to the ventricular chambers. The atrioventricular junction is characterized by the more apical insertion of the tricuspid valve than the mitral valve on the interventricular septum. This finding is useful in differentiating the morphologic right and left ventricle and in recognizing anomalies of the atrioventricular junction, such as the atrioventricular canal[11] (Fig. 4–2). The other important anatomic details in differenti-

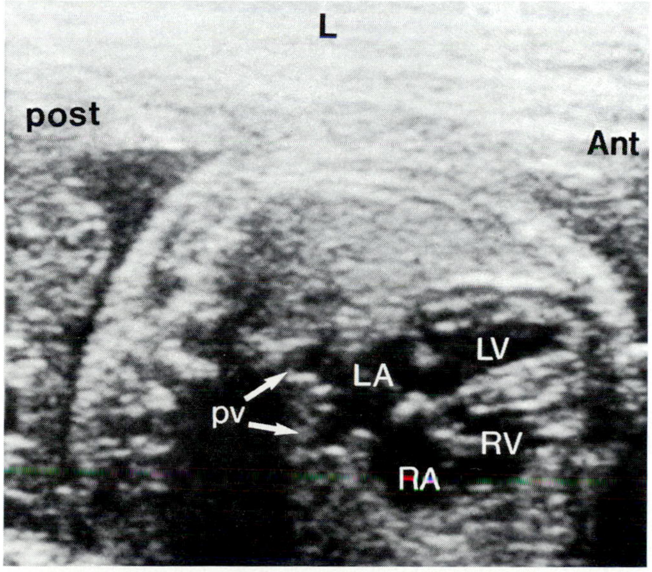

Figure 4–3. A subcostal four chamber view allows better definition of the integrity of the interventricular and interatrial septa. LV, left ventricle; RV, right ventricle; LA, left atrium; RA, right atrium; pv, pulmonary veins; Ant, anterior; Post, posterior; L, left.

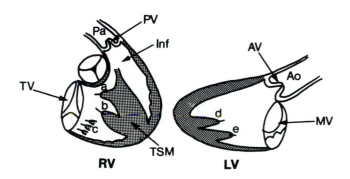

Figure 4–4. Schematic representation of the anatomic characteristics of the left and right ventricles (LV, RV). The right ventricle has a pyramidal shape, with an infundibulum (Inf) separating the tricuspid valve (TV) from the pulmonary valve (PV). The trabecular pattern is coarse and is characterized by the presence of the trabecula septomarginalis (TSM). The left ventricle is conical in shape, and the mitral valve (MV) and aortic valve (AV) are continuous. Pa, pulmonary artery; Ao, aorta; a,b,c,d,e, papillary muscles. *(Modified from Becker, Anderson: Pathology of Congenital Heart Disease. London, Butterworths, 1981.)*

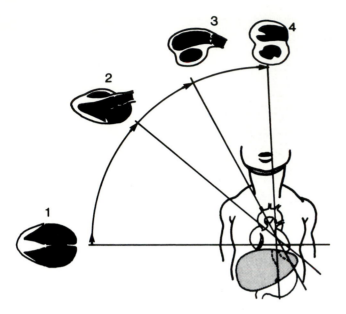

Figure 4–5. Schematic representation of the scanning planes employed in the echocardiographic examination of the fetal heart. 1. Four chamber view. 2. Long axis view of the left ventricle. 3. Long axis view of the right ventricle. 4. Short axis view of the ventricular cavities.

ating the morphologic right and left ventricle is the trabecular pattern. Whereas the left ventricle has a smooth internal surface on ultrasound studies, the right ventricle has a much coarser appearance. Particulary evident is the moderator band of the trabecula septomarginalis, which appears as a thickening of the interventricular septum at the level of the

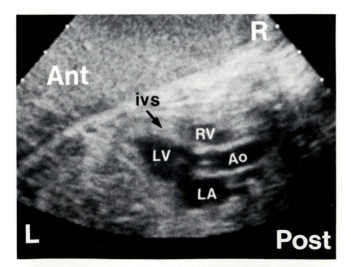

Figure 4–6. The long axis view of the left ventricle (LV) demonstrates the normal continuity between the anterior wall of the ascending aorta (Ao) and the interventricular septum (ivs) and between the posterior wall of the ascending aorta and the anterior leaflet of the mitral valve (unlabeled). Within the aortic root, the aortic valves can be seen. RV, right ventricle; LA, left atrium; R, right; L, left; Ant, anterior; Post, posterior.

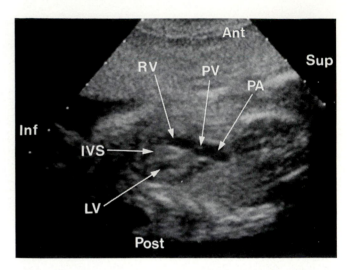

Figure 4–7. Long axis view of the right ventricle (RV). Note the posterior course of the pulmonary artery (PA). In the same scanning plane, a cross-section of the left ventricle (LV) is seen. IVS, interventricular septum; PV, pulmonary valve; Ant, anterior; Post, posterior; Sup, superior; Inf, inferior.

apex (Fig. 4–4). In the fetus, the right and left ventricular cavities are of similar size in the four chamber view.

Evaluation of all the anatomic details provided by the four chamber view often requires different approaches. The apical four chamber view allows optimal visualization of the atrioventricular junction and of the relative position of the atrioventricular valves, but the interventricular and interatrial septa are often inadequately imaged (Fig. 4–2). In this view, one may frequently observe an artifactual dropout of echoes at the level of the high portion of the interventricular septum and of the atrial septum secundum. These findings often create suspicion of a ventricular or atrial septal defect. With a subcostal approach, the leaflets of the atrioventricular valves are usually poorly visualized, but because of the angle of incidence of the sound beam, the integrity of the interatrial and interventricular septa can be optimally demonstrated (Fig. 4–3).

The ventriculoarterial connections can be studied by tilting the transducer in the direction of the outflow tract of the ventricles. Evaluation of the fetal heart can be carried out with a continuous sweep of the transducer because incomplete calcification of the rib cage and absence of air in the lungs do not interfere with the visualization of the fetal heart. In this fashion, it is possible to follow the outflow tracts to the great vessels. These can be subsequently identified by following their course to the aortic arch and bifurcation of the pulmonary artery.

In the neonatal period, cardiac anatomy is assessed by well-standardized echocardiographic views. These views can also be applied to a fetus.

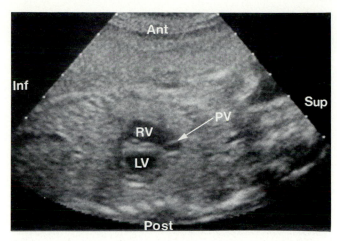

Figure 4–8. Short axis view of the ventricular chambers. The pulmonary valve (PV) is seen on top of the infundibulum of the right ventricle (RV). Note that the ventricular chambers have similar transverse diameters. LV, left ventricle; Ant, anterior; Post, posterior; Sup, superior; Inf, inferior.

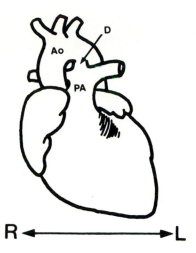

Figure 4–9. Normal course of the great vessels. PA, pulmonary artery; Ao, aorta; D, ductus arteriosus; R, right; L, left.

However, it should be stressed that it may be difficult to reproduce them accurately in an actively moving fetus. Furthermore, the fetal heart can be studied from a great number of angles. Rather than adhere strictly to a rigid scheme of a given set of views, we believe that the examination should be performed by using the scanning planes that are more convenient in relation to the position of the fetus.

Figure 4–5 illustrates an ideal evaluation of the fetal heart, in which a simple continuous rotation of the transducer from the transverse to the longitudinal plane enables visualization of the relevant cardiac anatomy.

In a fetus whose chest is directed toward the transducer, the left ventriculoarterial connection can be evaluated by tilting the medial portion of the transducer toward the head. In this plane, a long axis view of the left ventricle (Fig. 4–6), the typical conical shape of the left ventricular chamber can be seen. The left atrium is demonstrated posterior to the ventricle. The ascending aorta arises from the ventricle, resting on the left atrium and aiming upward. In this view, it is possible to verify the normal continuity between the anterior wall of the ascending aorta and the interventricular septum and between the posterior wall of the ascending aorta and the anterior leaflet of the mitral valve.

By further tilting of the transducer toward the longitudinal plane, the outflow tract of the right ventricle can be followed to the pulmonary artery, which is directed posteriorly. A cross-section of the left ventricle is seen posterior to the right ventricle. This plane is the long axis view of the right ventricle (Fig. 4–7).

A cross-section of the ventricular cavities is im-

aged (short axis view of the ventricles) by reaching the longitudinal axis of the fetus (Fig. 4–8).

Figure 4–9 shows the normal intrathoracic course of the great vessels. The pulmonary artery travels from the right to the left, encircling the ascending aorta. In the fetus, most of the right ventricular output is directed through the ductus arteriosus to the descending aorta. The normal course of the great arteries can be visualized by two longitudinal scans of the fetal torso (Fig. 4–10). One scan is directed from

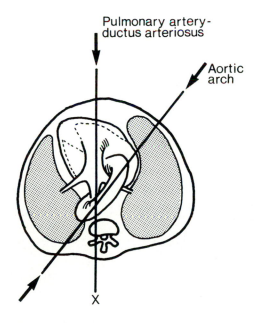

Figure 4–10. Schematic representation of the scanning planes used to demonstrate the aortic arch and the pulmonary artery–ductus arteriosus complex. Given the position of the spine, it is easy to see that the aortic arch can be imaged both from the anterior thoracic wall and from the shoulder of the fetus, whereas the pulmonary artery–ductus arteriosus view can usually be obtained only when scanning from the anterior thoracic wall.

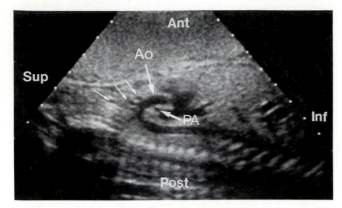

Figure 4–11. The aortic arch (Ao) as viewed from the anterior thoracic wall. The head and neck vessels are indicated by the small arrows. Below the arch, a cross-section of the right pulmonary artery (PA) is seen. Ant, anterior; Post, posterior; Sup, superior; Inf, inferior.

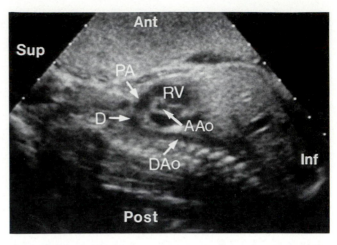

Figure 4–13. In this longitudinal view, the pulmonary artery (PA) can be followed to the ductus arteriosus (D) and to the descending aorta (DAo). In the same scanning plane, a cross-section of the ascending aorta (AAo) is seen. RV, right ventricle; Ant, anterior; Post, posterior; Sup, superior; Inf, inferior.

the left shoulder to the right hemithorax (Fig. 4–11), or vice versa (Fig. 4–12), and reveals the aortic arch, with the head and neck vessels. The second scan is directed along the anteroposterior axis of the thorax and reveals the pulmonary artery, which is continuous with the ductus arteriosus and descending aorta (Fig. 4–13). The complex formed by the pulmonary artery, the ductus, and the descending aorta frequently has been confused with the aortic arch. A distinction is important, since incorrect identification of the great arteries could lead to the erroneous diagnosis of transposition of the great vessels. Helpful hints are (1) the superior course of the arch when compared to the flattened, anteroposterior course of the pulmonary artery and ductus complex and (2)

demonstration of the head and neck vessels originating from the aortic arch.

Another important view of the fetal heart is the short axis view of the great vessels, which can be obtained easily by a transverse cross-section of the thorax oriented as in Figure 4–14. In this view, the pulmonary artery is seen arising from the right ventricle and passing anterior to and to the left of the ascending aorta (Fig. 4–15). This view (commonly referred to as "circle and sausage") demonstrates the normal criss-crossing of the great arteries and rules out a transposition.

The systemic venous return can be assessed

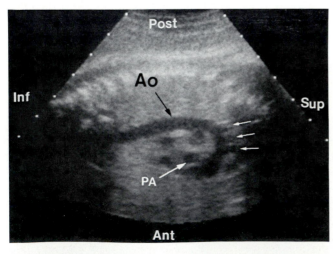

Figure 4–12. The aortic arch (Ao) as viewed from the back of the fetus. The head and neck vessels are indicated by the small arrows. PA, pulmonary artery; Ant, anterior; Post, posterior; Sup, superior; Inf, inferior.

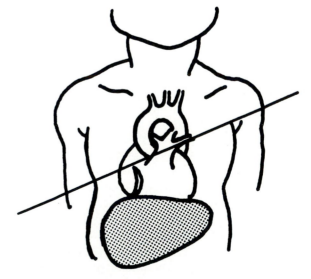

Figure 4–14. Schematic representation of the scanning plane for a short axis view of the great vessels.

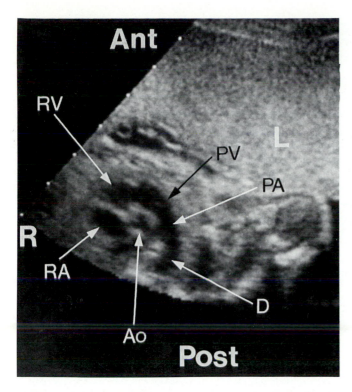

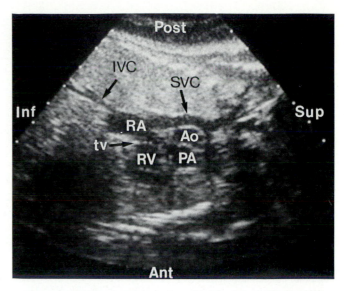

Figure 4–16. Right parasagittal scan of the fetal trunk demonstrating the inferior and superior venae cavae (IVC, SVC) entering the right atrium (RA). The tricuspid valve (tv) divides the right atrium from the right ventricle (RV). Ao, aorta; PA, pulmonary artery; Ant, anterior; Post, posterior; Sup, superior; Inf, inferior.

Figure 4–15. In the short axis view of the great vessels, the pulmonary artery (PA) is seen arising from the right ventricle (RV), passing anterior to and to the left of the ascending aorta (Ao) and bifurcating into the ductus arteriosus (D) and the right pulmonary artery (unlabeled). The tricuspid valve separates the right atrium (RA) from the right ventricle. Both aortic (unlabeled) and pulmonary valves (PV) can be seen within the roots of the great arteries. Ant, anterior; Post, posterior; L, left; R, right.

easily by a right parasagittal scan demonstrating the inferior and superior vena cava entering the right atrium (Fig. 4–16).

M-MODE ECHOCARDIOGRAPHY

M-mode is a modality of ultrasound in which the information derived from a single sound beam is displayed against time. This technique allows the movement of structures to be evaluated both quantitatively and qualitatively. M-mode was the first ultrasound modality employed in the study of the fetal heart.[20,26] Its major shortcoming was difficulty in blindly directing the sound beam toward the cardiac structures of a moving fetus. Recently, advances in ultrasound technology have resulted in the introduction of equipment with which the direction of the single beam can be selected on a bidimensional real-time image (Fig. 4–17). Fetal M-mode echocardiography is useful for measurement of cardiac chambers and great vessels and for assessment of cardiac arrhythmias.

M-mode tracings are provided with markers that indicate distance in the sound field on the vertical axis and time on the horizontal axis. With most equipment, the vertical distance between markers corresponds to 1 cm, and the horizontal distance corresponds to 0.5 second. This allows calculation of the fetal heart rate and biometry. Until a few years ago, these calculations were made off line, using calipers on a hard copy. Newer equipment is provided with software capable of on-screen measurements with electronic calipers.

The most relevant cardiac structures for M-mode examination are the atrial and ventricular chambers, atrioventricular valves, roots of the great vessels, and semilunar valves.

Examination of the ventricular chambers should be performed by directing the M-mode beam across the ventricles at a right angle to the interventricular septum and at the level of the atrioventricular valves. In Figure 4–17, the myocardium is externally lined by a bright linear echo that represents the pericardium. Inside the ventricular chambers, it is possible to observe the movement of the atrioventricular valves. The movement of the ventricular walls toward the interventricular septum indicates ventricular systole.

In Figure 4–18, the typical movement pattern of the mitral valve is shown. The anterior and posterior leaflets of the mitral valve are seen apposed during ventricular systole. At the beginning of ventricular filling, the valve opens, and the anterior leaflet moves toward the interventricular septum (point D). The point of maximal excursion of the leaflet is called

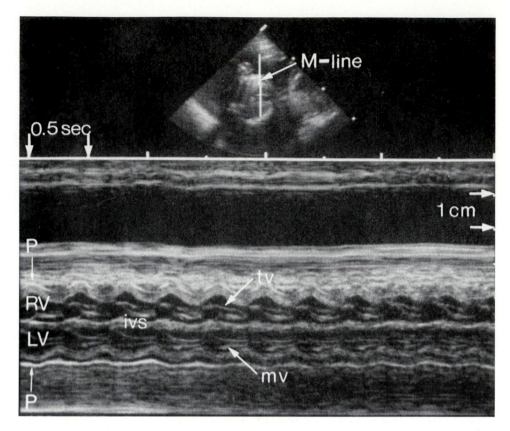

Figure 4–17. With ultrasound equipment that has the option of real-time-directed M-mode, the position of the cursor (M-line) can be easily selected during the real-time examination. An M-mode echocardiogram of the ventricular cavities (RV, LV) at the level of the atrioventricular valves (tv, mv) is shown. The undulations of free ventricular walls and of the interventricular septum (ivs) reflect systole and diastole. P, pericardium.

point E. After this, the leaflet moves away from the interventricular septum until it reaches the F point. The valve opens again with atrial systole (point A), and the leaflet moves away from the interventricular septum and presents a small undulation corresponding to the onset of ventricular systole (point B). At point C, the leaflets are apposed to each other. The movement of the posterior leaflet of the mitral valve is a mirror image of the movement of the anterior leaflet. The movement of the tricuspid valve closely resembles that of the mitral valve. Therefore, it is clear that by directing the M-mode beam across the

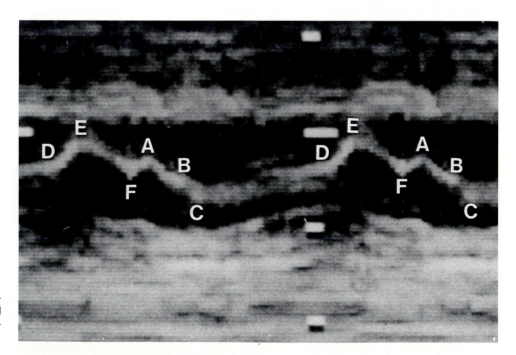

Figure 4–18. M-mode echocardiogram of the mitral valve in a second trimester fetus. See text for explanation of points A through F.

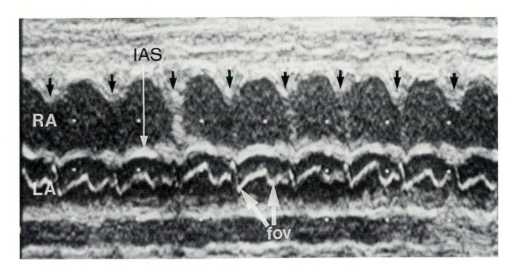

Figure 4–19. M-mode echocardiogram of the atria (RA, LA). To demonstrate the movement of the foramen ovale valve (fov), the cursor passes obliquely through the atrial chambers. This accounts for the discrepancy in size in the right and the left chambers. The undulation of the free wall of the right atrium *(arrowheads)* indicate atrial systole. IAS, interatrial septum.

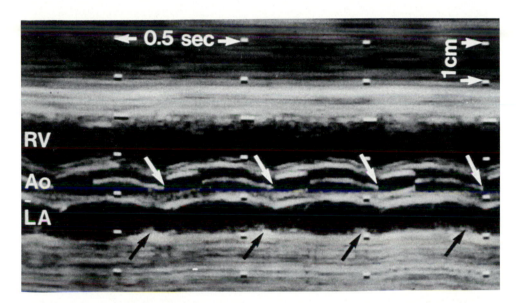

Figure 4–20. M-mode echocardiogram of the aortic root (Ao). Note the typical movement of the aortic valves. The opening of the aortic valves *(white arrows)* reflects ventricular systole, and the undulation of the posterior wall of the left atrium (LA) indicates atrial systole *(black arrows)*. RV, right ventricle. *(Reproduced with permission from Bovicelli L, Baccarani G, Picchio FM, Pilu G: Ecocardiografia Fetale. La Diagnosi e il Trattamento Prenatale delle Cardiopatie Congenite. Milan, Masson, 1985.)*

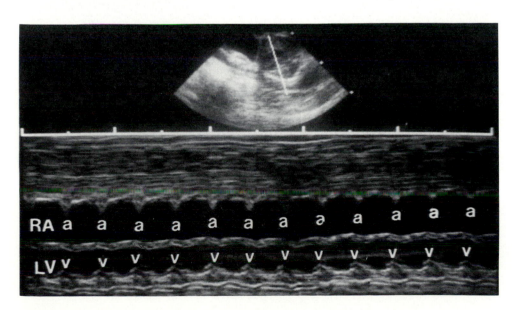

Figure 4–21. In this fetus, the atrioventricular contraction sequence can be easily demonstrated by positioning the cursor through the right atrium (RA) and left ventricle (LV). a, atrial contractions; v, ventricular contractions.

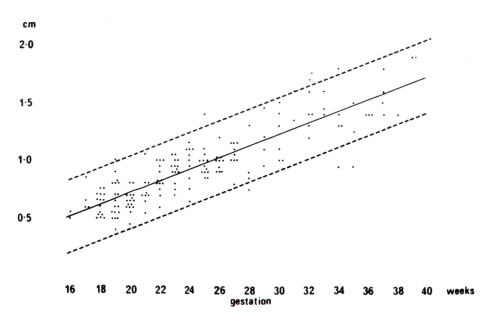

Figure 4–22. Normal dimensions of the left ventricle throughout gestation. *(Reproduced with permission from Allan et al.: Br Heart J 47:573, 1982.)*

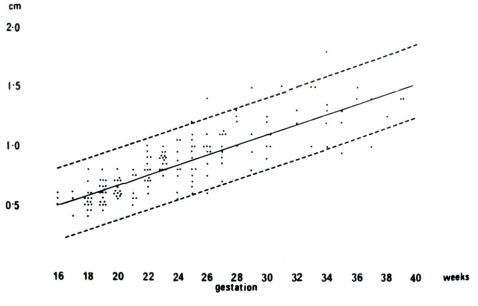

Figure 4–23. Normal dimensions of the right ventricle throughout gestation. *(Reproduced with permission from Allan et al.: Br Heart J 47:573, 1982.)*

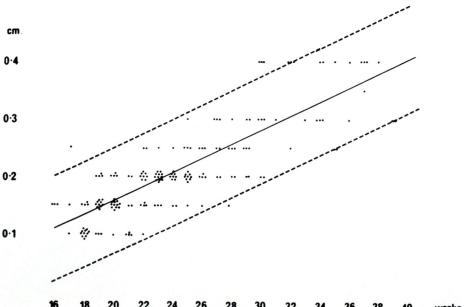

Figure 4–24. Normal dimensions of the interventricular septum throughout gestation. *(Reproduced with permission from Allan et al.: Br Heart J 47:573, 1982.)*

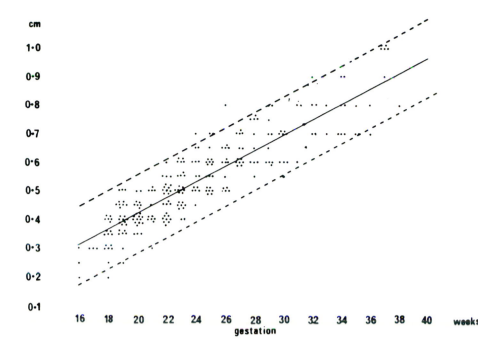

Figure 4–25. Normal dimensions of the aortic root throughout gestation. *(Reproduced with permission from Allan et al.: Br Heart J 47:573, 1982.)*

wall of the ventricular chambers and the atrioventricular valves, it is possible to simultaneously assess the atrial and ventricular contraction (the former corresponding to the A wave on the atrioventricular valves, the latter corresponding to the undulation of the ventricular wall). The sequence of excitation can be inferred by study of the contraction sequence. This information is of value in the assessment of cardiac dysrhythmias.

By directing the M-mode beam across the atrial chambers, it is possible to observe the undulation of the atrial walls, which reflect atrial systole. Inside the left atrium, the typical biphasic pattern of movement of the foramen ovale flap is seen. The flap moves toward the interatrial septum during atrial systole and again during ventricular systole[2] (Fig. 4–19).

The aortic root is best studied in a long axis view of the left ventricle. In this orientation, the M-mode beam passes through the right ventricle, ascending aorta, semilunar valves, and left atrium. The aortic root has a typical sinusoidal pattern of movement, which is due both to the blood flow inside the vessel and to the modification in the size of the left atrium during the cardiac cycle on which the vessel lies in its

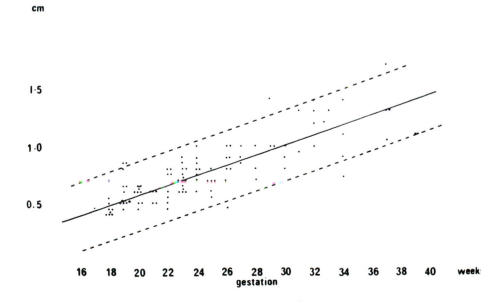

Figure 4–26. Normal dimensions of the left atrium throughout gestation. *(Reproduced with permission from Allan et al.: Br Heart J 47:573, 1982.)*

TABLE 4–1. DISTRIBUTION OF TYPES OF CONGENITAL HEART DISEASE AMONG AFFECTED LIVE-BORN INFANTS

Lesion	Frequency (%)
Ventricular septal defect	30.3
Patent ductus arteriosus	8.6
Pulmonary stenosis	7.4
Atrial septal defect (secundum)	6.7
Coarctation of the aorta	5.7
Aortic stenosis	5.2
Tetralogy of Fallot	5.1
Transposition of the great arteries	4.7
Atrioventricular defects	3.2
Hypoplastic right ventricle	2.2
Hypoplastic left heart syndrome	1.3
Total anomalous pulmonary venous return	1.1
Truncus arteriosus	1.0
Single ventricle	0.3
Double outlet right ventricle	0.2
Miscellaneous	17.1

Data derived from Hoffman, Christianson: Am J Cardiol 42:641, 1978.

TABLE 4–2. MONOGENIC INHERITANCE AND CONGENITAL HEART DISEASE

Specific Cardiac Lesions Transmitted as Single Gene Disorders

Lesion	Mode of Transmission
Supravalvular aortic stenosis	AR
Asymmetrical septal hypertrophy	AD
Wolff-Parkinson-White syndrome	AD
Complete heart block	AD
Endocardial fibroelastosis	AR (?), XLR
Hypoplastic left heart syndrome	AR (?)
Hypoplastic right ventricle	AD (?)

Syndromes with Monogenic Inheritance Featuring Cardiac Lesions with a Variable Degree of Penetrance

Syndrome	Mode of Transmission
Holt-Oram	AD
Noonan	AD
Apert	AD
Ehlers-Danlos	AD
Leopard	AD
Marfan	AD
Osteogenesis imperfecta	AD
Treacher Collins	AD
Tuberous sclerosis	AD
Carpenter	AR
Ellis-Van Creveld	AR
Friedreich ataxia	AR
Glycogenosis IIa, III, IV	AR
Ivemark	AR
Laurence-Moon-Biedl	AR
Meckel-Gruber	AR
Mucolipidosis II, III	AR
Mucopolysaccaridosis III, IS, IV, VI	AR
Refsum	AR
Smith-Lemli-Opitz	AR
Thrombocytopenia absent radius	AR
Mucopolysaccaridosis II	XLR
Duchenne and Dreifus muscular dystrophies	XLR

AR, autosomal recessive; AD, autosomal dominant; XLR, X-linked recessive.
Adapted from Nora, Nora: Genetics and Counseling in Cardiovascular Disease. Springfield, IL, Chas. C Thomas, 1978.

proximal tract. Inside the aortic root, the semilunar valves are seen. These are apposed during diastole and open briskly at the beginning of the ejection period, displaying a boxlike appearance. The undulation of the wall of the left atrium reflects atrial systole. Therefore, it is possible to correlate the atrial contraction with the ventricular contraction (opening of the aortic valve) and to infer the sequence of excitation (Fig. 4–20). The movement of the pulmonary valve closely resembles that of the aortic valve.

While evaluating a fetus with dysrhythmia, it is not always possible to obtain the views that have been described. It should be remembered that the sequence of excitation (which is the key to the differential diagnosis of arrhythmias) can be inferred from any orientation of the sound beam that allows the simultaneous demonstration of an atrial and a ventricular structure. Figure 4–21 shows how the atrioventricular contraction sequence can be easily demonstrated in a fetus by simply directing the sound beam across the right atrium and left ventricle. In this view, the atrial systole is reflected by the undulations of the atrial wall, and the ventricular systole is reflected by the movement of the ventricular wall.

M-mode echocardiography has been used to quantitate fetal cardiac structures.[2,18] In the nomograms reported by Allan et al.,[2] a short axis view of the ventricles below the level of the atrioventricular valve was used to measure the inner dimensions of the ventricular chambers at the end of diastole (Figs. 4–22, 4–23) and the thickness of the interventricular septum (Fig. 4–24). The ascending aorta was measured with an orientation that allowed a visualization of the boxlike pattern of the semilunar valves (Fig. 4–25). The left atrium was measured by using a long axis view of the left ventricle as the point of reference (Fig. 4–26).

It should be stressed that the variability range of many reported nomograms of cardiac dimensions is quite wide and the usefulness of nomograms in the assessment of enlargement or hypoplasia of cardiac chambers and vessels is limited. We have found that a subjective evaluation by an experienced operator has great value.

TABLE 4–3. CHROMOSOMAL ABNORMALITIES AND CONGENITAL HEART DISEASE (CHD)

Chromosomal Abnormality	Incidence of CHD (%)	Most Common Lesions
21 trisomy	50	VSD, AV canal, ASD, PDA
18 trisomy	99+	VSD, PDA, PS
13 trisomy	90	VSD, PDA, Dex
22 trisomy	67	ASD, VSD, PDA
22 partial trisomy (cat-eye)	40	TAPVR, VSD, ASD
4p–	40	ASD, VSD, PDA
5p– (cri-du-chat)	20	VSD, PDA, ASD
8 trisomy (mosaic)	50	VSD, ASD, PDA
9 trisomy (mosaic)	50	VSD, coarc, DORV
13q–	25	VSD
+14q–	50	PDA, ASD, Tet
18q–	50	VSD
XO Turner	35	coarc, AS, ASD
XXXXY	14	PDA, ASD, ARCA

ARCA, anomalous right coronary artery; AS, aortic stenosis; ASD, atrial septal defect; AV canal, atrioventricular canal; CHD, congenital heart disease; coarc, coarctation of the aorta; Dex, dextroversion; DORV, double outlet right ventricle; PDA, patent ductus arteriosus; PS, pulmonary stenosis; TAPVR, total anomalous pulmonary venous return; Tet, tetralogy of Fallot; VSD, ventricular septal defect.

Modified from Nora, Nora: Genetics and Counseling in Cardiovascular Disease. Springfield, IL, Chas. C Thomas, 1978.

TABLE 4–4. ENVIRONMENTAL FACTORS AND CONGENITAL HEART DISEASE (CHD)

	Frequency of CHD (%)	Most Common Lesions
Maternal alcoholism	25–30	VSD, PDA, ASD
Drugs		
Amphetamines	?5–10	VSD, PDA, TGA
Hydantoin	2–3	PS, AS, coarc, PDA
Trimethadione	15–30	TGA, Tet, HLHS
Lithium	10	Ebstein, tricuspid atresia, ASD
Thalidomide	5–10	Tet, VSD, ASD, truncus
Infections		
Rubella	35	Peripheral pulmonary stenosis, PS, PDA, VSD, ASD
Maternal conditions		
Diabetes	3–5 (30–50)	TGA, VSD, coarc (for cardiomegaly and cardiomyopathy)
Lupus erythematosus	?	Heartblock
Phenylketonuria	25–50	Tet, VSD, ASD

AS, aortic stenosis; ASD, atrial septal defect; coarc, coarctation of the aorta; Ebstein, Ebstein's anomaly; HLHS, hypoplastic left heart syndrome; PDA, patent ductus arteriosus; PS, pulmonary stenosis; Tet, tetralogy of Fallot; TGA, transposition of the great arteries; truncus, truncus arteriosus; VSD, ventricular septal defect.

Modified from Nora, Nora: Genetics and Counseling in Cardiovascular Disease. Springfield, IL, Chas. C Thomas, 1978.

INCIDENCE AND ETIOLOGY OF CONGENITAL HEART DISEASE

The true incidence of congenital heart disease is not easily assessed. Some anomalies, such as mitral valve prolapse and bicuspid aortic valve, which are probably the most common cardiac defects, are not usually recognized until late in infancy or childhood and, therefore, escape epidemiologic surveys at birth.

The largest series now available indicate an average incidence of 8 to 9 cases per 1000 live births, and their authors agree that this figure is an underestimation.[8,15] Ventricular septal defects, patent ductus arteriosus, pulmonary stenosis, and atrial septal defects are the most common anomalies (Table 4–1).

Some cardiac defects otherwise considered uncommon, such as hypoplastic left heart syndrome, have been seen frequently in fetuses since the advent of fetal echocardiography. The discrepancy between pediatric and prenatal series is probably because of the high lethality rate of some malformations in the perinatal period.

Congenital heart disease is believed to be a multifactorial disorder arising from the combined effect of a genetic predisposition and environmental factors in over 90 percent of cases.[16] In these cases, the recurrence risk after the birth of one affected child is 2 to 5 percent, and it rises to 10 to 15 percent after the birth of two affected siblings. The recurrence risk when the proband is one of the parents varies from defect to defect, but it is believed to range between 2 and 5 percent.[16] However, important exceptions have been recently reported,[7,25] suggesting that further investigation is required in this area.

A monogenic inheritance probably accounts for no more than 1 to 2 percent of affected infants. This figure includes both cases of isolated cardiac anomalies transmitted as single gene disorders and cases of congenital heart disease occurring with a variable degree of penetrance in syndromes with monogenic inheritance (Table 4–2).

In 4 to 5 percent of patients, a chromosomal abnormality, most commonly an autosomal trisomy, is found (Table 4–3). It is possible that the prevalence of associated chromosomal abnormalities is higher when the defect is detected in utero. In 1 to 2 percent of patients, environmental factors alone are thought to account for the anomalies (Table 4–4).

It has recently been demonstrated that fetal echocardiography is a valuable tool in the prenatal diagnosis of congenital heart disease. It should be stressed, however, that ultrasound investigation of the fetal heart requires both an experienced operator

TABLE 4–5. INDICATIONS FOR FETAL ECHOCARDIOGRAPHY

Maternal and familial indications
  Familial history of congenital heart disease
  Maternal diabetes
  Maternal drug exposure during pregnancy
  Maternal infections during pregnancy
  Maternal alcoholism
  Maternal lupus erythematosus
  Maternal phenylketonuria
Fetal indications
  Polyhydramnios
  Nonimmune hydrops
  Dysrhythmias
  Extracardiac abnormalities
  Chromosomal abnormalities
  Symmetrical intrauterine growth retardation

and meticulous scanning. Currently accepted indications for fetal echocardiographic evaluation are shown in Table 4–5.

REFERENCES

1. Allan LD, Crawford DC, Anderson RH, et al.: Echocardiographic and anatomical correlates in fetal congenital heart disease. Br Heart J 52:542, 1984.
2. Allan LD, Joseph MC, Boyd EGCA, et al.: M-mode echocardiography in the developing human fetus. Br Heart J 47:573, 1982.
3. Allan LD, Tynan M, Campbell S, et al.: Echocardiographic and anatomical correlates in the fetus. Br Heart J 44:444, 1980.
4. Allan LD, Tynan M, Campbell S, et al.: Identification of congenital cardiac malformations by echocardiography in midtrimester fetus. Br Heart J 46:358, 1981.
5. Becker AE, Anderson RH: Pathology of Congenital Heart Disease. London, Butterworths, 1981.
6. DeLuca I, Ianniruberto A, Colonna L: Aspetti ecografici del cuore fetale. G Ital Cardiol 8:778, 1978.
7. Emanuel R, Somerville J, Inns A, et al.: Evidence of congenital heart disease in the offspring of parents with atrioventricular defects. Br Heart J 49:144, 1983.
8. Hoffman JI, Christianson R: Congenital heart disease in a cohort of 19,502 births with long-term follow-up. Am J Cardiol 42:641, 1978.
9. Huhta JC, Smallhorn JF, Macartney FJ: Two-dimensional echocardiographic diagnosis of situs. Br Heart J 48:97, 1982.
10. Ianniruberto A, Iaccarino M, DeLuca I, et al.: Analisi delle strutture cardiache fetali mediante ecografia. Nota tecnica. In: Colagrande C, Ianniruberto A, Talia B (eds):

Proceedings of the 3rd National Congress of the SISUM. Terlizzi, September 24–25, 1977, pp 285–290.
11. Kleinman CS, Santulli TV: Ultrasonic evaluation of the fetal human heart. Semin Perinatol 7:90, 1983.
12. Kleinman CS, Donnerstein RL, DeVore GR, et al.: Fetal echocardiography for evaluation of in utero congestive heart failure: A technique for study of nonimmune fetal hydrops. N Engl J Med 306:568, 1982.
13. Kleinman CS, Hobbins JC, Jaffe CC, et al.: Echocardiographic studies of the human fetus: prenatal diagnosis of congenital heart disease and cardiac dysrhythmias. Pediatrics 65:1059, 1980.
14. Lange, LW, Sahn DJ, Allen HD, et al.: Qualitative real-time cross-sectional echocardiographic imaging of the human fetus during the second half of pregnancy. Circulation 62:799, 1980.
15. Mitchell SC, Korones SB, Berendes HW: Congenital heart disease in 56,109 births. Incidence and natural history. Circulation 43:323, 1971.
16. Nora JJ, Nora AH: Genetics and Counseling in Cardiovascular Diseases. Springfield, IL, Chas. C Thomas, 1978.
17. Pilu G, Rizzo N, Orsini LF, et al.: La diagnosi delle anomalie cardiache strutturali nel feto mediante ultrasonografia bidimensionale. Ultr Ost Gin 1:257, 1983.
18. Sahn DJ, Lange LW, Allen HD, et al.: Quantitative real-time cross-sectional echocardiography in the developing normal human fetus and newborn. Circulation 62:588, 1980.
19. Shinebourne EA, Macartney FJ, Anderson RH: Sequential chamber localization: Logical approach to diagnosis in congenital heart disease. Br Heart J 38:327, 1976.
20. Schulz Roczen R: Fetal echocardiography: Present and future applications. J Clin Ultrasound 9:223, 1981.
21. Silverman NH, Golbus MS: Echocardiographic techniques for assessing normal and abnormal fetal cardiac anatomy. J Am Coll Cardiol 5:20S, 1985.
22. Stewart PA, Tonge HM, Wladimiroff JW: Arrhythmia and structural abnormalities of the fetal heart. Br Heart J 50:550, 1983.
23. Stewart PA, Wladimiroff JW, Essed CE: Prenatal ultrasound diagnosis of congenital heart disease associated with intrauterine growth retardation. A report of 2 cases. Prenat Diagn 3:279, 1983.
24. Van Praagh R: The segmental approach to diagnosis in congenital heart disease. Birth Defects 8:4, 1972.
25. Whittemore R, Hobbins JC, Engle MA: Pregnancy and its outcome in women with and without surgical treatment of congenital heart disease. Am J Cardiol 50:641, 1982.
26. Winsberg F: Echocardiography of the fetal and newborn heart. Invest Radiol 7:152, 1972.
27. Wladimiroff JW, McGhie JS: M-mode ultrasonic assessment of fetal cardiovascular dynamics. Br J Obstet Gynaecol 88:1241, 1981.

Atrial Septal Defects

Embryology of the Atrial Septum

The separation of atrial cavities is initiated by the development of a membrane called "septum primum" (Fig. 4–27). This membrane grows from the atrial walls toward the endocardial cushions. The temporary orifice defined by these two structures is the ostium primum. As the septum primum grows toward the endocardial cushions, the foramen primum becomes progressively smaller and is obliterated by the end of the fifth week. Then, multiple small perforations occur in the central portion of the septum primum. The coalescence of these orifices results in the formation of the ostium secundum.

Another membrane called the "septum secundum" develops on the right side of the septum primum. This membrane covers part of the foramen secundum. The term "foramen ovale" refers to the orifice limited by the septum secundum and the septum primum. The foramen ovale is the anatomic communication between the two atria in utero and allows the passage of the oxygenated blood via the inferior vena cava from the umbilical vein to the left side of the heart. During intrauterine life, the lower edge of the septum primum acts as a valve (foramen ovalis flap). After birth, the increased pressure at the level of the left atrium apposes the flap against the rest of the septum. Anatomic closure takes place several months after birth.[5] However, a probe-patent foramen ovale is found in about 30 percent of normal adults.[6]

Pathology

Atrial septal defects (ASD) are commonly subdivided into:

1. Defects of the inlet atrial septum
2. Defects in the body of the atrial chambers
3. Defects of the outlet atrial septum

Defects of the inlet portion of the atrial septum are also commonly referred to as "sinus venosus defects." In these cases, the defect is located near the entrance of the superior vena cava. It is invariably associated with anomalous pulmonary venous return.

Defects in the body of the atrial chamber are also known as "ostium secundum" defects or "secundum" defects and are characterized by either absence or deficiency of the foramen ovale flap.

Defects of the outlet portion of the atrial septum are also referred to as "ostium primum" defects or "primum" defects. They are almost always associated

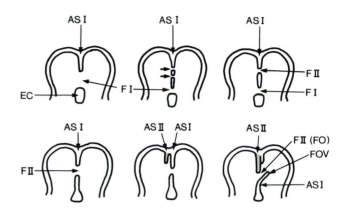

Figure 4–27. Embryology of the atrial septum. AS I, atrial septum primum; AS II, atrial septum secundum; F I, foramen primum; F II (FO), foramen secundum (foramen ovale); EC, endocardial cushion; FOV, foramen ovale valve.

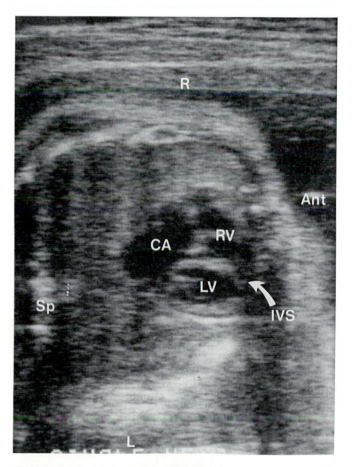

Figure 4–28. In this fetus with complete atrioventricular canal, both the septum primum and septum secundum are absent, resulting in a common atrium (CA). RV, right ventricle; LV, left ventricle; IVS, interventricular septum; Ant, anterior; Sp, spine; R, right; L, left.

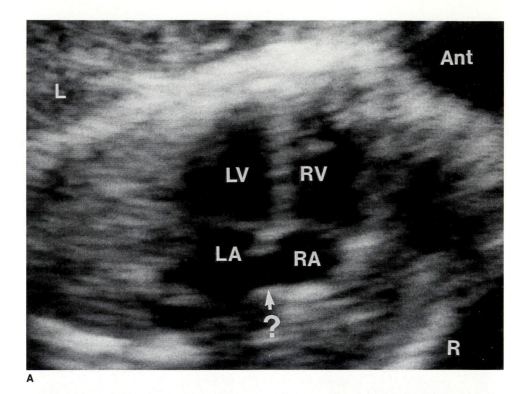

A

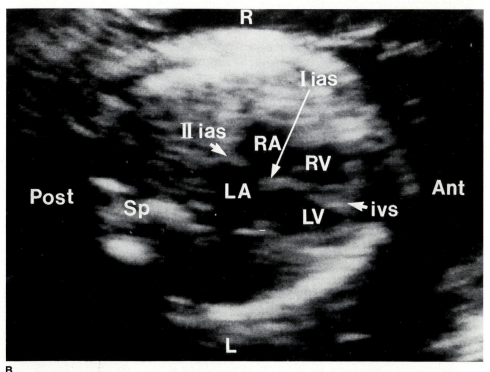

B

Figure 4–29. **A.** In this apical four chamber view, the lack of lateral resolution of the ultrasound equipment resulted in a dropout of echoes at the level of the septum secundum (?). LV, left ventricle; RV, right ventricle; LA, left atrium; RA, right atrium; Ant, anterior; L, left; R, right. **B.** Subcostal four chamber view of the patient, demonstrating normal septum secundum (II ias). I ias, septum primum; RV, right ventricle; LV, left ventricle; LA, left atrium; RA, right atrium; Sp, spine; Ant, anterior; Post, posterior; L, left; R, right; ivs, intact ventricular septum.

with anomalies of the atrioventricular junction and therefore, are discussed in the section on atrioventricular canal malformations (see p. 144).[2]

Hemodynamic Considerations

Since a large right-to-left shunt is physiologic during intrauterine life, neither defects of the inlet atrial septum nor defects at the level of the foramen ovale flap (secundum defects) are a cause of hemodynamic perturbance in the fetus. After birth, there is a physiologic increase in the pressure at the level of the left atrium, creating conditions for a left-to-right shunt. In time, the overload of the right ventricle may lead to dilatation and, in rare instances, to congestive heart failure. Pulmonary vascular bed damage can lead to pulmonary hypertension.

Symptomatic infants may suffer from repeated respiratory infections, feeding difficulties, arrhythmias, thromboembolism, and failure to thrive.[1]

Diagnosis

Diagnosis of an ASD relies on the demonstration of a dropout of echoes at the level of the atrial septum. Because of the presence of the foramen ovale and the rapidly flapping valve, it is unlikely that a small ostium secundum defect can be recognized in the fetus. The prenatal diagnosis of a defect of the inlet portion has not been reported, and it seems extremely difficult to recognize because of its location and size. Larger defects involving both the septum secundum and septum primum are easily recognizable (Fig. 4–28).

It should be stressed that the thin interatrial septum may be difficult to image properly with an apical four chamber view of the heart. For an adequate evaluation, the subcostal approach should be used (Fig. 4–29).

Prognosis

Campbell reported in 1970 his observations on the natural history of ASD.[3] He found that the mortality rates for the first two decades of life were 0.6 percent and 0.7 percent per year, respectively. The figures rose to 2.7 percent, 4.5 percent, 5.4 percent, and 7.5 percent in successive decades. The median age of death was 37 years. Cockerham et al.[4] have subsequently reported on the rate of spontaneous closure of ASDs. They studied 264 patients with ostium secundum and found that infants younger than 1 year of age with clinical symptoms had a rate of closure of 22 percent. The rate of closure in patients between the ages of 1 and 2 years was 33 percent. Patients older than 4 years of age had a spontaneous

closure rate of 3 percent. In view c authors suggested that infants syr years old should be initially treatec years of age, elective surgery v because of the unlikelihood of sp The mortality rate with surgery has been estimated to be about 1 percent.[4]

As with other cardiac defects, it should be stressed that these data have been generated from infants, children, and adults with ASD. They may not apply to the larger defects susceptible to antenatal diagnosis.

Obstetrical Management

ASDs are often associated with both cardiac and extracardiac anomalies. Therefore, a careful evaluation of the entire fetal anatomy and an amniocentesis for chromosomal analysis are recommended. In the presence of an isolated secundum ASD, standard obstetrical management is not altered.

REFERENCES

1. Adams CW: A reappraisal of life expectancy with atrial shunts of the secundum type. Dis Chest 48:357, 1965.
2. Becker AE, Anderson RH: Atrial septal defects. In: Pathology of Congenital Heart Disease. London, Butterworths, 1981, pp 67–75.
3. Campbell M: Natural history of atrial septal defect. Br Heart J 32:820, 1970.
4. Cockerham JT, Martin TC, Gutierrez FR, et al.: Spontaneous closure of secundum atrial septal defect in infants and young children. Am J Cardiol 52:1267, 1983.
5. Moore KL: The Developing Human: Clinically Oriented Embryology, 2d ed. Philadelphia, Saunders, 1977.
6. Patten BM: The closure of the foramen ovale. Am J Anat 48:19, 1931.

Ventricular Septal Defects

Pathology and Embryology

The ventricular septum originates from the fusion of the endocardial cushions with the muscular part of the septum and the conus ridges at the 7th week.

Ventricular septal defects (VSD) can be classified according to the position of the defect. The septum is commonly divided into a membranous and a muscular portion. The muscular portion is subdivided into three components: inlet, trabecular, and outlet or infundibular (Fig. 4–30). The most common location for the VSD is the membranous portion of the septum. Since most of these defects involve the muscular por-

tion as well, the term "perimembranous" has been suggested.[14]

VSDs are by far the most common cardiac lesion, accounting for 30 percent of all structural heart defects. Furthermore, they are found in many complex abnormalities, such as tetralogy of Fallot and transposition of the great arteries.[5]

Hemodynamic Considerations

The presence of an isolated VSD is not regarded as a cause of hemodynamic disturbances in utero. Since the pressure in both ventricular cavities is believed to

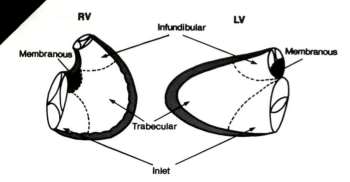

Figure 4–30. Diagram of the components of the interventricular septum viewed from the right ventricle (RV) and left ventricle (LV). *(Modified from Becker, Anderson: Pathology of Congenital Heart Disease. London, Butterworths, 1981.)*

be equal, it is possible that even large VSDs are only responsible for small bidirectional shunts.[12] This view seems to be supported by the observations that most infants are asymptomatic at birth.[7,8]

After birth, there is a decrease in the arterial pressure in the pulmonary vascular bed and an increase in the systemic arterial pressure. In the presence of a VSD, a left-to-right shunt occurs. Very small VSDs have little or no hemodynamic consequences because of the negligible magnitude of the shunt. With larger VSDs, some or all of the systemic pressure is transmitted to the pulmonary arteries. In time, this may lead to pulmonary vascular disease and pulmonary hypertension. Increased pressure in the right ventricle may eventually result in a reversal of the shunt, with cyanosis and congestive heart failure.[7,8] An exception to this course of events is an infant with a very large VSD, in whom a large portion of the left ventricular output is diverted into the right ventricle, with ventricular overload, thus possibly creating congestive heart failure soon after birth.[11]

Several studies have documented spontaneous closure of VSDs. Factors influencing this phenomenon include the size and location of the defect. Smaller defects and those located in the muscular septum have a higher tendency to close than do large and membranous defects. Hoffman and Rudolph[8,9] reported that 40 percent of VSDs are closed within 2 years of life and that 60 percent will close by 5 years. The incidence of closure for membranous defects is 25 percent by 5 years and that of muscular defects is 65 percent.[3]

The mechanisms of closure are different for perimembranous and muscular defects. The latter are closed by fibrous tissue originating from the septum,[8] whereas the former are closed either completely or partially with a variety of anatomic derivatives, in-

cluding reduplication of the tricuspid valve tissue, adhesion of tricuspid valve leaflets, and prolapse of an aortic valve leaflet.[4]

Diagnosis

The diagnosis depends on the demonstration of a dropout of echoes at the level of the interventricular septum[1,2,13] (Fig. 4–31). It should be stressed that a careful examination of the interventricular septum is necessary. Since a four chamber view of the heart will reveal only a small portion of the inlet and trabecular septum, it is obvious that a VSD can be missed easily by relying on this view. This is especially true if the defect is located in the outlet or membranous portion of the septum (Fig. 4–32). In addition to the four chamber view, the examination of the septum should include a long axis view of the left ventricle, a long axis view of the right ventricle, and an apex to base sweep along the short axis of the heart.[6]

The sonographer should be alerted to a potential pitfall. When an apical four chamber view of the heart is obtained, the limitations of lateral resolution of the sound beam could result in the creation of an artifactual hypoechogenic image in the higher portion of the inlet septum (Fig. 4–33). This pitfall is easily recognized by failure to demonstrate the defect in other views. Optimal examination is achieved when

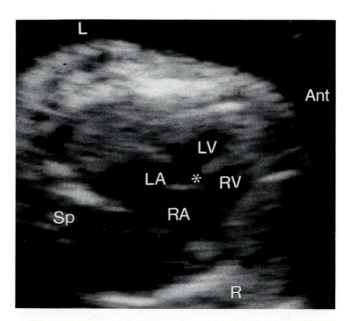

Figure 4–31. In this 25-week-old fetus, a four chamber view reveals a perimembranous ventricular septal defect (*). LV, left ventricle; RV, right ventricle; LA, left atrium; RA, right atrium; Sp, spine; Ant, anterior; L, left; R, right. *(Reproduced with permission from Bovicelli L, Baccarani G, Picchio FM, Pilu G: Ecocardiografia Fetale. La Diagnosi ed il Trattamento Prenatale delle Cardiopatie Congenite. Milan, Masson, 1985.)*

the sound beam is perpendicular to the septum. An artifactual "defect" often demonstrates a "fading-out" of the septum. A true defect is usually seen as a sharply terminating bright spot or area.

Since the resolution of current ultrasound equipment is limited to 1 to 2 mm, it is not surprising that some VSDs will escape detection prenatally.

Since VSDs are frequent components of more complex cardiac abnormalities, a careful examination of the entire cardiac morphology is mandatory.

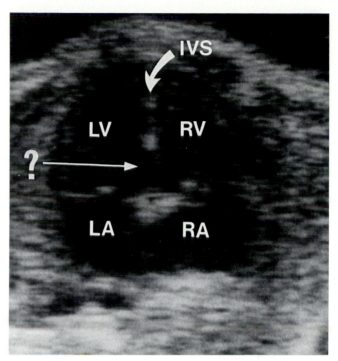

Figure 4–33. In this apical four chamber view, lack of lateral resolution and low gain settings result in a dropout of echoes (?) at the level of the perimembranous ventricular septum. LV, left ventricle; RV, right ventricle; LA, left atrium; RA, right atrium; IVS, interventricular septum.

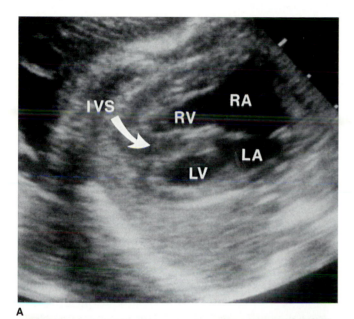

A

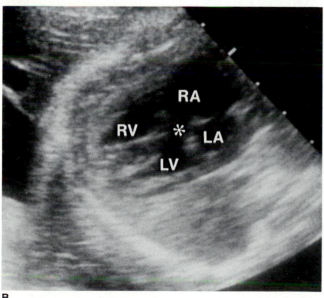

B

Figure 4–32. A. A four-chamber view in a 30-week fetus reveals a seemingly intact ventricular septum (IVS). LV, left ventricle; RV, right ventricle; LA, left atrium; RA, right atrium. **B.** In the same patient, a subaortic VSD (∗) is clearly demonstrated by a slight cephalic angulation of the transducer. LV, left ventricle; RV, right ventricle; LA, left atrium; RA, right atrium.

Prognosis

The prognosis of infants with VSD is good. It is difficult to provide precise figures because of ascertainment bias in old studies. However, most infants born with VSDs are asymptomatic, 40 percent of defects spontaneously close within 2 years, and 60 percent close within 5 years.[7-9] In a series of 428 symptomatic infants, 130 (30 percent) required surgery because of intractable congestive heart failure and failure to thrive.[10] In a group of 50 infants less than 18 months of age treated with primary closure of the VSD, there was a 6 percent postoperative mortality rate. In addition, 14 percent had seizures attributable to low cardiac output and hypoxic episodes, and 49 percent had rhythm disturbances (right bundle branch block isolated or associated with left hemiblocks).[10] Postoperative studies showed normal pressure in the pulmonary artery.[10]

Obstetrical Management

A careful search for other cardiac and extracardiac abnormalities is indicated if the prenatal diagnosis of VSD is made. An amniocentesis for chromosomal analysis is recommended. In the presence of an isolated VSD, standard obstetrical management is not altered. Infants should be delivered in a tertiary care center where a pediatric cardiologist is immediately available.

REFERENCES

1. Allan LD, Crawford DC, Anderson RH, et al.: Echocardiographic and anatomical correlations in fetal congenital heart disease. Br Heart J 52:542, 1984
2. Allan LD, Tynan M, Campbell S, et al.: Identification of congenital cardiac malformations by echocardiography in mid-trimester fetus. Br Heart J 46:358, 1981
3. Alpert BS, Mellits ED, Rowe RD: Spontaneous closure of small ventricular septal defects. Probability rates in the first five years of life. Am J Dis Child 125:194, 1973
4. Anderson RH, Lenox CC, Zuberbuhler JR: Mechanisms of closure of perimembranous ventricular septal defect. Am J Cardiol 52:341, 1983
5. Becker AE, Anderson RH: Pathology of Congenital Heart Disease. London, Butterworths, 1981.
6. Capelli H, Andrade JL, Somerville J: Classification of the site of ventricular septal defect by 2-dimensional echocardiography. Am J Cardiol 51:1474, 1983
7. Hoffman JIE: Natural history of congenital heart disease. Problems in its assessment, with special reference to ventricular septal defects. Circulation 37:97, 1968.
8. Hoffman JIE, Rudolph AM: The natural history of isolated ventricular septal defect. With special reference to selection of patients for surgery. Adv Pediatr 17:57, 1970.
9. Hoffman JIE, Rudolph AM: The natural history of ventricular septal defects in infancy. Am J Cardiol 16:634, 1965.
10. Rein JG, Freed MD, Norwood WI, et al.: Early and late results of closure of ventricular septal defect in infancy. Ann Thorac Surg 24:19, 1977.
11. Rowe RD, Freedom RM, Mehrizi A, et al.: The Neonate with Congenital Heart Disease, 2d ed. Philadelphia, Saunders, 1981.
12. Rudolph AM: Congenital Diseases of the Heart: Clinical-Physiologic Considerations in Diagnosis and Management. Chicago, Year Book, 1974.
13. Silverman NH, Golbus MS: Echocardiographic techniques for assessing normal and abnormal fetal cardiac anatomy. J Am Coll Cardiol 5:20S, 1985.
14. Soto B, Becker AE, Moulaert AJ, et al.: Classification of ventricular septal defects. Br Heart J 43:332, 1980.

Atrioventricular Septal Defects

Synonyms
Ostium primum atrial septal defect, atrioventricular canal malformation, endocardial cushion defects, and persistent ostium atrioventriculare commune.

Definition
Atrioventricular septal defects (AVSD) include a spectrum of cardiac anomalies involving to a different extent the atrial and ventricular septa and the atrioventricular valves.

Embryology
In the primitive heart, the atrium and common ventricle communicate through a single opening, the atrioventricular canal. The growth of the endocardial cushions divides this opening into two distinct orifices at the 6th week (Fig. 4–34). Subsequently, the fusion of the atrial and ventricular septum partitions the heart into four chambers. AVSDs result from the persistence of the primitive atrioventricular canal. Since the endocardial cushions participate in the development of the atrioventricular valves, anomalies at the level of the tricuspid and mitral valves are the rule in these defects.

Pathology
AVSDs are subdivided into complete and incomplete or partial forms (Fig. 4–35).[3]

Incomplete AVSDs (also known as "ostium primum atrial septal defects") are characterized by separate atrioventricular orifices. There is usually an interatrial communication or a communication between the left ventricle and the right atrium. Less frequently, an interventricular communication occurs. The right atrioventricular valve is often normal. The left atrioventricular valve has usually three leaflets, and there is a cleft between the anterior and posterior ones (Fig. 4–35).[3]

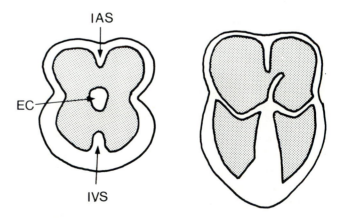

Figure 4–34. Embryology of the atrioventricular junction. The primitive atrioventricular canal is partitioned by the growth of the endocardial cushions (EC), interatrial septum (IAS), and interventricular septum (IVS).

LV   RV

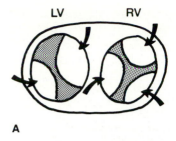   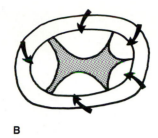   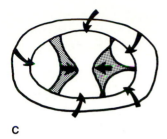

A   **B**   **C**

Figure 4–35. The atrioventricular junction as seen from above in the normal heart (**A**), in the atrioventricular canal with a single orifice (**B**), and in the atrioventricular canal with two orifices (**C**). The curved arrows indicate the leaflets of the atrioventricular valve. The straight arrows in C indicate the fused leaflets that partition the atrioventricular orifice. LV, left ventricle; RV, right ventricle.

Complete AVSDs are characterized by a common atrioventricular orifice guarded by a common valve with five leaflets (Fig. 4–35). The anterior and posterior leaflets are attached on both sides of the ventricular septum and are, therefore, called "bridging leaflets." There is a defect in the lower portion of the atrial septum and in the higher portion of the ventricular septum that assumes an oval configuration. The size of this defect may vary. According to Rastelli et al.,[13–15] the complete form of AVSD can be subdivided into three types according to the insertion of the tensor apparatus of the anterior leaflet. In type 1, the anterior bridging leaflet is attached by chordae tendinae to both sides of the ventricular septum. In type 2, the leaflet is unattached to the septum but attached medially to an anomalous papillary muscle in the right ventricle. In type 3, the leaflet is free floating or unattached to the septum. It is attached to the usual papillary muscles on both sides. This classification has surgical relevance.

It is a common finding in AVSDs that the atrial septum secundum is spared. Sometimes, especially when associated with atrial isomerism, the septum secundum is lacking. Such an anomaly is commonly defined as "common atrium."[3]

Complete AVSDs are frequently associated with malpositions of the heart, namely, mesocardia and dextrocardia.[6]

As a consequence of the AVSD, distortion of the conduction tissues is often seen and accounts for the frequently observed cardiac dysrhythmias (atrioventricular block).[3]

Associated Anomalies

AVSDs are frequently associated with other cardiac defects, including coarctation of the aorta, truncoconal abnormalities (tetralogy of Fallot, double outlet right ventricle, transposition of the great arteries), pulmonary stenosis or atresia, and many others. Of special relevance for prenatal diagnosis purposes is the association of AVSDs with Down syndrome[16] and asplenia and polysplenia syndromes.

Hemodynamic Considerations

The major problem in the fetus is the frequent incompetence of the atrioventricular valves due to their distorted anatomy. This may lead to regurgitation toward the atria and congestive heart failure.[11] The existence of other associated cardiac anomalies may further complicate the hemodynamic disturbance. In the neonatal period, the decrease in pulmonary vascular resistance rapidly leads to a large left-to-right shunt, which in turn leads to pulmonary hypertension.

Diagnosis

The diagnosis of complete AVSD relies on demonstration of the defect of the inferior portion of the atrial septum and of the superior portion of the ventricular septum. The presence of a common leaflet at the level of the atrioventricular valve can also be detected and allows differentiation between complete and incomplete forms[1,2,10–12,17] (Figs. 4–36, 4–37). In the incomplete form of AVSD, the only demonstrable echocardiographic finding may be the defect in the lower portion of the atrial septum. It has been demonstrated recently that pulsed Doppler ultrasound plays a major role in the diagnostic workup and intrauterine follow-up of fetal AVSDs by allowing the identification of atrioventricular valve insufficiency, which represents a poor prognostic factor.[18]

Careful evaluation of the entire cardiac anatomy is necessary to exclude the presence of associated anomalies that could complicate the prognosis for the infant.

Prognosis

The natural history of nonoperated infants with complete atrioventricular canal has been described by Berger et al.[5] They reported that the survival rate was 54 percent at 6 months of age, 35 percent at 12 months, 15 percent at 24 months, and 4 percent at 5 years. The first surgical approach to this defect was intended to deal with the problem of pulmonary hypertension by banding the pulmonary artery.[8]

More recently, intracardiac repair of the defect has been carried out in several centers. Berger et al.[5] reported a 91 percent long-term survival with primary intracardiac repair. Bender et al.[4] reported 2 operative and 1 postoperative deaths in 24 operated infants, for a mortality rate of 8 percent and 4 percent, respectively. Chin et al.[7] have described two consecutive groups of patients. The first group included 13 infants operated on between 1975 and 1977, with an operative mortality of 62 percent and late mortality of 7 percent. In the second group of 30 infants operated on between 1978 and 1980, the operative mortality decreased to 17 percent and late mortality was 6 percent. Prognostic factors related to the outcome of operative procedures include (1) deficiency of atrioventricular tissue, (2) presence of ventricular hypoplasia, (3) malalignment of the common atrioventricular valve, (4) the presence of double orifice mitral valve, (5) the presence of solitary left ventricular papillary muscle group, and (6) the presence of additional muscular septal defects.

Obstetrical Management

An amniocentesis is strongly recommended because of the association of this defect with Down syndrome. A careful ultrasound evaluation of the entire fetal anatomy is also mandatory. Diagnosis before

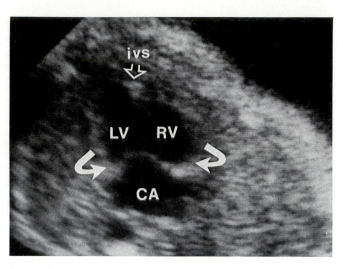

Figure 4–37. Four-chamber view in a 28-week fetus with complete atrioventricular canal. The curved arrows indicate the common atrioventricular valve. LV, left ventricle; RV, right ventricle; ivs, interventricular septum; CA, common atrium.

viability may allow the parents to opt for pregnancy termination. Diagnosis in the third trimester should not alter obstetrical management. Delivery in a tertiary care center where a pediatric cardiologist is immediately available is mandatory. Every effort should be made to prolong pregnancy to term because, at present, intracardiac surgery is exceedingly risky in preterm infants. In utero congestive heart failure is an ominous sign,[11,18] since it suggests profound valvular incompetence.

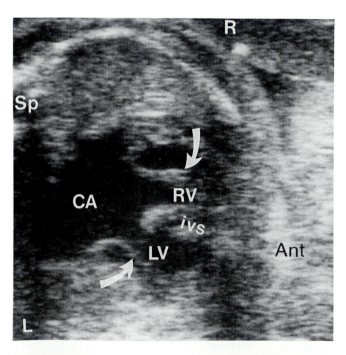

Figure 4–36. Four chamber view in a fetus with complete atrioventricular canal. The diastolic frame reveals the complete absence of the interatrial septum and the presence of a common atrioventricular valve (*arrows*). CA, common atrium; LV, left ventricle; RV, right ventricle; ivs, interventricular septum; Sp, spine; R, right; L, left; Ant, anterior.

REFERENCES

1. Allan LD, Crawford DC, Anderson RH, et al.: Echocardiographic and anatomical correlations in fetal congenital heart disease. Br Heart J 52:542, 1984.
2. Allan LD, Tynan M, Campbell S, et al.: Normal fetal cardiac anatomy: A basis for the echocardiographic detection of abnormalities. Prenatal Diagn 1:131, 1981.
3. Becker AE, Anderson RH: Pathology of Congenital Heart Disease. London, Butterworths, 1981.
4. Bender HW, Hammon JW, Hubbard SG, et al.: Repair of atrioventricular canal malformation in the first year of life. J Thorac Cardiovasc Surg 84:515, 1982.
5. Berger TJ, Blackstone EH, Kirklin JW, et al.: Survival and probability of cure without and with operation in complete atrioventricular canal. Ann Thorac Surg 27:104, 1979.
6. Bharati S, Lev M: Fundamentals of clinical cardiology. The spectrum of common atrioventricular orifice (canal). Am Heart J 86:553, 1973.
7. Chin AJ, Keane JF, Norwood WI, et al.: Repair of complete common atrioventricular canal in infancy. J Thorac Cardiovasc Surg 84:437, 1982.

8. Epstein ML, Moller JH, Amplatz K, et al.: Pulmonary artery banding in infants with complete atrioventricular canal. J Thorac Cardiovasc Surg 78:28, 1979.

9. Fisher EA, Doshi M, DuBrow IW, et al.: Effect of palliative and corrective surgery on ventricular volumes in complete atrioventricular canal. Pediatr Cardiol 5:159, 1984.

10. Kleinman CS, Santulli TV: Ultrasonic evaluation of the fetal human heart. Semin Perinatol 7:90, 1983.

11. Kleinman CS, Donnerstein RL, De Vore GR, et al.: Fetal echocardiography for evaluation of in utero congestive heart failure: A technique for study of nonimmune fetal hydrops. N Engl J Med 306:568, 1982.

12. Pilu G, Rizzo N, Orsini LF, et al.: La diagnosi delle anomalie cardiache strutturali nel feto mediante ultrasonografia bidimensionale. Ultr Ost Gin 1:257, 1983.

13. Rastelli GC, Kirklin JW, Kincaid OW: Angiocardiography of persistent common atrioventricular canal. Mayo Clin Proc 42:200, 1967.

14. Rastelli GC, Kirklin JW, Titus JL: Anatomic observations on complete form of persistent common atrioventricular canal with special reference to atrioventricular valves. Mayo Clin Proc 41:296, 1966.

15. Rastelli GC, Ongley PA, Kirklin JW, et al.: Surgical repair of the complete form of persistent common atrioventricular canal. J Thorac Cardiovasc Surg 55:299, 1968.

16. Rowe RD, Uchida IA: Cardiac malformation in mongolism. A prospective study of 184 mongoloid children. Am J Med 31:726, 1961.

17. Silverman NH, Golbus MS: Echocardiographic techniques for assessing normal and abnormal fetal cardiac anatomy. J Am Coll Cardiol 5:20S, 1985.

18. Silverman NH, Kleinman CS, Rudolph AM, et al.: Fetal atrioventricular valve insufficiency associated with nonimmune hydrops: A two-dimensional echocardiographic and pulsed Doppler ultrasound study. Circulation 72:825, 1985.

Univentricular Heart

Synonym
Single ventricle.

Definition
The definition of univentricular heart is controversial. According to some authors,[11] this term refers to a condition in which there are two atrioventricular valves or a common atrioventricular valve and a single ventricle (classic double inlet single ventricle). According to Becker and Anderson,[2] univentricular heart indicates a group of anomalies in which the entire atrioventricular junction is connected to only one chamber in the ventricular mass. This includes, by definition, the classic double inlet single ventricle and the absence of one atrioventricular connection.

Embryology
The double inlet univentricular heart seems to be related to failure of development of the interventricular septum. Absence of one atrioventricular connection results from mitral or tricuspid atresia.

Pathology
According to Van Praagh et al.,[11] the univentricular heart is classified as type A or C according to the presence or absence of outflow tract. Depending on the relationship between the aorta and pulmonary artery, three subtypes are defined: (1) normal relationship (the aorta is posterior and to the left of the pulmonary artery), (2) the aorta is anterior and to the right, and (3) the aorta is anterior and to the left. Six different varieties of univentricular heart are possible.

According to the elegant definition of Becker and Anderson,[2] the univentricular heart is "a generic term for a group of anomalies unified by their ventricular morphology. The unifying criterion is that the entire atrioventricular junction is connected to only one chamber in the ventricular mass." The chamber may be either of left ventricular, right ventricular, or undetermined type depending on the trabecular pattern. In 85 percent of patients, the chamber has a left ventricular morphology.

A second rudimentary ventricular chamber may be present. In these cases, a rudimentary ventricular septum that does not extend to the crux can be seen. The atrioventricular valves may straddle the septum. In a univentricular heart of left ventricular type, the rudimentary chamber is usually anterior. In a right univentricular heart, the rudimentary chamber is usually posterior, and a rudimentary ventricular septum extends to the crux.

The rudimentary chamber may or may not be connected to the great arteries. Aortic and pulmonic stenosis are frequently seen.

In the case of tricuspid atresia with absence of the right ventricular connection, the right atrium communicates with the main ventricular chamber through an atrial septal defect. An interatrial communication is equally necessary in cases of mitral atresia.

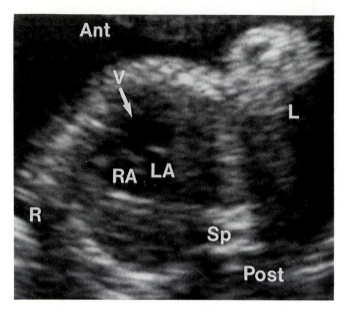

Figure 4–38. Double inlet univentricular heart. In this four chamber view, the two atrioventricular valves are seen emptying into a single ventricular chamber (V). LA, left atrium; RA, right atrium; Sp, spine; Ant, anterior; Post, posterior; L, left; R, right.

Conduction defects are frequent in univentricular heart. Most probably, this is related to the aberrant anatomy of the conduction system due to the anatomic absence or derangement of the ventricular septum.[2]

Hemodynamic Considerations

Univentricular heart per se is not expected to cause intrauterine congestive heart failure. Since the pressure in both ventricular cavities is believed to be equal in the fetus,[10] the presence of a single ventricular chamber should not be the cause of major hemodynamic perturbations, and the onset of congestive heart failure in utero is unlikely. Exceptions may be represented by those cases associated with obstructions to intracardiac blood flow (stenosis or atresia of the atrioventricular valves) or with incompetence of the atrioventricular valves.

After birth, the hemodynamics of univentricular heart depend largely on associated anomalies. The simultaneous decrease in the arterial pressure in the pulmonary vascular bed and increase in the systemic arterial pressure usually leads to a large left-to-right shunt at the level of the ventricle. However, the presence of pulmonic stenosis may lead to a severe reduction in pulmonary blood flow.

Diagnosis

The diagnosis of double inlet univentricular heart relies on the demonstration of two atrioventricular valves connected to a main ventricular chamber (Fig. 4–38). Ultrasound may also demonstrate the presence and position of a rudimentary chamber (Fig. 4–39) and the ventriculoarterial connection. Differential di-

agnoses include a large VSD and an AVSD. Recognition of a rudimentary chamber and study of the ventriculoarterial connection are helpful in differential diagnosis.[1] Furthermore, AVSDs are usually characterized by a defect in the atrial septum primum.

In the presence of tricuspid or mitral atresia, ultrasound can demonstrate the absence of one atrioventricular connection (Fig. 4–40).

Prognosis

The clinical course of unoperated patients with univentricular heart who survive the neonatal period has been described by Moodie et al.[8] They reported their data using a modification of Van Praagh's classification proposed by Hallerman et al.[5] Patients with type A had a 50 percent survival rate 14 years after the diagnosis, whereas patients with type C had a 50 percent survival rate 4 years after the diagnosis.

Palliative procedures include systemic pulmonary artery shunts and pulmonary artery banding. Using these procedures, a 5-year 70 percent survival rate after diagnosis has been reported for type A and 54 percent for type C.[9] Intracardiac repair of the univentricular heart has recently been suggested. McKay et al.[7] reported 16 patients having ventricular septation with double inlet univentricular heart. Seven hospital deaths occurred. The 9 survivors were followed for a period ranging from 2 months to 4 years. They were all in New York Heart Association functional class I.

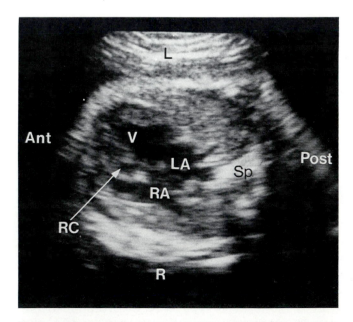

Figure 4–39. Univentricular heart. In this scanning plane, the main ventricular chamber (V) and an anterior rudimentary chamber (RC) are imaged. RA, right atrium; LA, left atrium; Sp, spine; Ant, anterior; Post, posterior, L, left; R, right. *(Reproduced with permission from Bovicelli L, Baccarani G, Picchio FM, Pilu G: Ecocardiografia Fetale. La Diagnosi ed il Trattamento prenatale delle Cardiopatie Congenite. Milan, Masson, 1985.)*

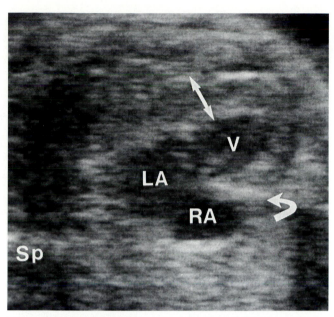

Figure 4—40. Tricuspid atresia. The left atrium (LA) is connected to a single ventricular chamber (V) with hypertrophic walls (*double arrow*). The right atrium (RA) lacks a connection with the ventricular mass. A bright linear echo arises from the atretic tricuspid plane (*curved arrow*). LA, left atrium. Sp, spine.

Obstetrical Management

When the diagnosis is made before viability, the option of pregnancy termination should be offered. In all pregnancies, a careful search for associated cardiac and extracardiac anomalies, including karyotype evaluation, is recommended.

Serial ultrasound examinations should be performed to search for signs of congestive heart failure. The association of hydrops with a structural cardiac defect is an ominous combination. Optimal management of these patients has not been established. The option of early delivery may be considered, but the parents should be aware that the mortality rate in these patients is extremely high.[6] In the absence of congestive heart failure, there is no indication to alter standard obstetrical management, but delivery in a tertiary care center where a pediatric cardiologist is immediately available is mandatory.

REFERENCES

1. Allan LD, Crawford DC, Anderson RH, et al.: Echocardiographic and anatomical correlations in fetal congenital heart disease. Br Heart J 52:542, 1984.
2. Becker AE, Anderson RH: Pathology of Congenital Heart Disease. London, Butterworths, 1981.
3. Bisset GS, Hirschfeld SS: The univentricular heart: Combined two-dimensional-pulsed Doppler (duplex) echocardiographic evaluation. Am J Cardiol 51:1149, 1983.
4. Goldberg HL, Sniderman K, Devereux RB, et al.: Prolonged survival (62 years) with single ventricle. Am J Cardiol 52:214, 1983.
5. Hallerman FJ, Davis GD, Ritter DG, et al.: Roentgenographic features of common ventricle. Radiology 87:409, 1966.
6. Kleinman CS, Donnerstein RL, DeVore GR, et al.: Fetal echocardiography for evaluation of in utero congestive heart failure: A technique for study of nonimmune fetal hydrops. N Engl J Med 306:568, 1982.
7. McKay R, Pacifico AD, Blackstone EH, et al.: Septation of the univentricular heart with left anterior subaortic outlet chamber. J Thorac Cardiovasc Surg 84:77, 1982.
8. Moodie DS, Ritter DG, Tajik AJ, et al.: Long-term follow-up in the unoperated univentricular heart. Am J Cardiol 53:1124, 1984.
9. Moodie DS, Ritter DG, Tajik AH, et al.: Long-term follow-up after palliative operation for univentricular heart. Am J Cardiol 53:1648, 1984.
10. Rudolph AM: Congenital Diseases of the Heart: Clinical-Physiological Considerations in Diagnosis and Management. Chicago, Year Book, 1974.
11. Van Praagh R, Ongley PA, Swan HJC: Anatomic types of single or common ventricle in man: Morphologic and geometric aspects of sixty necropsied cases. Am J Cardiol 13:367, 1964.

Ebstein's Anomaly

Definition

Ebstein's anomaly is a congenital defect usually characterized by downward displacement of the septal and posterior leaflets of the tricuspid valve, with dysplasia of this valve.

Etiology

Ebstein's anomaly of the tricuspid valve has been reported to occur in 10 percent of cases of chronic maternal lithium intake during pregnancy.[8]

Pathology

Displacement of the tricuspid valve leaflets leads to division of the right ventricle into two components: a superior or atrialized portion and an inferior, functional chamber. The walls of the right ventricle are generally thin.[4]

The tricuspid valve is most frequently insufficient, and this results in right atrial enlargement. Cardiomegaly is almost the rule in these patients.

Although the posterior and septal leaflets of the valve are displaced downward, the anterior leaflet may be normal.[4]

Associated Anomalies

ASDS (secundum type or patent foramen ovale), pulmonary atresia or stenosis, patent ductus arteriosus, tetralogy of Fallot, coarctation of the aorta, atrioventricular canal, and transposition of the great vessels[4] are possible associated anomalies.

Hemodynamic Considerations

Dysplasia and displacement of the tricuspid valve leads to tricuspid insufficiency, with blood regurgitation into the right atrium during systole. In turn, this may lead to congestive heart failure in utero. Congestive heart failure is found in 50 percent of affected newborns.[10]

Diagnosis

The main criterion for diagnosis is demonstration of downward displacement of the tricuspid valve into the right ventricle. The right atrium is generally extremely enlarged (Fig. 4–41).[2,13] Doppler studies may be helpful in assessing tricuspid valve regurgitation. An enlarged right atrium without valve displacement and regurgitation may be caused by "idiopathic giant right atrium."

Prognosis

In the absence of tricuspid regurgitation, this condition may be completely asymptomatic. Such patients do not develop symptoms until adolescence or adult life. On the other hand, symptomatic newborns often develop congestive heart failure. In a series of 23 patients, 12 died during the first month of life or later in infancy.[10] Advances in cardiovascular surgery have improved the prognosis for these patients. In a total of 147 cases reported in nine series,[1,3,5–7,9,11,12,14] there were 19 operative deaths (12.9 percent) and 11 late deaths (7.4 percent). In the largest available series,[5] cardiac surgery resulted in important improvements in the clinical condition of the patients. The majority of the 22 patients with long-term follow-up improved from New York Heart Association class III or IV to class I or II.

Obstetrical Management

When the diagnosis is made before viability, the option of pregnancy termination should be offered. A careful search for associated cardiac and extracardiac anomalies, including karyotype, is recommended for all cases.

Serial ultrasound examinations should be performed to search for signs of congestive heart failure. The association of hydrops with a structural cardiac defect is an ominous combination. The optimal man-

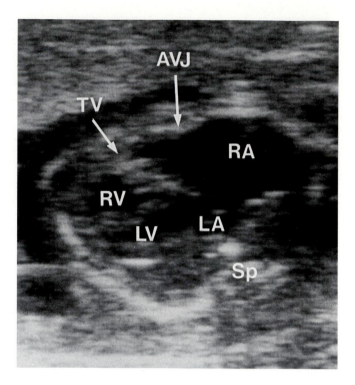

Figure 4–41. Four chamber view in a fetus with Ebstein's anomaly of the tricuspid valve. The right atrium (RA) is disproportionately enlarged. The sail-like tricuspid valve (TV) is displaced apically far away from the atrioventricular junction (AVJ). RV, right ventricle; LV, left ventricle; LA, left atrium; Sp, spine.

agement of these patients has yet to be established. The option of early delivery may be considered, but the parents should be aware that the mortality rate in these patients is extremely high.

In the absence of congestive heart failure, there is no indication to alter standard obstetrical management, but delivery in a tertiary care center where a pediatric cardiologist is immediately available is mandatory.

REFERENCES

1. Abe T, Komatsu S: Valve replacement for Ebstein's anomaly of the tricuspid valve. Early and long-term results of eight cases. Chest 84:414, 1983.
2. Allan LD, Crawford DC, Anderson RH, et al.: Echocardiographic and anatomical correlations in fetal congenital heart disease. Br Heart J 52:542, 1984.
3. Barbero-Marcial M, Verginelli G, Awad M, et al.: Surgical treatment of Ebstein's anomaly. Early and late results in twenty patients subjected to valve replacement. J Thorac Cardiovasc Surg 78:416, 1979.
4. Becker AE, Anderson RH: Pathology of Congenital Heart Disease. London, Butterworths, 1981.
5. Danielson GK: Ebstein's anomaly: Editorial comments

and personal observations. Ann Thorac Surg 34:396, 1982.

6. Danielson GK, Maloney JD, Devloo RA: Surgical repair of Ebstein's anomaly. Mayo Clin Proc 54:185, 1979.

7. Mattila S, Harjula A, Kyllonen KEJ, et al.: Surgical intervention in cases of Ebstein's anomaly. Abnormal origin and structure of the tricuspid valve. Scand J Thorac Cardiovasc Surg 16:223, 1982.

8. Nora JJ, Nora AH: Genetics and Counseling in Cardiovascular Diseases. Springfield, IL, Chas. C Thomas, 1978.

9. Raj-Behl P, Blesovsky A: Ebstein's anomaly: Sixteen years' experience with valve replacement without plication of the right ventricle. Thorax 39:8, 1984.

10. Rowe RD, Freedom RM, Mehrizi A, Bloom KR: The

11. Schmidt-Habelmann P, Meisner H, Struck E, et al.: Results of valvuloplasty for Ebstein's anomaly. Thorac Cardiovasc Surg 29:155, 1981.

12. Shigenobu M, Mendez MA, Zubiate P, et al.: Thirteen years' experience with the Kay-Shiley disc valve for tricuspid replacement in Ebstein's anomaly. Ann Thorac Surg 29:423, 1980.

13. Silverman NH, Golbus MS: Echocardiographic techniques for assessing normal and abnormal fetal cardiac anatomy. J Am Coll Cardiol 5:20S, 1985.

14. Westaby S, Karp RB, Kirklin JW, et al.: Surgical treatment in Ebstein's malformation. Ann Thorac Surg 34:388, 1982.

Neonate with Congenital Heart Disease, 2d ed. Philadelphia, Saunders, 1981.

Hypoplastic Left Heart Syndrome

Synonym
Aortic atresia.

Definition
Hypoplastic left heart syndrome (HLHS) is a condition characterized by the association of a diminutive left ventricle with aortic atresia and mitral hypoplasia or atresia.

Etiology
Shokeir[22] reported five families in which HLHS was transmitted as an autosomal recessive condition. Subsequently, Nora and Nora[15] disputed this view, although they suggested a rather high recurrence risk for this anomaly (4 percent after the birth of one affected infant and 25 percent after the birth of two).

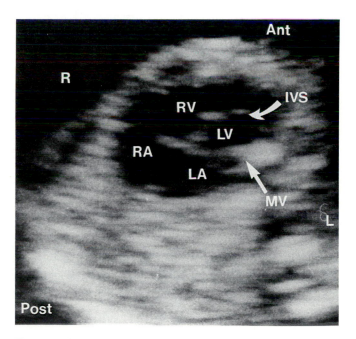

Figure 4–43. Hypoplastic left heart syndrome in a 21-week-old fetus. Note the diminutive left ventricle (LV) and the hyperechogenic atretic mitral valve (MV). RV, right ventricle; LA, left atrium; RA, right atrium; IVS, interventricular septum; Ant, anterior; Post, posterior; L, left; R, right. (*Reproduced with permission from Bovicelli L, Baccarani G, Picchio FM, Pilu G: Ecocardiografia Fetale. La Diagnosi ed il Trattamento Prenatale delle Cardiopatie Congenite. Milan, Masson, 1985.*)

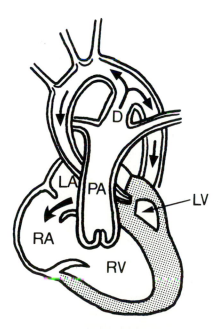

Figure 4–42. Schematic representation of the circulation in hypoplastic left heart syndrome. RV, right ventricle; LV, left ventricle; RA, right atrium; LA, left atrium; PA, pulmonary artery; D, ductus arteriosus.

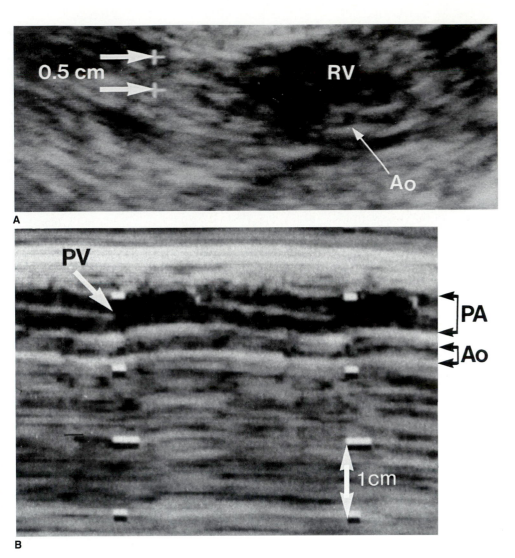

Figure 4–44. A. Note the hypoplastic ascending aorta (Ao) in the same patient as in Figure 4–43. RV, right ventricle. **B.** M-mode echocardiogram comparing the size of the roots of the aorta (Ao) and pulmonary artery (PA). Note the normal opening movement of the pulmonary valve (PV). *(Figure B reproduced with permission from Bovicelli L, Baccarani G, Picchio FM, Pilu G: Ecocardiografia Fetale. La Diagnosi ed il Trattamento Prenatale delle Cardiopatie Congenite. Milan, Masson, 1985.)*

Pathogenesis

The pathogenesis of HLHS is unknown. Development of the cardiac chambers is thought to be related to blood flow rather than to intracardiac blood pressure. HLHS is probably the consequence of decreased perfusion of the left ventricle and atrium. It has been postulated that this could result from premature closure of the foramen ovale. However, this hypothesis seems unlikely, since in the majority of cases, a large interatrial communication is present. A primary role may be played by atresia of the aortic valve, causing diminished right-to-left shunt at the level of the atria.

Pathology

The left atrium is either small or normal in size. An interatrial communication is almost always the rule in newborns and provides a path for oxygenated blood coming through the pulmonary veins into the right heart. Left-to-right shunting at the level of the atrium more frequently occurs through a communication created by herniation and prolapse of the valve of the foramen ovale into the right atrium. In the majority of cases, the mitral valve is hypoplastic and stenotic. In rare instances, an imperforate membrane is found (mitral atresia). The left ventricle is usually severely underdeveloped, although there is a broad spectrum of hypoplasia. The aortic valve is an imperforate membrane in the majority of cases. The ascending aorta and the aortic arch are hypoplastic.[2,18,21] Eighty percent of patients have an associated coarctation of the aorta.[7]

Hemodynamic Considerations

The right ventricle supplies both the pulmonary and systemic circulations. Pulmonary venous return is diverted from the left atrium to the right atrium through the interatrial communication. Through the pulmonary artery and the ductus arteriosus, the right ventricle supplies the descending aorta and, in a

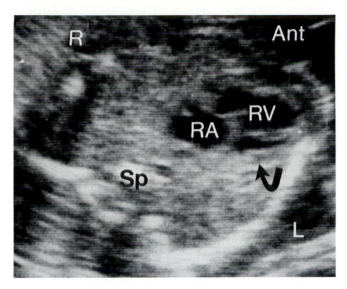

Figure 4–45. A. Hypoplastic left heart syndrome in a 21-week-old fetus. The left ventricular cavity cannot be visualized (*curved arrow*). RV, right ventricle; RA, right atrium; Sp, spine; Ant, anterior; L, left; R, right.

retrograde manner, the aortic arch, ascending aorta, and coronary circulation (Fig. 4–42).[8]

Work overload to the right ventricle may lead to intrauterine congestive heart failure.[12,20,23] Untreated infants with HLHS usually die within 6 weeks of life[4] from a combination of three problems: (1) cyanosis in patients with an inadequate left-to-right shunt at the level of the atria, (2) decreased perfusion of the aorta and coronary arteries, resulting in generalized tissue hypoxia and compromise of myocardial function, and

(3) congestive heart failure due to right ventricular volume and pressure overload.

Diagnosis

In the fetus, both ventricles should be of equal size. Logically, recognition of HLHS depends on demonstration of a small left ventricular cavity.[12,17,20,23] Nomograms of the inner dimensions of the ventricular chambers obtained from real-time[19] and M-mode[1] are available (see Fig 4–22). However, the reader should be aware of the limitations of biometry for prenatal diagnosis of congenital heart disease: (1) normal dimensions encompass a very wide range, and (2) the anatomic landmarks commonly used for standardization of measurements may be altered in malformed hearts. In some patients, the condition is obvious, and measurements are unnecessary. A useful "rule" to remember is that the apex of both ventricles should be at the same level. Even severe dilatation of one ventricle will not alter this because the ventricle will increase in diameter, but very little in length. Associated findings, such as atresia of the aortic valve and hypoplasia of the proximal portion of the ascending aorta,[10,17,23] should be looked for when suspicion arises (Figs. 4–43 to 4–45).

Prognosis

HLHS is responsible for 25 percent of cardiac deaths in the first week of life. Almost all of the affected infants die within 6 weeks if they are not treated.[4] An exceptional infant has survived 3.5 years without surgery.[14] Several palliative procedures, including atrial septectomy,[5] banding of the pulmonary ar-

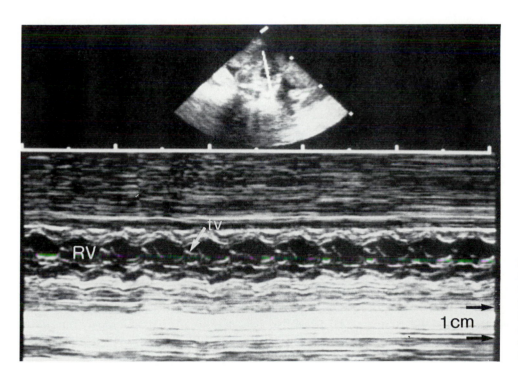

Figure 4–45. B. In the same patient as in Figure A, the M-mode echocardiogram directed through the atrioventricular junction demonstrates a large right ventricular (RV) cavity within which the tricuspid valve (tv) can be seen. The left ventricle cannot be demonstrated.

tery,[11] and creation of an aortopulmonary shunt[3,6,13] have been used. Patients undergoing these procedures either died at some time after the operation or have been followed for a very limited period of time. Norwood et al.[16] reported a 6-month survivor who had been treated with an initial palliative procedure and a modified Fontan operation that connected the left atrium to the tricuspid valve and the right atrium to the pulmonary artery. Subsequently, the same group reported 10 infants with HLHS who survived the palliative procedure. Three patients subsequently underwent a modified Fontan procedure, and two were alive 9 and 12 months after surgery. Three patients were awaiting repair at the time of the report.[9]

Notwithstanding this valuable experience, HLHS still has an extremely poor prognosis. The policy of cardiovascular surgeons varies, and reparative procedures for this condition are not available in every center. This consideration is relevant to obstetrical management. Transplant of a baboon heart to a newborn human infant has recently been attempted without success.

Obstetrical Management

When the diagnosis is made before viability, the option of pregnancy termination should be offered. After viability, a frank discussion with the parents is recommended. A careful search for associated anomalies, including fetal karyotyping, is recommended. The association of HLHS with in utero congestive heart failure is a sign of an extremely poor prognosis, and we believe that in these cases a conservative obstetrical approach should be followed. We would consider the option of not performing a cesarean section for fetal distress if the parents so desired under these circumstances. If the parents want every effort to be made to improve survival, delivery should occur in a tertiary care center where a cardiovascular team is prepared to undertake surgical care of the infant.

REFERENCES

1. Allan LD, Joseph MC, Boyd EGCA, et al.: M-mode echocardiography in the developing human fetus. Br Heart J 47:573, 1982.
2. Becker AE, Anderson RH: Pathology of Congenital Heart Disease. London, Butterworths, 1981.
3. Behrendt DM, Rocchini A: An operation for the hypoplastic left heart syndrome: Preliminary report. Ann Thorac Surg 32:284, 1981.
4. Doty DB: Aortic atresia. J Thorac Cardiovasc Surg 79:462, 1980.
5. Doty DB, Knott HW: Hypoplastic left heart syndrome. Experience with an operation to establish functionally normal circulation. J Thorac Cardiovasc Surg 74:624, 1977.
6. Doty DB, Marvin WJ, Schieken RM, et al.: Hypoplastic left heart syndrome. Successful palliation with a new operation. J Thorac Cardiovasc Surg 80:148, 1980.
7. Hawkins JA, Doty DB: Aortic atresia: Morphologic characteristics affecting survival and operative palliation. J Thorac Cardiovasc Surg 88:620, 1984
8. Kanjuh VI, Eliot RS, Edwards JE: Coexistent mitral and aortic valvular atresia. A pathologic study of 14 cases. Am J Cardiol 15:611, 1965.
9. Lang P, Norwood WI: Hemodynamic assessment after palliative surgery for hypoplastic left heart syndrome. Circulation 68:104, 1983.
10. Lange LW, Sahn DJ, Allen HD, et al.: Cross-sectional echocardiography in hypoplastic left ventricle: Echocardiographic–angiographic–anatomic correlations. Pediatr Cardiol 1:287, 1980.
11. Levitsky S, van der Horst RL, Hastreiter AR, et al.: Surgical palliation in aortic atresia. J Thorac Cardiovasc Surg 79:456, 1980.
12. Mandorla S, Narducci PL, Migliozzi L, et al.: Ecocardiografia fetale. Diagnosi prenatale di sindrome di cuore sinistro ipoplasico. G Ital Cardiol 14:517, 1984.
13. Mohri H, Horiuchi T, Haneda K, et al.: Surgical treatment for hypoplastic left heart syndrome. Case reports. J Thorac Cardiovasc Surg 78:223, 1979.
14. Moodie DS, Gallen WJ, Friedberg DZ: Congenital aortic atresia. Report of long survival and some speculations about surgical approaches. J Thorac Cardiovasc Surg 63:726, 1972.
15. Nora JJ, Nora AH: Genetics and Genetic Counseling in Cardiovascular Diseases. Springfield, IL, Chas. C Thomas, 1978.
16. Norwood WI, Lang P, Hansen DD: Physiologic repair of aortic atresia—Hypoplastic left heart syndrome. N Engl J Med 308:23, 1983.
17. Pilu G, Rizzo N, Orsini LF, et al.: La diagnosi prenatale delle anomalie cardiache strutturali nel feto mediante ultrasonografia bidimensionale. Ultr Ost Gin 1:257, 1983.
18. Roberts WC, Perry LW, Chandra RS, et al.: Aortic valve atresia: A new classification based on necropsy study of 73 cases. Am J Cardiol 37:753, 1976.
19. Sahn DJ, Lange LW, Allen HD, et al.: Quantitative real-time cross-sectional echocardiography in the developing normal human fetus and newborn. Circulation 62:588, 1980.
20. Sahn DJ, Shenker L, Reed KL, et al.: Prenatal ultrasound diagnosis of hypoplastic left heart syndrome in utero associated with hydrops fetalis. Am Heart J 104:1368, 1982.
21. Saied A, Folger GM: Hypoplastic left heart syndrome. Clinicopathologic and hemodynamic correlation. Am J Cardiol 29:190, 1972.
22. Shokeir MHK: Hypoplastic left heart syndrome: An autosomal recessive disorder. Clin Genet 2:7, 1971.
23. Silverman NH, Golbus MS: Echocardiographic techniques for assessing normal and abnormal fetal cardiac anatomy. J Am Coll Cardiol 5:20S, 1985.

Hypoplastic Right Ventricle

Synonyms
Pulmonary atresia with intact ventricular septum, pulmonary valve fusion with intact ventricular septum, and pulmonary atresia with normal aortic root.

Definition
The term "hypoplastic ventricle" refers to an underdeveloped ventricular chamber that is normally formed. Hypoplastic right ventricle (HRV) occurs in the majority of cases due to pulmonary atresia in the presence of an intact ventricular septum (PA:IVS). However, PA:IVS can occur with a normal or enlarged right ventricle.

Pathology
All the components of a normal ventricular chamber (inlet, trabecular, and outlet) are present but hypoplastic in HRV. The underdevelopment of the right ventricle is a consequence of the obstruction of the pulmonary outflow. The tricuspid valve is frequently small and the pulmonary infundibulum may be either atretic or patent. The proximal pulmonary artery is hypoplastic.[2] In cases of pulmonary atresia, a communication occurs between the dilated myocardial sinusoids and the coronary circulation. These sinusoids are the anatomic basis for a circular shunt that allows blood to flow from the right ventricle to the coronary circulation, to the right atrium, and back to the blind right ventricle.[7]

PA:IVS may exist with a small ventricular chamber (type I) or with a normal or large right ventricular chamber (type II).[3,8] The size of the ventricle seems to be related to the competence (type I) or incompetence (type II) of the tricuspid valve.[6] Type I is the most common variety. A secundum atrial septal defect is a frequent finding.

Hemodynamic Considerations
During intrauterine life, blood flow is diverted from the right atrium into the left atrium through the foramen ovale. The pulmonary vascular bed is supplied by retrograde flow through the ductus. At birth, closure of the ductus usually results in cyanosis and acidosis, frequently leading to neonatal death. Even if congestive heart failure is not usually seen before the postnatal circulatory changes, it is conceivable that this can occur during fetal life, especially in those cases associated with tricuspid insufficiency.

Diagnosis
In the fetus, both ventricles should be of equal size. Logically, recognition of HRV depends on the demonstration of a small right ventricular cavity. Nomograms of the inner dimensions of the ventricular chambers obtained with real-time[12] and M-mode[1] echocardiography are available (see Fig. 4–23). However, the reader should be aware of the limitations of biometry for prenatal diagnosis of congenital heart disease: (1) normal dimensions encompass a very wide range, and (2) the anatomic landmarks commonly used for standardization of measurements may be altered in malformed hearts. In some cases, the condition is obvious, and measurements are unnecessary (Fig. 4–46). A useful "rule" to remember is that the apex of both ventricles should be at the same level. Even severe dilatation of one ventricle will not alter this because the ventricle will increase in diameter, but very little in length. In other cases, associated findings, such as atresia of the pulmonary valve and hypoplasia of the proximal portion of the pulmonary artery, should be looked for when the suspicion arises (Fig. 4–47).

Prenatal identification of PA:IVS with a normal right ventricular cavity is a diagnostic challenge. In these cases, the diagnosis relies entirely on the demonstration of an atretic pulmonary valve.

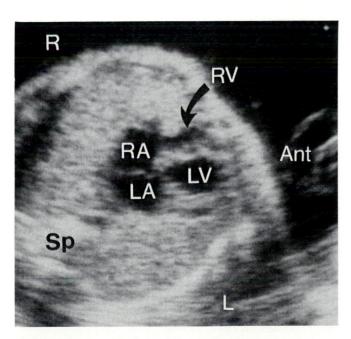

Figure 4–46. Four chamber view in a third trimester fetus with hypoplastic right ventricle (RV). LV, left ventricle; LA, left atrium; RA, right atrium; Sp, spine; R, right; L, left; Ant, anterior.

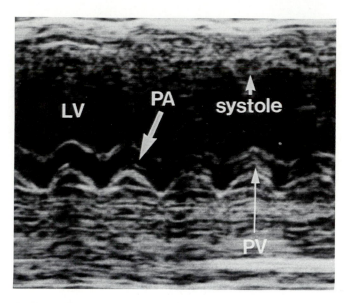

Figure 4–47. M-mode echocardiogram at the level of the root of the pulmonary artery (PA) shows failure of opening of the pulmonary valve (PV) during systole. LV, left ventricle.

recommended. A careful search for associated anomalies, including fetal karyotyping, is recommended.

In the absence of intrauterine congestive heart failure (hydrops), there is no indication to alter standard obstetrical management, but delivery in a tertiary care center where a pediatric cardiologist is immediately available is mandatory.

Optimal management of patients whose fetuses have congestive heart failure has not yet been established. A reasonable approach is to deliver the patient after fetal lung maturity is documented, because the mortality rate of respiratory distress syndrome associated with congestive heart failure is extremely high. For a further discussion of management issues concerning fetal well-being assessment and mode of delivery, see Nonimmune Hydrops Fetalis in Chapter 12.

Prognosis

HRV is a severe congenital anomaly that frequently occurs as a neonatal emergency when ductal closure stops pulmonary flow. Several series have been published about the prognosis of infants with HRV.[4,5,9–11] Moulton et al.[11] reported on the outcome of 30 infants who underwent palliative procedures. Six who underwent only pulmonary valvotomy died, as did 3 of 6 who had only a systemic pulmonary artery shunt. Of the 17 who had both valvotomy and shunt, 14 survived the operation. Among these patients, there were 9 long-term survivors, 5 of whom underwent corrective open heart surgery.

De Leval et al.[4] reported their experience with 60 patients observed between 1970 and 1980. The overall 5-year survival rate was 36 percent. However, an important decrease in early mortality occurred after 1977, when they introduced preoperative prostaglandin E_1 (PGE_1) infusions with valvotomy, and systemic pulmonary artery shunt as a palliative procedure in the neonatal period. Among 15 patients treated after this period, only 1 death occurred. Lewis et al.[10] reported 18 long-term survivors of 27 treated infants. It is of note that growth of the right ventricle has been documented after surgical correction.

Obstetrical Management

When the diagnosis is made before viability, the option of pregnancy termination should be offered. After viability, a frank discussion with the parents is

REFERENCES

1. Allan LD, Joseph MC, Boyd EGCA, et al.: M-Mode echocardiography in the developing human fetus. Br Heart J 47:573, 1982.
2. Becker AE, Anderson RH: Pathology of Congenital Heart Disease. London, Butterworths, 1981.
3. Celermajer JM, Bowdler JD, Gengos DC, et al.: Pulmonary valve fusion with intact ventricular septum. Am Heart J 76:452, 1968.
4. De Leval M, Bull C, Stark J, et al.: Pulmonary atresia and intact ventricular septum: Surgical management based on a revised classification. Circulation 66:272, 1982.
5. Dobell ARC, Grignon A: Early and late results in pulmonary atresia. Ann Thorac Surg 24:264, 1977.
6. Elliott LP, Adams P, Edwards JE: Pulmonary atresia with intact ventricular septum. Br Heart J 25:489, 1963.
7. Freedom RM, Harrington DP: Contributions of intramyocardial sinusoids in pulmonary atresia and intact ventricular septum to a right-sided circular shunt. Br Heart J 36:1061, 1974.
8. Greenwold WE, DuShane JW, Burchell HB, et al.: Congenital pulmonary atresia with intact ventricular septum: Two anatomic types. Circulation 14:945, 1956.
9. Laks H, Milliken JC, Perloff JK, et al.: Experience with the Fontan procedure. J Thorac Cardiovasc Surg 88:939, 1984.
10. Lewis AB, Wells W, Lindesmith GG: Evaluation and surgical treatment of pulmonary atresia and intact ventricular septum in infancy. Circulation 67:1318, 1983.
11. Moulton AL, Bowman FO, Edie RN, et al.: Pulmonary atresia with intact ventricular septum. Sixteen-year experience. J Thorac Cardiovasc Surg 78:527, 1979.
12. Sahn DJ, Lange LW, Allen HD, et al.: Quantitative real-time cross-sectional echocardiography in the developing normal human fetus and newborn. Circulation 62:588, 1980.

Tetralogy of Fallot

Synonyms
Fallot tetrad and pulmonary atresia with ventricular septal defect.

Definition
This defect consists of an association of four anatomic abnormalities: (1) VSD, (2) stenosis of the infundibulum of the pulmonary artery, (3) aortic valve overriding the interventricular septum, and (4) hypertrophy of the right ventricle.

Embryology
Tetralogy of Fallot is a defect basically caused by underdevelopment of the pulmonary infundibulum.

The fundamental problem seems to be unequal defective partitioning of the truncus conus (Fig. 4–48). Internal segmentation of the truncus conus is essential for the separation of the two great vessels and the formation of the ventricular outflow tracts, as well as part of the ventricular septum.[30] Incorrect alignment of the ascending aorta results in this vessel overriding the interventricular septum, a VSD, and narrowing of the right ventricular outflow tract.[4] Hypertrophy of the right ventricle does not seem to be present in the fetus.[14]

Pathology
Each of the components of the tetralogy offers a wide spectrum of severity.[3,13] The VSD generally is located in the perimembranous or superior portion of the septum, but it may involve the muscular part as well.[3] The outflow tract of the right ventricle may be mildly stenotic to atretic.[5,11] In the latter case, the anomaly is commonly referred to as "pulmonary atresia with a VSD." The overriding aorta is also a variable entity. This vessel may arise predominantly from the left and straddle both ventricles or emanate predominantly from the right ventricle. Anomalies of the pulmonary valve are frequently seen. The absence of the pulmonary valve (tetralogy of Fallot with absent pulmonary valve) is characterized by an aneurysmal dilatation of the pulmonary artery.[7,12,15,17,26,32]

Hemodynamic Considerations
Tetralogy of Fallot should not be a cause of hemodynamic compromise in the fetus. In utero, the blood pressure in the systemic and pulmonary vascular beds is thought to be equal.[24] Even in the presence of a tight pulmonic stenosis or atresia, right ventricular output could be diverted into the aorta and pulmonary blood flow supplied by retrograde flow through the ductus arteriosus.[9,16] This seems to be confirmed by the normal intrauterine growth of fetuses with tetralogy of Fallot and by the absence of right ventricular hypertrophy at birth.[14] Tetralogy of Fallot with absence of the pulmonic valve should be regarded as an exception because pulmonic regurgitation may cause congestive heart failure. These infants also experience respiratory distress as a consequence of the external compression of bronchi and trachea by the aneursymal dilatation of the main pulmonary artery and its branches.[7,12,15,17,26,29,32]

After birth, the hemodynamic problems are caused by the establishment of a right-to-left shunt at the level of the ascending aorta and the bypassing of the pulmonary circulation. The decreased oxygen saturation in the systemic circulation causes cyanosis. The association of pulmonic–infundibular stenosis and the systemic pressure in the aorta results in pressure overload and hypertrophy of the right ventricle.

The clinical problems of infants diagnosed with tetralogy of Fallot are cyanosis and the potential for the development of heart failure. Congestive heart failure is a rare occurrence in the neonatal period and is usually seen in infants with concomitant absence of the pulmonary valve.

Diagnosis
The diagnosis relies on demonstration of a dilated aorta overriding the interventricular septum (Fig. 4–49).[25] In our experience as well as that of others,[1,20] there is no sonographically detectable hypertrophy of the right ventricle in the midtrimester. Furthermore,

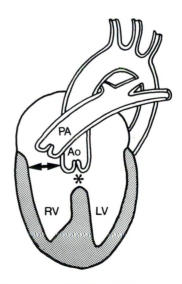

Figure 4–48. Diagram showing the features of tetralogy of Fallot. The aorta (Ao) overrides the interventricular septal defect (*), and there is stenosis of the infundibulum of the right ventricle (RV) (*double arrow*). LV, left ventricle; PA, pulmonary artery.

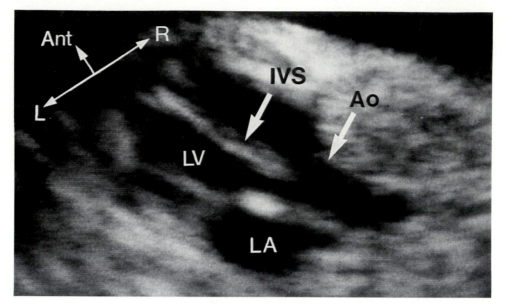

Figure 4–49. Overriding of the aorta (Ao) in a third trimester fetus with tetralogy of Fallot. IVS, interventricular septum; LV, left ventricle; LA, left atrium, Ant, anterior; L, left; R, right. *(Reproduced with permission from Bovicelli L, Baccarani G, Picchio FM, Pilu G: Ecocardiografia Fetale. La Diagnosi ed il Trattamento Prenatale delle Cardiopatie Congenite. Milan, Masson, 1985.)*

in early pregnancy, infundibular pulmonic stenosis may not be apparent.

If overriding of the aorta is identified and the pulmonary artery cannot be seen arising from the right ventricle, the differential diagnosis includes pulmonary atresia with VSD and truncus arteriosus communis. If the connection between the overriding artery and the pulmonary arteries can be demonstrated, a confident diagnosis of truncus arteriosus can be made[2] (see p. 168).

Aneurysmal dilatation of the pulmonary artery should prompt the diagnosis of absence of the pulmonary valve.[10]

Prenatal diagnosis of tetralogy of Fallot has been reported in several instances.[1,10,20]

The sonographer should be alerted to a frequent artifact that resembles overriding of the aorta. Incorrect orientation of the transducer may demonstrate septo-aortic discontinuity in a normal fetus (Fig. 4–50). The mechanism of this artifact is probably

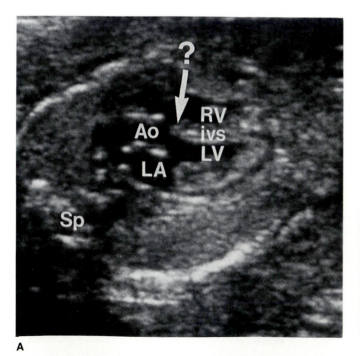

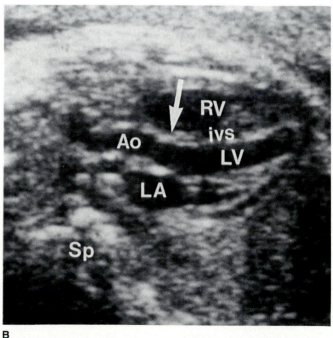

A   B

Figure 4–50. A. Incorrect alignment of the scanning plane reveals a false overriding of the aorta (Ao) in a normal fetus. **B.** A correct scanning plane in the same fetus demonstrates a normal septo-aortic continuity (*arrow*). ivs, interventricular septum; RV, right ventricle; LV, left ventricle; LA, left atrium; Sp, spine; Ant, anterior; Post, posterior.

related to the angle of incidence of the sound beam. Meticulous scanning is always required to evaluate the relationship between the interventricular septum and the ascending aorta.

Prognosis

The prognosis for infants with tetralogy of Fallot has changed significantly over the last 3 decades. The development of pediatric cardiothoracic surgery is responsible for the improved outlook for these infants.[22]

The first surgical approach to tetralogy of Fallot was intended to obviate the underperfusion of the lungs. The Blalock-Taussig shunt consisted of anastomosing the subclavian artery to the pulmonary artery. This procedure was used for many years. Results indicated that the survival rate with a successful anastomosis was 64 percent (441/685 patients) at 15 years and 55 percent (376/679) at 20 years.[27,28]

The development of extracorporeal circulation and rapid advances in cardiothoracic surgery permitted correction of the primary anatomic defects, namely, closure of the VSD and reconstruction of the right outflow tract.[23] Follow-up for 5 to 11 years in 311 patients indicated a survival rate of 85 percent.[21] Eighty-seven percent of the survivors had neither symptoms nor restriction of activity. Another study reported a survival rate of 82 percent for a follow-up period ranging from 1 month to 15 years. The author estimated that half of the treated patients would survive to the 4th decade of life. The major contributor to decreased survival was an early postoperative mortality rate (30 days after operation) of 11 percent.[8] These results refer to operations performed during adolescence or adulthood. In the last few years, intracardiac correction in infants of very early age has gained popularity. The first series indicated an early mortality rate ranging from 0[31] to 5 percent.[18] Operations in younger infants seem to significantly improve the mortality rate, as well as the hemodynamic response.[8]

The prognosis of tetralogy of Fallot with pulmonary atresia and tetralogy of Fallot with absence of the pulmonary valve is different. In a group of 38 patients with pulmonary atresia treated by right ventricular outflow construction, 3 deaths were recorded (mortality of 8 percent). The survivors had both clinical and hemodynamic improvement.[19]

Tetralogy of Fallot with an absent pulmonary valve may cause congestive heart failure in the fetus or newborn.[10,12] Aneurysmal dilatation of the pulmonary artery and its branches may be a cause of pulmonary distress. These findings should be considered as major prognostic factors.[7] In a review of the cases published before 1974, Lakier et al.[12] reported that infants with severe respiratory complications who received medical treatment had a mortality rate of 76 percent compared to a mortality rate of 41 percent in the group of infants treated surgically. Infants with mild or no pulmonary problems who underwent surgery had a mortality rate of 31 percent. Stafford et al.[26] reported 3 deaths (17 percent) in 18 surgically treated patients. Survivors were in good functional condition. Finally, in a series of 15 infants, 10 survived with relief of symptoms.[7]

Obstetrical Management

A careful search for other cardiac and extracardiac abnormalities is indicated whenever the prenatal diagnosis of tetralogy of Fallot is made. An amniocentesis for chromosomal analysis is recommended. The option of pregnancy termination should be offered before viability. In continuing pregnancies, no alteration of standard obstetrical management is required. However, infants should be delivered in a tertiary care center where a pediatric cardiologist is immediately available. Tetralogy of Fallot with an absent pulmonary valve requires careful monitoring to rule out the development of in utero congestive heart failure.

In the absence of intrauterine congestive heart failure (hydrops), there is no indication to alter standard obstetrical management, but delivery in a tertiary care center where a pediatric cardiologist is immediately available is mandatory.

Optimal management of patients whose fetuses have congestive heart failure has not yet been established. A reasonable approach is to deliver the patient after fetal lung maturity is documented, because the mortality rate of respiratory distress syndrome associated with congestive heart failure is extremely high. For a further discussion of management issues concerning fetal well-being assessment and mode of delivery, see Nonimmune Hydrops Fetalis in Chapter 12.

REFERENCES

1. Allan LD, Crawford CC, Anderson RH, et al.: Echocardiographic and anatomical correlations in fetal congenital heart disease. Br Heart J 52:542, 1984.
2. Barron JV, Sahn DJ, Attie F: Two-dimensional echocardiographic study of right ventricular outflow and great artery anatomy in pulmonary atresia with ventricular septal defects and in truncus arteriosus. Am Heart J 105:281, 1983.
3. Becker AE, Anderson RH: Pathology of Congenital Heart Disease. London, Butterworths, 1981.
4. De La Cruz MV, Da Rocha JP: An ontogenetic theory for the explanation of congenital malformations involving the truncus and conus. Am Heart J 51:782, 1956.
5. Edwards JE, McGoon DC: Absence of anatomic origin from heart of pulmonary arterial supply. Circulation 47:393, 1973.
6. Finnegan P, Haider R, Patel RG, et al.: Results of total correction of the tetralogy of Fallot. Long-term

haemodynamic evaluation at rest and during exercise. Br Heart J 38:934, 1976.

7. Fischer DR, Neches WH, Beerman LB, et al.: Tetralogy of fallot with absent pulmonic valve: Analysis of 17 patients. Am J Cardiol 53:1433, 1984.

8. Garson A, Nihill MR, McNamara DG, et al.: Status of the adult and adolescent after repair of tetralogy of fallot. Circulation 59:1232, 1979.

9. Jefferson K, Rees S, Somerville J: Systemic arterial supply to the lungs in pulmonary atresia and its relation to pulmonary artery development. Br Heart J 34:418, 1972.

10. Kleinman CS, Donnerstein RL, DeVore GR, et al.: Fetal echocardiography for evaluation of in utero congestive heart failure: A technique for study of nonimmune fetal hydrops. N Engl J Med 306:568, 1982.

11. LaFargue RT, Vogel JHK, Pryor R, et al.: Pseudotruncus arteriosus. A review of 21 cases with observations on oldest reported case. Am J Cardiol 19:239, 1967.

12. Lakier JB, Stanger P, Heymann MA, et al.: Tetralogy of Fallot with absent pulmonary valve. Natural history and hemodynamic considerations. Circulation 50:167, 1974.

13. Lev M, Eckner FAO: The pathologic anatomy of tetralogy of Fallot and its variations. Dis Chest 45:251, 1964.

14. Lev M, Rimoldi HJA, Rowlatt UF: The quantitative anatomy of cyanotic tetralogy of Fallot. Circulation 30:531, 1964.

15. Litwin SB, Rosenthal A, Fellows K: Surgical management of young infants with tetralogy of Fallot, absence of the pulmonary valve, and respiratory distress. J Thorac Cardiovasc Surg 65:552, 1973.

16. Macartney FJ, Scott O, Deverall PB: Haemodynamic and anatomical characteristics of pulmonary blood supply in pulmonary atresia with ventricular septal defect, including a case of persistent fifth aortic arch. Br Heart J 36:1049, 1974.

17. Osman MZ, Meng CCL, Girdany BR: Congenital absence of the pulmonary valve: Report of eight cases with review of the literature. AJR 106:58, 1969.

18. Pacifico AD, Bargeron LM, Kirklin JW: Primary total correction of tetralogy of Fallot in children less than four years of age. Circulation 48:1085, 1973.

19. Piehler JM, Danielson GK, McGoon DC, et al.: Management of pulmonary atresia with ventricular septal defect and hypoplastic pulmonary arteries by right

ventricular outflow construction. J Thorac Cardiovasc Surg 80:552, 1980.

20. Pilu G, Rizzo N, Orsini LF, et al.: La diagnosi delle anomalie cardiache strutturali nel feto mediante ultrasonografia bidimensionale. Ultr Ost Gin 1:257, 1983.

21. Poirier RA, McGoon DC, Danielson GK, et al.: Late results after repair of tetralogy of Fallot. J Thorac Cardiovasc Surg 73:900, 1977.

22. Rashkind WJ: Pediatric cardiology: A brief historical perspective. Pediatr Cardiol 1:63, 1979.

23. Richardson JP, Clarke CP: Tetralogy of Fallot. Risk factors associated with complete repair. Br Heart J 38:926, 1976.

24. Rudolph AM: Congenital Diseases of the Heart: Clinical-Physiologic Consideration in Diagnosis and Management. Chicago, Year Book, 1974.

25. Sanders SP, Bierman FZ, Williams RG: Conotruncal malformations: Diagnosis in infancy using subxiphoid 2-dimensional echocardiography. Am J Cardiol 50:1361, 1982.

26. Stafford EG, Mair DD, McGoon DC, et al.: Tetralogy of Fallot with absent pulmonary valve. Surgical considerations and results. Circulation 48 [Suppl III]:24, 1972.

27. Taussig HB: Tetralogy of Fallot: Early history and late results. AJR 133:423, 1979.

28. Taussig HB, Kallman CH, Nagel D, et al.: Long-time observations on the Blalock-Taussig operation VIII: 20 to 28 year follow-up on patients with a tetralogy of Fallot. Johns Hopkins Med J 137:13, 1975.

29. Thiene G, Frescura C, Bortolotti U, et al.: The systemic pulmonary circulation in pulmonary atresia with ventricular septal defect: Concept of reciprocal development of the fourth and sixth aortic arches. Am Heart J 101:339, 1981.

30. Van Praagh R, Van Praagh S, Nebesar R, et al.: Tetralogy of Fallot: Underdevelopment of the pulmonary infundibulum and its sequelae. Am J Cardiol 26:25, 1970.

31. Venugopal P, Subramanian S: Intracardiac repair of tetralogy of Fallot in patients under 5 years of age. Ann Thorac Surg 18:228, 1974.

32. Waldhausen JA, Friedman S, Nicodemus H, et al.: Absence of the pulmonary valve in patients with tetralogy of Fallot. Surgical management. J Thorac Cardiovasc Surg 57:669, 1969.

Complete Transposition of the Great Arteries

Synonyms
Complete transposition of the great vessels, D-transposition, and atrioventricular concordance with ventriculoarterial discordance.

Definition
The term "complete transposition of the great arteries" (TGA) refers to a condition in which the aorta is connected to the right ventricle and the pulmonary

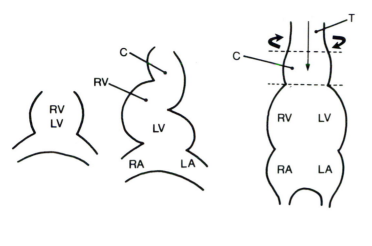

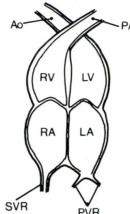

Figure 4–51. Schematic representation of the normal embryologic development of the heart according to de la Cruz et al.[3] RV, right ventricle; LV, left ventricle; LA, left atrium; RA, right atrium; C, conus; T, truncus; Ao, aorta; PA, pulmonary artery; PVR, pulmonary venous return; SVR, systemic venous return.

artery is connected to the left ventricle in the presence of a normal atrioventricular connection.

Embryology

According to the hypothesis suggested by de la Cruz et al.,[3] in the first stages of development, the embryonic heart is formed by the primordia of both ventricles. In a subsequent stage, the primordia of the ventricles form a loop, and the caudal atrial segment and the cephalic conus (the primordia of the outflow tracts) develop. Later, the truncus (arterial segment) appears. Opposing thickenings of subendocardial tissue arise in the conus (conal ridges) and meet with similar ridges that arise from the truncus. They form the aorticopulmonary septum, which has a spiral course and divides the truncus into aorta and pulmonary trunk. Later, the conus is incorporated into the walls of the ventricle. The normal relationship between the aorta and the pulmonary artery is such that the pulmonary artery is anterior and to the right of the aorta. This developmental sequence is depicted in Figure 4–51.

It has been proposed that transposition of the great vessels results from failure of the aorticopulmonary septum to follow a spiral course (Fig. 4–52), resulting in the aorta connecting with the right ventricle and the pulmonary artery with the left ventricle.

Pathology

Depending on the disorder in conotruncal segmentation, the relative positions of the aorta and pulmonary artery will vary. In most cases, the aorta is anterior and to the right of the pulmonary artery. Less frequently, the two arteries are side by side or the aorta is posterior.

Associated Anomalies

TGA can be associated with a number of other cardiac anomalies. According to Becker and Anderson,[2] three main varieties of TGA can be distinguished:

1. Complete TGA with intact interventricular septum. Pulmonic stenosis may be present, due either to a discrete membrane or bulging of the ventricular septum.

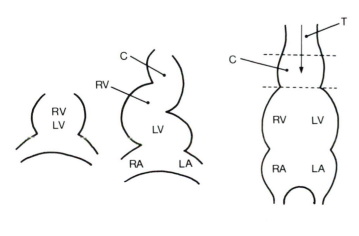

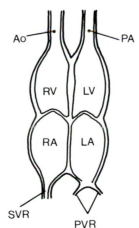

Figure 4–52. Schematic representation of the embryology of complete transposition of the great vessels. Failure of the aorticopulmonary septum to follow a spiral course results in the abnormal ventriculoarterial connection. RV, right ventricle; LV, left ventricle; LA, left atrium; RA, right atrium; C, conus; T, trunus; Ao, aorta; PA, pulmonary artery; PVR, pulmonary venous return; SVR, systemic venous return.

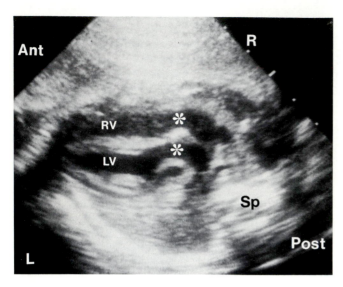

Figure 4–53. Long axis view of the ventricles in a fetus with TGA. The great arteries (*) are seen arising from the heart in a parallel fashion. RV, right ventricle; LV, left ventricle; Sp, spine; Ant, anterior; Post, posterior; R, right; L, left.

2. Complete TGA with VSD. The septal defect can be perimembranous, muscular, or infundibular.
3. Complete TGA with VSD and pulmonic stenosis, which is often due to the displacement of the ventricular septum into the left ventricle.

Other associated anomalies include ASDs, anomalies of the atrioventricular valves, and varying degrees of underdevelopment of either right or left

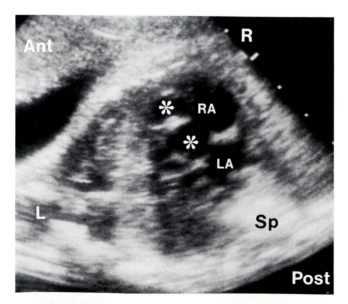

Figure 4–54. The abnormal side-by-side relationship of the great vessels (*) is further demonstrated by this short axis view of the patient in Figure 4–53. Compare with the normal appearance of this view, which is shown in Figure 4–15. RA, right atrium; LA, left atrium; Sp, spine; Ant, anterior; Post, posterior; R, right; L, left.

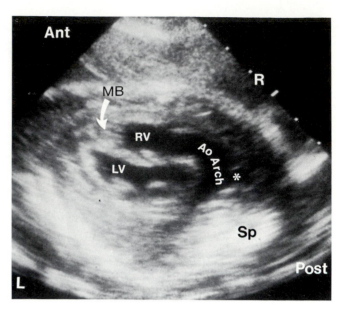

Figure 4–55. The morphologic right ventricle (RV) is identified by demonstration of the moderator band (MB) in the same patient as in Figure 4–53. The artery connected to the right ventricle can be positively identified as the aorta by observing its long upward course. The aortic arch (Ao Arch) is recognized by the connection with a brachiocephalic vessel (*). LV, left ventricle; Sp, spine; Ant, anterior; Post, posterior; L, left; R, right.

ventricles. Coarctation of the aorta can be found in 5 percent of patients.[12]

Hemodynamic Considerations

The fetus with uncomplicated TGA or with TGA and VSD should not have hemodynamic compromise because of the parallel model of intrauterine circulation. The oxygenated blood coming from the placenta via the umbilical vein and inferior vena cava reaches the right atrium. From there, two main pathways can be followed: (1) most of the blood will be diverted through the foramen ovale into the left atrium; much of the left ventricular output will then be distributed via pulmonary artery, ductus arteriosus, and descending aorta to the body, and (2) part of the blood will also enter the right ventricle directly and will be distributed via the aorta to the brachiocephalic district. The lack of significant hemodynamic compromise seems to be indirectly confirmed by the frequency of normal birth weight in this group of infants. An exception to this rule is represented by those infants in whom an obstructive lesion, such as pulmonary stenosis, is present.

After birth, survival depends on the amount and size of the mixing of the two otherwise independent circulations. Untreated infants with no communications die soon after the postnatal circulatory changes. The most frequent sites of communication include an open foramen ovale, an ASD, a VSD, or a patent ductus arteriosus.

Diagnosis

The diagnosis rests on the absence of the normal anatomic criss-crossing of the aorta and pulmonary arteries, which arise from the ventricles in a parallel fashion. This finding can be demonstrated either in a long axis view of the ventricles (Fig. 4–53) or a short axis view of the great vessels (Fig. 4–54). The aorta and pulmonary artery can be positively identified by following the course of the vessels to the arch (Fig. 4–55) and to the bifurcation into the left and right pulmonary artery, respectively (Fig. 4–56).

A prenatal diagnosis of TGA is a serious challenge to the sonographer, since a proper assessment of the ventriculoarterial connections is sometimes difficult because of fetal movement and position. A false negative diagnosis has been reported twice.[1,6] We have made the prenatal diagnosis of TGA in a third trimester fetus. However, difficulties in using echocardiography to differentiate complete TGA with VSD and other conotruncal malformations, such as double outlet right ventricle, are encountered in newborns[11] and probably in the fetus as well. Recognition of TGA should prompt a careful search for other associated cardiac anomalies.

Prognosis

The natural history of TGA has been outlined by Liebman et al.[7] on the basis of a review of 742 cases. Survival rate was 70 percent at 1 week, 50 percent at 1 month, and 11 percent at 1 year.

Several operative procedures have changed the life expectancy for infants with TGA. Since survival depends on the degree of mixture of the two circulations, a surgical approach consists of creating an ASD, either by intracardiac surgery or by balloon septostomy (Rashkind procedure).[10] An alternative is the Mustard operation,[8] which consists of the creation of an intraatrial baffle diverting the pulmonary venous return to the right ventricle and the systemic venous return to the left ventricle. Anatomic repair with arterial switch was first attempted by Mustard et al.[9] and had a very high mortality rate. This approach has recently gained interest because of the work of Jatene et al.[5] At present, the choice of procedure depends on the hemodynamic status of the infant and the presence or absence of associated cardiac anomalies.

The experience of the Baylor group in Houston[4] during the decade of 1968–1978 includes 112 patients with complete TGA; the group performed 46 palliative procedures and 71 corrective repairs on these patients. The 1-year and 5-year survival rates were 79

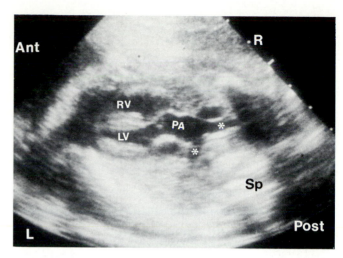

Figure 4–56. In the same patient as in Figure 4–53, the great artery connected to the left ventricle (LV) is identified as the pulmonary artery (PA) by following its course until it bifurcates into the left and right pulmonary arteries (*) RV, right ventricle; Sp, spine; Ant, anterior; Post, posterior; R, right; L, left.

percent and 64 percent, respectively. In the report from the Hospital for Sick Children of Toronto,[12] which includes 394 patients with TGA and intact interventricular septum, the 5-year survival rate was 89 percent. It should be stressed that the prognosis is influenced by the presence of associated cardiac anomalies that may not be detectable with ultrasound in utero (e.g., pulmonic stenosis and coarctation of the aorta). In a group of 32 patients with TGA and coartation of the aorta, the 5-year survival rate was only 57 percent.[12]

Obstetrical Management

When the diagnosis is made before viability, the option of pregnancy termination should be offered. A careful search for associated cardiac and extracardiac anomalies, including karyotype evaluation, is recommended. TGA is not associated per se with intrauterine congestive heart failure. However, the presence of associated anomalies, such as pulmonic stenosis, can represent exceptions to this rule. Therefore, we believe that serial ultrasound examinations should be performed. The association of hydrops with a structural cardiac defect is an ominous combination. The optimal management in these cases has not been established. The option of early delivery may be considered, but the parents should be aware that the mortality rate in these cases is extremely high.[6] In the absence of congestive heart failure, standard obstetrical management is not changed, but delivery in a tertiary care center where a pediatric cardiologist is immediately available is mandatory.

REFERENCES

1. Allan LD, Crawford DC, Anderson RH, et al.: Echocardiographic and anatomical correlations in fetal congenital heart disease. Br Heart J 52:542, 1984.
2. Becker AE, Anderson RH: Pathology of Congenital Heart Disease. London, Butterworths, 1981.
3. de la Cruz MV, Arteaga M, Espino-Vela J, et al.: Complete transposition of the great arteries: Types and morphogenesis of ventriculoarterial discordance. Am Heart J 102:271, 1981.
4. Gutgesell HP, Garson A, Park IS, et al.: Prognosis for the neonate and young infant with congenital heart disease (Abstr). Pediatr Cardiol 2:168, 1982.
5. Jatene AD, Fontes VF, Paulista PP, et al.: Anatomic correction of transposition of the great vessels. J Thorac Cardiovasc Surg 72:364, 1976.
6. Kleinman CS, Donnerstein RL, DeVore GR, et al.: Fetal echocardiography for evaluation of in utero congestive heart failure: A technique for study of nonimmune fetal hydrops. N Engl J Med 306:568, 1982.
7. Liebman J, Cullum L, Belloc NB: Natural history of transposition of the great vessels. Anatomy and birth and death characteristics. Circulation 40:237, 1969
8. Mustard WT: Successful two-stage correction of transposition of the great vessels. Surgery 55:469, 1964.
9. Mustard WT, Chute AL, Keith JD, et al.: A surgical approach to transposition of the great vessels with extracorporeal circuit. Surgery 36:39, 1954.
10. Rashkind WJ, Miller WW: Creation of an atrial septal defect without thoracotomy: A palliative approach to complete transposition of the great arteries. JAMA 196:991, 1966.
11. Sanders SP, Bierman FZ, Williams RG: Conotruncal malformations: Diagnosis in infancy using subxiphoid 2-dimensional echocardiography. Am J Cardiol 50:1361, 1982.
12. Vogel M, Freedom RM, Smallhorn JF, et al.: Complete transposition of the great arteries and coarctation of the aorta. Am J Cardiol 53:1627, 1984.

Corrected Transposition of the Great Arteries

Synonyms
L-Transposition and atrioventricular discordance with ventriculoarterial discordance.

Definition
Corrected transposition of the great arteries (TGA) refers to a condition in which the right atrium and left atrium are connected to the morphologic left and right ventricle, respectively, and the great arteries are transposed. These two defects cancel each other, and ideally there should not be any hemodynamic consequences. Corrected TGA may indeed be an occasional finding at autopsy. However, in the majority of cases, important associated anomalies alter the prognosis.

Embryology
According to the hypothesis suggested by de la Cruz et al.,[3] the embryonic heart in the first stages of development is formed by the primordia of both ventricles. In a subsequent stage, while the primordia of the ventricles form a loop, both the caudal atrial segment and the cephalic conus (the primordia to the outflow tracts) develop. Later, the truncus (arterial segment) appears. Opposing thickenings of subendocardial tissue arise in the conus (conal ridges) and meet with similar ridges arising from the truncus. They form the aorticopulmonary septum, which has a spiral course and divides the truncus into aorta and pulmonary trunk. Later, the conus is incorporated into the walls of the ventricle. The normal relationship between the aorta and the pulmonary artery is such that the pulmonary artery is anterior and to the right of the aorta. This developmental sequence is depicted in Figure 4–57.

It has been suggested that corrected transposition results from anomalous looping of the primordia of the ventricle. This is associated with the lack of spiral rotation of the truncoconal septum. In this fashion, the aorta is connected to the morphologic right ventricle and the pulmonary artery is connected to the morphologic left ventricle. Such an abnormality is functionally corrected, since the ventricles are attached to the anatomically anchored, and thus normally positioned, atria (Fig. 4–58).[3]

Pathology
Corrected TGA is frequently associated with malpositions of the heart and occasionally with situs inversus.[7] Because of the ventriculoarterial discordance, the aortic valve is separated from the tricuspid valve by a complete infundibulum, whereas there is fibrous continuity between the pulmonic and the mitral valve. In more than 50 percent of patients, there is a VSD, generally of the perimembranous type. The pulmonary artery may override the VSD, and pulmonic stenosis is seen in about 50 percent of cases studied.[1,2,7]

Anomalies of the atrioventricular valves are frequently found and include Ebsteinlike malformation and straddling of the tricuspid valve.[1,2,7]

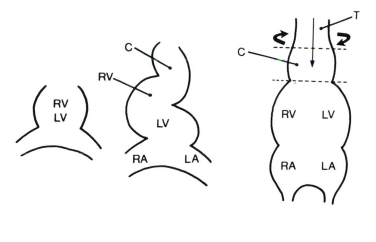

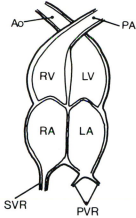

Figure 4–57. Schematic representation of the normal embryologic development of the heart according to de la Cruz et al.[3] RV, right ventricle; LV, left ventricle; LA, left atrium; RA, right atrium; C, conus; T, truncus; Ao, aorta; PA, pulmonary artery; PVR, pulmonary venous return; SVR, systemic venous return.

The derangement of the conduction tissue secondary to malalignment of the atrial and ventricular septa results in dysrhythmias, namely, atrioventricular block.[1]

Noncardiac associated anomalies are rare in corrected TGA.[7]

Diagnosis

Diagnosis of corrected TGA in the fetus is extremely complex, and we are not aware of any case described thus far. It is expected that ultrasound can recognize the absence of criss-crossing of the great arteries. The same findings described for the diagnosis of complete TGA are of value for corrected TGA as well. The study of the trabeculated pattern of the ventricular chambers may help in identifying the atrioventricular discordance. Nonetheless, it is likely that even if the truncoconal malformation can be detected, a differentiation with double outlet right ventricle will be extremely difficult.

The presence of atrioventricular block should increase the index of suspicion.

Prognosis

In the absence of any additional cardiac defect, corrected TGA could be asymptomatic even through adulthood. However, due to the frequency of other intracardiac defects (some of which may not be detected prenatally with ultrasound), the mortality rate in this group of infants appears to be high. The likelihood of survival as estimated by Friedberg and Nadas[4] in 1970 was almost 40 percent at 1 year of age and 30 percent at 10 years. Recently, Hwang et al.[5] reported the results of intracardiac repair of cardiac defects associated with corrected TGA in a group of 18 infants. The survival rate was 78 percent in a follow-up period of 4.5 years.

Obstetrical Management

If the diagnosis is made before viability, the option of pregnancy termination should be offered. A careful search for associated cardiac and extracardiac anomalies, including karyotype evaluation, is recommended. TGA is not associated per se with intrauterine congestive heart failure. However, the presence of associated anomalies, such as pulmonic stenosis, can represent an exception to this rule. Therefore, serial ultrasound ex-

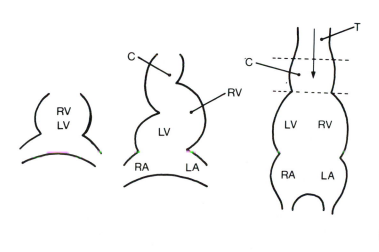

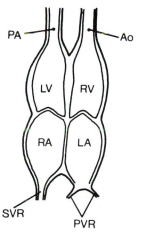

Figure 4–58. Schematic representation of the embryology of corrected transposition of the great arteries, according to de la Cruz et al.[3] The inverted ventricular loop results in the abnormal atrioventricular and ventriculoarterial connections. RV, right ventricle; LV, left ventricle; LA, left atrium; RA, right atrium; C, conus; T, truncus; Ao, aorta; PA, pulmonary artery; PVR, pulmonary venous return; SVR, systemic venous return.

aminations should be performed. The association of hydrops with a structural cardiac defect is an ominous combination. To date, the optimal management in these patients has yet to be established. The option of early delivery may be considered, but the parents should be aware that the mortality rate in these patients is extremely high.[6]

In the absence of congestive heart failure, there is no indication to alter standard obstetrical management, but delivery in a tertiary care center where a pediatric cardiologist is immediately available is mandatory.

REFERENCES

1. Becker AE, Anderson RH: Pathology of Congenital Heart Disease. London, Butterworths, 1981.
2. Bonfils-Roberts EA, Guller B, McGoon DC, et al.: Cor-
rected transposition. Surgical treatment of associated anomalies. Ann Thorac Surg 17:200, 1974.
3. de la Cruz MV, Arteaga M, Espino-Vela J, et al.: Complete transposition of the great arteries: Types and morphogenesis of ventriculoarterial discordance. Am Heart J 102:271, 1981.
4. Friedberg DZ, Nadas AS: Clinical profile of patients with congenital corrected transposition of the great arteries. A study of 60 cases. N Engl J Med 282:1053, 1970.
5. Hwang B, Bowman F, Malm J, et al.: Surgical repair of congenitally corrected transposition of the great arteries: Results and follow-up. Am J Cardiol 50:781, 1982.
6. Kleinman CS, Donnerstein RL, De Vore GR, et al.: Fetal echocardiography for evaluation of in utero congestive cardiac failure: A technique for study of nonimmune hydrops. N Engl J Med 306:568, 1982.
7. Schiebler GL, Edwards JE, Burchell HB, et al.: Congenital corrected transposition of the great vessels: A study of 33 cases. Pediatrics 27:851, 1961.

Double Outlet Right Ventricle

Synonyms
Syndromes of origin of both great arteries from the right ventricle; Taussig-Bing heart.

Definition
Double outlet right ventricle (DORV) describes a condition in which most of the aorta and the pulmonary artery arise from the right ventricle. In pathologic studies, a threshold of 50 percent is sufficient to fulfill the definition.[1] Some cardiovascular surgeons believe that a 90 percent threshold is more appropriate for clinical assessment.[6]

Embryology
DORV refers to a heterogeneous group of disorders that can be considered as arising from anomalies in conotruncal development[2] (see description of conotruncal development, Fig. 4–51 and page 161).

Pathology
The relevant pathology varies considerably from case to case. DORV simply describes a ventriculoarterial connection. According to the relationship of the great arteries, DORV may be subdivided into three types.[3] The first type is the most frequent: the aorta is situated posteriorly to the pulmonary root and the two vessels spiral around each other as they leave the base of the heart. The other two types are characterized by the great arteries ascending in a parallel

fashion, with either the aorta posterior to the pulmonary artery (second type) or vice versa (third type).[1,2] The second type is also commonly referred to as "Taussig-Bing heart." A VSD is the rule and may be subaortic, subpulmonic, noncommitted, or doubly committed. Associated defects include anomalies of the atrioventricular valves (atresia, stenosis, and straddling), anomalous venous return, coarctation of the aorta, and univentricular heart. Atrioventricular discordance is present in 5 percent of patients studied.[1]

By definition, DORV includes those cases of tetralogy of Fallot in which more than 50 percent or 90 percent of the aorta (depending upon the threshold used) is connected to the right ventricle.

Associated Extracardiac Anomalies
Ten of 80 infants (12.5 percent) with DORV reported in one series had severe anomalies, including trisomy 13, cardiosplenic syndrome, tracheoesophageal fistula, and cleft lip and palate.[7]

Hemodynamic Considerations
The hemodynamics are dependent on the anatomic type of DORV and the associated anomalies. Since the fetal heart functions as a single chamber where the blood is mixed and pumped, the presence of an uncomplicated DORV is not expected to be a cause of in utero congestive heart failure. Exceptions to this rule may occur in the presence of associated anoma-

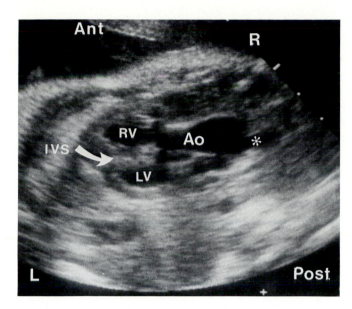

Figure 4–59. In this third trimester fetus, an enlarged aorta (Ao) overrides the ventricular septum (IVS), being predominantly connected to the right ventricle (RV). One of the brachiocephalic vessels (∗) is seen arising from the arch. LV, left ventricle; Ant, anterior; Post, posterior; R, right; L, left.

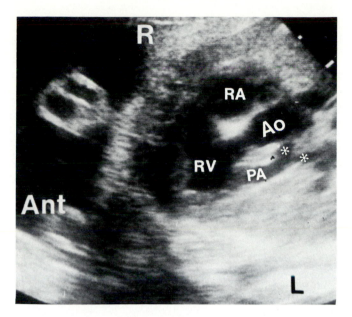

Figure 4–60. In the same patient as in Figure 4–59, both the enlarged aorta (Ao) and small pulmonary artery (PA) are seen arising from the right ventricle (RV), the aorta being posterior to the pulmonary artery. A confident diagnosis of DORV can be made. The common pulmonary trunk is seen dividing into the pulmonary arteries (∗). RA, right atrium; Ant, anterior; R, right; L, left.

lies obstructing the blood flow (e.g., pulmonic stenosis, mitral stenosis, and atresia).

With postnatal circulatory changes, the right ventricle assumes the burden of both the systemic and pulmonary circulations. In time, ventricular work overload may lead to congestive heart failure. The clinical course for infants with DORV is extremely variable depending on the accompanying defects.[7]

Diagnosis

The same sectional planes that have already been suggested for the diagnosis of tetralogy of Fallot and complete and corrected TGA are of value in this condition. However, a specific diagnosis of DORV is difficult, since the findings may closely resemble tetralogy of Fallot or TGA with VSD.

We have made a prenatal diagnosis of DORV in a fetus who subsequently proved to have a corrected TGA. We have also diagnosed tetralogy of Fallot in a fetus whose necropsy showed DORV. Similar difficulties in diagnosis have been reported by others.[4,8] More recently, we have been able to correctly identify DORV in three fetuses (Figs. 4–59 through 4–62). Stewart et al. have also reported the prenatal diagnosis of this condition in a 22-week fetus.[7a]

Prognosis

The outcome of infants with DORV depends largely on the associated anomalies. It is extremely difficult to obtain information about the natural history of this disease from the literature. Operative procedures may include primary repair or palliative surgery. The

presence of hypoplasia of the mitral valve or left ventricle has important implications for treatment, since these infants are not considered surgical candidates for definitive repair and will only undergo palliative repair.[6] Short-term results of surgical correction for classic DORV at the University of Alabama

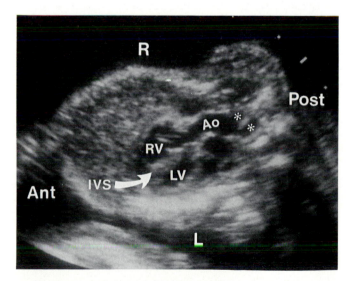

Figure 4–61. DORV in a second trimester fetus. The aorta (Ao) is seen overriding the ventricular septum (IVS) and is predominantly connected to the right ventricle (RV). Head and neck vessels (∗) arising from the arch are demonstrated in the same scanning plane. LV, left ventricle; Ant, anterior; Post, posterior; R, right; L, left.

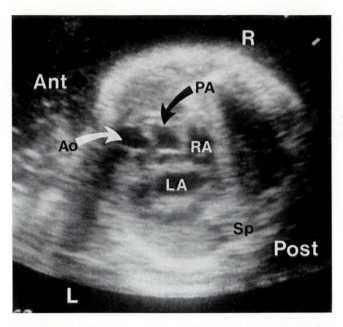

Figure 4–62. In the same patient as in Figure 4–61, a short axis view of the great vessels reveals an abnormal side-to-side relationship, the aorta (Ao) being anterior to the pulmonary artery (PA). A confident diagnosis of DORV third type can be made. RA, right atrium; LA, left atrium; Ant, anterior; Post, posterior; L, left; R, right.

show a 10 percent hospital mortality rate in the period between 1967 and 1982.[6]

Obstetrical Management

When the diagnosis is made before viability, the option of pregnancy termination should be offered. A careful search for associated cardiac and extracardiac anomalies, including karyotype evaluation, is recommended in all cases..

Serial ultrasound examinations should be performed to search for signs of congestive heart failure. The association of hydrops with a structural cardiac defect is an ominous combination. At present, the

optimal management in these patients has not been established. The option of early delivery may be considered, but the parents should be aware that the mortality rate in these cases is extremely high.[5]

In the absence of congestive heart failure, there is no indication to alter standard obstetrical management, but delivery in a tertiary care center where a pediatric cardiologist is immediately available is mandatory.

REFERENCES

1. Anderson RH, Becker AE, Wilcox BR, et al.: Surgical anatomy of double-outlet right ventricle—A reappraisal. Am J Cardiol 52:555, 1983.
2. Angelini P, Leachman RD: Spectrum of double outlet right ventricle: An embryologic interpretation. Cardiol Dis 3:127, 1976.
3. Becker AE, Anderson RH: Pathology of Congenital Heart Disease. London, Butterworths, 1981.
4. Kleinman CS, Santulli TV: Ultrasonic evaluation of the fetal human heart. Semin Perinatol 7:90, 1983.
5. Kleinman CS, Donnerstein RL, DeVore GR, et al.: Fetal echocardiography for evaluation of in utero congestive heart failure: A technique for study of nonimmune fetal hydrops. N Engl J Med 306:568, 1982.
6. Piccoli G, Pacifico AD, Kirklin JW, et al.: Changing results and concepts in the surgical treatment of double-outlet right ventricle: Analysis of 137 operations in 126 patients. Am J Cardiol 52:549, 1983.
7. Rowe RD, Freedom RM, Mehrizi A, Bloom KR: The Neonate with Congenital Heart Disease, 2d ed. Philadelphia, Saunders, 1981.
7a. Stewart PA, Wladimiroff JW, Becker AE: Early prenatal detection of double outlet right ventricle by echocardiography. Br Heart J 54:340, 1985.
8. Stewart PA, Wladimiroff JW, Essed CE: Prenatal ultrasound diagnosis of congenital heart disease associated with intrauterine growth retardation. A report of 2 cases. Prenatal Diagn 3:279, 1983.

Truncus Arteriosus

Synonym
Single outlet of the heart.

Definition
Truncus arteriosus is a congenital anomaly in which only one great artery arises from the base of the heart and gives rise to the coronary, pulmonary, and systemic arteries.

Embryology
This anomaly is thought to result from abnormal septation of the conotruncus, the portion of the embryonic heart that gives rise to the outflow tract of the ventricles and to the great arteries.[17]

The conus corresponds to the middle third of the bulbus cordis. It gives rise to the outflow tract of both ventricles and to the muscular portion of the ventricles located between the atrioventricular valves and the semilunar valves. The part of the conus giving rise to the ventricular free walls is referred to as the "parietal conus," and the portion responsible for the development of the septum is called the "conal septum."

The truncus is the distal part of the bulbus cordis. Through a process of rotation and internal septation, it gives origin to the semilunar valves and the two great arteries. Separation between the aorta and pulmonary arteries occurs by fusion of the truncal ridges (Fig. 4–51).

Septation of the conotruncus occurs between the 6th and 7th weeks of embryonic life and begins at the level of the 4th and 6th aortic arch, progressing toward the heart. The close temporal relationship of these two phenomena explains the frequent association between truncus arteriosus and aortic arch abnormalities, which has been reported to occur in 20 percent of cases studied.[2]

Pathology

The anomaly consists of a single arterial vessel with one semilunar valve arising from both ventricles.[3] A wide variety of intracardiac abnormalities is associated with this disorder. Most frequently, there is an infundibular VSD because of a failure in development of the proximal portion of the conotruncal septum.

According to Van Praagh and Van Praagh,[18] truncus arteriosus may be classified as type A or B depending on the presence or absence, respectively, of a VSD. Furthermore, type A can be subdivided into four types: A1, the aorticopulmonary septum is incompletely formed, resulting in a partially separated main pulmonary artery; A2, there is complete failure of development of the aorticopulmonary septum, resulting in pulmonary arteries arising directly from the truncus; A3, one lung is supplied by a pulmonary artery arising from the truncus, and the other lung is supplied by arteries derived from the descending aorta; A4, there is underdevelopment of the aortic arch, resulting in hypoplasia, coarctation, atresia, or interruption.[4,18]

In the classification suggested by Collett and Edwards,[5] truncus arteriosus is divided into four types: type I is characterized by the presence of a pulmonary trunk that bifurcates into right and left pulmonary arteries; type II is characterized by the presence of two pulmonary arteries arising from the back of the truncus; in type III, the two pulmonary arteries arise from the sides of the truncus; in type IV, the pulmonary arteries are absent, and the lungs are supplied by systemic pulmonic collateral arteries derived from the descending aorta (Fig. 4–63).

By definition, there is a single arterial valve (truncal valve). In the presence of a VSD, the truncal

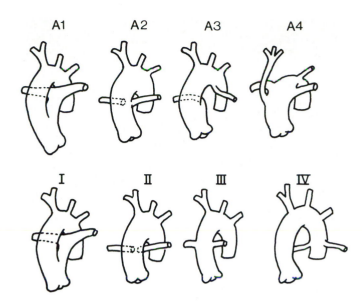

Figure 4–63. Schematic representations of the classification of truncus arteriosus according to Van Praagh and Van Praagh[18] (A1–A4) and to Collett and Edwards[5] (I–IV).

valve overrides the septum and is connected to both ventricular cavities in almost equal proportions. In most cases, the truncal valve has three leaflets (tricuspid), but it may have two to six leaflets. The truncal valve is frequently dysplastic and incompetent.[2]

Associated Anomalies

Cardiac defects include mitral atresia, ASD, univentricular heart, and aortic arch abnormalities.[2]

Hemodynamic Considerations

A crucial issue concerns the competence of the truncal valve. Since the fetal heart functions as a common chamber where the blood is mixed and pumped, truncus arteriosus with a competent valve is not expected to be a cause of significant hemodynamic perturbance. Conversely, truncal incompetence may lead to massive regurgitation from the truncus to the ventricles, which may result in congestive heart failure.

With postnatal circulatory changes, the decreased resistance of the pulmonary vascular bed leads to massive diversion of flow to the pulmonary district. This left-to-right shunt leads either to congestive heart failure due to ventricular overload or, in time, to pulmonary vascular damage and pulmonary hypertension.

Diagnosis

Truncus arteriosus is characterized by the presence of a single arterial vessel overriding the ventricular septum (Fig. 4–64). However, an identical finding is

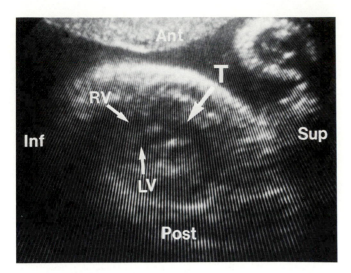

Figure 4–64. Truncus arteriosus in a third trimester fetus with multiple congenital anomalies. A single arterial trunk (T) with a long upward course is seen arising from the base of the heart. The pulmonary artery could not be demonstrated. This finding may be compatible with truncus arteriosus or tetralogy of Fallot with atresia of the pulmonary artery. Due to the presence of multiple intrathoracic cysts, the heart is malpositioned and the apex points inferiorly. LV, left ventricle; RV, right ventricle; Ant, anterior; Post, posterior; Sup, superior; Inf, inferior.

present in tetralogy of Fallot with pulmonary atresia. Differential diagnosis between these two conditions in the newborn can only be made by visualizing either a truncal valve with more than three leaflets or the origin of the pulmonary arteries from the truncus.[8,13] The latter finding could be demonstrated in the fetus.[1]

Prognosis
Most infants with truncus arteriosus develop heart failure within the first days or months of life. It has been estimated that the survival rate is less than 40 percent at 6 months and less than 20 percent at 1 year.[5,9,11,18] Survivors are affected by rapidly progressive pulmonary vascular disease, and at 4 years of age, 30 percent are no longer operable.[10]

The surgical treatment of truncus arteriosus consists of either palliation or physiologic correction. Attempts to palliate patients by reducing pulmonary blood flow with pulmonary artery banding, have resulted in uniformly poor outcomes with operative mortality rates of 60 percent.[12,14]

On the other hand, physiologic correction by a valved or valveless conduit connecting the right ventricle to the pulmonary artery showed better results, with a lower mortality rate.[6,10,15,16] The goal in these studies was to operate on the patients only when maximal medical therapy failed to control the congestive heart failure. Therefore, patients were operated on either in critical conditions or months after birth.

However, some adverse effects develop after birth in patients with truncus arteriosus, namely elevation of pulmonary vascular resistance, truncal valve insufficiency, and progressive ventricular dysfunction, which can compromise the outcome of the operation. A recent study reviewed the results of the infants who underwent physiologic correction prior to 6 months of age.[7] Out of 100 patients, there were 11 operative deaths. A 2-year follow-up showed 3 late deaths, 1 with bacterial endocarditis and 2 unrelated to their cardiac conditions. Fifty-five infants, as they grew older, required conduit change, which provided excellent results. The experience of these and other authors supports the need for early repair of truncus arteriosus.[6,7,15]

Obstetrical Management
When the diagnosis is made before viability, the option of pregnancy termination should be offered. A careful search for associated cardiac and extracardiac anomalies, including karyotype evaluation, is recommended. Serial ultrasound examinations should be performed to search for signs of congestive heart failure, which is frequently seen in patients with truncal valve incompetence. The association of hydrops with a structural cardiac defect is an ominous combination. The optimal management in these patients has not been established. The option of early delivery may be considered, but the parents should be aware that the mortality rate in these patients is extremely high.

In the absence of congestive heart failure, there is no indication to alter standard obstetrical management, but delivery in a tertiary care center where a pediatric cardiologist is immediately available is mandatory.

REFERENCES

1. Allan LD: Fetal cardiac ultrasound. In: Sanders RC, James AE (eds): The Principles and Practice of Ultrasonography in Obstetrics and Gynecology, 3d ed. E. Norwalk, CT, Appleton-Century-Crofts, 1985, pp 211–217.
2. Becker AE, Anderson RH: Pathology of Congenital Heart Disease. London, Butterworths, 1981.
3. Bharati S, McAllister HA, Rosenquist GC, et al.: The surgical anatomy of truncus arteriosus communis. J Thorac Cardiovasc Surg 67:501, 1974.
4. Calder L, Van Praagh R, Van Praagh S, et al.: Truncus arteriosus communis. Clinical, angiocardiographic, and pathologic findings in 100 patients. Am Heart J 92:23, 1976.
5. Collett RW, Edwards JE: Persistent truncus arteriosus: A classification according to anatomic types. Surg Clin North Am 29:1245, 1949.
6. Di Donato RM, Fyfe DA, Puga FJ, et al.: Fifteen-year

experience with surgical repair of truncus arteriosus. J Thorac Cardiovasc Surg 89:414, 1985.

7. Ebert PA, Turley K, Stanger P, et al.: Surgical treatment of truncus arteriosus in the first 6 months of life. Ann Surg 200:451, 1984.

8. Houston AB, Gregory NL, Murtagh E, et al.: Two-dimensional echocardiography in infants with persistent truncus arteriosus. Br Heart J 46:492, 1981.

9. Kidd BSL: Persistent truncus arteriosus. In: Keith JD, Rowe RD, Vlad P (eds): Heart Disease in Infancy and Childhood. New York, Macmillan, 1978, pp 457–469.

10. Musumeci F, Piccoli GP, Dickinson DF, et al.: Surgical experience with persistent truncus arteriosus in symptomatic infants under 1 year of age. Report of 13 consecutive cases. Br Heart J 46:179, 1981.

11. Nadas AS, Fyler DC: Pediatric Cardiology, 3d ed. Philadelphia, Saunders, 1972.

12. Poirier RA, Berman MA, Stansel HC: Current status of the surgical treatment of truncus arteriosus. J Thorac Cardiovasc Surg 69:169, 1975.

13. Riggs TW, Paul MH: Two-dimensional echocardiographic prospective diagnosis of common truncus arteriosus in infants. Am J Cardiol 50:1380, 1982.

14. Singh AK, DeLeval MR, Pincott JR, et al.: Pulmonary artery banding for truncus arteriosus in the first year of life. Circulation 54 [Suppl 3]:17, 1976.

15. Stanger P, Robinson SJ, Engle MA, et al.: "Corrective" surgery for truncus arteriosus in the first year of life (Abstr). Am J Cardiol 39:293, 1977.

16. Stark J, Gandhi D, de Leval M, et al.: Surgical treatment of persistent truncus arteriosus in the first year of life. Br Heart J 40:1280, 1978.

17. Thiene G, Bortolotti U, Gallucci V, et al.: Anatomical study of truncus arteriosus communis with embryological and surgical considerations. Br Heart J 38:1109, 1976.

18. Van Praagh R, Van Praagh S: The anatomy of common aorticopulmonary trunk (truncus arteriosus communis) and its embryologic implications. A study of 57 necropsy cases. Am J Cardiol 16:406, 1965.

Coarctation and Tubular Hypoplasia of the Aortic Arch

Definition
Coarctation of the aorta is a discrete shelflike lesion present at any point along the aortic arch. Tubular hypoplasia is characterized by a segmental narrowing of a portion of the aortic arch.

Pathogenesis
The pathogenesis of coarctation of the aorta is controversial.[2–5,8,9,16,18,20,22] Three main hypotheses have been suggested to explain the origin of the anomaly. In 1828 Reynaud proposed that coarctation is a primary developmental defect of the aortic arch. This theory has recently been revived by Rosenberg,[16] who suggested that aortic coarctation may result from failure of connection of the fourth and sixth aortic arches with the descending aorta.

The second hypothesis, commonly known as Skodaic theory, relates coarctation of the aorta to the presence of aberrant ductal tissue at the level of the aortic arch. This would result in a narrowing of the vessel at the time of ductal closure. This view has been strongly supported by some authors[3,5,8,22] and disputed by others.[2,4,9]

The third hypothesis proposes that coarctation is the result of decreased blood flow in the ascending aorta and increased flow in the ductus. Following this hemodynamic perturbance, the major blood flow pathway occurs through the ductus arteriosus and the descending aorta. The increased flow entering the aorta leads to the formation of an aortic ridge opposite to the ductus. The decreased flow through the isthmus creates conditions favoring the development of narrowing.[9,18,20]

Pathology
Coarctation of the aorta was traditionally classified as infantile or preductal and adult or postductal form. However, this classification has been abandoned because of its lack of clinical and surgical relevance.

Coarctation of the aorta is most frequently seen as a shelflike lesion located in the juxtaductal portion of the aortic arch. The isthmus above the lesion tends to be narrow. In postnatal life, a dilatation of the aorta distal to the coarctation is seen.[3]

A bicuspid aortic valve is found in 25 to 50 percent of the patients studied. In those patients in whom a bicuspid aortic valve is accompanied by a patent ductus arteriosus (after birth), there is a high incidence of intracardiac anomalies that divert blood away from the aorta and into the pulmonary arterial system (left-sided obstructive lesions).[3]

Associated Anomalies
Intracardiac associated malformations are present in 87 to 90 percent of cases. They include aortic stenosis, aortic insufficiency, VSD, ASD, TGA, ostium primum defects, truncus arteriosus, and double outlet right ventricle.[6,7,12]

Noncardiac malformations have been observed in up to 13 percent of patients.[6] Coarctation of the

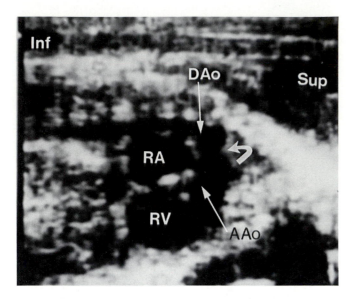

Figure 4–65. Coarctation of the aorta in a third trimester fetus with congestive heart failure. Isthmal narrowing (*curved arrow*) and enlargement of the ascending and descending aorta (AAo, DAo) are demonstrated. RV, right ventricle; RA, right atrium; Sup, superior; Inf, inferior. *(Courtesy of Professor A. Ianniruberto.)*

aorta and VSD are the most common cardiac defects in Turner's syndrome.

Hemodynamic Considerations

Since the blood flowing through the aortic isthmus represents only 10 percent of the total fetal cardiac output,[17] it seems unlikely that coarctation of the aorta can cause significant hemodynamic perturbance in utero. However, in a recent case of coarctation of the aorta diagnosed in a fetus, enlargement and hypertrophy of the right ventricle were found. This suggests that obstruction to isthmal flow may alter hemodynamics.[1]

After birth, hemodynamics are determined by how rapidly the ductus closes and by the presence or absence of associated cardiovascular anomalies. A wide variety of clinical manifestations may result. Approximately half of the patients have congestive heart failure in the neonatal period or shortly thereafter. In these patients, the preductal coarctation complex (isthmus hypoplasia and patent ductus) is generally present. Associated intracardiac anomalies are frequently found. In the remaining patients (juxtaductal and postductal types), the anomaly is an incidental finding later on in life. In patients with an intact ventricular septum, left ventricular overload may lead to congestive heart failure in early life.

Diagnosis

The diagnosis of coarctation of the aorta relies on demonstration of a narrowing of the vessel in the isthmal region, which may be associated with proximal or distal dilatation (Fig. 4–65). However, prenatal

recognition of this condition appears extremely difficult. In fact, in some cases coarctation of the aorta is a postnatal event related to ductal closure. Furthermore, the ultrasound detection of a shelflike lesion in the aortic lumen even during the neonatal period requires a meticulous scanning technique.[19] This quality of examination is hard to achieve in utero.

Notwithstanding these difficulties, coarctation of the aorta has been identified in the fetus,[1,10] thus demonstrating that the prenatal diagnosis of this anomaly is feasible in some cases.

Prognosis

Eleven percent of symptomatic infants presenting before 6 months of age die before surgery.[7] Perioperative mortality for infants operated on within the first 3 to 6 months of life ranges from 3.6 to 11.4 percent.[7,12] Five-year follow-up studies suggest excellent long-term function.[7,12] However, a 32 percent rate of residual coarctation has been reported.[7]

An important prognostic factor is the presence of associated intracardiac anomalies. In a series of 97 symptomatic infants, no deaths occurred over a mean follow-up period of 6 years in those with isolated coarctation. The mortality rate for those with associated anomalies was 39 percent.[7] When comparing the infants operated on before and after 1 year of age, a 100-fold increase in operative mortality was found (43 versus 0.4 percent).[13] In recent years, an important decrease in operative mortality in the symptomatic infant has been reported, with figures ranging from 3.6[12] to 14 percent.[15]

Obstetrical Management

At the time of echocardiographic examination, parents should be informed that coarctation of the aorta may be impossible to diagnose in the fetus for the previously discussed considerations. As a rule, isolated coarctation of the aorta has a better prognosis than coarctation associated with intracardiac anomalies. In the former case, there does not appear to be a need to modify standard obstetrical management. In the presence of associated anomalies, the obstetrical management should be changed according to the severity and nature of the intracardiac defect.

Fetal karyotype and serial ultrasound examinations for the detection of signs of congestive heart failure are recommended. The association of hydrops with a structural cardiac defect is an ominous combination. The optimal management of these patients has yet to be established. The option of early delivery may be considered, but the parents should be aware that the mortality rate in these patients is extremely high.[11] In the absence of congestive heart failure, there is no need to modify standard obstetrical management, but delivery in a tertiary care center where a pediatric cardiologist is immediately available is recommended.

REFERENCES

1. Allan LD, Crawford DC, Tynan M: Evolution of coarctation of the aorta in intrauterine life. Br Heart J 52:471, 1984.
2. Balis JU, Chan AS, Conen PE: Morphogenesis of human aortic coarctation. Exp Mol Pathol 6:25, 1967.
3. Becker AE, Anderson RH: Pathology of Congenital Heart Disease. London, Butterworths, 1981.
4. Berry CL, Tawes RL: Mucopolysaccharides of the aortic wall in coarctation and recoarctation. Cardiovasc Res 4:224, 1970.
5. Bruins C: Competition between aortic isthmus and ductus arteriosus: Reciprocal influence of structure and flow. Eur J Cardiol 8:87, 1978.
6. Campbell M, Polani PE: Etiology of coarctation of the aorta. Lancet 1:473, 1961.
7. Hesslein PS, Gutgesell HP, McNamara DG: Prognosis of symptomatic coarctation of the aorta in infancy. Am J Cardiol 51:299, 1983.
8. Ho SY, Anderson RH: Coarctation, tubular hypoplasia and the ductus arteriosus: Histological study of 35 specimens. Br Heart J 41:268, 1979.
9. Hutchins GM: Coarctation of the aorta explained as a branch point of the ductus arteriosus. Am J Pathol 63:203, 1971.
10. Ianniruberto A, Tajani E: Ecocardiografia fetale e diagnosi prenatale di malformazioni congenite. In: Zulli P, Catizone FA, Ianniruberto A (eds): Esperienze di Ultrasonografia in Ostetricia e Ginecologia. Cosenza, Bios, 1983, pp 117–127.
11. Kleinman CS, Donnerstein RL, DeVore GR, et al.: Fetal echocardiography for evaluation of in utero congestive cardiac failure: A technique for study of nonimmune fetal hydrops. N Engl J Med 306:568, 1982.
12. Korfer R, Meyer H, Kleikamp G, et al.: Early and late results after resection and end-to-end anastomosis of coarctation of the thoracic aorta in early infancy. J Thorac Cardiovasc Surg 89:616, 1985.
13. Lerberg DB, Hardesty RL, Siewers RD, et al.: Coarctation of the aorta in infants and children: 25 years of experience. Ann Thorac Surg 33:159, 1982.
14. Macmanus Q, Starr A, Lambert LE, et al.: Correction of aortic coarctation in neonates. Mortality and late results. Ann Thorac Surg 24:544, 1977.
15. Moulton AL, Brenner JI, Roberts G, et al.: Subclavian flap repair of coarctation of the aorta in neonates. Realization of growth potential. J Thorac Cardiovasc Surg 87:220, 1984.
16. Rosenberg H: Coarctation of the aorta: Morphology and pathogenesis considerations. In: Rosenberg HS, Bolande RP (eds): Perspectives in Pediatric Pathology, vol. 1. Chicago, Year Book, 1973.
17. Rudolph AM: Congenital Diseases of the Heart: Clinical-Physiologic Considerations in Diagnosis and Management. Chicago, Year Book, 1974.
18. Rudolph AM, Heymann MA, Spitznas U: Hemodynamic considerations in the development of narrowing of the aorta. Am J Cardiol 30:514, 1972.
19. Smallhorn JF, Huhta JC, Adams PA, et al.: Cross-sectional echocardiographic assessment of coarctation in the sick neonate and infant. Br Heart J 50:349, 1983.
20. Talner NS, Berman MA: Postnatal development of obstruction in coarctation of the aorta: Role of the ductus arteriosus. Pediatrics 56:562, 1975.
21. Tawes RL, Aberdeen E, Waterston DJ, et al.: Coarctation of the aorta in infants and children. A review of 333 operative cases including 179 infants. Circulation 39–40 [Suppl 1]:173, 1969.
22. Wielenga G, Dankmeijer J: Coarctation of the aorta. J Pathol Bacteriol 95:265, 1968.

Pulmonic Stenosis

Definition
Pulmonic stenosis is an obstructive lesion of the right outflow tract.

Pathology
Pulmonic stenosis is generally the result of fusion of the commissures of the pulmonary cusps. In 10 percent of cases, the stenosis occurs at the level of the infundibulum of the right ventricle. Hypertrophy of the right ventricle is a frequent finding, and the right ventricular chamber is reduced in size. The pulmonary artery is often enlarged (poststenotic dilatation). An interatrial communication (patent foramen ovale or a secundum defect) is a common finding.[1]

Hemodynamic Considerations
The obstruction of the outflow tract puts excessive demands on the right ventricle. Pulmonic stenosis is not generally a neonatal emergency. In severe instances, this lesion may lead to congestive heart failure soon after birth[9,10] and in utero as well.

Associated Anomalies
Intracardiac associated anomalies include atrial septal defects, total anomalous pulmonary venous return, and supravalvar aortic stenosis. Furthermore, pulmonic stenosis is the most common cardiac defect in Noonan's syndrome and may be part of the maternal rubella syndrome.

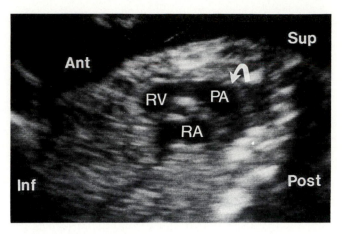

Figure 4–66. Enlargement of the pulmonary artery (PA) in a third trimester fetus. The pulmonary valve opening appeared normal on both real-time and M-mode examination. Nevertheless, the infant was found at birth to have moderate to severe valvular pulmonic stenosis. RV, right ventricle; RA, right atrium; Sup, superior; Inf, inferior; Ant, anterior; Post, posterior. *(Reproduced with permission from Bovicelli L, Baccarani G, Picchio FM, Pilu G: Ecocardiografia Fetale. La Diagnosi e il Trattamento Prenatale delle Cardiopatie Congenite. Milan, Masson, 1985.)*

Diagnosis

A prenatal diagnosis is extremely difficult. The condition should be suspected when there is either enlargement of the pulmonary artery or reduction in size of the right ventricle (Figs. 4–23, 4–66).

In the newborn, the valvular form of pulmonic stenosis is diagnosed by demonstrating the systolic doming (incomplete opening) of the pulmonary valve. The identification of this finding in a fetus is extremely difficult because of the small size of the pulmonary valve and its distance from the transducer. It should be stressed that M-mode echocardiography is not a reliable tool in the recognition of semilunar valve stenosis.[4] Indeed, demonstration of the apparently normal opening of the pulmonic valve with this technique does not rule out stenosis. Doppler echocardiography is a useful technique in the newborn. Its diagnostic value depends on the detection of poststenotic turbulent flow in the pulmonary trunk. However, because of the small size of the fetal pulmonary artery, it is doubtful that a turbulence in the flow at this level can be reliably detected. Doppler echocardiography may play a major role by demonstrating the tricuspid regurgitation that is seen in the most severe cases.

Prognosis

Pulmonic stenosis encompasses a wide spectrum of severity. An autopsy study has reported that the mean age of death in untreated patients is 21 years.[6] In a large series of 221 patients operated on between 1 day of life and 61 years of age, there were 9 operative deaths (4 percent) and 2 late deaths (1 percent).[2]

However, severe pulmonic stenosis may be a neonatal emergency. Luke reported a 17 percent preoperative mortality rate in a group of critically ill infants diagnosed between birth and 2 years of age.[9] Operative mortality for these patients ranged between 12.5 percent[11] and 16 percent.[3] However, Litwin et al.[8] reported no perioperative deaths on 29 patients.

The most relevant data available for prenatal counseling is that of Freed et al.[5] who reported no deaths in a group of 13 critically ill neonates diagnosed within 2 days of birth and who had a diminutive right ventricle.

Obstetrical Management

For every congenital cardiac lesion, careful scanning of the entire fetal anatomy and karyotyping are recommended. The option of pregnancy termination should be offered before viability. Serial ultrasound examinations to rule out early signs of congestive heart failure are indicated. The association of hydrops with a structural cardiac defect is an ominous combination. The optimal management in these patients has yet to be established. The option of early delivery may be considered, but the parents should be aware that the mortality rate in these patients is extremely high.[7]

In the absence of congestive heart failure, there is no indication to alter standard obstetrical management, but delivery in a tertiary care center where a pediatric cardiologist is immediately available is mandatory.

REFERENCES

1. Becker AE, Anderson RH: Pathology of Congenital Heart Disease. London, Butterworths, 1981.
2. Danielson GK, Exarhos ND, Weidman WH, et al.: Pulmonic stenosis with intact ventricular septum. Surgical considerations and results of operation. J Thorac Cardiovasc Surg 61:228, 1971.
3. Daskalopoulos DA, Pieroni DR, Gingell RL, et al.: Closed transventricular pulmonary valvotomy in infants. Long-term results and the effect of the size of the right ventricle. J Thorac Cardiovasc Surg 84:187, 1982.
4. Feigenbaum H: Echocardiography, 3d ed. Philadelphia, Lea & Febiger, 1981.
5. Freed MD, Rosenthal A, Bernhard WF, et al.: Critical pulmonary stenosis with a diminutive right ventricle in neonates. Circulation 48:875, 1973.
6. Keith JD, Rowe RD, Vlad P: Heart Disease in Infancy and Childhood, 3d ed. New York, Macmillan, 1978.
7. Kleinman CS, Donnerstein RL, De Vore GR, et al.: Fetal echocardiography for evaluation of in utero congestive heart failure: A technique for study of nonimmune fetal hydrops. N Engl J Med 306:568, 1982.
8. Litwin SB, Williams WH, Freed MD, et al.: Critical pulmonary stenosis in infants: A surgical emergency. Surgery 74:880, 1973.

9. Luke MJ: Valvular pulmonic stenosis in infancy. J Pediatr 68:90, 1966.
10. Mustard WT, Jain SC, Trusler GA: Pulmonary stenosis in the first year of life. Br Heart J 30:255, 1968.
11. Srinivasan V, Konyer A, Broda JJ, et al.: Critical pulmonary stenosis in infants less than three months of age: A reappraisal of closed transventricular pulmonary valvotomy. Ann Thorac Surg 34:46, 1982.

Aortic Stenosis

Definition

Aortic stenosis is an obstructive lesion of the left outflow tract. Depending on the site of the lesion, this entity is classified as supravalvar, valvar, or subvalvar. The term includes aortic valvar stenosis, aortic supravalvar stenosis, aortic subvalvar stenosis, subaortic stenosis, asymmetric septal hypertrophy (ASH), and idiopathic hypertrophic subaortic stenosis (IHSS).

Etiology and Pathology

Supravalvar aortic stenosis can be due to one of three anatomic defects: a membrane (usually placed above the sinuses of Valsalva), a localized narrowing of the ascending aorta (hourglass deformity), or a diffuse narrowing involving the aortic arch and branching arteries (tubular variety).[2] Isolated supravalvar aortic stenosis can be inherited with an autosomal recessive pattern.[12] The Williams syndrome is a sporadic disease that is characterized by the association of supravalvar aortic or pulmonic stenosis, elfin facies, and idiopathic hypercalcemia. Maternal hypervitaminosis D has been implicated as a cause of this condition.[3]

The valvar form of aortic stenosis can be due to dysplastic, thickened aortic cusps or fusion of the commissures between the cusps.[2]

The subvalvar form of aortic stenosis is commonly divided into two subgroups: fixed and dynamic. The fixed form can be due to either a membrane (discrete subaortic stenosis) or a fibromuscular tunnel (diffuse subaortic stenosis). The dynamic form is due to a muscular thickening of the septal surface.[2] Many of these cases are inherited in an autosomal dominant fashion,[5] and they are commonly referred to as asymmetric septal hypertrophy (ASH), idiopathic hypertrophic subaortic stenosis (IHSS), or hypertrophic obstructive cardiomyopathy (HOCM). A transient form of dynamic obstruction of the left outflow tract is seen in infants of diabetic mothers. This condition is commonly attributed to the association of fetal hyperglycemia and hyperinsulinemia.[8]

The left ventricle is usually of normal size or enlarged. In some instances, the ventricular cavity may be small. In severe forms of aortic stenosis, the endocardium may be thickened (secondary endocardial fibroelastosis). In these patients, mitral insufficiency is a frequent finding.[2]

Associated Anomalies

Supravalvar aortic stenosis may be related to the Williams syndrome. Subaortic stenosis has been described in patients with Turner's syndrome, Noonan's syndrome, and congenital rubella.[14]

Hemodynamic Considerations

Aortic stenosis causes obstruction of the left ventricular outflow tract. Depending on the severity of the stenosis, the pressure in the left ventricle is increased. Although subvalvar and supravalvar forms are not generally manifested in the neonatal period, the valvar type can be a cause of congestive heart failure in the newborn and the fetus as well.[10] Of all congenital cardiac abnormalities, aortic stenosis is the one most frequently found in association with intrauterine growth retardation.[13]

Diagnosis

A prenatal diagnosis is extremely difficult. The condition should be suspected when there is either enlargement or hypoplasia of the left ventricle or ascending aorta.[1]

The prenatal diagnosis of supravalvar aortic stenosis has not been reported. Even if the ascending aorta can be well visualized in utero, it is doubtful that a discrete membrane or an hourglass deformity can be identified. It should be stressed that this condition is not usually manifested in the neonatal period.

In the newborn, the valvar form of aortic stenosis is diagnosed by demonstrating the systolic doming (incomplete opening) of the aortic valve. Identification of this finding in a fetus is extremely difficult due to the small size of the aortic valve and its distance from the transducer. It should be stressed that M-mode echocardiography is not a reliable tool in the recognition of semilunar valvar stenosis.[6] Indeed, demonstration of the apparently normal opening of the aortic valve with this technique does not rule out

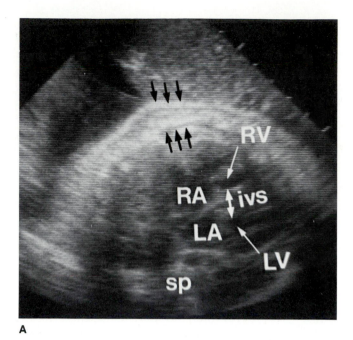

A

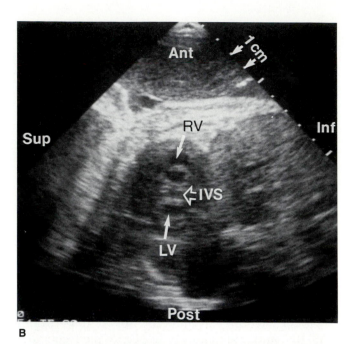

B

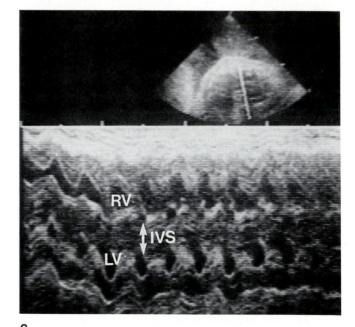

C

Figure 4–67. Hypertrophic cardiomyopathy in a 35-week fetus of a diabetic mother. A four chamber view (**A**), short axis view (**B**), and an M-mode echocardiogram (**C**) of the ventricles reveals a disproportionately thick interventricular septum (14 mm) and a small left ventricular cavity. Note the thickness of the soft tissues overlying the rib cage (*black arrows*). RV, right ventricle; LV, left ventricle; RA, right atrium; LA, left atrium; IVS, interventricular septum; Sp, spine; Sup, superior; Inf, inferior; Ant, anterior; Post, posterior. (Fig. 4–24 is a nomogram for the size of the IVS; see p 134.)

stenosis. Pulsed Doppler echocardiography is a useful technique in the newborn. Its diagnostic value depends on the detection of poststenotic turbulent flow in the ascending aorta. However, because of the small size of the fetal ascending aorta, it is doubtful that turbulence at this level can be reliably detected. Doppler echocardiography may play a diagnostic role by demonstrating the mitral regurgitation that is frequently seen in severe cases.

For the fixed forms of subaortic stenosis, the same considerations formulated for the supravalvar form apply. ASH and hypertrophic cardiomyopathy of infants of diabetic mothers can be diagnosed by demonstrating an abnormal thickening of the ventricular septum (Fig. 4–67). We have been able to docu-

ment the latter condition on several occasions. Prenatal diagnosis of ASH has been reported.[13a] Although there is evidence that ASH is a progressive disease, it is usually not present at birth.[14]

Prognosis

Supravalvar and subvalvar aortic stenosis are rarely a cause of severe hemodynamic compromise in the neonatal period. Among the infants with valvar aortic stenosis, two groups should be considered. In some patients, severe obstruction to the left outflow tract results in congestive heart failure in the first days or weeks of life. Other patients are asymptomatic at birth, and the condition is recognized only later in infancy and childhood.

Delineating the natural history of congenital aortic stenosis, Campbell[4] estimated that the mortality rate in the first year of life was 23 percent and fell to 1.2 percent for the rest of the first two decades. It then rose again to about 3 percent, 3.5 percent, 6 percent, and 8.5 percent in the third to sixth decades, respectively. According to this estimation, 60 percent of the patients were living at 30 years of age and 40 percent were living at 40 years. Sudden death accounts for a significant proportion of losses in this condition.

Jones et al.[9] reported the results of corrective surgery in infants with either valvar or subvalvar aortic stenosis. The operative mortality rate was 1.9 percent in the patients with valvar aortic stenosis, 6 percent in those with fixed subaortic stenosis, and 5.5 percent in those with ASH. Late survival rates with an average follow-up duration of 5 years were 90 percent, 86 percent, and 82 percent, respectively. It was estimated that 54 percent, 54 percent, and 70 percent, respectively, of patients in the three groups had satisfactory late results 5 to 14 years after operation. These data refer mainly to patients who were not critically ill at birth.

The newborn with symptomatic aortic stenosis usually has severe dyspnea and intractable congestive heart failure. In these patients, an operative mortality of 29 to 71 percent has been reported. Recently, Messina et al.[11] described a much lower mortality rate (9 percent). The only death in their series occurred in an infant with a small left ventricle. The authors suggested that the association between aortic stenosis and an underdeveloped left ventricular cavity is a poor prognostic indicator.

A wide range of clinical and morphologic expression is expected from patients with supravalvar aortic stenosis. Flaker et al.[7] reported a series of 16 patients who underwent patch aortoplasty. Three surgical deaths occurred, and 2 of these patients had a diffuse narrowing of the aorta. Ten patients were asymptomatic 1 to 12 years after operation, one had angina, and one died from cancer.

The hypertrophic cardiomyopathy of infants of diabetic mothers is a transient condition that is, in most cases, asymptomatic. Less frequently, cyanosis and congestive heart failure may occur.[8]

Obstetrical Management

If the diagnosis is made, careful scanning of the entire fetal anatomy and karyotyping are recommended. The option of pregnancy termination should be offered before viability. Serial ultrasound examinations to rule out early signs of congestive heart failure are indicated. The association of hydrops with a structural cardiac defect is an ominous combination. The optimal management of these patients has not been established. The option of early delivery may be considered, but the parents should be aware that the mortality rate in these patients is extremely high.[10] In the absence of congestive heart failure, there is no indication to alter standard obstetrical management, but delivery in a tertiary care center where a pediatric cardiologist is immediately available is mandatory.

The diagnosis of septal hypertrophy in a fetus of a diabetic mother is an indication for a careful examination of the metabolic control of the patient.

REFERENCES

1. Allan L, Little D, Campbell S, et al.: Fetal ascites associated with congenital heart disease: Case report. Br J Obstet Gynaecol 88:453, 1981.
2. Becker AE, Anderson RH: Pathology of Congenital Heart Disease. London, Butterworths, 1981.
3. Beuren AJ: Supravalvular aortic stenosis: A complex syndrome with and without mental retardation. Birth Defects 8:45, 1972.
4. Campbell M: The natural history of congenital aortic stenosis. Br Heart J 30:514, 1968.
5. Clark CE, Henry WL, Epstein SE: Familial prevalence and genetic transmission of idiopathic hypertrophic subaortic stenosis. N Engl J Med 289:709, 1973.
6. Feigenbaum H: Echocardiography, 3d ed. Philadelphia, Lea & Febiger, 1981.
7. Flaker G, Teske D, Kilman J, et al.: Supravalvular aortic stenosis. A 20-year clinical perspective and experience with patch aortoplasty. Am J Cardiol 51:256, 1983.
8. Gutgesell HP, Mullins CE, Gillette PC, et al.: Transient hypertrophic subaortic stenosis in infants of diabetic mothers. J Pediatr 89:120, 1976.
9. Jones M, Barnhart GR, Morrow AG: Late results after operations for left ventricular outflow tract obstruction. Am J Cardiol 50:569, 1982.
10. Kleinman CS, Donnerstein RL, De Vore GR, et al.: Fetal echocardiography for evaluation of in utero congestive heart failure: A technique for study of nonimmune fetal hydrops. N Engl J Med 306:568, 1982.
11. Messina LM, Turley K, Stanger P, et al.: Successful aortic valvotomy for severe congenital valvular aortic stenosis in the newborn infant. J Thorac Cardiovasc Surg 88:92, 1984.
12. Nora JJ, Nora AH: Genetics and Counseling in Cardiovascular Diseases. Springfield, IL, Chas. C Thomas, 1978.
13. Reynolds JL: Intrauterine growth retardation in children with congenital heart disease—Its relation to aortic stenosis. Birth Defects 8:143, 1972.
13a. Stewart PA, Buis-Liem T, Verwey RA, Wladimiroff JW: Prenatal ultrasonic diagnosis of familial asymmetric septal hypertrophy. Prenat Diagn 6:249, 1986.
14. Wright GB, Keane JF, Nadas AS, et al.: Fixed subaortic stenosis in the young: Medical and surgical course in 83 patients. Am J Cardiol 52:830, 1983.

Cardiomyopathies

Definition
Cardiomyopathies are a heterogeneous group of disorders of the heart muscle.

Etiology and Pathogenesis
A wide variety of etiologic factors can cause damage to the myocardium. Infectious agents, such as viruses and bacteria, can lead to myocarditis. Cardiomyopathies are a part of several inborn errors of metabolism. The list includes glycogenosis, mucolipidosis, and mucopolysaccharidosis. Involvement of the myocardium is seen in muscular dystrophies.[6] Endocardial fibroelastosis has been linked in the past to congenital infection by various viral agents (Coxsackie viruses[4] mumps virus[8]). Familial cases have often been reported, suggesting either an autosomal recessive or X-linked transmission.[5,9] Asymmetric septal hypertrophy (ASH) and the hypertrophic cardiomyopathy of infants of diabetic mothers have been discussed previously (see section on aortic stenosis). Another cause of cardiomyopathy is myocardial ischemia. Entities such as transient myocardial ischemia, anomalous origin of the left coronary artery, and coronary calcinosis are probably due to an ischemic mechanism. Cardiomyopathies can also be of idiopathic etiology.

Pathology
Pathologic findings differ according to the etiology. Myocarditis is characterized by necrosis and destruction of myocardial cells, as well as an inflammatory infiltrate. In endocardial fibroelastosis, a thickened

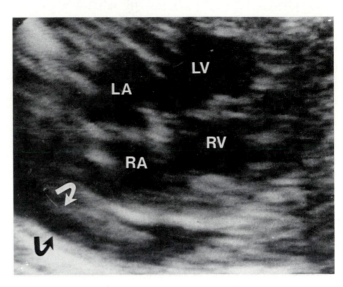

Figure 4–68. Endocardial fibroelastosis in a third trimester fetus. The cardiac chambers appear greatly enlarged, and the ventricular walls are thickened. At real-time examination, poor contractility of the ventricular walls was noted. A noticeable pleural effusion is visible (*arrows*). LV, left ventricle; RV, right ventricle; RA, right atrium; LA, left atrium. *(Reproduced with permission from Bovicelli et al.: Prenat Diagn 4:67, 1984.)*

grayish endocardium lines either the left or both ventricular cavities. The left ventricle may be either large (dilated form) or small (contracted form). With Pompe's disease or glycogenosis type IIa, the myocardium is hypertrophic with large myocardial cells containing accumulations of glycogen. Similar findings are expected in other storage diseases. Isch-

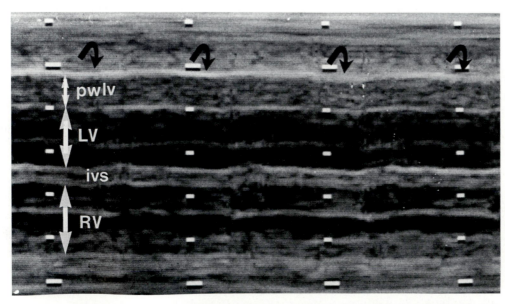

Figure 4–69. In the same patient as in Figure 4–68, an M-mode echocardiogram of the ventricular chambers reveals severely reduced contractility (*curved arrows*) and thickening of the posterior wall of the left ventricle (pwlv). LV, left ventricle; RV, right ventricle; ivs, interventricular septum.

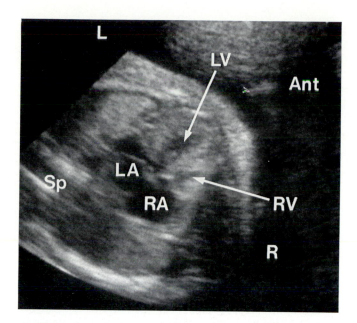

Figure 4–70. Hypertrophic cardiomyopathy in a second trimester fetus. Note the abnormal thickness of the ventricular walls and the slitlike ventricles. LV, left ventricle; RV, right ventricle; LA, left atrium; RA, right atrium; Sp, spine; Ant, anterior; L, left; R, right.

emic lesions can be caused by an obstruction of the coronary arteries or retrograde flow in the presence of a left coronary artery arising from the pulmonary artery. Valvar insufficiency is a frequent finding in cardiomyopathies. It is usually due to the enlargement of the valvar ring secondary to dilatation of the cardiac chambers.[7]

Hemodynamic Considerations

The most prominent clinical feature of cardiomyopathies is a tendency toward congestive heart failure. The mechanisms responsible are pump failure or valvar insufficiency (nonobstructive forms) or ob-

struction to ventricular outflow. The severity of these disorders depends largely on the etiology. The clinical spectrum ranges between forms that become symptomatic in childhood and infancy and forms that lead to intrauterine congestive heart failure.

Diagnosis

The diagnosis of nonobstructive cardiomyopathy depends on demonstration of cardiomegaly and poor contractility of the ventricular wall.[1,3] Biometry of the cardiac chambers, including ventricular wall thickness, has been reported by several investigators.[2,10,11] Contractility can be assessed by calculation of the fractional shortening, which is the percentage of shortening of the cardiac chamber in relation to the end-diastolic diameter.[10,11] The formula is the following:

$$\text{Fractional shortening (\%)} = \left(ED - \frac{ES}{ED} \right) \times 100$$

where ED is the end-diastolic diameter and ES is the end-systolic diameter of the ventricular wall. In severe cases, the ultrasound appearance is obvious, and measurements are unnecessary[3] (Figs. 4–68, 4–69). Obstructive cardiomyopathies are characterized by thickened ventricular walls (Figs. 4–70, 4–71).

ASH and hypertrophic cardiomyopathy of fetuses of diabetic mothers were discussed in the section on aortic stenosis (pp. 175–176).

Prognosis

There is extreme variability in the presentation and course of the different forms. No figures are available to predict fetal outcome. However, if the disease is evident in utero, the prognosis is probably poor.

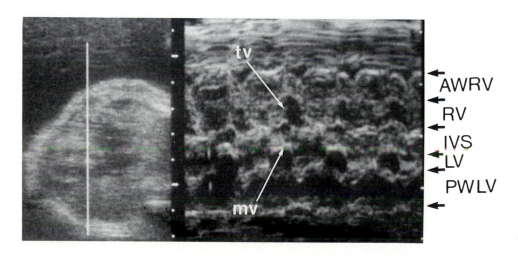

Figure 4–71. M-mode echocardiogram in the same patient as in Figure 4–70, demonstrating the reduction in size of the ventricular cavity and extreme thickness and hypercontractility of the ventricular walls. LV, left ventricle; RV, right ventricle; IVS, interventricular septum; AWRV, anterior wall of the right ventricle; PWLV, posterior wall of the left ventricle; tv, tricuspid valve; mv, mitral valve.

Obstetrical Management

When the diagnosis is made before viability, the option of pregnancy termination should be offered. Serial ultrasound examinations should be performed to search for signs of congestive heart failure. The association of hydrops with a cardiomyopathy is an ominous combination. The optimal management of these patients has not been established. The option of early delivery may be considered, but the parents should be aware that the mortality rate in these patients is extremely high. Delivery in a tertiary care center is mandatory.

REFERENCES

1. Allan LD, Crawford DC, Anderson RH, et al.: Echocardiographic and anatomical correlations in fetal congenital heart disease. Br Heart J 52:542, 1984.
2. Allan LD, Joseph MC, Boyd EGCA, et al.: M-mode echocardiography in the developing human fetus. Br Heart J: 47:573, 1982.
3. Bovicelli L, Picchio FM, Pilu G, et al.: Prenatal diagnosis of endocardial fibroelastosis. Prenat Diagn 4:67, 1984.
4. Brown GC, Evans TN: Serologic evidence of Coxsackie virus etiology of congenital heart disease. JAMA 199:183, 1967.
5. Chen S, Thompson MW, Rose V: Endocardial fibroelastosis: Family studies with special reference to counselling. J Pediatr 79:385, 1971.
6. Nora JJ, Nora AH: Genetics and Counseling in Cardiovascular Diseases. Springfield, IL, Chas. C Thomas, 1978.
7. Rowe RD, Freedom RM, Mehrizi A, Bloom KR: The Neonate with Congenital Heart Disease, 2d ed Philadelphia, Saunders, 1981.
8. St. Geme JW, Noren GR, Adams P Jr.: Proposed embryopathic relation between mumps virus and primary endocardial fibroelastosis. N Engl J Med 275:339, 1966.
9. Westwood M, Harris R, Burn JL, et al.: Heredity in primary endocardial fibroelastosis. Br Heart J 37:1077, 1975
10. Wladimiroff JW, Mc Ghie JS: M-mode ultrasonic assessment of fetal cardiovascular dynamics. Br J Obstet Gynaecol 88:1241, 1981.
11. Wladimiroff JW, Vosters R, Mc Ghie JS: Normal cardiac ventricular geometry and function during the last trimester of pregnancy and early neonatal period. Br J Obstet Gynaecol 89:839, 1982.

Total Anomalous Pulmonary Venous Return

Definition

Total anomalous pulmonary venous return (TAPVR) is characterized by drainage of the pulmonary veins into the right atrium.

Embryology

During early stages of development, the intraparenchymal or primary pulmonary veins are connected to the veins of the systemic circulation. In a later stage, an anastomosis between the intraparenchymal pulmonary veins and the primary pulmonary vein (derived from the left atrium) is established. At the same time, the communication with the systemic circulation is lost (Fig. 4–72). Failure of reabsorption of the communication between the intraparenchymal pulmonary veins and the systemic circulation results in anomalous pulmonary venous return.[1]

Pathology

The pulmonary veins normally drain into the left atrium. TAPVR occurs when part or all of the blood flow from these vessels returns to the right atrium.

Anomalous pulmonary venous return may be classified as total or partial according to whether all the blood coming from one lung (unilateral) or both lungs (bilateral) drains inside the right atrium. We discuss here only the total bilateral variety.

Depending on the site of the drainage, TAPVR is classified as supradiaphragmatic or infradiaphragmatic. The former can be subclassified into supracardiac or cardiac (Fig. 4–73). The supracardiac drainage follows the course of the left innominate vein, right and left persistent superior vena cava, hemiazygos and azygos veins. The cardiac drainage may end directly into the right atrium or into the coronary sinus. The infradiaphragmatic drainage is characterized by the presence of a venous channel that is normally connected either to the inferior vena cava or to the portal veins.[1] In some instances, the pulmonary venous return is obstructed. This has important prognostic implications.[9]

Hemodynamic Considerations

TAPVR is not thought to be a cause of significant hemodynamic perturbances in the fetus, because there is normally a right-to-left shunt at the level of the atrial chambers. Exceptions may exist in those

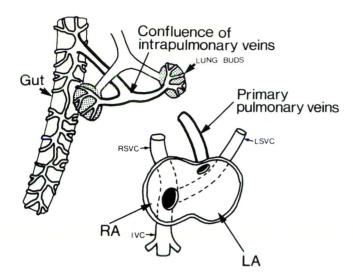

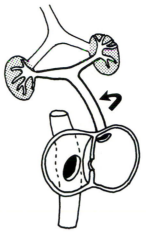

Figure 4–72. Schematic representation of the embryology of the pulmonary veins. In the early stages, the intrapulmonary veins are connected to the veins of the systemic circulation. In a later stage, the intrapulmonary veins connect with the primary pulmonary veins, which arise from the atria. RA, right atrium; LA, left atrium; RSVC, LSVC, IVC, right superior, left superior, and inferior venae cavae. *(Modified with permission from Becker, Anderson: Pathology of Congenital Heart Disease. London, Butterworths, 1981.)*

cases associated with obstruction of the pulmonary veins. After birth, the two major problems that arise are volume overload of the right ventricle and mixture of systemic and pulmonary venous blood at the level of the right atrium. Most of these infants experience congestive heart failure a few days or months after birth.

Diagnosis

Recognition of TAPVR is not easy in the fetus, since it is difficult to identify the abnormal venous communications between the right atrium and the pulmonary circulation. It is especially difficult in supracardiac or infradiaphragmatic types.

However, the presence of TAPVR should be suspected in all patients in whom the sonographer is

unable to demonstrate the entrance of the pulmonary veins in the left atrium. Due to the absent connection of the pulmonary veins, the left atrium is usually smaller than normal. Such a finding should raise the index of suspicion (Fig. 4–74).

Echocardiographic findings of TAPVR in the newborn often include a small left heart.[9] This is not to be expected to be prominent in utero because of the physiologic right-to-left shunt.

TAPVR should be suspected in all cases of

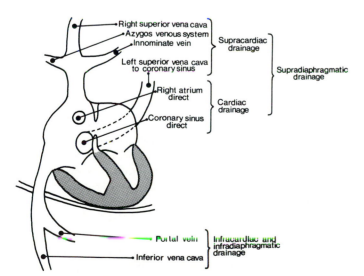

Figure 4–73. Schematic representation of the classification of anomalous pulmonary venous return. See text for a description. *(Modified with permission from Becker, Anderson: Pathology of Congenital Heart Disease. London, Butterworths, 1981.)*

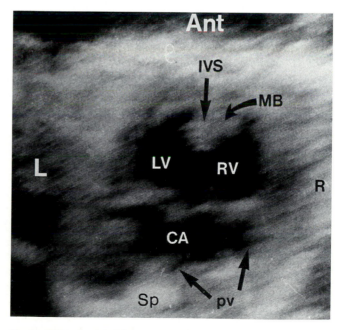

Figure 4–74. In this fetus with asplenia syndrome, mesocardia, and complete atrioventricular canal, the pulmonary veins (pv) are seen entering on the right side of the common atrium (CA). Note that the left side of the common atrium is indented at the level of the normal entry of the pulmonary veins. LV, left ventricle; RV, right ventricle; IVS, interventricular septum; MB, moderator band; Sp, spine; Ant, anterior; L, left; R, right.

atrioventricular septal defects and asplenia and polysplenia syndromes.

Prognosis

Seventy-five percent of untreated infants with TAPVR die within 1 year of birth, and the others usually die before reaching adulthood.[2–4,5–8] Operative procedures are intended to restore the anatomy of the pulmonary vein drainage.[8] In a series of 25 infants, the operative mortality was 20 percent, and all deaths occurred in critically ill infants with pulmonary venous obstruction. No late death was observed, and the hemodynamic condition of the survivors was good.[8] The most important prognostic factor was the presence of pulmonary venous obstruction.[10]

Obstetrical Management

TAPVR can be suspected in certain cases, but it is not clear yet if a specific prenatal diagnosis can be made with confidence. However, it should be stressed that if associated anomalies are absent and the infant is promptly assisted in the neonatal period, the prognosis after survival with surgical repair is excellent. Obstetrical management would not be altered by the prenatal diagnosis of TAPVR. It is unclear if TAPVR associated with pulmonary venous obstruction can result in congestive heart failure in utero. Serial ultrasound monitoring of these fetuses is, therefore, recommended. Delivery in a tertiary care center where a pediatric cardiologist is immediately available is suggested.

REFERENCES

1. Becker AE, Anderson RH: Pathology of Congenital Heart Disease. London, Butterworths, 1981.
2. Behrendt DM, Aberdeen E, Waterson DJ, et al.: Total anomalous pulmonary venous drainage in infants. I. Clinical and hemodynamic findings, methods, and results of operation in 37 cases. Circulation 46:347, 1972.
3. Bonham Carter RE, Capriles M, Noe Y: Total anomalous pulmonary venous drainage: A clinical and anatomical study of 75 children. Br Heart J 31:45, 1969.
4. Brody H: Drainage of the pulmonary veins into the right side of the heart. Arch Pathol 33:221, 1942.
5. El-Said G, Mullins CE, McNamara, DG: Management of total anomalous pulmonary venous return. Circulation 45:1240, 1972.
6. Gathman GE, Nadas AS: Total anomalous pulmonary venous connection. Clinical and physiologic observations of 75 pediatric patients. Circulation 42:143, 1970.
7. Gomes MMR, Feldt RH, McGoon DC, et al.: Total anomalous pulmonary venous connection. Surgical considerations and results of operation. J Thorac Cardiovasc Surg 60:116, 1970.
8. Hammon JW, Bender HW, Graham TP, et al.: Total anomalous pulmonary venous connection in infancy. Ten years' experience including studies of postoperative ventricular function. J Thorac Cardiovasc Surg 80:544, 1980.
9. Hawker RE, Celermajer JM, Gengos DC, et al.: Common pulmonary vein atresia. Premortem diagnosis in two infants. Circulation 46:368, 1972.
10. Lima CO, Valdes-Cruz LM, Allen HD, et al.: Prognostic value of left ventricular size measured by echocardiography in infants with total anomalous pulmonary venous drainage. Am J Cardiol 51:1155, 1983.

Tumors of the Heart

Pathology

Congenital cardiac tumors are extremely rare lesions. It has been estimated that their overall frequency is 1 in 10,000 autopsies in individuals of all ages. Most of these tumors are benign. In infants, the most common tumors are rhabdomyomas (58 percent) and teratomas (20 percent). Less common lesions include fibroma, myxoma (which predominates in adults), hemangioma, and mesothelioma.[14] Malignancy occurs in less than 10 percent of all cases.[10] Size and location of the tumors vary considerably. Rhabdomyomas tend to be multiple and to involve the septum. Teratomas may be both intrapericardic and extracardiac.[2] Fibromas account for 12 percent of the tumors in the neonatal period and until 1 year of age. Fibromas may be pedunculated and may calcify.

Associated Anomalies

Cardiac tumors are generally isolated anomalies. An exception to this is the association between tuberous sclerosis (TS) and rhabdomyomas: TS has been reported in 50 to 86 percent of patients with cardiac rhabdomyomas.[3,4] TS is generally a familial disease inherited as an autosomal dominant trait with a high degree of penetrance and variable expressivity. Rarely, it may be a sporadic event. However, the diagnosis of TS in the first child in the absence of a positive family tree does not allow distinguishing whether the event is sporadic or results from transmission from a mutation-bearing parent. TS is diagnosed when at least one of the following lesions is present: cortical tubers, subependymal hamartomas, multiple retinal hamartomas, and skin lesions

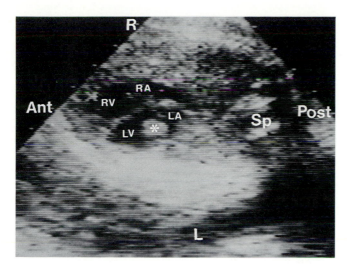

Figure 4–75. Four-chamber view of the heart in a third trimester fetus with a cardiac rhabdomyoma (∗) of the free wall of the left ventricle (LV). RV, right ventricle; RA, right atrium; LA, left atrium; Sp, spine; Ant, anterior, Post, posterior, R, right, L, left. *(Courtesy of Dr. Tullia Todros, University of Turin.)*

(adenoma sebaceum or periungual fibroma). Secondary or presumptive diagnostic criteria include hypomelanotic macules in the skin, subependymal or cortical calcifications, multiple renal tumors, and cardiac rhabdomyomas. Rhabdomyomas are also frequently associated with supraventricular tachycardia. Accessory conductive pathways within the tumor are thought to be responsible for this association.[6,13,15]

Hemodynamic Considerations

The mechanisms by which cardiac tumors become symptomatic include obstruction of the inflow or outflow of the cardiac chambers and cardiac dysrhythmias, both possibly leading to congestive heart failure.[11,13,14]

Diagnosis

Recognition of an intracardiac tumor depends on visualization of a mass-occupying lesion impinging upon the cardiac cavities.[1,5,7–9] The demonstration of multiple cardiac tumors suggests a diagnosis of rhabdomyomas (Fig 4–75).[4] Given the strong association between rhabdomyomas and TS, visualization of multiple cardiac tumors in a fetus should prompt a careful search to detect the other stigmata of TS (concentrating in particular on the CNS and kidneys). Review of the family history, focusing on the presence of mental retardation or seizures in the relatives, is also indicated. First degree relatives should have an eye examination and inspection of the skin with Wood's light.[8a]

Prognosis

The prognosis depends on the number, size, location, and histologic type of the tumors. The clinical spectrum varies from completely asymptomatic to severely ill. In a review of the surgical literature, rhabdomyomas operated on within the first year of life were associated with a 29 percent mortality rate. About one fourth of the patients with TS present by the age of 2 years with seizures or mental retardation. However, presentation may be delayed until adulthood or the disease may remain clinically absent. Since surgical excision is possible, the prenatal identification of congenital tumors is important for earlier referral and treatment.[3,12]

Obstetrical Management

When the diagnosis of a cardiac tumor is made before viability, the option of pregnancy termination should be offered. Serial ultrasound examinations should be performed to search for signs of congestive heart failure. The association of hydrops with a structural cardiac defect is an ominous combination. The optimal management of these patients has not been established. The option of early delivery may be considered, but the parents should be aware that the mortality rate in these patients is extremely high.[9] In the absence of congestive heart failure, there is no need to modify standard obstetrical management, but delivery in a tertiary care center where a pediatric cardiologist is immediately available is mandatory.

REFERENCES

1. Allan LD, Crawford DC, Anderson RH, et al.: Echocardiographic and anatomical correlations in fetal congenital heart disease. Br Heart J 52:542, 1984.
2. Arciniegas E, Hakimi M, Farooki ZQ, et al.: Primary cardiac tumors in children. J Thorac Cardiovasc Surg. 79:582, 1980.
3. Corno A, de Simone G, Catena G, et al.: Cardiac rhabdomyoma: Surgical treatment in the neonate. J Thorac Cardiovasc Surg. 87:725, 1984.
4. Dennis MA, Appareti K, Manco-Johnson ML, et al.: The echocardiographic diagnosis of multiple fetal cardiac tumors. J Ultrasound Med 4:327, 1985.
5. DeVore GR, Hakim S, Kleinman C, et al.: The in utero diagnosis of an interventricular septal cardiac rhabdomyoma by means of real-time directed M-mode echocardiography. Am J Obstet Gynecol 143:967, 1982.
6. Engle MA, Ito T, Ehlers KH, et al.: Rhabdomyomatosis of heart. Diagnosis during life with clinical and pathologic findings. Circulation 26:712, 1962.
7. Fischer DR, Beerman LB, Park SC, et al.: Diagnosis of intracardiac rhabdomyoma by two-dimensional echocardiography. Am J Cardiol 53:978, 1984.
8. Gladden JR, Dreiling RJ, Gollub SB, et al.: Two-dimensional echocardiographic features of multiple right atrial myxomas. Am J Cardiol 52:1364, 1983.
8a. Journel H, Roussey M, Plais MH, et al.: Prenatal diagnosis of familial tuberous sclerosis following detection of cardiac rhabdomyoma by ultrasound. Prenat Diagn 6:283, 1986.
9. Kleinman CS, Donnerstein RL, DeVore GR, et al.: Fetal

echocardiography for evaluation of in utero congestive heart failure. A technique for study of nonimmune fetal hydrops. N Engl J Med 306:568, 1982.

10. McAllister H: Primary tumors of the heart and pericardium. Pathol Annu 7:339, 1982.
11. Reece IJ, Cooley DA, Frazier OH, et al.: Cardiac tumors: Clinical spectrum and prognosis of lesions other than classical benign myxoma in 20 patients. J Thorac Cardiovasc Surg 88:439, 1984.
12. Semb BKH: Surgical considerations in the treatment of cardiac myxoma. J Thorac Cardiovasc Surg 87:251, 1984.
13. Shaher RM, Mintzer J, Farina M, et al.: Clinical presentation of rhabdomyoma of the heart in infancy and childhood. Am J Cardiol 30:95, 1972.
14. Schmaltz AA, Apitz J: Primary heart tumors in infancy and childhood. Report of 4 cases and review of literature. Cardiology 67:12, 1981.
15. Van der Hauwaert LG: Cardiac tumours in infancy and childhood. Br Heart J 33: 125, 1971.

Cardiosplenic Syndromes

Synonyms
Heterotaxy syndromes, including asplenia syndrome and polysplenia syndrome.

Definition
Cardiosplenic syndromes are sporadic disorders characterized by a tendency toward symmetrical development of normally asymmetrical organs or organ systems. Even though the term refers to the striking abnormalities of the heart and spleen, many other organs, including the lungs, intestines, and venous system, are involved.

Pathology
Cardiosplenic syndromes are commonly subdivided into asplenia syndrome and polysplenia syndrome. The two conditions are characterized by lack of the normal asymmetry of the visceral organs. The trunk tends to have two halves that are mirror images of one another. Asplenia syndrome could be thought of as a condition of bilateral right sidedness and polysplenia syndrome as bilateral left sidedness. Exceptions to this have been reported, however. Cases with left atrial isomerism and asplenia have occurred.[4a]

With asplenia syndrome, the spleen is usually absent, the lungs are bilaterally trilobed, and morphologic right bronchi are found on both sides. The liver is often in a central position, and it is symmetrical. The stomach may be either on the right, on the left, or in a central position. Malrotation of the gut is frequent. Bilateral superior venae cavae are found in the majority of patients, and the inferior vena cava may run either on the right or on the left of the spine. The relationship between the abdominal aorta and inferior vena cava is typical of asplenia syndrome and is relevant for diagnosis of this condition: the aorta and vena cava, which normally run on both sides of the spine (see section on normal anatomy of the heart), are always seen on the same side (either the right or the left).[2,5] Therefore, it is clear that asplenia syndrome, as well as polysplenia syndrome, are classic examples of situs ambiguous. The association between asplenia syndrome and congenital heart disease is striking. In a review of 145 patients, Van Mierop et al.[5] found total anomalous pulmonary venous return in almost all patients, AVSD in 85 percent, a single ventricle in 51 percent, TGA in 58 percent, and pulmonary stenosis or atresia in 70 percent. Dextrocardia was found in 42 percent of the patients studied. The atria resemble a morphologic right atrium (right atrial isomerism).

Polysplenia syndrome is usually characterized by the presence of two or more spleens (usually two major ones and an indefinite number of smaller ones) located on both sides of the mesogastrium.[3-5] Bilateral morphologic left lungs and bronchi are found in 68 percent of patients. Liver and stomach may be either on the right or on the left side. Malrotation of the bowel is found in 80 percent of patients. Bilateral superior vena cava occurs in 50 percent, and in 70 percent, the inferior vena cava is absent and blood is drained by an azygos vein that may be on either the left or the right. Cardiac malformations are frequent, although they are less frequent than seen with asplenia syndrome. In Van Mierop's series,[5] anomalous pulmonary venous return (usually pulmonary veins connected to both sides of the atria) was found in 70 percent of patients, dextrocardia in 37 percent, ASDs in 37 percent, AVSD in 43 percent, TGA in 17 percent, and double outlet right ventricle in 20 percent.

Asplenia syndrome is twice as common in males as in females, whereas polysplenia syndrome affects both sexes equally.[5]

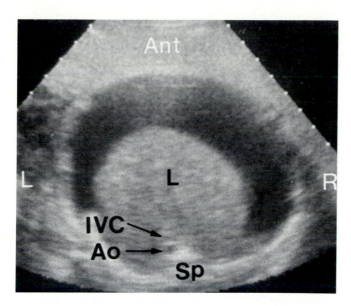

Figure 4–76. Transverse scan of the upper abdomen in a fetus with asplenia syndrome, congenital heart disease, and congestive heart failure. Posteriorly to the central liver (L), the abdominal aorta (Ao) and inferior vena cava (IVC) are seen on the same side of the spine (Sp). A large layer of ascitic fluid is seen. Ant, anterior; L, left; R, right.

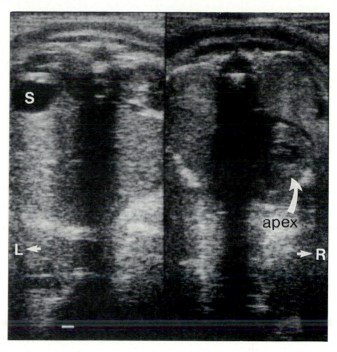

Figure 4–77. Dextrocardia. The apex of the heart points to the right (R) opposite to the position of the stomach (S). L, left.

Diagnosis

The recognition of a cardiosplenic syndrome relies on the demonstration of both the abnormal relationship between abdominal organs and the associated cardiovascular abnormalities. The key to the diagnosis is the identification of the visceral situs (see section on normal anatomy of the heart, p. 126).

Cardiosplenic syndromes are characterized by the presence of situs ambiguous. However, it is not easy to recognize hepatic isomerism, asplenia, or polysplenia with prenatal ultrasound. The position of the stomach is not a valuable parameter in assessing situs ambiguous, since it may be on the right or on the left as well. Huhta et al.[2] demonstrated that ultrasound allows a reliable diagnosis of situs by examining the relationship among the inferior vena cava, abdominal aorta, and spine in newborns. Such an approach can be used in the fetus as well. In situs solitus, the aorta is seen to the left of the spine and the inferior vena cava to the right (see section on normal anatomy of the heart). With asplenia syndrome, the descending aorta and inferior vena cava run on the same side of the spine (either to the left or to the right), the aorta being usually posterior. This typical configuration of the abdominal vessels can be easily demonstrated by a transverse cross-section of the fetal abdomen below the level of the diaphragm (Fig. 4–76). Inferior vena cava and aorta can be further identified by following their course to the atria and to the thoracic aorta and aortic arch, respec-

tively. In polysplenia syndrome, the inferior vena cava is often interrupted. Usually the aorta runs on the midline anterior to the spine. An azygos vein can be seen either to the left or to the right of the spine. It should be stressed that the presence of aorta and vena cava running on the same side of the spine has also been documented in cases of polysplenia syndrome. Therefore, this finding does not allow a specific diagnosis of these two conditions. Cardiac malposition is a frequent finding in both asplenia and polysplenia syndromes and can be easily recognized by ultrasound (Fig. 4–77).

Fetal echocardiography allows identification of the intracardiac anomalies associated with cardiosplenic syndromes. The reader should refer to the specific sections.

Prognosis

The outcome for infants with cardiosplenic syndrome depends primarily on the severity of the cardiac abnormalities.[4,5] In a series of 25 cases diagnosed under 6 months of age undergoing palliative or corrective surgery, the 1-year survival rate was 54 percent.[1]

Obstetrical Management

Management depends on the severity of the associated cardiac malformation. In fetuses without congenital heart disease, there is no indication to change standard obstetrical management. Nevertheless, delivery should take place in a tertiary care center.

REFERENCES

1. Gutgesell HP, Garson A, Park IS, et al.: Prognosis for the neonate and the young infant with congenital heart disease (Abstr). Pediatr Cardiol 2:168, 1982.
2. Huhta JC, Smallhorn JF, Macartney FJ: Two-dimensional echocardiographic diagnosis of situs. Br Heart J 48:97, 1982.
3. Moller JH, Nakib A, Anderson RC, et al.: Congenital cardiac disease associated with polysplenia. A develop-ment complex of bilateral "left-sidedness." Circulation 36:789, 1967.
4. Peoples WM, Moller JH, Edwards JE: Polysplenia: a review of 146 cases. Pediatr Cardiol 4:129, 1983.
4a. Stewart PA, Becker, AE, Wladimiroff JW, et al.: Left atrial isomerism associated with asplenia: Prenatal echo-cardiographic detection of complex congenital cardiac malformations. J Am Coll Cardiol 4:1015, 1984.
5. Van Mierop LHS, Gessner IH, Schiebler GL: Asplenia and polysplenia syndrome. Birth Defects 8:36, 1972.

Ectopia Cordis

Embryology and Pathology

The primitive heart is positioned outside the embryonic disc in the initial stages of development. With folding of the embryo, the heart comes to lie in the ventral and cranial part of the foregut and is infolded inside the pericardial cavity. At the same time, the septum transversum (primordium of the diaphragm) comes to lie caudal to the heart. The sternum begins to develop at the 5th week of intrauterine life. It derives bilaterally from mesenchymal cells that are converted into precartilage and converge in the midline where they fuse. The fusion is complete by the 9th week.[4]

According to the position of the heart, four types of ectopia cordis can be distinguished. The most frequently observed is the thoracic type, accounting for 60 percent of patients. The heart is displaced outside the thoracic cavity, protruding through a defect in the sternum. In the abdominal type, which accounts for 30 percent of patients, the primary defect is thought to be a gap in the diaphragm through which the heart protrudes inside the abdominal cavity. The thoracoabdominal type, which accounts for 7 percent of patients, is the variety present in the pentalogy of Cantrell (see p. 220). The cervical type accounts for 3 percent of all cases of ectopia cordis. This type is characterized by the displacement of the heart inside the cervical region.[4]

Associated Anomalies

Associated anomalies are very frequent and include facial and skeletal deformities, ventral wall defects, and central nervous system malformations (i.e., meningocele and cephaloceles). Intracardiac abnormalities are frequently seen and are the rule in the thoracoabdominal type, in which conotruncal malformations, such as tetralogy of Fallot and TGA, are prevalent.[4] Ectopia cordis is a frequent feature of amniotic band syndrome. We are aware of only one

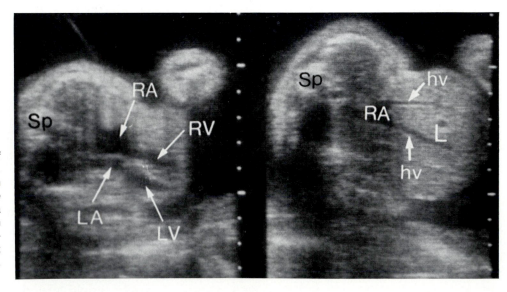

Figure 4–78. The diagnosis of ectopic cordis is obvious in this fetus. Note the heart displaced outside an abnormally small thoracic cavity. The ectopia cordis was associated with a large ventral wall defect through which most of the liver (L) was herniated. Sp, spine; RV, right ventricle; LV, left ventricle; RA, right atrium; LA, left atrium; hv, hepatic veins.

patient in whom a chromosomal aberration (45X/46XX) was found.[2]

Diagnosis

The diagnosis of ectopia cordis is easy and relies on demonstration of a displaced heart (Fig. 4–78). Several cases of prenatal diagnosis of either thoracic or thoracoabdominal types have been reported.[3,5–7] Identification of either the abdominal or the cervical type has not been reported yet, but attention to the anatomic relationships of the heart within the body would make this diagnosis possible.

Prognosis

The prognosis is generally poor, and infants are either stillborn or die in the first hours or days of life. Replacement of the heart inside the thoracic cavity has been successful in only a few cases.[1] Long-term survivors have only been reported for the abdominal type.

Obstetrical Management

A careful search for associated anomalies, including a detailed evaluation of the entire fetal anatomy and fetal echocardiography, is recommended. Fetal karyo-type should be considered. Given the extremely high mortality rate, the option of pregnancy termination should be offered before viability. In the third trimester, nonaggressive management should be considered and discussed with the parents.

REFERENCES

1. Asp K, Sulamaa M: Ectopia cordis. Acta Chir Scand Supp 283:52, 1961.
2. Garson A, Hawkins EP, Mullins CE, et al.: Thoracoabdominal ectopia cordis with mosaic Turner's syndrome: Report of a case. Pediatrics 62:218, 1978.
3. Haynor DR, Shuman WP, Brewer DK, et al.: Imaging of fetal ectopia cordis. Roles of sonography and computed tomography. J Ultrasound Med 3:25, 1984.
4. Kanagasuntheram R, Verzin JA: Ectopia cordis in man. Thorax 17:159, 1962.
5. Mercer LJ, Petres RE, Smeltzer JS: Ultrasonic diagnosis of ectopia cordis. Obstet Gynecol 61:523, 1983.
6. Todros T, Presbitero P, Montemurro D, et al.: Prenatal diagnosis of ectopia cordis. J Ultrasound Med 3:429, 1984.
7. Wicks JD, Levine MD, Mettler FA: Intrauterine sonography of thoracic ectopia cordis. AJR 137:619, 1981.

Premature Atrial and Ventricular Contractions

Synonyms

Atrial extrasystoles and ectopic atrial beats, ventricular extrasystoles and ectopic ventricular beats.

Definition

Premature atrial and ventricular contractions (PAC, PVC) arise from electrical impulses generated outside the cardiac pacemaker (sinus node).

Etiopathogenesis

Unknown. In the adult, PACs and PVCs may be stimulated by the ingestion of caffeine, alcohol, or smoking. Electrolyte imbalance and hyperthyroid states have also been implicated. The relevance of these factors to fetal PACs and PVCs is purely speculative. Immaturity or instability of the conducting tissue may be an etiologic factor.

Diagnosis

A disturbance in fetal heart rate can be detected either by direct auscultation or Doppler examination. These techniques provide information only about the ventricular rate, whereas accurate diagnosis of a fetal arrhythmia requires assessment of both atrial and ventricular activity. The fetal electrocardiogram is capable of determining both P and QRS waves corresponding to atrial and ventricular depolarization. However, a satisfactory fetal electrocardiogram can be obtained in a small number of patients. At present, the best available technique for the assessment of the fetal dysrhythmias is M-mode echocardiography. We have previously described how the simultaneous visualization of the atrial and ventricular contractions allows us to infer the atrioventricular activation sequence. By using this technique, the origin of an ectopic beat can be easily established (see pp. 131–133).

PACs and PVCs may give rise to complex rhythm patterns. PACs may either be conducted to the ventricles or blocked, depending on the moment of the cardiac cycle in which they occur. Thus, repeated PACs may lead to either an increased or a decreased ventricular rate. Blocked PACs must be differentiated from atrioventricular block. The dis-

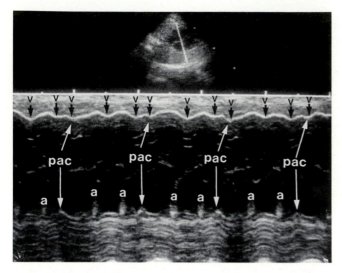

Figure 4–79. M-mode echocardiogram passing through the left ventricle and right atrium in a term fetus. Undulations of the atrial (a) and ventricular (v) walls reflect atrial and ventricular activity, respectively. Repeated premature atrial contractions (pac) conducted to the ventricles are seen.

tinction relies on demonstration of an atrial contraction that appears prematurely (Fig. 4–79). PVCs are characterized by a PVC that is not preceded by an atrial contraction.

Prognosis and Obstetrical Management

Neither PACs nor PVCs are associated with an increased incidence of congenital heart disease. There is unanimity in considering these rhythmic disturbances benign conditions that, in the vast majority of patients, disappear either in utero or shortly after birth.[1-4] However, PACs were detected in two fetuses that subsequently developed supraventricular tachycardia.[3] It is suggested that the heart rate of fetuses with PACs be serially monitored through pregnancy. There is no harm in asking patients to restrain from caffeine, nicotine, and alcohol and to verify the electrolyte balance of patients ingesting diuretics. There is no need to deliver these fetuses in a tertiary center.

REFERENCES

1. Allan LD, Anderson RH, Sullivan ID, et al.: Evaluation of fetal arrhythmias by echocardiography. Br Heart J 50:240, 1983.
2. Gleicher N, Elkayam U: Intrauterine dysrhythmias. In: Gleicher N, Elkayam U (eds): Cardiac Problems in Pregnancy: Diagnosis and Management of Maternal and Fetal Disease. New York, Alan R. Liss, 1982, pp 535–564.
3. Kleinman CS, Copel JA, Weinstein EM, et al.: In utero diagnosis and treatment of fetal supraventricular tachycardia. Semin Perinatol 9:113, 1985.
4. Kleinman CS, Donnerstein RL, Jaffe CC, et al.: Fetal echocardiography: A tool for evaluation of in utero cardiac arrhythmias and monitoring in utero therapy. Analysis of 71 patients. Am J Cardiol 51:237, 1983.

Supraventricular Tachyarrhythmias

Definition

Supraventricular tachyarrhythmias (SVT) include paroxysmal supraventricular tachycardia, paroxysmal atrial tachycardia, atrial flutter, and atrial fibrillation. SVT is characterized by an atrial frequency of 180 to 300 beats per minute (bpm) and a conduction rate of 1:1. In atrial flutter, the atrial rate ranges from 300 to 460 bpm. Due to variable degrees of atrioventricular block, the ventricular rate usually ranges between 60 and 200 bpm. Atrial fibrillation is characterized by an atrial rate of more than 400 bpm and a ventricular rate ranging from 120 to 200 bpm.[25]

Pathogenesis

SVT occurs by one of two mechanisms: automaticity and reentry.[7,21] In cases of automatic induced tachyarrhythmias, an irritable ectopic focus discharges at high frequency. The reentry mechanism consists of an electrical impulse reentering the atria, giving rise to repeated electrical activity. Reentry may occur at the level of the sinoatrial node, inside the atrium, the atrioventricular node, and the His Purkinje system. Reentry may also occur along an anomalous atrioventricular connection such as the Kent Bundle in the Wolff-Parkinson-White (WPW) syndrome.

Atrial flutter and fibrillation often alternate and are thought to result from a similar mechanism. Four theories have been postulated to explain such conditions: (1) circus movement of the electrical impulse, (2) ectopic formation of electrical impulses, (3) multiple reentry, and (4) multifocal impulse formation.[21]

SVT is by far the most frequent tachyarrhythmia in children, with an incidence of about 1:25,000.[21] Within SVT, the most commonly observed form is the

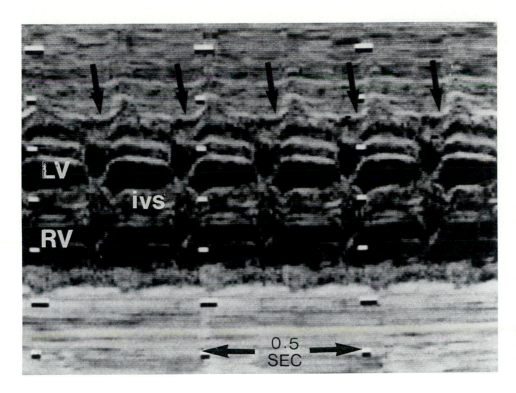

Figure 4–80. M-mode echocardiogram of the ventricular cavities (LV,RV) in a fetus with supraventricular tachycardia. A fast rate of 240 bpm is inferred by the movement of the posterior wall of the left ventricle. ivs, interventricular septum. *(Reproduced with permission from Bovicelli L, Baccarani G, Picchio FM, Pilu G: Ecocardiografia Fetale. La Diagnosi ed il Trattamento Prenatale delle Cardiopatie Congenite. Milan, Masson, 1985.)*

one caused by atrioventricular nodal reentry.[7,21] Viral infections may cause tachyarrhythmias. Hypoplasia of the sino-atrial tract has been implicated in three patients.[13a]

Hemodynamic Consequences

The association between supraventricular tachyarrhythmias and fetal nonimmune hydrops has been established.[17] It has been postulated that a fast ventricular rate results in suboptimal filling of the ventricles. This would lead to a decreased cardiac output, right atrial overload, and congestive heart failure. The frequency of this association is variable. SVT is a frequent cause of hydrops. Atrial flutter and fibrillation may be associated with variable ventricular rates, and if these are within normal limits, the tachyarrhythmia will be well tolerated.

Diagnosis

A disturbance in fetal heart rate can be detected either by direct auscultation or Doppler examination. How-

ever, these techniques provide information only about the ventricular rate, whereas accurate diagnosis of a fetal tachyarrhythmia requires assessment of both atrial and ventricular activity. The fetal electrocardiogram is capable of determining both P and QRS waves corresponding to atrial and ventricular depolarization. However, a satisfactory fetal electrocardiogram can be obtained in a small number of cases. At present, the best available technique for the assessment of the fetal dysrhythmias is M-mode echocardiography. We have previously described how the simultaneous visualization of the atrial and ventricular contractions allows one to infer the atrioventricular activation sequence (see p. 131). By using this technique, the ventricular and atrial rate and the atrioventricular conduction rate are easily established.[1,16,17,28]

SVT is characterized by an atrial rate of 180 to 300 bpm with a ventricular response of 1:1 (Fig. 4–80). M-mode echocardiography does not allow differenti-

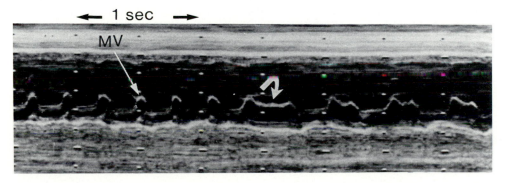

Figure 4–81. Spontaneous conversion to a normal heart rate and rhythm in a fetus with episodes of supraventricular tachyarrythmia. The sudden cessation of the tachycardia *(curved arrow)* indicates reentry as a pathogenic mechanism. The fetus was found at birth to have Wolff-Parkinson-White syndrome. MV, mitral valve.

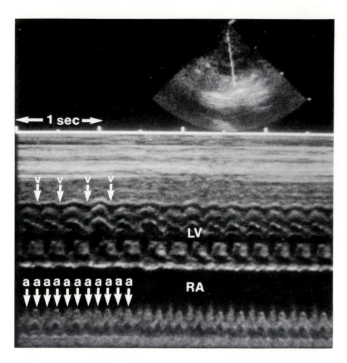

Figure 4–82. Atrial flutter. The rapid undulation of the posterior wall of the right atrium (RA) indicates an atrial rhythm of 420 bpm. The ventricular response, with a rate of about 200 bpm, indicates 2:1 atrioventricular block. LV, left ventricle; a, atrial contractions; v, ventricular contractions.

ation of the automatic from the reentry mechanism. Automatic SVT tends to be monotonous, whereas reentry SVT tends to be characterized by sudden onset and cessation of tachycardia (Fig. 4–81). However, it is not always possible to document such a finding.[16]

Atrial flutter and fibrillation are characterized by an atrial rate of 300 to 400 bpm and 400 to 700 bpm, respectively. The ventricular rate is variable. Usually, there is a second degree heart block with 2:1 conduction, but the ventricular rate may be as low as 60 bpm (Fig. 4–82).

Associated Anomalies
Cardiac anomalies are seen in 5 to 10 percent of patients with SVT. These include ASDs, congenital mitral valve disease, cardiac tumors, and WPW syndrome.[9,25] Atrial flutter and fibrillation have been described in patients with WPW syndrome, cardiomyopathies, and thyrotoxicosis.

Prognosis
A tachyarrhythmia is a serious condition in a fetus because it is frequently associated with congestive heart failure. The prognostic figures derived in the neonatal period do not apply to the fetus. In a series of 21 cases treated in utero, including 16 cases of SVT, 3 cases of atrial flutter, and 2 cases of atrial fibrillation, 2 deaths were observed. They occurred in 2 of

the 3 fetuses with atrial flutter, one of whom had a 7:1 or 8:1 heart block.[16]

Obstetrical Management
Obstetrical management is related to the gestational age at which the diagnosis is made. Generally, identification of a tachyarrhythmia in a term fetus is best managed by delivery and postnatal treatment. An exception may be the severely hydropic fetus who could pose serious difficulties in resuscitation. In these patients, an attempt to achieve intrauterine cardioversion can be considered.[16]

Intrauterine pharmacologic cardioversion is recommended before lung maturity. There is controversy in the literature about which fetuses should be treated. In the opinion of several authors, all fetuses with supraventricular tachyarrhythmias (regardless of the presence or absence of congestive heart failure) should receive antiarrhythmic agents.[1,16]

Among the antiarrhythmic agents, digoxin is the drug of choice because it is effective in treating neonatal tachyarrhythmias, is safe for both mother and fetus, and has been shown to cross the placenta.[2,4,23,26] The doses administered in different case reports have varied from 0.25 to 1 mg/day given orally to the mother.[1,6,12,14–16,28,31] Some authors have used a loading dose of 1.0 to 2.5 mg orally[11,14–17] or of 0.5 to 2 mg intravenously.[16] There is no evidence of superiority of slow versus rapid digitalization. However, it seems reasonable to use a loading dose in patients with hydrops in the attempt to achieve a more rapid response. Oral absorption of digoxin may vary in pregnancy, and it is usually lower than that seen in nonpregnant women.[23] Fetal levels have ranged between 50 and 100 percent of maternal levels.[4,16,23]

The goal of therapy is to achieve fetal cardioversion without causing digitalis toxicity in the mother. A maternal serum level of 2 ng/ml has been suggested as a reasonable target. Digoxin is contraindicated in fetuses with outlet ventricular obstructions, such as asymmetrical septal hypertrophy and tetralogy of Fallot. Furthermore, the use of digoxin in cases of supraventricular tachyarrhythmias associated with WPW syndrome is at present an unresolved issue. The drug may cause shortening of the refractory period in the accessory pathway, leading to ventricular fibrillation. WPW syndrome has been found in association with fetal supraventricular tachyarrhythmias in 4 of 27 cases reviewed by Gleicher and Elkayam.[9] Since this condition cannot be prenatally diagnosed at present, the use of digoxin may require revision in the future.

Second line agents include propranolol, verapamil, procainamide, and quinidine. One of these agents can be added to digoxin when this drug fails.

Transplacental crossage of propranolol has been reported to vary between 20 and 127 percent.[6,24,30] Fetal side effects have been described. In a review of 153 mothers receiving propranolol for different indications, 15 percent of infants had growth retardation, 9 percent had hypoglycemia, 8 percent had bradycardia, and 4 percent had respiratory distress at birth.[3] The drug has been given orally in doses of 160 mg/day.[15,30] A loading dose of 0.5 mg intravenously can be considered.

Transplacental crossage of verapamil has been documented.[29,31] Umbilical cord levels at birth have been reported to be 30 to 40 percent of maternal levels.[16] Fetal side effects have not been clearly established. Doses as high as 300 mg/day have been used for the treatment of pregnancy-related hypertension without demonstrable fetal toxicity.[19] A loading dose of 5 to 10 mg intravenously and a maintenance dose of 80 to 120 mg orally every 6 to 8 hours have been suggested. Since verapamil induces a decrease in digoxin clearance, a reduction of 33 to 50 percent of the dose of digoxin may be required when these two medications are used simultaneously.[16]

Transplacental crossage of procainamide has been reported to vary, with cord to maternal levels ranging from 25 percent to 130 percent.[6,8,16] This medication has been administered in combination with other antiarrhythmic agents, such as digoxin, verapamil, and propranolol, in daily dosages of 4 grams.[6,28]

Very limited experience is available with the administration of quinidine to control fetal supraventricular tachyarrythmias. Placental crossage has been demonstrated with a cord to maternal level ranging from 25 to 100 percent.[27] Neonatal thrombocytopenia has been reported in association with maternal administration of this drug.[5] Quinidine has been succesfully used in association with digoxin in three cases of fetal supraventricular tachyarrhythmias in dosages of 300 mg every 6 hours orally.[27]

In a review of 45 cases of supraventricular tachyarrhythmias treated in utero,[1,6,8,10–15,16,18,22,27,28,31] digoxin alone was successful in 16 cases (37 percent) and digoxin in association with another antiarrhythmic agents was successful in 18 cases (41 percent). An equivocal result was obtained in one case (2.6 percent), and failure of intrauterine treatment occurred in 10 cases (23 percent). One case of fetal supraventricular tachyarrhythmia has been successfully treated with propranolol alone.[30] It has been suggested that fetuses with severe congestive heart failure are less responsive to treatment.[1,16]

A nonpharmacologic approach to cardioversion has been attempted, with success, by intrauterine compression of the umbilical cord.[20]

When treating a fetal supraventricular tachyarrhythmia, digoxin alone is the first step. If this drug is ineffective, combination therapy with either verapamil or propranolol should be considered. Quinidine and procainamide should be the last alternatives.[6]

REFERENCES

1. Allan LD, Anderson RH, Sullivan ID, et al.: Evaluation of fetal arrhythmias by echocardiography. Br Heart J 50:240, 1983.
2. Allonen H, Kanto J, Iisalo E: The foeto-maternal distribution of digoxin in early human pregnancy. Acta Pharmacol Toxicol 39:477, 1976.
3. Briggs GG, Bodendorfer TW, Freeman RK, Yaffe SJ: Propranolol. In: Drugs in Pregnancy and Lactation: A Reference Guide to Fetal and Neonatal Risk. Baltimore, Williams & Wilkins, 1983, pp 310–313.
4. Chan V, Tse TF, Wong V: Transfer of digoxin across the placenta and into breast milk. Br J Obstet Gynaecol 85:605, 1978.
5. Domula VM, Weissbach G, Lenk H, et al.: Uber die auswirkung medikamentoser behandlung in der schwangerschaft auf das gerinnungspotential des neugeborenen. Zentralbl Gynaekol 99:473, 1977.
6. Dumesic DA, Silverman NH, Tobias S, et al.: Transplacental cardioversion of fetal supraventricular tachycardia with procainamide. N Engl J Med 307:1128, 1982.
7. Garson A, Gillette PC: Electrophysiologic studies of supraventricular tachycardia in children. I. Clinical-electrophysiologic correlations. Am Heart J 102:233, 1981.
8. Given BD, Phillippe M, Sanders SP, et al.: Procainamide cardioversion of fetal supraventricular tachyarrhythmia. Am J Cardiol 53:1460, 1984.
9. Gleicher N, Elkayam U: Intrauterine dysrhythmias. In: Elkayam U, Gleicher N (eds): Cardiac Problems in Pregnancy: Diagnosis and Management of Maternal and Fetal Disease. New York, Alan R. Liss, 1982, pp 535–564.
10. Guntheroth WG, Cyr DR, Mack LA, et al.: Hydrops from reciprocating atrioventricular tachycardia in a 27-week fetus requiring quinidine for conversion. Obstet Gynecol 66:29S, 1985.
11. Harrigan JT, Kangos JJ, Sikka A, et al.: Successful treatment of fetal congestive heart failure secondary to tachycardia. N Engl J Med 304:1527, 1981.
12. Heaton FC, Vaughan R: Intrauterine supraventricular tachycardia: Cardioversion with maternal digoxin. Obstet Gynecol 60:749, 1982.
13. Hill LM, Breckle R, Driscoll DJ: Sonographic evaluation of prenatal therapy for fetal supraventricular tachycardia and congestive heart failure: A case report. J Reprod Med 28:671, 1983.
13a. Ho SY, Mortimer G, Anderson RH, et al.: Conduction system defects in three perinatal patients with arrhythmia. Br Heart J 53:158, 1985.
14. Kerenyi TD, Gleicher N, Meller J, et al.: Transplacental

cardioversion of intrauterine supraventricular tachycardia with digitalis. Lancet 2:393, 1980.

15. Klein A, Holzman IR, Austin EM: Fetal tachycardia prior to the development of hydrops. Attempted pharmacologic cardioversion: Case report. Am J Obstet Gynecol 134:347, 1979.
16. Kleinman CS, Copel JA, Weinstein EM, et al.: In utero diagnosis and treatment of fetal supraventricular tachycardia. Sem Perinatol 9:113, 1985.
17. Kleinman CS, Donnerstein RL, DeVore GR, et al.: Fetal echocardiography for evaluation of in utero congestive heart failure: A technique for study of nonimmune fetal hydrops. N Engl J Med 306:568, 1982.
18. Lingman G, Ohrlander S, Ohlin P: Intrauterine digoxin treatment of fetal paroxysmal tachycardia. Case report. Br J Obstet Gynaecol 87:340, 1980.
19. Marlettini MG, Labriola M, Trabatti MR, et al.: Il verapamil nel trattamento dell'ipertensione in gravidanza. Proceedings of the 62nd National Congress of the Italian Society of Gynecology and Obstetrics. Bologna, Monduzzi, 1984, pp 307–310.
20. Martin CB, Nijhuis JG, Weijer AA: Correction of fetal supraventricular tachycardia by compression of the umbilical cord. Report of a case. Am J Obstet Gynecol 150:324, 1984.
21. Mehta AV, Casta A, Wolff GS: Supraventricular tachycardia. In: Roberts NK, Gelband H (eds): Cardiac Arrhythmias in the Neonate, Infant, and Child, 2d ed. E. Norwalk, CT, Appleton-Century-Crofts, 1983, pp 105–137.

22. Newburger JW, Keane JF: Intrauterine supraventricular tachycardia. J Pediatr 95:780, 1979.
23. Rogers MC, Willerson JT, Goldblatt A, et al.: Serum digoxin concentrations in the human fetus, neonate and infant. N Engl J Med 287:1010, 1972.
24. Schroeder JS, Harrison DC: Repeated cardioversion during pregnancy. Treatment of refractory paroxysmal atrial tachycardia during three successive pregnancies. Am J Cardiol 27:445, 1971.
25. Shenker L: Fetal cardiac arrhythmias. Obstet Gynec Surv 34:561, 1979.
26. Soyka LF: Digoxin: Placental transfer, effects on the fetus and therapeutic use in the newborn. Clin Perinatol 2:23, 1975.
27. Spinnato JA, Shaver DC, Flinn GS, et al.: Fetal supraventricular tachycardia. In utero therapy with digoxin and quinidine. Obstet Gynecol 64:730, 1984.
28. Stewart PA, Tonge HM, Wladimiroff JW: Arrhythmia and structural abnormalities of the fetal heart. Br Heart J 50:550, 1983.
29. Strigl R, Gastroph G, Hege HG, et al.: Nachweis von verapamil im mutterlichen und fetalen blut des menschen. Geburtshilfe Frauenheilkd 40:496, 1980.
30. Teuscher A, Bossi E, Imhof P, et al.: Effect of propranolol on fetal tachycardia in diabetic pregnancy. Am J Cardiol 42:304, 1978.
31. Wolff F, Breuker KH, Schlensker KH, et al.: Prenatal diagnosis and therapy of fetal heart rate anomalies: With a contribution on the placental transfer of verapamil. J Perinat Med 8:203, 1980.

Atrioventricular Block

Definition
Atrioventricular block (AV block) is a condition in which transmission of the electrical impulse from the atria to the ventricles is impaired.

Incidence
Congenital heart block affects 1:20,000 live births and is present in 4 to 9 percent of all infants with congenital heart disease.[8]

Etiology
The disorder could result from immaturity of the conduction system, absence of connection to the AV node, or abnormal anatomic position of the AV node.[6,8,9] It has been estimated that 50 percent of infants with congenital third degree heart block have associated structural anomalies, including corrected transposition, univentricular heart, cardiac tumors, and cardiomyopathies.[3] In the remaining 50 percent the cause remains obscure. Growing evidence suggests an association between maternal antinuclear antibodies against SSA and SSB antigens and congenital heart block. The SSA and SSB antibodies (also known as Ro and La, respectively) are directed against two saline-soluble ribonucleoprotein antigens from cell nuclei. Transplacental passage of the antibodies is thought to lead to inflammation in the heart conduction system and heart block. Anti-SSA antibodies have been reported in 83 percent of mothers who delivered infants with heart block even though only 30 percent had clinical evidence of connective tissue disease. The most common connective tissue disease associated with congenital heart block is lupus erythematosus.[2,7,11,13]

Pathophysiology
The normal propagation of the electrical impulse occurs from the sinoatrial node to the atrioventricular node and, from there, to the Purkinje system and the ventricles.

Atrioventricular block is commonly classified into three types. First degree heart block corresponds

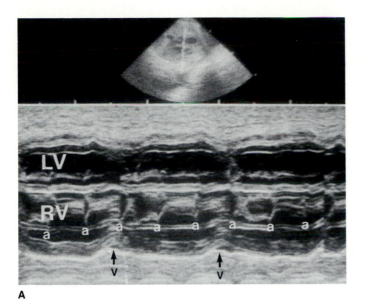 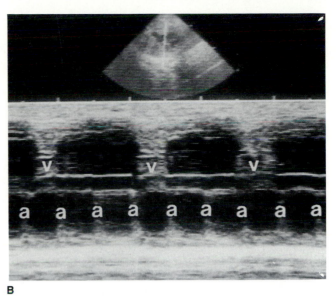

A

B

Figure 4–83. A. M-mode echocardiogram passing through the ventricles (LV,RV) of a third trimester fetus with complete AV block. The *a* waves seen on the tricuspid valve indicate a normal atrial rate of about 120 bpm. Undulation of the ventricular walls (v) indicate a ventricular rate of less than 50 bpm. **B.** This M-mode echocardiogram passing through the left ventricle and right atrium clearly demonstrates both the discrepancy and the dissociation between atrial (a) and ventricular (v) activity.

to a simple conduction delay, which on the electrocardiogram is manifested as a prolongation of the PR interval. Second degree block is subdivided into Mobitz types I and II. Mobitz type I consists of a progressive prolongation of the PR interval that finally leads to the block of one atrial impulse (Luciani-Wenckebach phenomenon). In Mobitz type II, there is intermittent conduction with a ventricular rate that is a submultiple of the atrial rate (e.g., 2:1, 3:1). Third degree heart block or complete heart block is characterized by a complete dissociation of atria and ventricles, usually with independent and slow activation of the ventricles.[10,12]

Hemodynamic Consequences

First and second degree AV block are not usually associated with any significant hemodynamic perturbance. Complete AV block may result in important bradycardia, leading to decreased cardiac output and congestive heart failure during fetal life.[5]

Diagnosis

A disturbance in fetal heart rate can be detected either by direct auscultation or Doppler examination. However, these techniques provide information only about the ventricular rate, whereas accurate diagnosis of a fetal arrhythmia requires assessment of both atrial and ventricular activity. Fetal electrocardiogram is capable of determining both P and QRS waves,

corresponding to atrial and ventricular depolarization. However, a satisfactory fetal electrocardiogram can be obtained in a small number of cases. At present, the best available technique for the assessment of the fetal dysrhythmias is M-mode echocardiography. We have previously described how the simultaneous visualization of the atrial and ventricular contractions allows one to infer the atrioventricular activation sequence (see p. 131). By using this technique, the ventricular and atrial rate and the atrioventricular conduction rate are easily established.

Since first degree heart block results in an entirely normal heart rate and rhythm, it is not surprising that this diagnosis has not been reported in the human fetus. Blockage of the normal atrial impulse can be diagnosed by demonstration of a normally timed atrial contraction that is not followed by a ventricular contraction.

Mobitz type I, type II, and third degree heart block may be differentiated by observing the relationship between atrial and ventricular rate. In Mobitz type I block, only a few atrial impulses are not conducted. In Mobitz type II, a submultiple of atrial impulses are transmitted. In third degree or complete heart block, atrial and ventricular rates are independent of each other and the atrial rate is generally slow (Fig. 4–83). Given the strong correlation between fetal heart block, maternal antinuclear antibodies, and connective tissue disease, appropriate workup is indicated.

Prognosis

The two most important prognostic factors are the presence or absence of congenital heart disease and the onset of congestive heart failure. These two factors are interrelated as congestive heart failure is rarely seen in infants without underlying heart disease.[4]

Obstetrical Management

The diagnosis of an atrioventricular block demands a careful search for associated intracardiac anomalies. Isolated second degree heart block does not require any change in clinical management. In the presence of Mobitz type II, serial ultrasound monitoring is suggested, since a transition to complete heart block may occur. Complete heart block may lead to congestive heart failure. Only very few cases of this condition with intrauterine congestive heart failure have been reported in the literature[1,3,5,7] and prognostic figures cannot be provided at present. In these cases, premature delivery may be considered to permit postnatal treatment and prevent intrauterine fetal demise. Steroid administration should be considered before the delivery of a preterm infant with an immature lung profile. Mothers of infants with congenital heart block should be followed prospectively because they are at high risk of developing a connective tissue disorder.

REFERENCES

 1. Allan LD, Anderson RH, Sullivan ID, et al.: Evaluation of fetal arrhythmias by echocardiography. Br Heart J 50:240, 1983.
 2. Chameides L, Truex RC, Vetter V, et al.: Association of maternal systemic lupus erythematosus with congenital complete heart block. N Engl J Med 297:1204, 1977.
 3. Gleicher N, Elkayam U: Intrauterine dysrhythmias. In: Elkayam U, Gleicher N (eds): Cardiac Problems in Pregnancy: Diagnosis and Management of Maternal and Fetal Disease. New York, Alan R. Liss, 1982, pp 535–564.
 4. Griffiths SP: Congenital complete heart block. Circulation 43:615, 1971.
 5. Kleinman CS, Donnerstein RL, Jaffe CC, et al.: Fetal echocardiography: A tool for evaluation of in utero cardiac arrhythmias and monitoring of in utero therapy. Analysis of 71 patients. Am J Cardiol 51:237, 1983.
 6. Lev M, Cuadros H, Paul MH: Interruption of the atrioventricular bundle with congenital atrioventricular block. Circulation 43:703, 1971.
 7. McCue CM, Mantakas ME, Tingelstad JB, et al.: Congenital heart block in newborns of mothers with connective tissue disease. Circulation 56:82, 1977.
 8. McHenry MM, Cayler GG: Congenital complete heart block in newborns, infants, children and adults. Med Times 97 (10):113, 1969.
 9. Reemtsma K, Copenhaver WM: Anatomic studies of the cardiac conduction system in congenital malformations of the heart. Circulation 17:271, 1958.
10. Roberts NK: Atrioventricular conduction: Disorders of atrioventricular conduction and intraventricular conduction. In: Roberts NK, Gelband H: (eds): Cardiac Arrhythmias in the Neonate, Infant and Child, 2d ed. E. Norwalk, CT, Appleton-Century-Crofts, 1983, pp 233–252.
11. Scott JS, Maddison PJ, Taylor PV, et al.: Connective-tissue disease, antibodies to ribonucleoprotein, and congenital heart block. N Engl J Med 309:209, 1983.
12. Shenker L: Fetal cardiac arrhythmias. Obstet Gynecol Surv 34:561, 1979.
13. Singsen BH, Akhter JE, Weinstein MM, et al.: Congenital complete heart block and SSA antibodies: Obstetric implications. Am J Obstet Gynecol 152:655, 1985.

5

The Lungs

Fetal Lung Congenital Anomalies

During fetal life, the lungs are not inflated and are visualized as solid structures that fill the space between the heart and the rib cage. Interest in these organs has increased in an attempt to recognize sonographic changes related to pulmonic maturity.

Fetal lungs appear as two paracardiac structures whose uniform echogenicity varies in comparison to that of fetal liver along gestation. Some authors have proposed that these differences may be helpful in the assessment of fetal lung maturity. They have reported that the lung becomes more reflective than the liver with advancing gestational age.[3] Other investigators have found that these changes do not correlate with the L:S ratio and phosphatylglycerol measurements.[2]

On the other hand, preliminary reports suggest that lung compressibility—assessed subjectively from the passive movements of the lung adjacent to the cardiac ventricular walls during diastole—varies throughout gestation and correlates with lung maturity. In a report of 54 infants delivered within 36 hours of ultrasound dynamic lung studies, a fetal lung stiff pattern was associated with respiratory distress syndrome (RDS), whereas fetuses with compliant lungs had no RDS.[2] These observations need confirmation.

This chapter focuses on the four most common thoracic anomalies diagnosed with ultrasound: chylothorax, cystic adenomatoid tumor, lung sequestration, and bronchogenic cysts. A nomogram for thoracic dimensions is displayed on p. 330. It is helpful in the assessment of pulmonary hypoplasia.

REFERENCES

1. Birnholz JC, Farrell EE: Fetal lung development: Compressibility as a measure of maturity. Radiology 157:495, 1985.
2. Fried AM, Loh FK, Umer MA, et al.: Echogenicity of fetal lung: Relation to fetal age and maturity. AJR 145:591, 1985.
3. Reeves GS, Garrett WJ, Warren PS, Fisher CC: Observations of fetal lung reflectivity using real-time ultrasound. Aust NZ J Obstet Gynaecol 24:91, 1984.

Chylothorax

Definition
Chylothorax is an accumulation of chyle in the pleural cavity.

Incidence
Chylothorax is a common cause of pleural effusion during the first days of neonatal life.[5] Its prevalence has been estimated to be 1:10,000 deliveries.[15] The male to female ratio is 2:1.[4,25]

Etiology
Accumulation of lymph within the pleural cavity can result from overproduction or impaired reabsorption of lymph. The latter could be due to either an obstruction

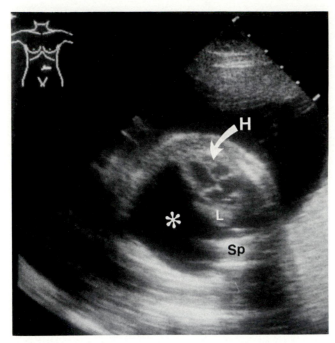

Figure 5–1. Transverse scan of a patient with congenital chylothorax. A predominantly left chylothorax (*) deviates the heart (H) toward the right. L, Lung; Sp, spine.

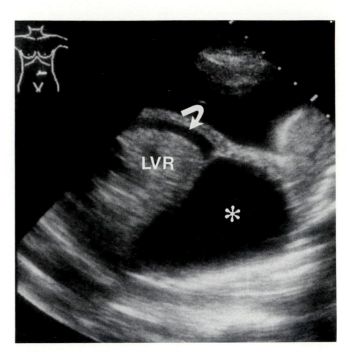

Figure 5–2. Longitudinal scan of the fetus shown in Figure 5–1. The arrow points to the presence of ascites. *, chylothorax; LVR, liver.

to pulmonary lymph drainage or abnormal lymphatic vessels.

Pathology

Pediatric series indicate that chylothorax occurs as a unilateral pleural effusion involving the right side of the lung in most instances. In rare cases, pleural effusions can be bilateral.[4,8] Chylothorax may lead to lung compression and the development of pulmonary hypoplasia. Unilateral pleural effusion can also shift the mediastinum, impair venous return, and lead to congestive heart failure and hydrops. There is a paucity of information about the histopathology of congenital chylothorax. In one autopsy series, dilated distal lymphatics that apparently failed to communicate with the more proximal lymphatic vessels were demonstrated, but this may be a nonspecific finding.[19]

Associated Anomalies

Chylothorax may be associated with trisomy 21.[6,24,26] Anomalies reported in association with chylothorax include congenital pulmonary lymphangiectasis,[13] tracheoesophageal fistula,[11] extralobar lung sequestration,[3,9,12] and a multiple malformation complex (anemia, tracheoesophageal fistula, Klippel-Feil deformity).[18]

Diagnosis

Chylothorax should be suspected in the presence of a pleural effusion (Figs. 5–1, 5–2, 5–3). A specific diagnosis of chylothorax is not possible on the basis of the

gross appearance of the fluid. Indeed, lymph looks serous at birth and becomes lactescent only after oral feedings.[8,10,15–17,20,21,24,25] It has been suggested that identification of abundant lymphocytes (>60 percent) in pleural fluid indicates chylothorax, since these are the predominant cells in lymph.[2,24]

The prenatal diagnosis of chylothorax has been reported in several instances.[7,10,14,17,21–23] However, documentation of these cases is generally poor. A definitive diagnosis can be made by demonstrating a change in the character of the pleural fluid after feedings. The value of lymphocyte counts in the differential diagnosis of intrauterine-diagnosed pleural effusions has not been established. In severe cases, this condition may be associated with nonimmune hydrops (Fig. 5–2).[1,7,14,22,24] Polyhydramnios has been noted in all cases prenatally diagnosed and registered in many neonatal series.[1,8,11,15,16,25,26] It may be the result of esophageal compression by the pleural effusion.

The differential diagnosis of congenital chylothorax is problematic. The condition can appear as isolated pleural effusions or as nonimmune hydrops. It is not known if biochemical or cytologic examination of the pleural fluid can permit a differential diagnosis between the effusion seen in congenital chylothorax and that seen in other causes of nonimmune hydrops.

Prognosis

It is extremely difficult to provide prognostic figures for congenital chylothorax diagnosed in utero because of the limited experience with this condition and the uncertainty surrounding its diagnosis. Of all cases claimed to have been prenatally diagnosed, 5 of 11 died perinatally; 2 were stillbirths and 3 were neonatal deaths. Hydrops was present in 3 of the dead infants and in only 1 of the survivors. The survivor was treated in utero with thoracentesis.[22]

In pediatric series in which the diagnosis is made postnatally, symptoms of respiratory distress are present at birth in 40 percent of infants and become manifest within 24 hours in 64 percent and within the first week in 79 percent.[4] The mortality rate is 15 percent.[4] Weight loss is a sign of wastage and can lead to death. Treatment consists of pleural drainage (repeated thoracentesis or continuous thoracic drainage), careful replacement of the nutritional losses, and reduction of the volume of lymph flow. A diet composed of medium-chain triglycerides, which are absorbed into the portal system rather than through the lymphatic system, has been used.[6,24] In most cases, chylothorax resolves spontaneously with time. If control of the chylous effusion is not achieved within 3 to 4 weeks, surgical ligature of the thoracic duct is performed.[1] At an average follow-up of 15 months, 19 of 20 patients were normal.[4]

Obstetrical Management

When a diagnosis is made before viability, the option of pregnancy termination can be offered. Karyotyping is indicated, since this condition has been associated with chromosomal anomalies, such as trisomy 21. After viability, the management depends on the gestational age and the development of signs of hydrops or mediastinal shift. In term infants, a thoracentesis should be considered before delivery to avoid respiratory failure due to a large pleural effusion. Decompression may also prevent rupture or inversion of the diaphragm secondary to pressure on the fetal thorax as it passes through the birth canal.[17]

The management of preterm infants depends on the degree of mediastinal shift present. If the pleural effusion is small and no mediastinal shift is demonstrated, intervention is not justified. Serial scans are required to monitor the evolution of the pleural effusion. If mediastinal shift and signs of hydrops develop, we would consider intervening to prevent pulmonary hypoplasia. It must be emphasized that fluid reaccumulation occurs rapidly, and repeated thoracentesis will probably be required. Two cases successfully managed with repeated thoracenteses have been reported.[2,21] The uncontrolled nature of these observations prevents firm conclusions about the benefit of this type of intervention. In one fetus, weekly thoracenteses were initiated at the 19th week and carried out until the 23d week of intrauterine life, at which time the effusion spontaneously disappeared.[2] The procedure may have prevented the development of pulmonary hypoplasia. There is little

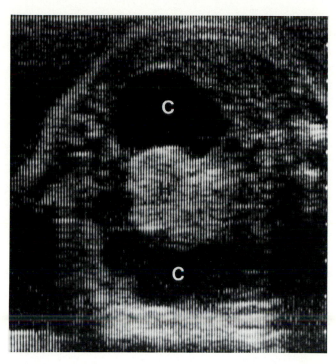

Figure 5–3. Transverse scan of the chest in a fetus with bilateral chylothorax (C). H, heart.

information to document the natural history of intra-uterine chylothorax. Spontaneous resolution of chylothorax in utero has not been reported. We have seen only one patient in whom a bilateral pleural effusion resolved spontaneously. This could have been explained by a viral infection rather than by transient chylothorax.

In our opinion, a chylothorax is not an indication for altering the delivery route. A cesarean section would be indicated for standard obstetrical reasons only. Infants should be delivered when pulmonic maturity is present, since the association of respiratory distress syndrome, pulmonary hypoplasia, and restrictive lung disease due to the pleural effusion would worsen the prognosis.

REFERENCES

1. Andersen EA, Hertel J, Pedersen SA, et al.: Congenital chylothorax: Management by ligature of the thoracic duct. Scand J Thorac Cardiovasc Surg 18:193, 1984.
2. Benacerraf BR, Frigoletto FD: Mid-trimester fetal thoracentesis. J Clin Ultrasound 13:202, 1985.
3. Bliek AJ, Mulholland DJ: Extralobar lung sequestration associated with fatal neonatal respiratory distress. Thorax 26:125, 1971.
4. Brodman RF: Congenital chylothorax. Recommendations for treatment. NY State J Med 75:553, 1975.
5. Chernick V, Reed MH: Pneumothorax and chylothorax in the neonatal period. J Pediatr 76:624, 1970.

6. Craenen JM, Williams Jr. TE, Kilman JW: Simplified management of chylothorax in neonates and infants. Ann Thoracic Surg 24:275, 1977.

7. Defoort P, Thiery M: Antenatal diagnosis of congenital chylothorax by gray scale sonography. J Clin Ultrasound 6:47, 1978.

8. Doolittle WM, Ohmart D, Egan EA: Congenital bilateral pleural effusions: A cause for respiratory failure in the newborn. Am J Dis Child 125:435, 1973.

9. Dresler S: Massive pleural effusion and hypoplasia of the lung accompanying extralobar pulmonary sequestration. Hum Pathol 12:862, 1981.

10. Dubos JP, Bouchez MC, Kacet N, et al.: Anasarque non immunologique et chylothorax congenital. Arch Fr Pediatr 42:537, 1985.

11. Harvey JG, Houlsby W, Sherman K, et al.: Congenital chylothorax: Report of unique case associated with "H"-type tracheo-oesophageal fistula. Br J Surg 66:485, 1979.

12. Horowitz RN: Extralobar sequestration of lung in a newborn infant. Am J Dis Child 110:195, 1965.

13. Hunter WS, Becroft DMQ: Congenital pulmonary lymphangiectasis associated with pleural effusions. Arch Dis Child 59:278, 1984.

14. Jaffa AJ, Barak S, Kaysar N, et al.: Case report. Antenatal diagnosis of bilateral congenital chylothorax with pericardial effusion. Acta Obstet Gynecol Scand 64:455, 1985.

15. John E: Pleural effusion in the newborn. Med J Aust 1:102, 1974.

16. Koffler H, Papile LA, Burstein RL: Congenital chylothorax: Two cases associated with maternal polyhydramnios. Am J Dis Child 132:638, 1978.

17. Lange IR, Manning FA: Antenatal diagnosis of congenital pleural effusions. Am J Obstet Gynecol 140:839, 1981.

18. Lazarus KH, McCurdy FA: Multiple congenital anomalies in a patient with Diamond-Blackfan syndrome. Clin Pediatr 23:520, 1984.

19. McKendry JBJ, Lindsay WK, Gerstein MC: Congenital defects of the lymphatics in infancy. Pediatrics 19:21, 1957.

20. Perry RE, Hodgman J, Cass AB: Pleural effusion in the neonatal period. J Pediatr 62:838, 1963.

21. Petres RE, Redwine FO, Cruikshank DP: Congenital bilateral chylothorax. Antepartum diagnosis and successful intrauterine surgical management. JAMA 248:1360, 1982.

22. Schmidt W, Harms E, Wolf D: Successful prenatal treatment of nonimmune hydrops fetalis due to congenital chylothorax. Case report. Br J Obstet Gynecol 92:685, 1985.

23. Thomas DB, Anderson JC: Antenatal detection of fetal pleural effusions and neonatal management. Med J Aust 2:435, 1979.

24. Van Aerde J, Campbell AN, Smyth JA, et al.: Spontaneous chylothorax in newborns. Am J Dis Child 138:961, 1984.

25. Yancy WS, Spock A: Spontaneous neonatal pleural effusion. J Pediatr Surg 2:313, 1967.

26. Yoss BS, Lipsitz PJ: Chylothorax in two mongoloid infants. Clin Genet 12:357, 1977.

Congenital Cystic Adenomatoid Malformation of the Lung

Synonym
Adenomatoid hamartoma.

Definition
Congenital cystic adenomatoid malformation of the lung (CCAML) is a hamartoma of the lung characterized by overgrowth of terminal bronchioles (adenomatoid) at the expense of saccular spaces. The term "hamartoma" refers to a benign tumorlike malformation which reproduces, in a disorderly manner, the mature structure of the organ from which it is derived.

Embryology
The respiratory tract includes the conducting airways and the respiratory component. They have different embryologic origins. The conducting airways are derived from the foregut (endoderm), whereas the respiratory component arises from mesenchyma that concentrate around the tips of the growing bronchi. The embryonic problem responsible for CCAML is thought to be an arrest of the connection of the two systems and subsequent overgrowth of the terminal bronchioles.[21,24] The insult seems to occur before the 5th week of conceptional age.

Incidence
CCAML is a rare malformation of the lung, and about 200 cases have been reported in the literature to date. There is no sex predilection.

Pathology
The lesion is almost always unilateral with no preference of right or left lung.[18] Only a few cases of bilateral involvement have been reported.[21] The disease generally affects one lobe, and the tumor appears as a mass of variable size that deforms the lung. It is often large enough to cause a shift of the

TYPE I   TYPE II   TYPE III

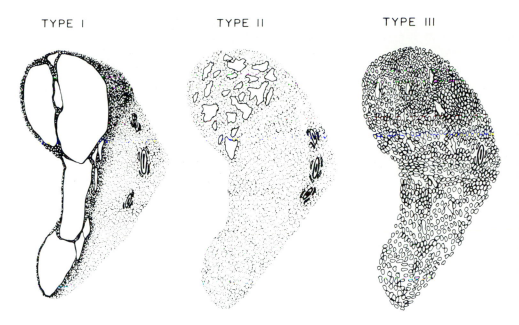

Figure 5–4. Classification of congenital cystic adenomatoid malformation. Type I is composed of a small number of large cysts with thick smooth muscle and elastic tissue walls. Relatively normal alveoli are seen between and adjacent to these cysts. Mucous glands may be present. Type II contains numerous smaller cysts (<1 cm in diameter), with a thin muscular coat beneath the ciliated columnar epithelium. The area between the cysts is occupied by large alveoluslike structures. The lesion blends with the normal parenchyma. Type III occupies the entire lobe or lobes and is composed of regularly spaced bronchiolelike structures separated by masses of cuboidal epithelium-lined alveoluslike structures. *(Reproduced with permission from Stocker et al.: Hum Pathol 8:155, 1977.)*

mediastinal structures and to compress the contralateral lung.

Stocker et al. proposed a classification of CCAML into three subtypes according to the size of the cysts[24]: type I has large cysts, type II has multiple small cysts of less than 1.2 cm in diameter, and type III consists of a noncystic lesion producing mediastinal shift (Fig. 5–4). The worst prognosis is seen in type III lesions. Associated anomalies are frequently present in type II. Another classification suggests that lesions are separated into two groups: macrocystic tumors with cysts of at least 5 mm in

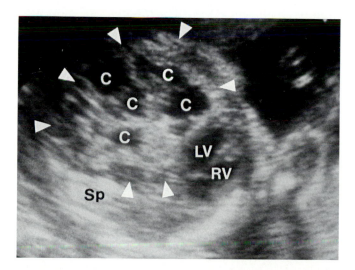

Figure 5–5. Transverse scan of the chest of a fetus with congenital cystic adenomatoid malformation of the lung type I. The heart is displaced toward the right hemithorax. Sp, spine; LV, left ventricle; RV, right ventricle; C, cysts; arrow heads point to pulmonary parenchyma.

diameter and microcystic lesions with cysts less than 5 mm in diameter. The latter lesion would be less common but almost invariably fatal.[1]

Polyhydramnios and nonimmune hydrops are frequently present in the cases detected antenatally or neonatally.[13,16] Fetal hydrops can result from decreased venous return due to vascular compression by the pulmonary mass or decreased myocardial contractility.[15,21] Fetal hydrops has been shown to subside after surgical decompression.[2] Polyhydramnios in the absence of hydrops is probably related to esophageal compression. Previously suggested explanations, such as decreased absorption of amniotic fluid by the malformed lung[16] or increased fluid production by the normal[3] or abnormal[17] lung, seem inconsistent with amniotic fluid dynamics and the anatomy of CCAML. Pulmonary hypoplasia results when the mass or the pleural effusion compresses the normal lung parenchyma.

Associated Anomalies

In most reports, CCAML is not associated with other anomalies. However, Stocker et al. reported anomalies in 10 of 38 patients, including bilateral renal agenesis, renal dysplasia, truncus arteriosus, tetralogy of Fallot, hydrocephalus, jejunal atresia, diaphragmatic hernia, deformity of clavicle and spine, and sirenomelia.[4,19,24] Cachia and Sobonya reported associated bronchial abnormalities in 9 patients.[5] Two reports have appeared in the literature of CCAML associated with prune-belly syndrome; in one case the massive ascites was thought to be responsible for the prune belly.[26,27]

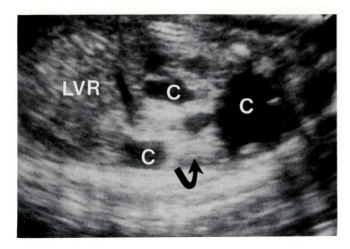

Figure 5–6. Longitudinal scan of the same fetus shown in Figure 5–5. Multiple large cysts (C) are visualized. Arrow points to pulmonary parenchyma. LVR, liver.

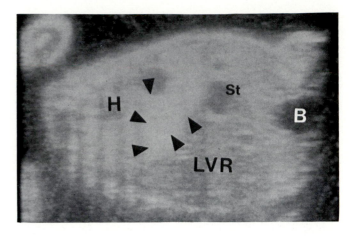

Figure 5–7. Longitudinal scan of an infant with congenital cystic malformation of the lung of the microcystic variety (type III). H, heart; LVR, liver; B, bladder; St, stomach; arrowheads point to the microcystic lesion.

Diagnosis

The diagnosis of CCAML relies on the demonstration of a nonpulsatile intrathoracic lung tumor that may be solid or cystic. The appearance of the macrocystic variety is demonstrated in Figures 5–5 and 5–6. A significant shift in the mediastinum can occur and be detected by displacement of the cardiac silhouette (Fig. 5–5). The microcystic variety appears as a solid tumor (Fig. 5–7). Hydrops is more commonly associated with the microcystic lesion.[1] Eleven different publications have reported a prenatal diagnosis of CCAML.[1,6,7,8,10,11,15,19,21–23] The earliest diagnosis was made at 24 weeks.[1]

Differential diagnosis includes thoracic lesions, such as diaphragmatic hernia and other congenital cystic lesions of the lung, like bronchogenic cysts and pulmonary sequestration. Peristalsis of the bowel within the thoracic cavity is helpful in distinguishing some macrocystic CCAML from diaphragmatic hernia. Extralobar pulmonary sequestration can be differentiated because it appears as a solid lesion without cysts, with a pyramidal shape.

Prognosis

Severe prematurity (before 34 weeks) is a common feature of the patients diagnosed antenatally or in the neonatal period,[8,15,16,21] and it appears to complicate the respiratory distress from pulmonary hypoplasia and heart failure. The prognosis for in utero-diagnosed cases depends on the variety of CCAML. Of 12 reported patients reviewed by Adzick et al.,[1] 5 of the 7 patients with macrocystic lesions survived, whereas only 1 of the 5 with microcystic lesions survived. Patients with microcystic lesions were more likely to have hydrops and polyhydramnios.

Some authors have reported a stillbirth rate of 30 percent and suggested that the presence of polyhydramnios and fetal hydrops is associated with poor prognosis.[13,16,21] A much better outcome has been reported for those diagnosed after the first day of life without associated anomalies.[2,4,9,12–14,18,20]

The most common symptom in the newborn is progressive respiratory distress, whereas older infants show repeated pulmonary infections. In rare cases, CCAML can be an incidental finding in patients with no respiratory impairment,[18] and small lesions may be asymptomatic for years.[20]

Treatment of the lesion consists of lobectomy rather than segmentectomy. Surgical removal of asymptomatic lesions seems justified because of the risk of growth and superimposed infection with respiratory compromise.[9,13,18] For this reason, most authors suggest that treatment be carried out without delay after the diagnosis is made in neonates and infants. Furthermore, in one reported case, a rhabdomyosarcoma was detected in an asymptomatic CCAML infant at age 18 months.[25]

In one study, eight patients were followed from 3 to 11 years after surgery for CCAML. Despite surgical removal of 20 percent of the total lung volume, total lung capacity, vital capacity and ventilatory capacity (measured as forced expiratory volume in 1 second) were on the average only 10 percent lower than the normal values, indicating a partial compensation of the remaining lung tissue. The subjective physical performance of the patients was equal to that of their playmates.[9]

Obstetrical Management

If this diagnosis is made before viability, the option of pregnancy termination should be offered. After viability, management and prognosis depend on the presence of associated hydrops. In patients without hydrops, delivery can wait until fetal and pulmonic maturity is reached. Serial scans are recommended to monitor the growth of the lesion and to look for early signs of hydrops. To date, fetuses with hydrops have had a 100 percent mortality rate. Nonaggressive management may be offered to the parents in these cases. Repeated thoracenteses do not seem to guarantee long-lasting decompression of the chest. In utero surgery for fetuses with hydrops and large lesions in early pregnancy has been suggested but has not been carried out at the time of this writing.[1] Antenatal diagnosis of CCAML mandates delivery in a tertiary care center, where immediate thoracic surgery can be performed.

REFERENCES

1. Adzick NS, Harrison MR, Glick PL, et al.: Fetal cystic adenomatoid malformation: Prenatal diagnosis and natural history. J Pediatr Surg 20:483, 1985.
2. Aslam PA, Korones SB, Richardson RL, et al.: Congenital cystic adenomatoid malformation with anasarca. JAMA 212:622, 1970.
3. Bates HR Jr: Fetal pulmonary hypoplasia and hydramnios. Am J Obstet Gynecol 91:295, 1965.
4. Birdsell DC, Wentworth P, Reilly BJ, et al.: Congential cystic adenomatoid malformation of the lung: A report of eight cases. Can J Surg 9:350, 1966.
5. Cachia R, Sobonya RE: Congenital cystic adenomatoid malformation of the lung with bronchial atresia. Hum Pathol 12:947, 1981.
6. Dibbins AW, Curci MR, McCrann DJ: Prenatal diagnosis of congenital anomalies requiring surgical correction. Am J Surg 149:528, 1985.
7. Diwan RV, Brennan JN, Philipson EH, et al.: Ultrasonic prenatal diagnosis of type III congenital cystic adenomatoid malformation of lung. J Clin Ultrasound 11:218, 1983.
8. Donn SM, Martin JN Jr, White SJ: Antenatal ultrasound findings in cystic adenomatoid malformation. Pediatr Radiol 10:180, 1981.
9. Frenckner B, Freyschuss U: Pulmonary function after lobectomy for congenital lobar emphysema and congenital cystic adenomatoid malformation: A follow-up study. Scand J Thorac Cardiovasc Surg 16:293, 1982.
10. Garrett WJ, Kossoff G, Lawrence R: Gray scale echography in the diagnosis of hydrops due to fetal lung tumor. J Clin Ultrasound 3:45, 1975.
11. Graham D, Winn K, Dex W, et al.: Prenatal diagnosis of cystic adenomatoid malformation of the lung. J Ultrasound Med 1:9, 1982.
12. Haller JA, Golladay ES, Pickard LR, et al.: Surgical management of lung bud anomalies: Lobar emphysema, bronchogenic cyst, cystic adenomatoid malformation, and intralobar pulmonary sequestration. Ann Thorac Surg 28:33, 1979.
13. Halloran LG, Silverberg SG, Salzberg AM: Congenital cystic adenomatoid malformation of the lung. Arch Surg 104:715, 1972.
14. Hartenberg MA, Brewer WH: Cystic adenomatoid malformation of the lung: Identification by sonography. AJR 140:693, 1983.
15. Johnson JA, Rumack CM, Johnson ML, et al.: Cystic adenomatoid malformation: Antenatal demonstration. AJR 142:483, 1984.
16. Kohler HG, Rymer BA: Congenital cystic malformation of the lung and its relation to hydramnios. J Obstet Gynaecol Br Commonw 80:130, 1973.
17. Krous HF, Harper PE, Perlman M: Congenital cystic adenomatoid malformation in bilateral renal agenesis: Its mitigation of Potter's syndrome. Arch Pathol Lab Med 104:368, 1980.
18. Madewell JE, Stocker JT, Korsower JM: Cystic adenomatoid malformation of the lung. AJR 124:436, 1975.
19. Mayden KL, Tortora M, Chervenak FA, et al.: The antenatal sonographic detection of lung masses. Am J Obstet Gynecol 148:349, 1984.
20. Moncrieff MW, Cameron AH, Astley R, et al.: Congenital cystic adenomatoid malformation of the lung. Thorax 24:476, 1969.
21. Oestoer AG, Fortune DW: Congenital cystic adenomatoid malformation of the lung. Am J Clin Pathol 70:595, 1978.
22. Pezzuti RT, Isler RJ: Antenatal ultrasound detection of cystic adenomatoid malformation of lung: Report of a case and review of the recent literature. J Clin Ultrasound 11:342, 1983.
23. Stauffer UG, Savoldelli G, Mieth D: Antenatal ultrasound diagnosis in cystic adenomatoid malformation of the lung. Case report. J Pediatr Surg 19:141, 1984.
24. Stocker JT, Madewell JE, Drake RM: Congenital cystic adenomatoid malformation of the lung. Classification and morphologic spectrum. Hum Pathol 8:155, 1977.
25. Ueda K, Gruppo R, Unger F, et al.: Rhabdomyosarcoma of lung arising in congenital cystic adenomatoid malformation. Cancer 40:383, 1977.
26. Weber ML, Rivard G, Perreault G: Prune-belly syndrome associated with congenital cystic adenomatoid malformation of the lung. Am J Dis Child 132:316, 1978.
27. Wilson SK, Moore GW, Hutchins GM: Congenital cystic adenomatoid malformation of the lung associated with abdominal musculature deficiency (prune belly). Pediatrics 62:421, 1978.

Lung Sequestration

Synonyms
Bronchopulmonary sequestration and accessory lung.

Definition
Lung sequestration is a congenital anomaly in which a mass of pulmonary parenchyma is separated from the normal lung. It usually does not communicate with an airway and receives its blood supply from the systemic circulation.

Embryology
The normal tracheobronchial tree derives from an outpouching of the foregut. A sequestered lung either originates from a separate outpouching of the foregut or is a segment of developing lung that has lost its connection with the rest of the tracheobronchial tree. Timing of the separation is critical. If the accessory lung bud arises before the formation of the pleura, the sequestered lung will be adjacent to the normal lung and surrounded by the same pleura (intralobar sequestration). If the accessory lung bud arises after formation of the pleura, the sequestered lung will have its own pleura (extralobar sequestration).[20]

Lung sequestration is one of the bronchopulmonary foregut malformations, a term that refers to a group of anomalies of the respiratory and gastrointestinal tracts that originate from the embryonic foregut. Besides lung sequestration, these anomalies include tracheoesophageal fistula, esophageal duplications, neurenteric cysts, esophageal diverticulum, esophageal cysts, and bronchogenic cysts.[5,6,8,9,16]

In some cases, the sequestered lung connects to the gastrointestinal tract. This occurs when the pedicle of the accessory lung bud does not involute. If a segment of the pedicle containing bronchial epithelium does not involute but loses its connection with the foregut, a bronchogenic cyst will result.

The circulatory supply of the sequestered lung derives from the aorta rather than the usual pulmonary artery. Therefore, the disturbance in lung development responsible for this anomaly must take place before the origin of separate pulmonary and aortic circulations.

Incidence
Lung sequestration is a rare anomaly without familial predisposition.[21] In the extralobar variety, a male predominance has been noted, with a male to female ratio of 3:1.[3,22]

Pathology
Lung sequestration can be classified into two types: intralobar and extralobar. In the intralobar variety, the sequestered lung and the normal lung share a common pleura. In the extralobar variety, the sequestered lung is covered by its own visceral pleura in a way similar to an accessory lobe. The most common variety in newborn infants is extralobar sequestration.[1,19] It is rare for sequestration to be present in both forms simultaneously,[21] involve an entire lung,[12] or be present bilaterally.[25]

Extralobar lung sequestration is located between the lower lobe and the diaphragm in 77.4 percent of patients (Fig. 5–8). The other locations include

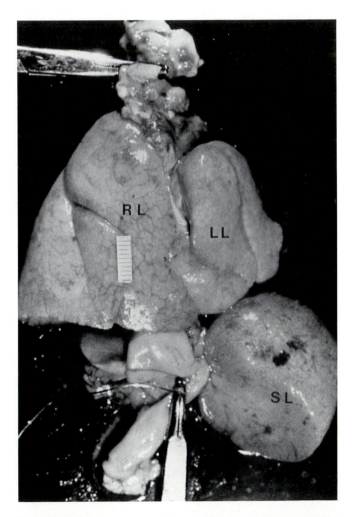

Figure 5–8. Autopsy specimen from a case of extralobar pulmonary sequestration. RL, right lung; LL, left lung; SL, sequestered lung. *(Reproduced with permission from Romero et al.: J Ultrasound Med 1:131, 1982.)*

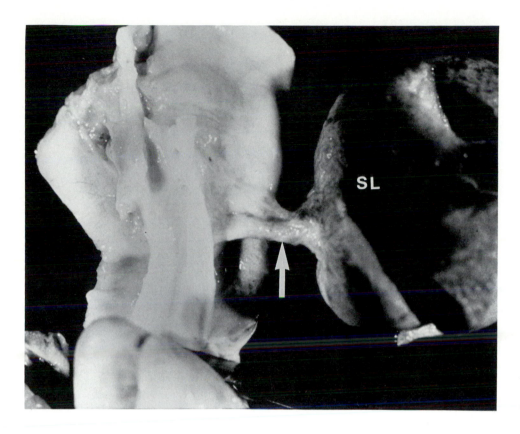

Figure 5–9. The blood supply to the sequestered lung (SL) is derived from the systemic circulation. The arrow points to the vascular supply to an extralobar sequestered lung.

paracardiac, mediastinal, infrapericardial, infradiaphragmatic, and abdominal sites.[21] The arterial supply and venous drainage are provided primarily by systemic vessels (Fig. 5–9). The size of the sequestered lung is variable.[22] Macroscopically, the parenchyma may resemble normal lung or be firm like thymus.[22]

In intralobar lung sequestration, either side is involved with similar frequency. The lower lobes are the most commonly affected (98 percent). The arterial supply is usually from the thoracic or abdominal aorta (93 percent), and the venous drainage terminates in the pulmonary veins (96 percent).[21] Macroscopically, the sectioned areas may show a wide spectrum of appearances, ranging from the most frequent cystic pattern (with a solitary cyst or polycysts) to the rare pseudotumorous form.[11,21]

Associated Anomalies

Lung sequestration is one of the bronchopulmonary foregut malformations. These foregut anomalies share a common embryologic pathogenesis and are associated with each other more frequently than would be expected by chance.[5,6,8,9,16] The other bronchopulmonary foregut malformations include tracheoesophageal fistula, esophageal duplications, neurenteric cysts, esophageal diverticulum, esophageal cysts, and bronchogenic cysts.

Extrapulmonary anomalies occur in 10 percent of patients with intralobar lung sequestration[21] and include skeletal deformities (funnel chest, polydactyly),[10] diaphragmatic hernias, congenital heart disease (tricuspid atresia, transposition of great vessels, subvalvular aortic stenosis),[24] and renal and cerebral anomalies (hydrocephalus).[10,21]

In contrast, the incidence of extrapulmonary anomalies in the extralobar variety is 59 percent, including diaphragmatic hernia, heart anomalies (atrial and ventricular septal defects, congenital absence of pericardium, truncus arteriosus),[1,22] funnel chest, vertebral defects,[2] and megacolon.[21] Often, several anomalies are present in the same patient.[22] Diaphragmatic hernia constitutes 50 percent of the anomalies associated with extralobar lung sequestration.[21]

The anomalous blood supply to the sequestered lung can cause a left-to-right shunt, leading in some patients to cardiac failure after birth.[4,7,8,14,17] Lung sequestration has been associated with nonimmune hydrops.

Diagnosis

Extralobar lung sequestration has been identified antenatally on several occasions.[13,15,18,23a] The sequestered lung appears as an echogenic, intra-

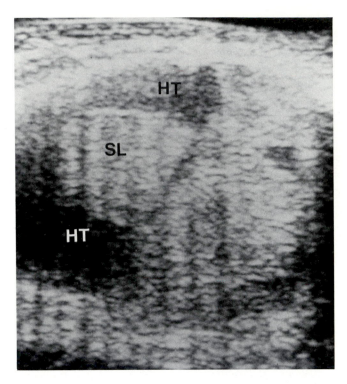

Figure 5–10. Longitudinal scan of an infant with extralobar pulmonary sequestration and nonimmune hydrops. Hydrothorax (HT) is present. SL, sequestered lung. *(Reproduced with permission from Romero et al.: J Ultrasound Med 1:131, 1982.)*

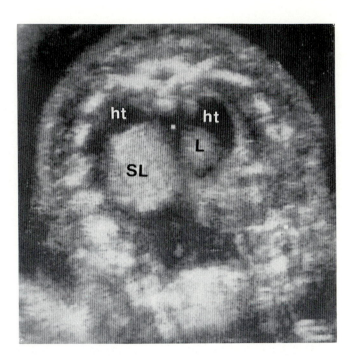

Figure 5–11. Transverse scan of the thorax demonstrates bilateral hydrothorax (ht), the right lung (L), and the sequestered lung (SL). *(Reproduced with permission from Romero et al.: J Ultrasound Med 1:131, 1982.)*

thoracic, or intraabdominal mass (Figs. 5–10, 5–11). Both the two fetuses with intrathoracic lung sequestration had nonimmune hydrops.[13,18] Polyhydramnios is frequently reported as well.[13,18,22] The prenatal diagnosis of intralobar pulmonary sequestration has not been reported thus far and would seem quite difficult, since even in the postnatal period, a preoperative diagnosis is made in only 39 percent of patients.[21]

Differential diagnosis should include mediastinal teratomas, whose high density usually causes an acoustic shadowing behind the mass, and other intrathoracic masses, such as cystic adenomatoid tumor of the lung, which will appear either multicystic or solid. In some cases, it is possible to have a high index of suspicion for lung sequestration when the echogenicity of the mass is homogeneous and identical to that of the adjacent normal lung. In addition, extralobar sequestration may simulate the pyramidal shape of a lower lobe. Extralobar lung sequestration should also be considered in the differential diagnosis of intraabdominal solid masses, such as mesonephroma.

Prognosis

Only 1 of the 4 patients with lung sequestration detected antenatally survived. The other 3 had nonimmune hydrops and intrathoracic sequestration.

The survivor had an intraabdominal sequestration and no signs of hydrops. The prognosis for extralobar lung sequestration derived from pediatric series is generally poor. In one report of 30 neonates, 23 died shortly after the diagnosis, and the majority had multiple anomalies.[21] In another series of 15 neonates, all infants diagnosed the first day of life died.[22]

The spectrum of the disease is wide, and some infants are asymptomatic until later in life, when recurrent pulmonary infection or hemorrhage, gastrointestinal symptoms, or heart failure from left-to-right shunt may occur.[1,4,8,11,22–24] Treatment consists of surgical resection of the sequestered lung. Patients subsequently do well.

Obstetrical Management

This condition will most often occur as a tumor of unknown etiology in the fetal chest. A certain diagnosis is difficult without histologic study. Before viability, the option of pregnancy termination should be offered. After viability, prognosis is probably related to the development of hydrops. The section on nonimmune hydrops discusses management in further detail (see pp. 422–423). A case treated with thoracentesis was reported recently.[23a] Although the infant died postnatally, drainage of the chest was associated with resolution of the hydrops. In the absence of hydrops, there is no apparent reason to change standard obstetrical care. Delivery in a tertiary center is recommended. Immediate respiratory support may be required.

REFERENCES

1. Buntain WL, Woolley MM, Mahour GH, et al.: Pulmonary sequestration in children: A twenty-five year experience. Surgery 81:413, 1977.
2. Canty TG: Extralobar pulmonary sequestration. Unusual presentation and systemic vascular communication in association with a right-sided diaphragmatic hernia. J Thorac Cardiovasc Surg 81:96, 1981.
3. Carter R: Pulmonary sequestration. Ann Thorac Surg 7:68, 1969.
4. Choplin RH, Siegel MJ: Pulmonary sequestration: Six unusual presentations. AJR 134:695, 1980.
5. Demos NJ, Teresi A: Congenital lung malformations. A unified concept and a case report. J Thor Cardiovasc Surg 70:260, 1975.
6. Gerle RD, Jaretzki A, Ashley CA, et al.: Congenital bronchopulmonary–foregut malformation: Pulmonary sequestration communicating with the gastrointestinal tract. N Engl J Med 278:1413, 1968.
7. Goldblatt E, Vimpani G, Brown JH: Extralobar pulmonary sequestration. Presentation as an arteriovenous aneurysm with cardiac failure in infancy. Am J Cardiology 29:100, 1971.
8. Haller JA, Golladay ES, Pickard LR, et al.: Surgical management of lung bud anomalies: Lobar emphysema, bronchogenic cyst, cystic adenomatoid malformation, and intralobar pulmonary sequestration. Ann Thorac Surg 28:33, 1979.
9. Heithoff KB, Sane SM, Williams HJ, et al.: Bronchopulmonary foregut malformations. A unifying etiological concept. AJR 126:46, 1976.
10. Iwa T, Watanabe Y: Unusual combination of pulmonary sequestration and funnel chest. Chest 76:3, 1979.
11. Iwai K, Shindo G, Hajikano H, et al.: Intralobar pulmonary sequestration, with special reference to developmental pathology. Am Rev Respir Dis 107:911, 1973.
12. Jona JZ, Raffensperger JG: Total sequestration of the right lung. J Thorac Cardiovasc Surg 69:361,1975.
13. Jouppila P, Kirkinen P, Herva R, et al.: Prenatal diagnosis of pleural effusions by ultrasound. J Clin Ultrasound 11:516, 1983.
14. Khalil KG, Kilman JW: Pulmonary sequestration. J Thorac Cardiovasc Surg 70:928, 1975.
15. Mariona F, McAlpin G, Zador I, et al.: Sonographic detection of fetal extrathoracic pulmonary sequestration. J Clin Ultrasound 5:283, 1986.
16. O'Connell DJ, Kelleher J: Congenital intrathoracic bronchopulmonary foregut malformations in childhood. J Can Assoc Radiol 30:103, 1979.
17. Ransom JM, Norton JB, Williams GD: Pulmonary sequestration presenting as congestive heart failure. J Thorac Cardiovasc Surg 76:378, 1978.
18. Romero R, Chervenak FA, Kotzen J, et al.: Antenatal sonographic findings of extralobar pulmonary sequestration. J Ultrasound Med 1:131, 1982.
19. Ryckman FC, Rosenkrantz JG: Thoracic surgical problems in infancy and childhood. Surg Clin North Am 65:1423, 1985.
20. Sade RM, Clouse M, Ellis FH Jr: The spectrum of pulmonary sequestration. Ann Thorac Surg 18:644, 1974.
21. Savic B, Birtel FJ, Tholen W, et al.: Lung sequestration: Report of seven cases and review of 540 published cases. Thorax 34:96, 1979.
22. Stocker JT, Kagan-Hallet K: Extralobar pulmonary sequestration. Analysis of 15 cases. Am J Clin Pathol 72:917, 1979.
23. Symbas PN, Hatcher CR, Abbott OA, et al.: An appraisal of pulmonary sequestration: Special emphasis on unusual manifestations. Am Rev Respir Dis 99:406, 1969.
23a. Weiner C, Varner M, Pringle K, et al.: Antenatal diagnosis and palliative treatment of nonimmune hydrops fetalis secondary to pulmonary extralobar sequestration. Obstet Gynecol 68:275, 1986.
24. White JJ, Donahoo JS, Ostrow PT, et al.: Cardiovascular and respiratory manifestations of pulmonary sequestration in childhood. Ann Thorac Surg 18:286, 1974.
25. Wimbish KJ, Agha FP, Brady TM: Bilateral pulmonary sequestration: Computed tomographic appearance. AJR 140:689, 1983.

Bronchogenic Cyst

Definition
A bronchogenic cyst is a cystic structure lined by bronchial epithelium.

Incidence
The incidence of bronchogenic cysts is unknown, since a large number of them are asymptomatic. They are extremely rare in the neonatal period.

Embryology
Bronchogenic cysts result from an abnormal budding of the foregut. They may remain attached to the primitive tracheobronchial tree, in which case they are found along the trachea, in the mediastinum, or within the pulmonary parenchyma. If the outpouching separates from its site of origin, the cyst may migrate into the mediastinum, neck, pericardium, vertebrae, subpleurae, and other locations.

Pathology

The cyst is lined by a ciliated columnar epithelium similar to that covering normal bronchi. It may contain cartilage, muscle, and mucous glands. The size and location are extremely variable. Although most cysts are considered mediastinal, this has been challenged recently by a study in which the majority of cysts were pulmonary in location (Fig. 5–12).[18] Multiple cysts can be found as well.[17]

Associated Anomalies

Bronchogenic cysts are one of the bronchopulmonary foregut malformations, a group of foregut anomalies that share a common embryologic pathogenesis and are associated with each other more frequently than expected by chance.[2,6,7,9,16] The other bronchopulmonary foregut malformations include tracheoesophageal fistula, esophageal duplications, neurenteric cysts, esophageal diverticulum, esophageal cysts, and lung sequestration. Vertebral abnormalities (hemivertebrae) are often associated with bronchogenic cysts of mediastinal origin.[4] Isolated reports have documented the occurrence of this condition in trisomy 21 and in association with congenital heart disease, including dextrocardia.[18]

Diagnosis

We are aware of only one prenatal diagnosis of bronchogenic cyst.[14] This lesion was identified as a single hypoechogenic mass in the upper part of the right lung and measured 15 × 19 mm at 36 weeks of

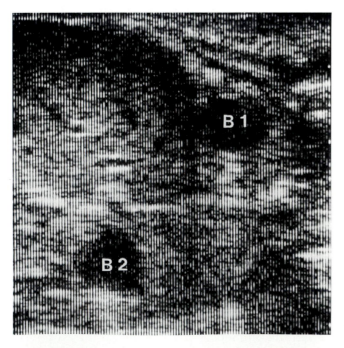

Figure 5–12. A fetus with two bronchogenic cysts. One is located in the apex of the right lung (B1), and the other (B2) is located in the opposite lung.

TABLE 5–1. DIAGNOSIS OF MEDIASTINAL MASSES

Prevalently Solid	Cystic
Anterior mediastinum	
Teratoma	Bronchogenic cyst
Thymus neoplasm	Lymphangioma
Germ cell tumor	Hemangioma
Intrathoracic goiter	Pericardial cyst
	Diaphragmatic hernia
Middle mediastinum	
Thymus	Bronchogenic cyst
	Pericardial cyst
Posterior mediastinum	
Neurogenic tumor [8,11,13]	Enteric cyst [10,15]
Thymus	Esophageal duplication
Pulmonary sequestration	Diaphragmatic hernia
	Anterior meningocele

gestation. No hydrops was present. The diagnosis was confirmed at a thoracotomy performed 8 days postpartum.

The differential diagnosis includes other mediastinal masses (Table 5–1).[1,5] A definitive differential diagnosis of cystic chest masses depends on histologic examination.

Prognosis

A bronchogenic cyst may be a completely asymptomatic lesion that is discovered during a radiograph of the chest. In other cases, the masses may compress the airway and cause respiratory distress, recurrent respiratory infections, and, on rare occasions, malignant transformation.[3] The treatment is surgical extirpation. Large cysts may require lobectomy and even pneumonectomy. The optimal management of asymptomatic lesions has not been established. When surgery is not contraindicated,[17] several authors have proposed resection to establish a histologic diagnosis and to avoid complications, such as infection.

Obstetrical Management

A diagnosis of an intrathoracic cyst should probably not alter standard obstetrical management. Every effort should be made to delay delivery until lung maturity is present. Immediate respiratory assistance may be required at birth, and delivery in a tertiary care center is recommended.

REFERENCES

1. Bower RJ, Kiesewetter WB: Mediastinal masses in infants and children. Arch Surg 112:1003, 1977.
2. Demos NJ, Teresi A: Congenital lung malformations. A unified concept and a case report. J Thorac Cardiovasc Surg 70:260, 1975.

3. Eraklis AJ, Griscom NT, McGovern JB: Bronchogenic cysts of the mediastinum in infancy. N Engl J Med 281: 1150, 1969.

4. Fallon M, Gordon ARG, Lendrum AC: Mediastinal cysts of foregut origin associated with vertebral abnormalities. Br J Surg 41:520, 1954.

5. Felman AH: The Pediatric Chest. Radiological, Clinical and Pathological Observations. Springfield, IL, Chas. C Thomas, 1983, p 167.

6. Gerle RD, Jaretzki A, Ashley CA, et al.: Congential bronchopulmonary–foregut malformation: Pulmonary sequestration communicating with the gastrointestinal tract. N Engl J Med 278:1413, 1968.

7. Haller JA, Golladay ES, Pickard LR, et al.: Surgical management of lung bud anomalies: Lobar emphysema, bronchogenic cyst, cystic adenomatoid malformation, and intralobar pulmonary sequestration. Ann Thorac Surg 28:33, 1979.

8. Halperin DS, Oberhansli I, Siegrist CA, et al.: Intrathoracic neuroblastoma presenting with neonatal cardiorespiratory distress. Chest 85:822, 1984.

9. Heithoff KB, Sane SM, Williams HJ, et al.: Bronchopulmonary foregut malformations. A unifying etiological concept. AJR 126:46, 1976.

10. Hobbins JC, Grannum PAT, Berkowitz RL, et al.: Ultrasound in the diagnosis of congenital anomalies. Am J Obstet Gynecol 134:331, 1979.

11. Illescas FF, Williams RL: Neonatal neuroblastoma pre senting with respiratory distress. J Assoc Can Radiol 35:310, 1984.

12. Knochel JQ, Lee TG, Melendez MG, et al.: Fetal anomalies involving the thorax and abdomen. Radiol Clin North Am 20:297, 1982.

13. Massad M, Haddad F, Slim M, et al.: Spinal cord compression in neuroblastoma. Surg Neurol 23:567, 1985.

14. Mayden KL, Tortora M, Chervenak FA, et al.: The antenatal sonographic detection of lung masses. Am J Obstet Gynecol 148:349, 1984.

15. Newnham JP, Crues JV, Vinstein AL, et al.: Sonographic diagnosis of thoracic gastroenteric cyst in utero. Prenat Diagn 4:467, 1984.

16. O'Connell DJ, Kelleher J: Congenital intrathoracic bronchopulmonary foregut malformations in childhood. J Can Assoc Radiol 30:103, 1979.

17. Phelan PD, Landau LI, Olinsky A: Respiratory Illness in Children, 2d ed. Oxford, Blackwell Scientific, 1982, pp 397–416.

18. Ramenofsky ML, Leape LL, McCauley RGK: Bronchogenic cyst. J Pediatr Surg 14:219, 1979.

6

The Abdominal Wall

Normal Anatomy of the Abdominal Wall

The superior wall of the abdominal cavity is formed by the diaphragm. This muscle can be seen as a hypoechogenic line separating the lung and fetal liver (Fig. 6–1). In cases of severe hydrops, the structure appears as a hyperechogenic sheet between the pleural effusion and the ascites. When a massive pleural effusion is present, the muscle can be inverted.

The floor of the abdominal cavity is formed by the pelvic diaphragm. The pelvic bones (iliac crests, ischial ossification centers) and pelvic muscles can be imaged with ultrasound but have limited diagnostic interest (Fig. 6–2).

The anterior abdominal wall is formed by the skin, subcutaneous tissue, and muscles. The muscles are visible as hypoechogenic structures (Fig. 6–3). In the past, the image of the muscles has been confused with ascites and referred to as "pseudoascites."[1,2] The entrance of the umbilical cord into the fetal abdomen should always be imaged to screen for the presence of an omphalocele (Fig. 6–4). Examination of the anterior abdominal wall should include visualization of its infraumbilical portion in order to rule out caudal fold defects (e.g., bladder exstrophy). Figure 6–5 shows the normal contours of the lower portion of the anterior abdominal wall.

The posterior wall of the abdomen can be easily imaged. Structures that can be identified include the spine and the paraspinal muscles.

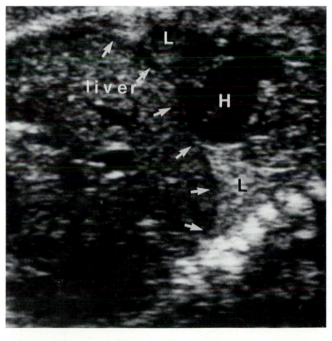

Figure 6–1. Coronal section of a third trimester fetus. The diaphragm appears as a hypoechogenic line between the thorax and the abdomen. L, lung; H, heart.

REFERENCES

1. Rosenthal SJ, Filly RA, Callen PW, et al.: Fetal pseudoascites. Radiology 131:195, 1979.
2. Hashimoto BE, Filly RA, Callen PW: Fetal pseudoascites: Further anatomic observations. J Ultrasound Med 5:151, 1986.

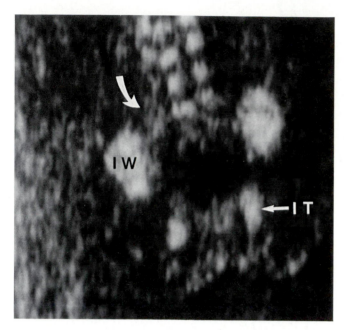

Figure 6–2. Coronal scan of a male fetal pelvis. A curved arrow points to the right ileopsoas muscle. IW, iliac wings; IT, ischial tuberosities.

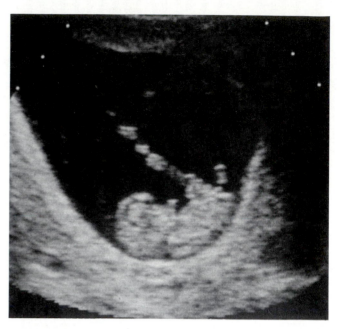

Figure 6–4. Longitudinal scan showing the insertion of the umbilical cord in the abdomen of a first trimester fetus.

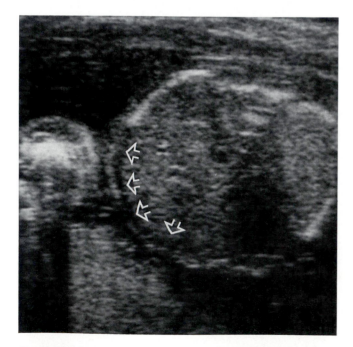

Figure 6–3. Transverse section of the abdomen of a third trimester fetus. The abdominal muscles appear as hypoechogenic structures (*arrowheads*).

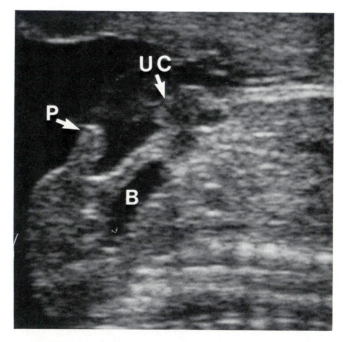

Figure 6–5. Longitudinal scan of the fetal abdomen between the insertion of the umbilical cord (UC) and the gender. B, bladder; P, penis.

Diaphragmatic Hernia

Definition

Diaphragmatic hernia consists of protrusion of the abdominal organs into the thoracic cavity through a diaphragmatic defect. It includes posterolateral diaphragmatic hernia, Bochdalek hernia, retrosternal diaphragmatic hernia, Morgagni hernia, and eventration of the diaphragm.

Incidence

The incidence of diaphragmatic hernia varies depending on the type of study. The best estimates vary from 0.033 to 0.05 percent of births.[11,19,31,47] Neonatal surgical series report a frequency of 0.012 percent.[67] This difference is due to an underestimation of the incidence of the disease because of its association with stillbirths and early neonatal deaths.[36] The male to female ratio in the two largest series to date varies between 0.67 and 0.77.[11,19]

Etiology and Risk of Recurrence

Congenital diaphragmatic hernia can be both a sporadic and a familial disorder. The pattern of inheritance for familial cases is unknown, but a multifactorial type of inheritance has been suggested,[17,57,58] indicating a recurrence risk for siblings of 2 percent.[57] Familial cases have a higher male to female ratio (M:F = 2.10 versus 0.67), a higher incidence of bilateral defects (20 percent versus 3 percent), and a lower incidence of life-threatening malformations than sporadic cases.[17] However, no specific features allow identification of a familial case. Diaphragmatic hernia has been associated with Fryns syndrome,[49] Beckwith-Wiedemann syndrome (see p. 221),[68] Pierre Robin syndrome, and congenital choanal atresia.[22] The defect has been associated with chromosomal defects (see section on associated anomalies).

The etiology of sporadic cases is largely unknown. Maternal ingestion of bendectin,[10] thalidomide,[43] quinine,[46] and antiepileptic drugs[40] has been reported in association with diaphragmatic hernia. In animal models, hypovitaminosis A was able to induce diaphragmatic hernia in rats.[1,72] The etiologic role of diabetes is considered weak.[45]

Embryology and Anatomy of the Diaphragm

The diaphragm is a dome-shaped septum dividing the thoracic and abdominal cavities. It consists of a central or aponeurotic segment and a peripheral or muscular one. It is formed by the fusion of four different structures: (1) the septum transversum, (2) the dorsal esophageal mesentery, (3) the pleuroperitoneal membrane, and (4) the body wall.[25,55,65] The septum tranversum is a mesodermal structure that migrates from the cranial portion of the embryo to the definitive location of the diaphragm. It gives origin to the central tendon of the diaphragm. The dorsal esophageal mesentery contributes to the median portion of the organ. The pleuroperitoneal membranes are structures that close the pleuroperitoneal cavity. Although they form a large segment of the embryonal diaphragm, their contribution to the final and fully developed diaphragm is relatively small. The participation of the body wall is limited to a narrow peripheral segment corresponding to the insertion of the muscle to the ribs and sternum (Fig. 6–6). The diaphragm is completely formed by the end of the 8th week of conceptional age. However, modeling continues throughout gestation. Expansion of the lungs results in the formation of the costodiaphragmatic recesses, which have a dome-shaped configuration.

The normal diaphragm allows the passage of organs, vessels, and nerves from the thoracic to the abdominal cavity. This is accomplished by three main orifices, allowing passage for the aorta, esophagus, and inferior vena cava (Fig. 6–7). The thoracic duct and azygos vein cross through the aortic foramen, and the vagal nerves use the esophageal foramen. The right phrenic nerves cross through the inferior vena cava orifice. Congenital diaphragmatic hernias occur when a diaphragmatic defect allows the protrusion of abdominal visceral content into the thoracic cavity. The spectrum of embryologic defects is wide, ranging from complete absence of the diaphragm through pathologic orifices (Bochdaleck foramen) to congenital hiatal hernia, in which the viscera protrude through a physiologic orifice.

Congenital diaphragmatic hernias are classified according to the location of the diaphragmatic defect:

1. Posterolateral defect, or Bochdaleck hernia, occurring through the primitive communication of the pleuroperitoneal canal or foramen of Bochdaleck
2. Parasternal defect, or Morgagni hernia, located in the anterior portion of the diaphragm between the costal and the sternal origins of the muscle (foramen of Morgagni or sternocostal hiatus)
3. Septum transversum defects, occurring because of a defect of the central tendon
4. Hiatal hernias, occurring through a congenitally large esophageal orifice

Another pathologic entity, eventration of the diaphragm, is frequently considered with congenital diaphragmatic hernias because they have a similar pathophysiologic sequence. However, eventration of

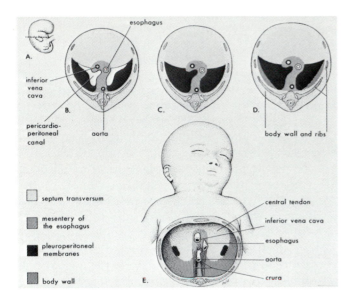

Figure 6–6. Development of the diaphragm (viewed from below). **A.** sketch of a lateral view of a 5-week embryo (actual size), indicating the level of the section. **B.** Transverse section showing the pleuroperitoneal membranes not yet fused. **C.** Same section at the end of the 6th week; the pleuroperitoneal membranes have fused with the other two diaphragmatic components. **D.** Same section at 12 weeks; the fourth diaphragmatic component has formed from the body wall. **E.** view in the newborn, indicating the probable embryologic origin of the different components. *(Reproduced from Moore: The Developing Human, 3d ed. Philadelphia, Saunders, 1982.)*

the diaphragm consists of an upward displacement of the abdominal content into the thoracic cavity because of a congenitally weak diaphragm, which is virtually reduced to an aponeurotic sheet.

The mechanisms responsible for the origin of a diaphragmatic hernia are unknown. The two main hypotheses are (1) delayed fusion of the diaphragm and (2) a primary diaphragmatic defect. The bowel normally returns to the abdominal cavity between the 10th and 12th weeks of gestation, at which time formation of the diaphragm should be completed. Delayed closure of the communication between the abdomen and the thorax would allow part of the abdominal contents to pass into the thorax, and

abdominal viscera would prevent complete closure of the diaphragm. An alternative hypothesis suggests that a primary defect occurs in the formation of the diaphragm, and this creates the condition for a subsequent migration of the abdominal organs into the thoracic cavity. The negative pressure created by fetal thoracic wall movements (fetal breathing) could be responsible for migration of the viscera into the thorax. Two observations support the first hypothesis. (1) In some cases, organs firmly attached to the abdomen in late fetal life, such as the pancreas, can be found in the thorax. This implies a precocious migration of abdominal organs into the thoracic cavity. (2) The discrepancy between the size of the defect and the dimensions of the herniated organs also suggests an early migration of the viscera and secondary partial closure of the defect.

The main cause of death of infants with congenital diaphragmatic hernia without associated anomalies is respiratory failure due to pulmonary hypoplasia. This can be easily understood if it is considered that development of the normal lung is an active process from the 5th week of gestation.[44,61] The fetal lung goes through four different stages (Figs. 6–8, 6–9): (1) embryonic period, from conception to the 5th week, (2) pseudoglandular period, from the 5th to the 17th week, (3) canalicular period, from the 17th to the 24th week, and (4) terminal sac period, from the 24th week until term. By the 16th week of gestation, the development of the conductive part of the airways is completed (from trachea to terminal bronchioles). From this time until birth, respiratory airways are fully developed. This includes respiratory bronchioles and saccules. Most alveolar development is a postnatal event. Their number increases until the age of 7 years, and their size keeps up with changes in thoracic volume until maturity. The development of the pulmonary circulation follows that of the airways. The total adult complement of blood vessels irrigating the conducting portion of the airways (also known as preacinar) is completed by 20 weeks of gestation. The alveolar or intraacinar portion devel-

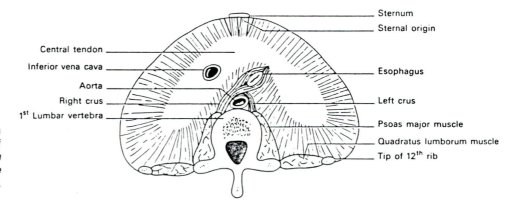

Figure 6–7. View of a diaphragm from below, showing the position of the normal orifices. *(Reproduced with permission from Thompson: Core Textbook of Anatomy. Philadelphia, Lippincott, 1977.)*

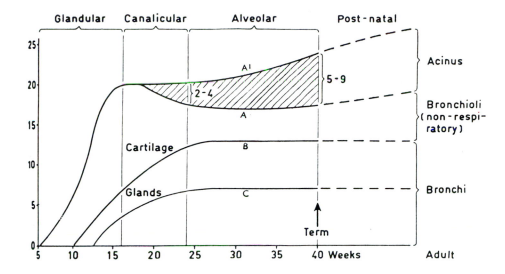

Figure 6–8. Development of the bronchial tree. Lobar bronchi appear at 6 weeks of gestation, and by 16 weeks all nonrespiratory airways are present. Most respiratory airways appear between 16 weeks and birth. Cartilage and glands appear later, with extension complete by 24 weeks of gestation. On the vertical axis: number of generations. *(Reproduced with permission from Bucher, Reid: Development of intrasegmental bronchial tree: The pattern of branching and development of cartilage at various stages of intrauterine life. Thorax 16:207, 1961.)*

ops postnatally. Knowledge of changes in the thickness and extension of the muscular component of the media is important in order to understand the development of postsurgical pulmonary hypertension. The muscle of these vessels is limited to the terminal bronchioles during fetal life. Postnatally, there is progressive extension peripherally to the respiratory bronchioles, alveolar ducts, and alveolar vessels. There is also a progressive decrease in the thickness of the muscle wall (Figs. 6–10, 6–11).

Infants with diaphragmatic hernia have profound changes in both the respiratory and the vascular components of the lungs. These are more pronounced in the ipsilateral than in the contralateral lung, depending on the timing and the degree of herniation.[20] An early insult (before 16 weeks) could reduce the number of conducting airways. After this time, it also impairs the development of respiratory airways. After surgical correction, gains can be achieved in respiratory airways as their normal development continues postnatally. However, catchup growth cannot occur in conducting airways, and therefore, the total number of alveoli is diminished (pulmonary hypoplasia). The vascular changes in congenital diaphragmatic hernia include a reduction in the number of vessels, an increase in arterial medial wall thickness, and an extension of muscle peripherally into smaller preacinar arteries.[39,48,56] These morphologic changes are the basis for the occurrence of pulmonary hypertension in the postoperative period, which can be triggered even by mild acidosis, hypoxia, or hypercapnia and can lead to right-to-left shunt and persistent fetal circulation.[7,16,20,21,24,53,62,64] The presence of a transitory, postoperative, asymptomatic period shows that the cause of death is not lung hypoplasia but intense pulmonary vasospasm. Survival in these cases is related to surgical ligation of the ductus arteriosus[15,16]

and on a thorough pharmacologic treatment aimed at dilating the pulmonary vascular bed and at preventing acidosis and hypoxia.[7,16,31,54,73]

Pathology
Among the previously described varieties of congenital diaphragmatic hernia, the three most common are posterolateral or Bochdalek type, parasternal or

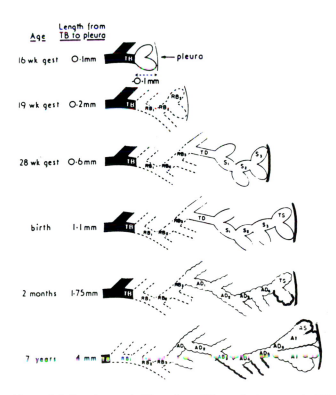

Figure 6–9. Development of the acinus. TB, terminal bronchiole; RB, respiratory bronchiole; TD, transitional duct; S, saccule; TS, terminal saccule; AD, alveolar duct; At, atrium; AS, alveolar sac. *(Reproduced with permission from Hislop, Reid: Development of the acinus in the human lung. Thorax 29:90, 1974.)*

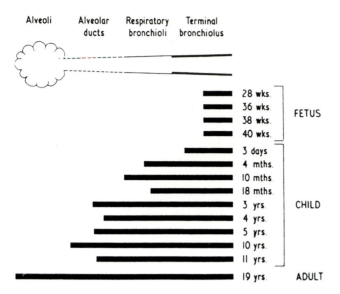

Figure 6–10. Bar graph showing progression of muscle in the walls of arteries within the acinus. In fetuses, there is no muscle within the acinus. With age, there is gradual extension into the acinar region, but, even at 11 years, muscular arteries have not reached the alveolar wall, where they are found in adults. *(Reproduced with permission from Reid: AJR 129:777, 1977.)*

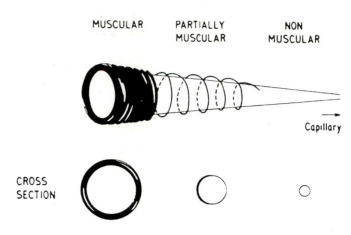

Figure 6–11. Pulmonary artery structure at distal end. Complete muscle coat (muscular artery) gives way to spiral of muscle (partially muscular artery) before it completely disappears, leaving nonmuscular artery. In cross-section, vessels within the spiral region have a crescent of muscle. *(Reproduced with permission from Reid: AJR 129:777, 1977)*

Morgagni type, and eventration. Hiatal hernia has little relevance for prenatal diagnosis.

Bochdalek type is the most common, accounting for 85 to 90 percent of all congenital diaphragmatic defects found in the neonatal period.[11,19] It occurs in the left side in 80 percent of cases, in the right side in 15 percent of cases, and is bilateral in the rest.[11,19,28] An explanation for this predominance is that the right pleuroperitoneal canal closes before the left. A true sac is present in only 5 to 10 percent of patients. The small bowel is involved in about 90 percent of cases, the stomach in 60 percent, the spleen in 54 percent, and the colon in 56 percent. Less frequently, the pancreas (24 percent), liver, adrenal glands, and even kidneys (12 percent) may be found.[11] In the chest, the heart and mediastinum are shifted generally to the right. When the hernia is located in the right side, the main organs include the liver and gallbladder. Incomplete rotation of the intestine and anomalous mesenteric attachment are the rule.

Morgagni hernia accounts for only 1 to 2 percent of congenital diaphragmatic hernias.[19] It is most frequently located in the right side and can also be bilateral.[52] This type of hernia is considered to be the result of failure of muscle to develop from the transverse septum. The content of the hernia is usually liver; other organs, such as colon, small bowel, and stomach, may follow as well. The hernia is usually small because the liver may limit the degree of herniation. A peritoneal sac is always present, al-

though on occasion rupture occurs, leaving little trace of the sac. Herniation into the pericardial cavity has been reported rarely. The heart may herniate through the foramen of Morgagni into the epigastric area.[4]

Eventration of the diaphragm occurs in 5 percent of diaphragmatic defects.[19] It is five times more common in the right side than in the left, and some bilateral instances have been reported. All or part of the hemidiaphragm is involved. The disorder can be considered a failure of muscularization of the diaphragm, which appears thin and lacks, either partially or totally, muscle fibers. Acquired eventration can be caused by paralysis of the phrenic nerve, and injury of this nerve during delivery may account for some cases of eventration in the neonatal period. In congenital eventration, the phrenic nerve is normal. The frequency of malrotation of the intestine in congenital eventration suggests that this disorder can occur during fetal life.

Associated Anomalies

Congenital diaphragmatic hernia has been associated consistently with a high incidence of other anomalies, excluding lung hypoplasia and gut malrotation, which are implied in the diaphragmatic hernia sequence. Three major studies have reported a remarkably similar incidence of major anomalies, ranging from 50 to 57 percent.[11,19,47] These studies have included both stillbirths and neonatal deaths. The incidence of anomalies is much lower in survivors.[9,28] Congenital diaphragmatic hernia has been considered as part of the schisis type of abnormalities, which include neural tube defects (anencephaly, cephaloceles, spina bifida), oral cleft (lip and palate),

TABLE 6–1. ASSOCIATED ANOMALIES IN DIAPHRAGMATIC HERNIA

Nervous system	Genitourinary system
Spina bifida	Hydronephrosis
Hydrocephalus	Renal agenesis (unilateral or
Anencephaly	bilateral)
Occipital bone defect	Polycystic kidney
Encephalocele	Horseshoe kidney
Iniencephaly	Bicornuate uterus
Defect of falx or tentorium	Hydroureter
Absence of corpus callosum	Duplex kidney
Gastrointestinal system	Ectopic kidney
Malrotation	Vaginal atresia
Accessory spleen	Unilateral absence of tube
Rectal atresia	and ovary
Esophageal atresia	Male pseudohermaphroditism
Meckel's diverticulum	Cardiovascular system
Duodenal band	Single umbilical artery
Exomphalos	Atrial septal defect
Gastrojejunal fistula	Ventricular septal defect
Abdominal situs inversus	Tetralogy of Fallot
Hepatic cyst	Complex anomalies
Duodenal atresia	Hypoplastic left heart
Skeletal system	Transposition
Talipes equinovarus	Persistent ductus arteriosus
Scoliosis	Other defects
Rib defects	Abnormal ears
Radial limb defect	Incomplete division of lobes of
Lower limb defect	lung
Polydactyly	Harelip
Abnormal fingers and toes	Cleft palate
Short sternum	Bilateral inguinal hernia
Flexion deformities of fingers	Hygromatous cysts in neck
	Fused adrenals
	Anophthalmia
	Coloboma of left eyelid

Reproduced with permission from David, Illingworth: J Med Genet 13:253, 1976.

and omphalocele. It is associated with these anomalies more frequently than is expected by chance.[18,57] However, other anomalies have also been reported. Table 6–1 illustrates the associated anomalies in the largest reported series in the literature. The central nervous system is the most frequently involved. Cardiovascular abnormalities have been found in 23 percent of newborn babies with congenital diaphragmatic hernias excluding eventration.[26] Ventricular septal defects and tetralogy of Fallot were the most common anomalies. Less frequent anomalies include coarctation of the aorta, ectopia cordis, atrial septal defects, absence of pericardium, and tricuspid atresia. Half of the infants with cardiac anomalies (5 of 11) had other extracardiac anomalies compared to those without cardiac disease (1 of 37, $p < 0.05$).

Congenital diaphragmatic hernia has been reported in association with chromosomal abnormalities. Hansen reported one trisomy 21, one trisomy 18, and one ring 4 in 75 newborns.[28] Harrison reported 2 cases (trisomies 18 and 13) in 20 patients with con-

genital diaphragmatic hernia.[33] Greenwood et al. found 2 cases of trisomy 21 in 48 patients.[26] David and Illingworth reported 3 cases (2 trisomy 18 and 1 trisomy 21) in 143 patients.[19] Boles and Anderson found 3 genetic anomalies (including 2 Down syndrome babies) in 58 infants.[9] Other reports have suggested an association between trisomy 21 and Morgagni congenital diaphragmatic hernia.[2,19] It is controversial whether eventration of the diaphragm is associated with a higher incidence of trisomy 18.[3,71]

Diagnosis

The diagnosis of congenital diaphragmatic hernia has been made in utero several times.[5,12,14,23,33,42,51] A definitive diagnosis can be made if abdominal organs are seen in the thoracic cavity. Visualization of fluid-filled bowel at the level of the four chamber view of the heart is diagnostic (Figs. 6–12, 6–13, 6–14). The ribs and the inferior margin of the scapula can be used as landmarks when trying to establish the intrathoracic location of viscera. The visualization of these organs in the chest is difficult in early pregnancy. In late pregnancy, they can be seen as fluid-filled cystic structures that may peristalte in the thoracic cavity.

We have found that the most sensitive sign of the presence of a congenital diaphragmatic hernia is a shift in the position of the heart within the chest. Polyhydramnios is common and thought to be secondary to bowel obstruction. However, this mechanism does not explain the presence of polyhydram-

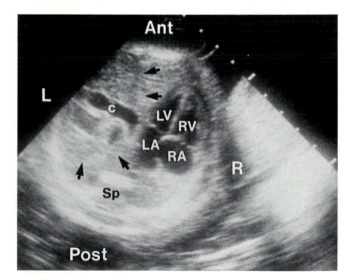

Figure 6–12. Transverse scan at the level of the heart in a fetus with diaphragmatic hernia. There is a striking mediastinal shift with deviation of the heart to the right. The left hemithorax is occupied by a complex mass (*arrows*) with cystic components (c). Sp, spine; LV, left ventricle; RV, right ventricle; LA, left atrium; RA, right atrium; Ant, anterior; Post, posterior; L, left; R, right.

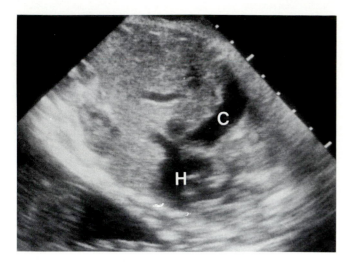

Figure 6–13. Longitudinal scan of the fetus shown in Figure 6–12. The diagnosis is suspected by the visualization of a cystic mass (C) at the level of the heart (H).

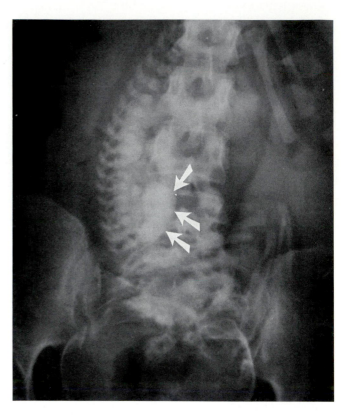

Figure 6–15. Amniogram of a fetus with a diaphragmatic hernia. The fetus has swallowed the contrast medium, which is visualized as dilated loops of bowel in the fetal chest (*arrows*).

nios in right hernias or left hernias in which intestinal transit is not impaired.

The diagnosis of right diaphragmatic hernia is extremely difficult because of the similar echogenicity of liver and lung. A helpful hint is the identification of the gallbladder, which is frequently herniated into the chest. The presence of a pleural effusion and ascites may also aid in the differentiation between lung and liver. The mechanism for fluid accumulation in serous cavities is thought to be related to an obstruction of venous return. We made the diagnosis of right diaphragmatic hernia in one patient with a

duodenal atresia by realizing that there was malrotation of the stomach (see Fig. 7.5).

Small congenital diaphragmatic hernias may not be detected in utero. Presumably, these would have a better prognosis. In cases of uncertainty, other diagnostic maneuvers, such as amniography (Fig. 6–15)[5,17] and computed tomography,[14,33] can be used. This would be helpful in the differential diagnosis of cystic lesions of the chest, such as cystic adenomatoid malformation of the lung and mediastinal cystic processes (neuroenteric cysts, bronchogenic cysts) (see Table 5.1). The presence of a normally placed stomach can help to distinguish these two conditions.

A diagnosis of diaphragmatic hernia mandates a careful examination of the fetal anatomy.

Prognosis

The prognosis of congenital diaphragmatic hernia is poor. Infants with congenital diaphragmatic hernia are at risk for antepartum and neonatal death.[36] In a retrospective review of such infants, 35 percent were stillbirths.[11] Associated anomalies are thought to be responsible for most antenatal deaths, and they were present in 90 percent of stillbirths. An earlier study noted that abnormalities severe enough to account

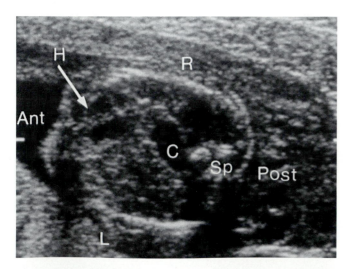

Figure 6–14. Diaphragmatic hernia in a 23-week-old fetus. Transverse scan of the chest shows deviation of the heart (H) and a cystic structure (C). Sp, spine; Ant, anterior; Post, posterior; L, left; R, right.

for death were most frequently located in the CNS (anencephalus, iniencephalus, Dandy-Walker malformation, Arnold-Chiari malformation).[11] The other frequent location of lethal anomalies is the cardiovascular system.[53] A significant number of infants die within the first few hours of life. In Butler's series, 35 percent of all neonatal deaths occurred 1 hour after birth.[11] The causes of immediate neonatal death are severe pulmonary insufficiency and associated congenital anomalies.[11,53] Of infants who survive the immediate neonatal period and go to surgery, the mortality rate varies between 29 percent[50] and 53 percent.[69] The following are prognostic factors.

Age in Hours at Time of Operation. Infants who clinically manifest respiratory failure immediately after birth have a poor prognosis. In fact, the survival rate is almost 100 percent in infants operated on 24 hours after birth,[15,50,63,73] but it drops to 38 to 64 percent in infants less than 24 hours old.[9,28,50,63,64,69,73] Unfortunately, most of the babies treated surgically are in the latter group.[53,63,64]

Blood Gas Data. Infants with acidosis, hypercapnia, and hypoxemia have a poor prognosis.[8,9,15,29,53,63,69] The predictive value of blood gas determinations does not seem to be purely dependent on the volume of lung parenchyma, since no correlation has been found between lung weight and blood gas data in dead infants.[59,63]

Chest X-ray Data. The presence of a pneumothorax, location of the stomach above the diaphragm, and volume of aerated ipsilateral and contralateral lungs have prognostic value.[69] On the other hand, the degree of mediastinal shift and the amount of visceral distention have not been found to be statistically different between surviving and nonsurviving groups.

Associated Anomalies. The presence of additional major malformations, excluding gut malrotation and patent ductus arteriosus, which are often part of the disease process, portends a poorer outcome.[28] In one series, the postsurgery mortality rate was significantly higher ($p < 0.02$) in infants with cardiac abnormalities (73 percent) than in those without cardiac disease (27 percent).[26] In another series, the death rate among infants with associated serious congenital anomalies was higher (70.6 percent) than the overall mortality rate (36 percent).[9]

After excluding infants with associated anomalies, fetuses with congenital diaphragmatic hernia do not seem to be at higher risk for preterm delivery and intrauterine growth retardation.[17,33]

Overall, the prognosis for infants with congenital diaphragmatic hernia diagnosed in utero is extremely poor. Harrison reported a mortality of 100 percent in nine consecutive patients.[33] We have made 10 prenatal diagnoses of diaphragmatic hernia and have had only 1 survivor, in whom diagnosis was made at 23 weeks of gestation. The poor prognosis for infants diagnosed in utero may reflect a selection bias, as smaller hernias may not be detectable with ultrasound.

Abnormally low lecithin:sphingomyelin (L:S) ratios have been reported in infants with congenital diaphragmatic hernia.[5,6,33,41] Such observation has been attributed to decreased surfactant production by a hypoplastic lung.[41] However, it has not been established whether a mature L:S ratio has prognostic value for infants diagnosed in utero.

One study provided information in long-term follow-up of 21 infants with congenital diaphragmatic hernia operated on within 24 hours of life.[9] Infants were followed for an average of 8 1/2 years, and they were found to be in good health, vigorous, active, and without evidence of growth failure. Although some infants had respiratory problems in the first 3 to 4 years of life (2 had pneumonia, 2 had recurrent upper respiratory infections, 1 was said to have "chronic asthma"), all complaints subsequently disappeared. Other authors have performed pulmonary function tests in infants with congenital diaphragmatic hernia and have found residual defects in ventilatory function[13] and impaired blood flow to the lung in the side of the hernia, but normal airway resistance and distribution of ventilation.[75] Interpretation of some long-term follow-up studies is difficult because they have included infants operated on at different ages.[13,60,75] In one study involving 30 infants, 3 had evidence of mental retardation that was attributed to hypoxia after birth, although no evidence was presented to support this contention.[60]

Obstetrical Management

Before viability the option of pregnancy termination should be offered to the parents. Karyotype determination and echocardiography should be performed in each infant in whom a diagnosis of diaphragmatic hernia is made. There are no data to justify delivery before fetal maturity or to alter the mode of delivery. Labor should occur in a tertiary center where a neonatologist and a pediatric surgeon are immediately available.

Diaphragmatic hernia is one of the conditions for which there is solid experimental basis for in utero surgery.[32,35,70] An animal model for this condition has been developed in the fetal lamb by inflating an intrathoracic balloon[27,34,37] or by producing a diaphragmatic defect surgically.[30,35,66] The ventilatory and hemodynamic changes observed in the lamb are similar to those seen in affected human fetuses.[27,34,37,66] Furthermore, intrauterine correction by deflation of the intrathoracic balloon[37] or by closure of the defect[30,35] has been associated with a favorable outcome. This procedure has been attempted in the human fetus at the time of this writing, with poor results.

REFERENCES

1. Andersen DH: Effect of diet during pregnancy upon the incidence of congenital hereditary diaphragmatic hernia in the rat. Am J Pathol 25:163, 1949.
2. Baran EM, Houston HE, Lynne HB, et al.: Foramen of Morgagni hernias in children. Surgery 62:1076, 1967.
3. Barash BA, Freedman L, Optiz JM: Anatomic studies in the 18-trisomy syndrome. Birth Defects 6:3, 1970.
4. Behrman RE, Vaughn VC: Nelson's Textbook of Pediatrics, 11th ed. Philadelphia, Saunders, 1983, pp 988–990.
5. Bell MJ, Ternberg JL: Antenatal diagnosis of diaphragmatic hernia. Pediatrics 60:738, 1977.
6. Berk C, Grundy M: "High-risk" lecithin/sphingomyelin ratios associated with neonatal diaphragmatic hernia. Case Reports. Br J Obstet Gynaecol 89:250, 1982.
7. Bloss RS, Aranda JV, Beardmore HE: Congenital diaphragmatic hernia: Pathophysiology and pharmacologic support. Surgery 89:518, 1981.
8. Boix-Ochoa J, Natal A, Canals J, et al.: The important influence of arterial blood gases on the prognosis of congenital diaphragmatic hernia. World J Surg 11:783, 1977.
9. Boles ET, Anderson G: Diaphragmatic hernia in the newborn: Mortality, complications, and long term follow up observations. In: Kiesewetter WB (ed). Long Term Follow Up in Congenital Anomalies. Pediatric Surgical Symposium, September 14–15, 1979, Pittsburgh, PA, pp 13–22.
10. Bracken MB, Berg A: Bendectin (Debendox) and congenital diaphragmatic hernia. Lancet 1:586, 1983.
11. Butler NR, Claireaux AE: Congenital diaphragmatic hernia as a cause of perinatal mortality. Lancet 1:659, 1962.
12. Campbell S, Pearce JM: The prenatal diagnosis of fetal structural anomalies by ultrasound. Clin Obstet Gynaecol 10:475, 1983.
13. Chatrath RR, El Shafie M, Jones RS: Fate of hypoplastic lung after repair of congenital diaphragmatic hernia. Arch Dis Child 46:633, 1971.
14. Chinn DH, Filly RA, Callen PW: Congenital diaphragmatic hernia diagnosed prenatally by ultrasound. Radiology 148:119, 1983.
15. Collins DL, Marks L, Edwards D: Management of infants with diaphragmatic hernia. West J Med 127:479, 1977.
16. Collins DL, Pomerance JJ, Travis KW, et al.: A new approach to congenital posterolateral diaphragmatic hernia. J Pediatr Surg 12:149, 1977.
17. Crane JP: Familial congenital diaphragmatic hernia: Prenatal diagnostic approach and analysis of twelve families. Clin Genet 16:244, 1979.
18. Czeizel A: Schisis association. Am J Med Genet 10:25, 1981.
19. David TJ, Illingworth CA: Diaphragmatic hernia in the south-west of England. J Med Genet 13:253, 1976.
20. Dibbins AW: Congenital diaphragmatic hernia, hypoplastic lung, and pulmonary vasoconstriction. Clin Perinatol 5:93, 1978.
21. Dibbins AW, Wiener ES: Mortality from neonatal diaphragmatic hernia. J Pediatr Surg 9:633, 1974.
22. Evans JNG, MacLachlan RF: Choanal atresia. J Laryngol 85:903, 1971.
23. Fleischer AC, Killam AP, Boehm FH, et al.: Hydrops fetalis: Sonographic evaluation and clinical implications. Radiology 141:163, 1981.
24. Geggel RL, Reid LM: The structural basis of PPHN. Clin Perinatol 2:525, 1984.
25. Gray SW, Skandalakis JE: The diaphragm. In: Embryology for Surgeons. The Embryological Basis for the Treatment of Congenital Defects. Philadelphia, Saunders, 1972, pp 359–385.
26. Greenwood RD, Rosenthal A, Nadas AS: Cardiovascular abnormalities associated with congenital diaphragmatic hernia. Pediatrics 57:92, 1976.
27. Haller JA, Signer RD, Golladay ES, et al.: Pulmonary and ductal hemodynamics in studies of simulated diaphragmatic hernia of fetal and newborn lambs. J Pediatr Surg 11:675, 1976.
28. Hansen J, James S, Burrington J, et al.: The decreasing incidence of pneumothorax and improving survival of infants with congenital diaphragmatic hernia. J Pediatr Surg 19:385, 1984.
29. Hardesty RL, Griffith BP, Debski RJ, et al.: Extracorporeal membrane oxygenation. Successful treatment of persistent fetal circulation following repair of congenital diaphragmatic hernia. J Thorac Cardiovasc Surg 81:556, 1981.
30. Hardy KJ, Auldist AW, Shulkes A: Congenital diaphragmatic hernia. Intrauterine repair in fetal sheep. Med J Aust 2:223, 1982.
31. Harrison MR, de Lorimier AA: Congenital diaphragmatic hernia. Surg Clin North Am 61:1023, 1981.
32. Harrison MR, Golbus MS, Filly RA: Management of the fetus with a correctable congenital defect. JAMA 246:774, 1981.
33. Harrison MR, Golbus MS, Filly RA: The Unborn Patient. Prenatal Diagnosis and Treatment. Orlando, FL, Grune & Stratton, 1984, pp 257–275.
34. Harrison MR, Jester JA, Ross NA: Correction of congenital diaphragmatic hernia in utero. I. The model: Intrathoracic balloon produces fatal pulmonary hypoplasia. Surgery 88:174, 1980.
35. Harrison MR, Ross NA, de Lorimier AA: Correction of congenital diaphragmatic hernia in utero. III. Development of a successful surgical technique using abdominoplasty to avoid compromise of umbilical blood flow. J Pediatr Surg 16:934, 1981.
36. Harrison MR, Bjordal RJ, Langmark F, et al.: Congen-

ital diaphragmatic hernia: The hidden mortality. J Pediatr Surg 13:227, 1978.

37. Harrison MR, Bressack MA, Churg AM, et al.: Correction of congenital diaphragmatic hernia in utero. II. Simulated correction permits fetal lung growth with survival at birth. Surgery 88:260, 1980.

38. Harrison MR, Golbus MS, Filly RA, et al.: Fetal surgical treatment. Pediatr Ann 11:896, 1982.

39. Haworth SG, Reid L: Persistent fetal circulation: Newly recognized structural features. J Pediatr 88:614, 1976.

40. Hill RM, et al.: Infants exposed in utero to antiepileptic drugs. Am J Dis Child 127:645, 1974.

41. Hisanaga S, Shimokawa H, Kashiwabara S, et al.: Unexpectedly low lecithin/sphingomyelin ratio associated with fetal diaphragmatic hernia. Am J Obstet Gynecol 149:905, 1984.

42. Hobbins JC, Grannum PAT, Berkowitz RL, et al.: Ultrasound in the diagnosis of congenital anomalies. Am J Obstet Gynecol 134:331, 1979.

43. Hobolth N: Drugs and congenital abnormalities. Lancet 2:1332, 1962.

44. Inselman LS, Mellins RB: Growth and development of the lung. J Pediatr 98:1, 1981.

45. Kucera J: Rate and type of congenital anomalies among offspring of diabetic women. J Reprod Med 7:73, 1971.

46. Kup J: Zwerchfelldefekt nach Abtreibungsversuch mit Chinin. Munch Med Wschr 27:2582, 1967.

47. Leck I, Record RG, McKeown T, et al.: The incidence of malformations in Birmingham, England, 1950–1959. Teratology 1:263, 1959.

48. Levin DL: Morphologic analysis of the pulmonary vascular bed in congenital left-sided diaphragmatic hernia. J Pediatr 92:805, 1978.

49. Lubinsky M, Severn C, Rapoport JM: Fryns syndrome: A new variable multiple congenital anomaly (MCA) syndrome. Am J Med Genet 14:461, 1983.

50. Marshall A, Sumner E: Improved prognosis in congenital diaphragmatic hernia: Experience of 62 cases over 2-year period. J Roy Soc Med 75:607, 1982.

51. Marwood RP, Davison OW: Antenatal diagnosis of diaphragmatic hernia. Case report. Br J Obstet Gynaecol 88:71, 1981.

52. Merten DF, Bowie JD, Kirks DR, et al.: Anteromedial diaphragmatic defects in infancy: Current approaches to diagnostic imaging. Radiology 142:361, 1982.

53. Mishalany HG, Nakada K, Wooley MW: Congenital diaphragmatic hernias. Eleven years' experience. Arch Surg 114:1118, 1979.

54. Moodie DS, Telander RL, Kleinberg F, et al.: Use of tolazoline in newborn infants with diaphragmatic hernia and severe cardiopulmonary disease. J Thorac Cardiovasc Surg 75:725, 1978.

55. Moore KL: The Developing Human. Clinically Oriented Embryology, 3d ed. Philadelphia, Saunders, 1982, pp 172–175.

56. Naeye RL, Shochat SJ, Whitman V, et al.: Unsuspected pulmonary vascular abnormalities associated with diaphragmatic hernia. Pediatrics 58:902, 1976.

57. Norio R, Kaariainen H, Rapola J, et al.: Familial congenital diaphragmatic defects: Aspects of etiology, prenatal diagnosis, and treatment. Am J Med Genet 17:471, 1984.

58. Pollack LD, Hall JG: Posterolateral (Bochdalek's) diaphragmatic hernia in sisters. Am J Dis Child 133:1186, 1979.

59. Raphaely RC, Downes JJ Jr: Congenital diaphragmatic hernia: Prediction of survival. J Pediatr Surg 8:815, 1973.

60. Reid IS, Hutcherson RJ: Long-term follow-up of patients with congenital diaphragmatic hernia. J Pediatr Surg 11:939, 1976.

61. Reid L: The lung: Its growth and remodeling in health and disease. AJR 129:777, 1977.

62. Rudolph AM: Fetal and neonatal pulmonary circulation. Annu Rev Physiol 41:383, 1979.

63. Ruff SJ, Campbell JR, Harrison MW, et al.: Pediatric diaphragmatic hernias. An 11-year experience. Am J Surg 139:642, 1980.

64. Shochat SJ, Naeye RL, Ford WDA, et al.: Congenital diaphragmatic hernia. New concept in management. Ann Surg 190:332, 1979.

65. Snell RS: Clinical Embryology for Medical Students, 3d ed. Boston, Little, Brown, 1983, pp 177–194.

66. Starret RW, de Lorimer AA: Congenital diaphragmatic hernia in lambs: Hemodynamic and ventilatory changes with breathing. J Pediatric Surg 10:575, 1975.

67. Stauffer UG, Rickham PP: Congenital diaphragmatic hernia and eventration of the diaphragm. In: Rickham PP, Lister JP, Irving IM (eds): Neonatal Surgery, 2d ed. London, Butterworths, 1978, pp 163–178.

68. Thorburn MJ, Wright ES, Miller CG, et al.: Exomphalos-macro-glossia-gigantism syndrome in Jamaican infants. Am J Dis Child 119:316, 1970.

69. Touloukian RJ, Markowitz RI: A preoperative x-ray scoring system for risk assessment of newborns with congenital diaphragmatic hernia. J Pediatr Surg 19:252, 1984

70. Turley K, Vlahakes GJ, Harrison MR, et al.: Intrauterine cardiothoracic surgery: The fetal lamb model. Presented at the Eighteenth Annual Meeting of the Society of Thoracic Surgeons, January 11–13, 1982.

71. Warkany J: Congenital Malformations. Notes and Comments. Chicago, Year Book, 1971, pp 10, 303–310, 751–757.

72. Warkany J, Roth CB: Congenital malformations induced in rats by maternal vitamin A deficiency. J Nutr 35:1, 1948.

73. Wiener ES: Congenital posterolateral diaphragmatic hernia: New dimensions in management. Surgery 92:670, 1982.

74. Williams R: Congenital diaphragmatic hernia: A review. Heart Lung 11:532, 1982.

75. Wohl MEB, Griscom NT, Strieder DJ, et al: The lung following repair of congenital diaphragmatic hernia. J Pediatr 90:405, 1977.

Omphalocele

Synonym
Exomphalos.

Definition
Omphalocele is a ventral wall defect characterized by herniation of the intraabdominal contents into the base of the umbilical cord, with a covering amnioperitoneal membrane (Fig. 6–16).

Pentalogy of Cantrell is a term used to describe the association of five anomalies: (1) midline supraumbilical abdominal defect, (2) defect of the lower sternum, (3) deficiency of the diaphragmatic pericardium, (4) deficiency of the anterior diaphragm, and (5) intracardiac abnormality.[27]

The Beckwith-Wiedemann syndrome is characterized by the association of macroglossia, visceromegaly, and omphalocele.

Incidence
Omphalocele is estimated to occur in 1 in 5800 to 1 in 5130 live births.[2,15] Beckwith-Wiedemann syndrome has an incidence of 1 in 13,700 live births.[3] Pentalogy of Cantrell is a very rare disorder.

Etiology
Most cases of omphalocele are sporadic. Often the condition is associated with chromosomal aberrations, such as trisomies 13 and 18.

The familial occurrence of this anomaly with a sex-linked or autosomal pattern of inheritance has been reported.[10,20,23] The recurrence risk for isolated omphalocele cases appears to be less than 1 percent. However, when an omphalocele is identified in association with trisomies, a careful evaluation of the karyotype should exclude the possibility of a balanced translocation, which increases the recurrence risk.

Although most cases of Beckwith-Wiedemann syndrome are sporadic, familial occurrence has been described, suggesting autosomal dominant, recessive, sex-linked, and polygenic patterns.[3,20] Cantrell's pentalogy is also a sporadic condition.

Embryology
The development of the anterior abdominal wall depends on the fusion of four ectomesodermic folds (cephalic, caudal, and two laterals). Failure of the cephalic fold to fuse with the other folds usually results in the association of omphalocele with ectopia cordis and sternal and diaphragmatic defects. Failure of the lateral folds to meet in the midline (between the 3d and 4th weeks) leads to the formation of an isolated omphalocele. Defective fusion of the caudal fold results in cloacal exstrophy of the bladder.

Pathology
The defect is located in the midline, and the protrusion of the intraabdominal contents occurs through the base of the umbilical cord. Bowel loops, stomach, and liver are the most frequently herniated organs and are covered by a membrane made up of two layers: internally the peritoneum and externally the amnion. The umbilical cord inserts into the sac. The size of these defects is variable, ranging from a very small hernia containing a few bowel loops to a very large mass containing most of the visceral organs.

With pentalogy of Cantrell, the diaphragmatic defect is embryologically different from the hernia of Morgagni. The lesion is located in the anterior portion of the diaphragm and is rarely associated with

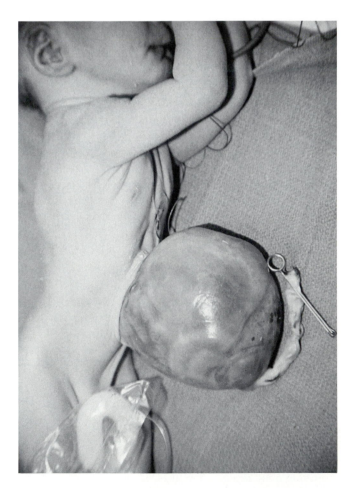

Figure 6–16. Typical omphalocele in a newborn. The lesion occurs in the midline and is covered by a membrane. *(Courtesy of Dr. Robert Touloukian.)*

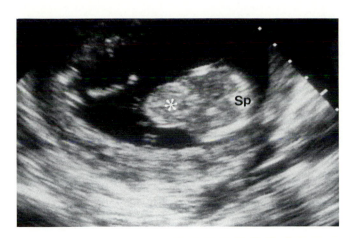

Figure 6–17. Prenatal diagnosis of an omphalocele at 15 weeks of gestation. Transverse scan of the abdomen at the level of the umbilicus demonstrating the lesion (∗) Sp, spine.

herniation of intraabdominal organs into the thoracic cavity, although bowel loop protrusion inside the pericardial sac has been documented.[27] The most frequent cardiac abnormalities are atrioventricular septal defects, ventricular septal defects, and tetralogy of Fallot. In a review of 36 patients, the incidence of these three cardiac defects was 50 percent, 18 percent, and 11 percent, respectively.[27]

The Beckwith-Wiedemann syndrome is a constellation of clinical abnormalities, including combinations of omphalocele, macroglossia, natal or postnatal gigantism, nephromegaly, facial flame nevus, hepatomegaly, ear lobe abnormalities, hemihypertrophy, and neonatal polycythemia. The most prominent features are exomphalos (E), macroglossia (M), and gigantism (G); hence, the condition is also known as "EMG syndrome."[25] Neonatal hypoglycemia is found in 50 percent of patients. Cardiac abnormalities occurred in 12 of 13 patients reported by Greenwood et al.[7] Seven of the 12 patients (58 percent) had structural abnormalities, and 5 had isolated cardiomegaly. No specific pattern of congenital heart disease has been described. Ten percent of infants with Beckwith-Wiedemann syndrome may develop malignant tumors, including nephroblastoma, hepatoblastoma, and adrenal tumor.[26] In a review of cases of omphalocele, Irving estimated that 11.7 percent of all cases were associated with the Beckwith-Wiedemann syndrome.[12]∗ The syndrome has no obligatory anomalies and has been diagnosed in the absence of macroglossia or omphalocele.[3]

Associated Anomalies

The frequency of trisomies in infants with omphalocele varies between 35 and 58 percent.[4,9,16,17,19] Chromosomal aberrations include trisomy 13 and 18. Car-

diac anomalies (ventricular and atrial septal defects, tetralogy of Fallot) are found in up to 47 percent of patients,[4,6,19] genitourinary abnormalities in up to 40 percent,[19,23] and neural tube defects in up to 39 percent.[2,16] Gastrointestinal anomalies, either primary or secondary (e.g., bowel obstruction), are a frequent finding. Intrauterine growth retardation has been reported in 20 percent of patients.[2]

Diagnosis

The diagnosis of omphalocele relies on the demonstration of a mass adjacent to the anterior ventral wall representing the herniated visceral organs (Figs. 6–17 through 6–20). Differential diagnosis is mainly with gastroschisis.[21] Omphaloceles are located in the midline. The umbilical cord enters into the hernia, and the herniated organs are covered by a membrane that is continuous with the umbilical cord. Gastroschisis is a lateral defect, devoid of a surrounding membrane and separated from the umbilical cord insertion. These signs permit an accurate differential diagnosis in almost all patients. A possible exception may be those cases of omphalocele in which rupture of the amnioperitoneal sac occurs in utero, an exceedingly rare complication.[8] Pentalogy of Cantrell can be suspected in the presence of ectopia cordis.[24] In many cases, the defect in the diaphragm at the level of the pericardium is small and cannot be demonstrated by prenatal sonography. Suspicion should arise when the apex of the heart deviates inferiorly (under nor-

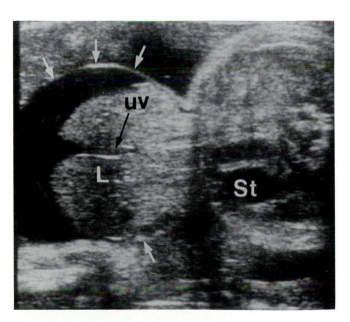

Figure 6–18. A large omphalocele in a third trimester fetus. Transverse scan of the abdomen at the level of the umbilicus. The amniotic peritoneal membrane is seen covering the lesion (*white arrows*). The liver (L) is herniated into the sac. The umbilical vein (uv) is visible. St, stomach.

∗ Our review of the literature indicates that this syndrome accounts for 4 percent of all cases of omphalocele.

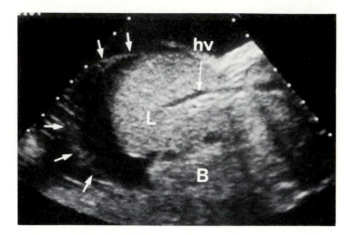

Figure 6–19. Omphalocele in a third trimester fetus. The herniated organs are the liver (L) and bowel (B). The amniotic peritoneal membrane is seen (*arrows*). hv, hepatic vein.

mal circumstances, the heart is horizontal within the thoracic cavity) and bulges under the skin of the chest due to the sternal defect.

A specific prenatal diagnosis of Beckwith-Wiedemann syndrome has not been reported. The condition should be suspected when an omphalocele is associated with visceromegaly and macroglossia. Nomograms are available for assessing the size of kidneys, heart, and spleen. However, the value of these measurements in the diagnosis of Beckwith-Wiedemann syndrome has not been tested. This condition has been prenatally visualized twice,[14,28] but a specific diagnosis of Beckwith-Wiedemann syndrome was not made before birth. Polyhydramnios is a frequent finding and is probably responsible for the increased incidence of premature labors.

Ventral wall defects may result in an elevation of the maternal serum alpha-fetoprotein (MSAFP). It has been reported that MSAFP screening has a sensitivity of 52 percent in the detection of anterior wall defects and 42 percent for omphaloceles.[16] Therefore, the evaluation of the anterior abdominal wall is an important part of the sonographic assessment of pregnancies with elevated AFP. Since an increased incidence of neural tube defects has been found in infants with omphalocele, identification of the latter lesion should not result in overlooking the fetal spine.

Prognosis

A small defect can be repaired in a one-stage operation. Larger defects usually require a two-stage operation, generally using a Silastic or Teflon membrane to cover and reduce the herniation of the intraabdominal organs.[22]

Prognosis of omphalocele depends largely on the presence of associated anomalies. Losses are mainly due to cardiac abnormalities, chromosomal aberra-

tions, and prematurity. Kirk and Wah have reported 38 cases of omphaloceles, with a mortality rate of 29 percent.[13] Of the 11 deaths, 5 occurred in infants with multiple congenital anomalies and 3 in infants with associated congenital heart disease. Carpenter et al. reported an overall mortality rate of 40 percent.[2] Among the infants who died, two had trisomies, two had other severe anomalies (esophageal atresia, tetralogy of Fallot, pulmonary hypoplasia), and three had pentalogy of Cantrell.

Cephalic fold defects carry a worse prognosis than do the lateral and caudal fold defects. In the series by Carpenter et al., the mortality rate among cephalic fold defects was 78 percent versus 19 percent in the lateral fold defects.[2] In a review of the literature by Toyama, the survival rate among individuals with pentalogy of Cantrell was only 20 percent.[27] Since this report is based on data collected before 1970, it is quite likely that the outcome for infants with this condition has improved due to advances in cardiothoracic surgery.

Infants with Beckwith-Wiedemann syndrome have respiratory and feeding difficulties because of the large tongue. The oral cavity may grow with time, and the tongue eventually fits inside the mouth. In some patients, glossectomy has been required. The excessive rate of growth often slows down after the first few years.[27] Neonatal hypoglycemia is a serious complication, which has been implicated in the mild to moderate mental deficiency noted in some of these infants. Steroids have been used to control hypoglycemia. Ten percent of these infants develop neoplasms. In a review of 17 cases of Beckwith-

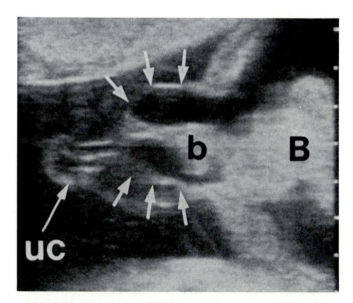

Figure 6–20. Small omphalocele in a fetus with hydrops. The insertion of the umbilical cord (uc) in the abdomen is interrupted by a lesion that contains small bowel (b). The amniotic peritoneal membrane is outlined by the short arrows. Ascites is present in the peritoneal cavity. B, intraabdominal bowel loops.

Wiedemann syndrome associated with tumors, a 47 percent mortality rate was reported.[26]

Obstetrical Management

Identification of a fetal omphalocele should prompt a careful search for associated anomalies. Fetal karyotyping[18] and echocardiography are indicated. Diagnosis before viability may allow parents to opt for pregnancy termination. In continuing pregnancies and in those cases diagnosed after viability, serial ultrasound monitoring is indicated to look for signs of intestinal obstruction and intrauterine growth retardation. In recent years, the optimal mode of delivery of fetuses with omphalocele has been a subject of debate. Some authors have suggested that delivery of these infants should be performed by cesarean section to avoid birth injury with rupture of the amnioperitoneal sac. However, in two large retrospective and uncontrolled series, no benefits of cesarean section versus vaginal delivery could be documented.[2,13]

The major limitation of these studies is their design. The incidence of complications in infants delivered vaginally seems to be small. However, we believe that there is a subgroup of patients who may benefit from a cesarean section. An example of this is the large omphalocele with external protrusion of a large part of the liver.[1] A careful search for associated anomalies is indicated also in those cases diagnosed in the third trimester. Omphalocele may be accompanied by anomalies incompatible with life (e.g., trisomies 13 and 18), and the recognition of such disorders could alter obstetrical management.

REFERENCES

1. Bartolucci L: Discussion in Kirk EP, Wah RM: Obstetric management of the fetus with omphalocele or gastroschisis: A review and report of one hundred twelve cases. Am J Obstet Gynecol 146:512, 1983.
2. Carpenter MW, Curci MR, Dibbins AW, et al.: Perinatal management of ventral wall defects. Obstet Gynecol 64:646, 1984.
3. Cohen MM, Ulstrom RA: Beckwith-Wiedemann syndrome. In: Bergsma D (ed): Birth Defects Compendium, 2d ed. New York, Alan R. Liss, 1979, pp 140–141.
4. Crawford DC, Chapman MG, Allan LD: Echocardiography in the investigation of anterior abdominal wall defects in the fetus. Br J Obstet Gynecol 92:1034, 1985.
5. Gosden C, Brock DJH: Prenatal diagnosis of extrophy of the cloaca. Am J Med Genet 8:95, 1981.
6. Greenwood RD, Rosenthal A, Nadas AS: Cardiovascular malformations associated with omphalocele. J Pediatr 85:818, 1974.
7. Greenwood RD, Sommer A, Rosenthal A, et al.: Cardiovascular abnormalities in the Beckwith-Wiedemann syndrome. Am J Dis Child 131:293, 1977.
8. Harrison MR, Golbus MS, Filly RA: Management of the fetus with an abdominal wall defect. In: The Unborn Patient. Prenatal Diagnosis and Treatment. Orlando, FL, Grune & Stratton, 1984, pp 217–234.
9. Hauge M, Bugge M, Nielsen J: Early prenatal diagnosis of omphalocele constitutes indication for amniocentesis. Lancet 2:507, 1983.
10. Havalad S, Noblett H, Speidel BD: Familial occurrence of omphalocele, suggesting sex-linked inheritance. Arch Dis Child 54:142, 1979.
11. Hoyme HE, Jones MC, Jones KL: Gastroschisis: Abdominal wall disruption secondary to early gestational interruption of the omphalomesenteric artery. Sem Perinatol 7:294, 1983.
12. Irving I: Exomphalos with macroglossia: A study of 11 cases. J Pediatr Surg 2:499, 1967.
13. Kirk EP, Wah RM: Obstetric management of the fetus with omphalocele or gastroschisis: A review and report of one hundred twelve cases. Am J Obstet Gynecol 146:512, 1983.
14. Koontz WL, Shaw LA, Lavery JP: Antenatal sonographic appearance of Beckwith-Wiedemann syndrome. J Clin Ultrasound 14:57, 1986.
15. Lindham S: Omphalocele and gastroschisis in Sweden 1965–1976. Acta Paediatr Scand 70:55, 1981.
16. Mann L, Ferguson-Smith MA, Desai M, et al.: Prenatal assessment of anterior abdominal wall defects and their prognosis. Prenat Diagn 4:427, 1984.
17. Mayer T, Black R, Matlak ME, et al.: Gastroschisis and omphalocele. An eight-year review. Ann Surg 192:783, 1980.
18. Nicolaides KH, Rodeck CH, Gosden CM: Rapid karyotyping in non-lethal fetal malformations. Lancet 1:283, 1986.
19. Nivelon-Chevallier A, Mavel A, Michiels R, et al.: Familial Beckwith-Wiedemann syndrome: Prenatal echography diagnosis and histologic confirmation. J Genet Hum 5:397, 1983.
20. Osuna A, Lindham S: Four cases of omphalocele in two generations of the same family. Clin Genet 9:354, 1976.
21. Redford DHA, McNay MB, Whittle MJ: Gastroschisis and exomphalos: Precise diagnosis by midpregnancy ultrasound. Br J Obstet Gynaecol 92:54, 1985.
22. Rickham PP: Exomphalos and gastroschisis. In: Rickham PP, et al. (eds): Neonatal Surgery. New York, Appleton-Century-Crofts, 1969, p 254.
23. Rott HD, Truckenbrodt H: Familial occurrence of omphalocele. Hum Genet 24:259, 1974.
24. Seeds JW, Cefalo RC, Lies SC, et al.: Early prenatal sonographic appearance of rare thoraco-abdominal eventration. Prenat Diagn 4:437, 1984.
25. Smith DW: Recognizable Patterns of Human Malformations. Genetic, Embryologic and Clinical Aspects, 3d ed. Philadelphia, Saunders, 1982, p 130.
26. Sotelo-Avila C, Gooch M: Neoplasms associated with the Beckwith-Wiedemann syndrome. Perspect Pediatr Pathol 3:255, 1977
27. Toyama WM: Combined congenital defects of the anterior abdominal wall, sternum, diaphragm, pericardium and heart: A case report and review of the syndrome. Pediatrics 50:778, 1972.
28. Weinstein L, Anderson C: In utero diagnosis of Beckwith-Wiedemann syndrome by ultrasound. Radiology 134:474, 1980.

Gastroschisis

Definition
Gastroschisis is a paraumbilical defect of the anterior abdominal wall associated with evisceration of abdominal organs.

Incidence
The incidence of gastroschisis ranges from 1:10,000 to 1:15,000 live births.[1,2,8]

Etiology
Most cases are sporadic. Familial occurrence has been documented in five families.[1,9,10,13,15] The findings in two families indicate the possibility of an autosomal dominant inheritance, with variable expressivity.

Embryology and Pathogenesis
Gastroschisis is a defect resulting from vascular compromise of either the umbilical vein or the omphalomesenteric artery.[5,6]

Human embryos initially bear both left and right umbilical veins. Involution of the right umbilical vein occurs between the 28th and the 32d day after conception. Premature involution may lead to ischemia and to the resultant mesodermal and ectodermal defects.

The omphalomesenteric arteries (OMAs) branch from the primitive dorsal aorta and extend to the right along the omphalomesenteric duct toward the yolk sac. The left OMA involutes, whereas the right one is transformed into the superior mesenteric artery. The terminal portion extends into the extraembryonic coelom, which is now located in the body stalk. Disruption of the distal segment could result in right-sided periumbilical ischemia and the paramedian defect characteristic of gastroschisis. Ischemic injury to the territory of the superior mesenteric artery may account for the high incidence of jejunal atresia found in association with gastroschisis.[5,6,11]

Pathology
Gastroschisis is characterized by a full-thickness defect of the abdominal wall, usually located to the right of the umbilical cord, which has a normal insertion. The defect in the abdominal wall is generally quite small (3 to 5 cm). The herniated organs include mainly bowel loops covered by an inflammatory exudate possibly resulting from chemical irritation by exposure to amniotic fluid.[3] They appear edematous and are not protected by a membrane. Hepatic herniation is less frequent with gastroschisis than with omphaloceles. Meconium is frequently found in the amniotic fluid of these fetuses. Its presence probably reflects intestinal irritation.[2,14] At birth, infants have low serum albumin and total protein levels, which probably indicate intestinal chronic sclerosing peritonitis.

Associated Anomalies
In contrast to omphalocele, gastroschisis is not associated with an increased incidence of other anomalies. However, in 25 percent of patients, gastrointestinal problems secondary to the vascular impairment and adhesions are found, including bowel malrotation, atresia, and stenosis.[3] Intrauterine growth retardation has been reported in up to 77 percent of infants.[2]

Diagnosis
The diagnosis of gastroschisis relies on the demonstration of a mass adjacent to the anterior ventral wall representing the herniated visceral organs. Differential diagnosis from omphalocele can be made in almost all cases because, in gastroschisis, (1) the defect is usually located in the right paraumbilical area, (2) the umbilical cord is normally connected to the abdominal wall, and (3) the herniated organs are not covered by a membrane but float freely in the amniotic cavity (Figs. 6–21, 6–22). An omphalocele is a central defect surrounded by a membrane on which the umbilical cord is inserted.[12] A possible exception may be those cases of omphalocele in which rupture of the amnioperitoneal sac occurs in utero, an exceed-

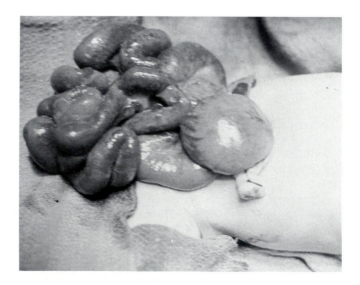

Figure 6–21. Newborn with gastroschisis. There is no covering membrane, and the defect is on the right paraumbilical area. *(Courtesy of Dr. Robert Touloukian.)*

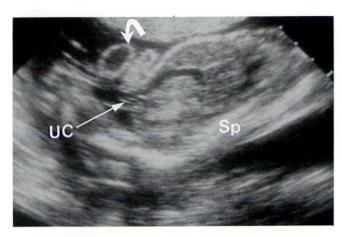

Figure 6–22. Sagittal scan of a 20-week fetus with a gastroschisis. Bowel is seen floating in the amniotic cavity (*curved arrow*). The normal insertion on the umbilical vessels is demonstrated. UC, umbilical cord inserting into the anterior abdominal wall; Sp, spine.

ingly rare complication.[4] Polyhydramnios is a frequent finding, and it is probably related to impaired gastrointestinal transit.

Ventral wall defects may result in elevation of the MSAFP. It has been reported that MSAFP screening will identify 77 percent of these fetuses.[10] Therefore, examination of the anterior abdominal wall is an important part of the sonographic evaluation of pregnancies with elevated AFP.

Prognosis

In three different series, the mortality rate ranged from 7.6 percent to 28 percent.[2,7,14] Death was caused by prematurity, sepsis, and intraoperative complications. In one series, herniation of the liver was associated with a higher mortality rate (50 percent versus 7 percent).[7]

Obstetrical Management

The critical issue is the differential diagnosis from an omphalocele, since this defect is associated with a higher incidence of associated anomalies and carries a worse prognosis. In the past, the consensus was that fetal karyotyping was not indicated in gastroschisis. We have recently seen two cases with karyotype abnormalities. When the diagnosis is made before viability, the parents may opt for termination of pregnancy. In continuing pregnancies and in those cases diagnosed in the third trimester, serial ultrasound examinations are recommended to detect intrauterine growth retardation and early signs of bowel obstruction. Polyhydramnios is a frequent finding and may contribute to the onset of premature labor. In this situation, tocolytic agents and amniotic fluid drainage are indicated to prolong the gestation.

In recent years, the optimal mode of delivery of fetuses with ventral wall defects has been a subject of debate. Some authors have suggested that delivery of these infants should be performed by cesarean section to avoid birth injury to the herniated visceral organs. However, in two large series, no benefits of cesarean section versus vaginal delivery could be documented.[2,7] The major limitation with such studies is their retrospective and uncontrolled design. The incidence of complications in infants delivered vaginally seems to be small. Delivery in a tertiary care center is recommended.

REFERENCES

1. Baird PA, MacDonald EC: An epidemiologic study of congenital malformations of the anterior abdominal wall in more than half a million consecutive live births. Am J Hum Genet 33:470, 1981.
2. Carpenter MW, Curci MR, Dibbins AW, et al.: Perinatal management of ventral wall defects. Obstet Gynecol 64:646, 1984.
3. Grybowski J, Walker WA: Gastrointestinal problems in the infant. Philadelphia, Saunders, 1983, pp 284–287.
4. Harrison MR, Golbus MS, Filly RA: Management of the fetus with an abdominal wall defect. In: The Unborn Patient. Prenatal Diagnosis and Treatment. Orlando, FL, Grune & Stratton, 1984, pp 217–234.
5. Hoyme HE, Higginbotton MC, Jones KL: The vascular pathogenesis of gastroschisis: Intrauterine interruption of the omphalomesenteric artery. J Pediatr 98:228, 1981.
6. Hoyme HE, Jones MC, Jones KL: Gastroschisis: Abdominal wall disruption secondary to early gestational interruption of the omphalomesenteric artery. Semin Perinat 7:294, 1983.
7. Kirk EP, Wah RM: Obstetric management of the fetus with omphalocele or gastroschisis: A review and report of one hundred twelve cases. Am J Obstet Gynecol 146:512, 1983.
8. Lindham S: Omphalocele and gastroschisis in Sweden 1965–1976. Acta Paediatr Scand 70:55, 1981.
9. Lowry RB, Baird PA: Familial gastroschisis and omphalocele. Am J Hum Gen 34:517, 1982.
10. Mann L, Ferguson-Smith MA, Desai M, et al.: Prenatal assessment of anterior abdominal wall defects and their prognosis. Prenat Diagn 4:427, 1984.
11. Moore TC: Gastroschisis and omphalocele: Clinical differences. Surgery 82: 561, 1977.
12. Redford DHA, McNay MB, Whittle MJ: Gastroschisis and exomphalos: Precise diagnosis by midpregnancy ultrasound. Br J Obstet Gynaecol 92:54, 1985.
13. Salinas CF, Bartoshesky L, Othersen HB, et al.: Familial occurrence of gastroschisis. Am J Dis Child 133:514, 1979.
14. Seashore JH: Congenital abdominal wall defects. Clin Perinatol 5:61, 1978.
15. Ventruto V, Stabile M, Lonardo F, et al.: Gastroschisis in two sibs with abdominal hernia in maternal grandfather and great-grandfather. Am J Med Genet 21:405, 1985.

Body Stalk Anomaly

Definition
This is a severe abdominal wall defect due to failure of formation of the body stalk and characterized by absence of the umbilicus and umbilical cord.

Incidence
The incidence of body stalk anomaly is 1 in 14,273 births.[2]

Embryology
During the third week of embryonic life the flat trilaminar embryo is transformed into a cylindrical fetus by a parallel set of contiguous body folds: cephalic, lateral, and caudal. Folding separates the intraembryonic coelom (peritoneal cavity) from the extraembryonic coelom (chorionic cavity). The amnion then fuses with the chorion peripherally and forms the covering of the umbilical cord centrally. Body stalk anomaly results from severe maldevelopment of cephalic, caudal, and lateral embryonic body folds. The failure of complete extraembryonic coelom obliteration accounts for the absence of umbilical cord formation and the wide-based insertion of the amnioperitoneal membrane onto the placental chorionic plate. The intraabdominal contents persist in the extraembryonic coelom. Fusion of the amnion and chorion takes place only at the margin of the placenta.

Pathology
The abdominal organs lie in a sac outside the abdominal cavity (Fig. 6–23). This sac is covered by amnion and placenta and is attached directly to the placenta.

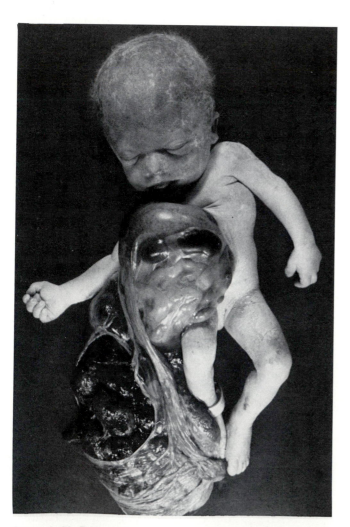

Figure 6–23. Body stalk anomaly. The placenta is attached to the herniated viscera without an intervening umbilical cord.

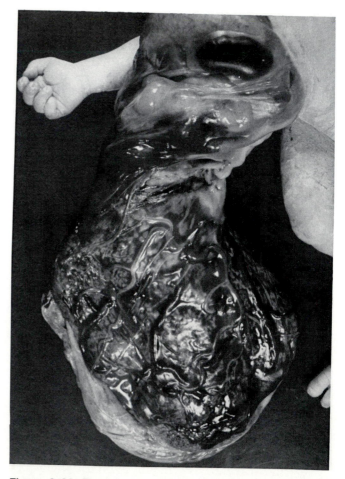

Figure 6–24. The umbilical vessels run along the wall of the sac.

The umbilical vessels are short and run along the sac walls (Fig. 6–24). The absence of the umbilical cord results in the fetus lying directly against the placenta and the uterine wall. This may lead to malposition and skeletal deformities, including kyphosis and scoliosis (Fig. 6–25).

Etiology

The disorder is sporadic in most cases, but concordance for this anomaly has been noted in twins.[2]

Diagnosis

This diagnosis should be suspected when the fetus is attached to the placenta and uterine wall and a large defect of the anterior abdominal wall allows protrusion of the viscera (Fig. 6–26). Prenatal diagnosis of this condition has been reported using MSAFP and ultrasound.[1,2]

Associated Anomalies

Anomalies, including neural tube defects, intestinal atresias, genitourinary and skeletal defects, anoma-

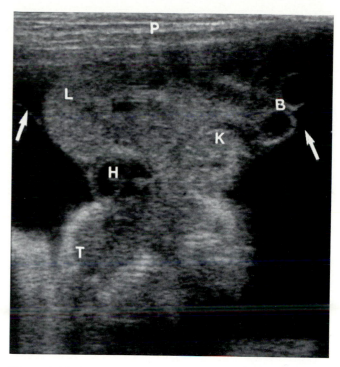

Figure 6–26. Sonogram of the fetus shown in Figures 6–24 and 6–25. Note that the viscera is herniated and in proximity with the placenta. The condition was suspected because the infant was constantly apposed to one uterine wall. L, liver; K, kidney; B, bowel loops; H, heart; T, thorax; P, placenta. *(Reproduced with permission from Lockwood et al.: Am J Obstet Gynecol 155:1049, 1986.)*

lies of the chest wall, pericardium, heart, liver, and lungs, are nearly always present. One umbilical artery is usually absent.[3]

Prognosis

Potter and Craig[3] and Mann et al.[2] have stated that this condition is uniformly fatal.[2,3]

Obstetrical Management

The option of pregnancy termination for this uniformly lethal condition could be offered to the parents anytime the diagnosis is made.

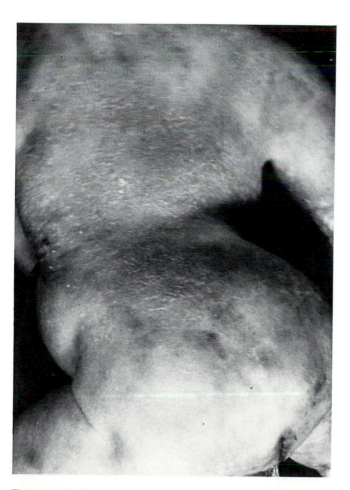

Figure 6–25. Severe scoliosis in a fetus with body stalk anomaly.

REFERENCES

1. Lockwood CJ, Scioscia AL, Hobbins JC: Congenital absence of the umbilical cord resulting from maldevelopment of embryonic body folding. Am J Obstet Gynecol 155:1049, 1986.
2. Mann L, Ferguson-Smith MA, Desai M, et al.: Prenatal assessment of anterior abdominal wall defects and their prognosis. Prenat Diagn 4:427, 1984.
3. Potter EL, Craig JM: Pathology of the Fetus and the Infant, 3d ed. Chicago, Year Book, 1975, p 388.

Bladder Exstrophy and Cloacal Exstrophy

Definition
Exstrophic anomalies are a group of disorders derived by a maldevelopment of the caudal fold of the anterior abdominal wall. In bladder exstrophy, the anterior wall of the bladder is absent, and the posterior wall of this organ is exposed. Cloacal exstrophy is a more complex anomaly in which there is involvement of both the urinary and intestinal tracts caused by a defect in the formation of the urorectal septum.

Incidence
Exstrophy of the bladder occurs in 1:30,000 deliveries, with a male to female ratio of 2.3:1.[5] Exstrophy of the cloaca has an incidence of 1:200,000 live births without a sex preponderance.[2,11]

Etiology
Most cases of bladder exstrophy are sporadic. Familial cases have been reported, and the risk of recurrence in a given family is 1 percent.[4] The risk of having an affected offspring if one parent has bladder exstrophy is 1 in 70 live births, which is 500 times greater than the risk of the general population.[10] Presumably, cloacal exstrophy is also a sporadic disorder, although affected individuals have not reproduced.

Embryology
The cloaca is a blind pouch that receives the midgut and the allantoic duct. The anterior wall of the cloaca is formed by the cloacal membrane, which extends from the two lateral mesodermal ridges to the body stalk (the primordium of the umbilical cord). By the 6th week of conception, the cloaca is divided by a proliferating mesodermal ridge (the urorectal septum) into a urogenital sinus anteriorly and a hindgut posteriorly. The urorectal septum divides the cloacal membrane in an anterior portion, or urogenital membrane, and a posterior one, or anal membrane (Fig. 6–27).

Normally, the two mesodermal ridges fuse in the midline to form the genital tubercle, and the cloacal membrane retracts downward toward the perineum. The lower portion of the anterior abdominal wall is reinforced by the tissues derived from the mesodermal ridges (Fig. 6–28A). If the cloacal membrane does not retract normally, the two mesodermal ridges fuse inferiorly, and the cloacal membrane becomes the anterior wall of the bladder. By the 9th week, the cloacal membrane disappears and the posterior wall of the bladder is exposed, giving rise to bladder exstrophy (Figs. 6–28B, 6–29). If the membranes disappear before the urorectal septum divides the primitive cloaca, both bladder and rectum will be exposed, leading to cloacal exstrophy (Fig. 6–30).

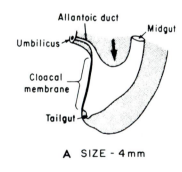

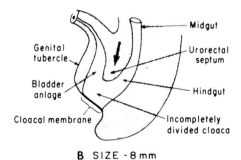

A SIZE - 4 mm

B SIZE - 8 mm

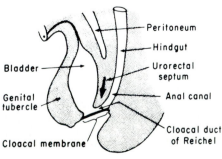

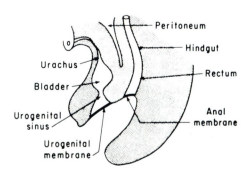

Figure 6–27. A–D. Developmental changes of the cloaca and cloacal membrane in the 4 to 16 mm embryo. Arrows show the direction of growth of the urorectal septum. *(Reproduced with permission from Muecke: In Campbell's Urology. Philadelphia, Saunders, 1986, pp 1856–1880.)*

C SIZE - 12 mm

D SIZE - 16 mm

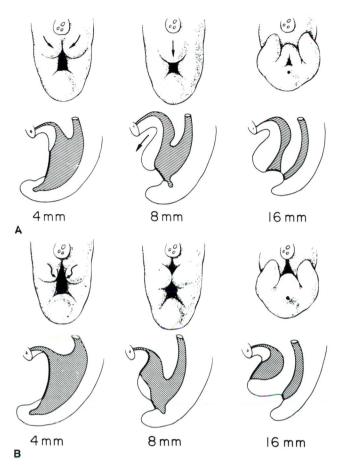

A

B

Figure 6–28. Schematic view of regression of cloacal membrane and formation of the primitive phallus. **A.** Normal sequential events. **B.** Genesis of the exstrophy group of anomalies by a persistent cloacal membrane impeding mesodermal flow. The paired genital folds fuse inferiorly, carrying the thin cloacal membrane along the anterior surface of the enlarging phallus. A weak, membranous anterior body wall persists, leading to the eventual catastrophic event of exstrophy. *(Reproduced with permission from Muecke: In Campbell's Urology. Philadelphia, Saunders, 1986, pp 1856–1880.)*

Pathology

In bladder exstrophy, there are protrusion of the posterior vesical wall, separation of pubic bones, low set umbilicus, incomplete descent of the testes, short penis pointing upward and epispadias in males, and cleft clitoris in females (Fig. 6–31). The size of the everted bladder is quite variable, ranging from a small area of the trigone to complete eversion of the posterior wall of the organ. The perineum is short and broad. Divergent elevator ani- and puborectal muscles may result in rectal incontinence and anal prolapse.

In cloacal exstrophy, there are two hemibladders, each with its own ureteral orifice, separated by an area of intestine. This bowel mucosa probably corresponds to the cecum, since it receives the ileum superiorly. Other structures that can be observed include an umbilical hernia and diphallus (separation of the two corpora) (Figs. 6–32, 6–33).

Associated Anomalies

Associated anomalies are rare in bladder exstrophy. In contrast, associated anomalies are very frequent in cloacal exstrophy.[9] Renal anomalies (renal agenesis, hydronephrosis, multicystic kidney, hydroureter, ureteric atresia) are present in 60 percent of patients. Skeletal defects other than separation of pubic bones were noted in 72 percent of patients. Spina bifida is by far the most common.[11] Anomalies of the cardiovascular and gastrointestinal tract occur in 16 percent and 10.5 percent, respectively. Omphaloceles are present in 87 percent of patients. A double vena cava is also frequent.[9]

Diagnosis

The prenatal diagnosis of bladder exstrophy has been reported.[8] This condition was suspected because of the presence of a solid mass (47 mm in diameter) in the lower part of the fetal abdomen (Fig. 6–34). The mass did not contain cystic areas, and the bladder could not be identified. The penis was extremely short, and a normal amount of amniotic fluid was present. The diagnosis should be suspected any time a bladder cannot be visualized in a fetus with a

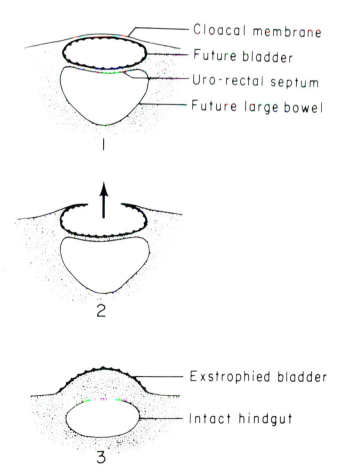

Figure 6–29. Diagram of events leading to classic exstrophy. *(Reproduced with permission from Muecke: In Campbell's Urology. Philadelphia, Saunders, 1986, pp 1856–1880.)*

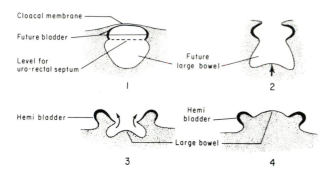

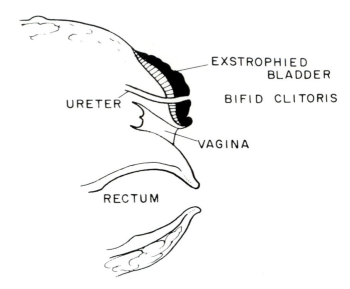

Figure 6–30. Diagram of eventration of the cloaca, forming cloacal exstrophy. *(Reproduced with permission from Muecke: In Campbell's Urology. Philadelphia, Saunders, 1986, pp 1856–1880.)*

Figure 6–32. Descriptive drawing of classic exstrophy of the bladder in a female child. *(Reproduced with permission from Muecke: In Campbell's Urology. Philadelphia, Saunders, 1986, pp. 1856–1880.)*

normal amount of amniotic fluid. The differential diagnosis includes omphalocele, gastroschisis, and cloacal exstrophy. Visualization of a normal bladder and the relationship of the mass to the fetal abdomen are helpful hints in the differentiation of bladder exstrophy from the first two defects. A prenatal diagnosis of cloacal exstrophy with ultrasound has not been reported. Elevated amniotic fluid AFP has been reported in one case of exstrophy cloaca.[1]

Prognosis

The main problems of bladder exstrophy are urinary incontinence, presence of an abdominal wall defect, and the cosmetic consequences of the lesion in the male genitalia. These problems can be treated surgi-

cally by the performance of a primary bladder closure, reconstruction of the bladder neck, and epispadias repair. Alternatively, the approach may consist of a urinary diversion, cystectomy, and epispadias repair. An optimal surgical treatment between these two alternatives has not been established, and there are merits to both approaches. The genital defects in the male are quite serious, and sex reassignment may be required in 1 in 50 to 1 in 100 patients in whom an adequately functional penis cannot be created.[5] Genital defects in the female are less complex. Approximation of the hemiclitoris can generally be accomplished. Vaginal dilatation and perineoplasty may be required for satisfactory sexual intercourse.

Patients with bladder exstrophy grow into adulthood and have an acceptable social adjustment.[7,13] Fertility is decreased in both males and females.[10] Pregnancy is possible, although there is an increased likelihood of uterine prolapse postpartum.[6] This complication is due to hypoplasia of the cardinal ligaments.

Cloacal exstrophy is a very serious anomaly associated with a 55 percent mortality rate.[3] The most common associated anomaly is a neural tube defect. Untreated infants frequently die from sepsis, short bowel syndrome, or renal or central nervous system defects. The correct surgical approach consists of a series of operations including repair of the omphalocele, functional bladder closure (neonatal period), antiincontinence and antireflux surgery at age 2 to 3 years, and vaginal reconstruction at age 14 to 18 years. Tank and Lindenauer[12] have recommended the conversion of males to females because of the

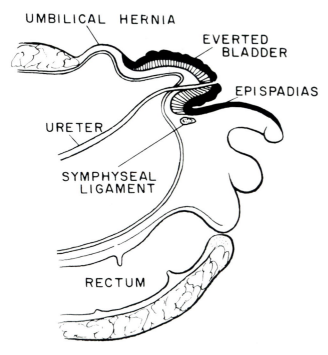

Figure 6–31. Descriptive drawing of classic exstrophy of the bladder in a male child. *(Reproduced with permission from Muecke: In Campbell's Urology. Philadelphia, Saunders, 1986, pp 1856–1880.)*

uniformly disappointing results when trying to create a functionally acceptable penis. Gonadectomy is performed when sexual reassignment has been selected.[12]

Obstetrical Management

If a diagnosis of bladder exstrophy is suspected before viability, the option of pregnancy termination should be offered. After this point, no change in standard obstetrical management is required. There is no evidence that altering the mode of delivery changes the prognosis for these infants. After birth, the exposed bladder mucosa is very friable and easily denuded. Jeffs and Lepor[5] have recommended that the umbilical cord be tied closely to its area of

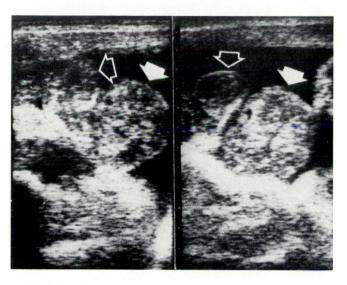

Figure 6–34. Sonogram of a fetus with bladder exstrophy. Oblique and longitudinal scans through the caudal aspect of the fetus, demonstrating fetal genitalia (*closed arrow*), with a solid mass (*open arrow*) projecting anteriorly. *(Reproduced with permission from Mirk et al.: J Ultrasound Med 5:291, 1986.)*

insertion so that a long cord does not add trauma to the bladder mucosa. It is preferable to tie the cord with a suture as opposed to the standard clamp, which may also traumatize the defect. The bladder mucosa may be covered with a nonadherent film of plastic wrap to prevent the mucosa from sticking to clothing. The traditional petroleum jelly gauze should be avoided, since it may lift the bladder epithelium when removed.

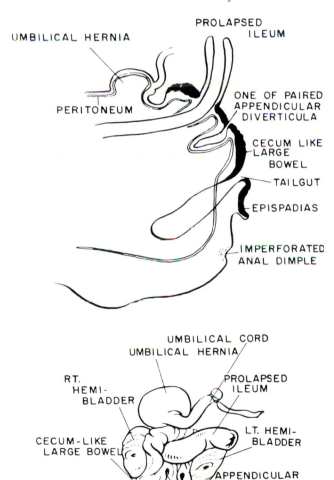

Figure 6–33. Diagrams of cloacal exstrophy in the newborn emphasizing characteristic anatomic features: two hemibladders with their ureteral orifices, cecumlike exstrophied intestine receiving the terminal ileum superiorly and the tailgut inferiorly, paired appendiceal diverticula, two hemipenises or corpora cavernosa. *(Reproduced with permission from Muecke: In Campbell's Urology. Philadelphia, Saunders, 1986, pp 1856–1880.)*

REFERENCES

1. Gosden C, Brock DJH: Prenatal diagnosis of exstrophy of the cloaca. Am J Med Genet 8:95, 1981.
2. Gravier L: Exstrophy of the cloaca. Am Surg 34:387, 1968.
3. Howell C, Caldamone A, Snyder H, et al.: Optimal management of cloacal exstrophy. J Pediatr Surg 18:365, 1983.
4. Ives E, Coffey R, Carter CO: A family study of bladder exstrophy. J Med Genet 17:139, 1980
5. Jeffs RD, Lepor H: Management of the exstrophy–epispadias complex and urachal anomalies. In Walsh PC (ed): Campbell's Urology, 5th ed. Philadelphia, Saunders, 1986, pp 1882–1921.
6. Krisiloff M, Puchner PJ, Tretter W, et al.: Pregnancy in women with bladder exstrophy. J Urol 119:478, 1978.
7. Lattimer JK, Beck L, Yeaw S, et al.: Long-term follow-up after exstrophy closure. Late improvement and good quality of life. J Urol 119:664, 1978.
8. Mirk P, Calisti A, Fileni A: Prenatal sonographic diagnosis of bladder exstrophy. J Ultrasound Med 5:291, 1986.

9. Muecke EC: Exstrophy, epispadias and other anomalies of the bladder. In Walsh PC (ed): Campbell's Urology, 5th ed. Philadelphia, Saunders, 1986, pp 1856–1880.
10. Shapiro E, Lepor H, Jeffs RD: The inheritance of the exstrophy epispadias complex. J Urol 132:308, 1984.
11. Soper RT, Kilger K: Vesico-intestinal fissure. J Urol 92:490, 1964.
12. Tank ES, Lindenauer SM: Principles of management of exstrophy of the cloaca. Am J Surg 119:95, 1970.
13. Woodhouse CRJ, Ransley PC, Williams DI: The patient with exstrophy in adult life. Br J Urol 55:632, 1983.

7

The Gastrointestinal Tract and Intraabdominal Organs

Normal Anatomy of the Gastrointestinal Tract and the Anterior Abdominal Wall

The stomach forms at about 4 weeks after conception by the development of a spindle-shaped dilatation of the foregut caudal to the esophagus. The stomach descends into the abdomen at about 6 to 7 weeks after conception, and by 11 weeks the muscles in its wall are developed. Visualization with ultrasound is possible as early as the 9th week of menstrual age. Different parts of the gastric anatomy (greater curvature, fundus, body, and pylorus) can be seen by the 14th week. Peristalsis is rarely visible before the 16th week. Table 7–7 (see p. 254) displays data on fetal stomach dimensions. Observations of this organ over a 3-hour period of time have demonstrated that there are no dramatic changes in size and therefore these dimensions should be useful in evaluating stomach size.[3] On occasion, an echogenic mass (fetal gastric pseudomass) is seen within the fetal stomach. The origin of this sonographic image is not clear. If it disappears on subsequent examinations, it has no proven pathologic significance.[1]

The small and large bowels can be distinguished from each other. The small bowel is centrally located, and it changes its position and appearance with peristalsis, which is visible as early as the 18th week of menstrual age. Early in gestation, peristaltic waves are characterized by vigorous and fleeting movements with a duration of less than 3 seconds. Later in gestation, peristaltic waves are more vigorous, ubiquitous, and of longer duration. A small bowel loop of more than 7 mm in internal diameter should raise the index of suspicion for bowel obstruction.[4] Generally, segments of small bowel measure less than 15 mm in length. Meconium formation begins at 16 to 20 weeks of menstrual age. Sonographically, meconium appears hypoechogenic in comparison to the bowel wall. The large bowel appears as a large tubular structure in the periphery of the fetal abdomen. Haustral clefts are sonographically apparent at 30 weeks in 87 percent of the fetuses and in all cases at 31 weeks of menstrual age. Table 7–8 (see p. 254) shows the correlation between transverse colonic diameter and gestational age. The echogenicity of the colon is assessed and graded in comparison with bladder and liver echogenicity. Grade 0 means the abdomen is uniform in appearance and the colon is not identified. Grade 1, the colonic appearance is hypoechogenic and essentially identical to the stomach and bladder. Haustra may be identified. Grade 2, the echogenicity of the colon is greater than the bladder, but less than the liver. Grade 3, colonic content has echogenicity similar to the liver. Grade 2 appears at 29 weeks and Grade 3 begins after 34 weeks of menstrual age.[2]

The pancreas can be seen in the third trimester in fetuses with the spine down. It can be found behind the stomach and in front of the splenic vein.

The gallbladder is a hypoechogenic structure in the middle right of the abdomen. It is often confused with the umbilical vein. They can be differentiated because (1) the gallbladder is right-sided and not median, (2) the umbilical vein can be traced outside the fetus into the umbilical cord and inside the liver to the portal system, and (3) the gallbladder neck is thinner than its bottom, and, therefore, the gallbladder is conical, which contrasts with the cylindrical umbilical vein. Absence of the gallbladder occurs in rare chromosomal syndromes (G syndrome) and in about 20 percent of patients with biliary atresia.

The size of the liver is affected by fetal nutrition. There are four ductal systems in the liver: the portal circulation, the hepatic veins, the hepatic arteries, and the biliary ducts. The last two cannot be seen under normal circumstances. The umbilical vein courses cephalically after entering the abdomen, then follows the falciform ligament and enters the liver, where it receives blood from the venae advehentes. It anastomoses with the left portal vein. The umbilical vein is, in fact, the left umbilical vein, since the right umbilical vein regresses around the 6th to 7th week. From the junction with the left portal vein, the umbilical vein is called the "umbilical part of the left portal vein." The oxygenated blood may reach the heart through the ductus venosus or the hepatic sinusoids and hepatic veins. The sphincter at the origin of the ductus venosus is believed to protect the fetal heart from overload when uterine contractions increase the placental venous return. This also explains why the

ductus venosus is inconsistently visible in physiologic circumstances. The ductus venosus drains into the left hepatic vein or directly into the inferior vena cava.

The portal system is best seen in transverse scans of the fetus, whereas the hepatic veins are better visualized in longitudinal or oblique scans. The hepatic veins can be seen when they enter the distal inferior vena cava near the right atrium.

The aorta and its bifurcation into the common iliac vessels are usually visible. The internal iliac vessels are more difficult to visualize, but their main branches, the umbilical arteries, can commonly be seen along the fetal bladder. The external iliac arteries can be followed into the femoral artery.

The inferior vena cava is visible adjacent to the aorta. In the higher abdomen, the inferior vena cava can be observed to be more anterior than the aorta. This is because the inferior vena cava bends anteriorly to enter the right atrium, whereas the aorta comes from the posterior aspect of the chest after ending the arch. The major collaterals of the inferior vena cava, visible with ultrasound, are the renal, hepatic, and iliac veins.

REFERENCES

1. Fakhry J, Shapiro LR, Schechter A, et al.: Fetal gastric pseudomasses. J Ultrasound Med. 6:177, 1987.
2. Goldstein I, Lockwood C, Hobbins, JC: Ultrasound assessment of fetal intestinal development in the evaluation of gestational age. Obstet Gynecol (in press), 1987.
3. Goldstein I, Reece EA, Yarkoni S, et al.: Growth of the fetal stomach in normal pregnancies. Obstet Gynecol 70:(in press), 1987.
4. Nyberg DA, Mack LA, Patten RM, Cyr DR: Fetal bowel: Normal sonographic findings. J Ultrasound Med 6:3, 1987.

Esophageal Atresia with and without Tracheoesophageal Fistula

Definition

Esophageal atresia is the absence of a segment of the esophagus. In most cases, this condition is associated with a fistula between the gastrointestinal and respiratory tracts.

Etiology

Unknown. There is no demonstrable genetic predisposition, and the disease occurs sporadically.

Epidemiology

The incidence of esophageal atresia varies between 1:800[1] and 1:5,000 live births.[7,11] There is no established sex preponderance.

Embryology

The esophagus and trachea develop from a common diverticulum of the primitive pharyngeal cavity. The diverticulum is subsequently partitioned by the tra-

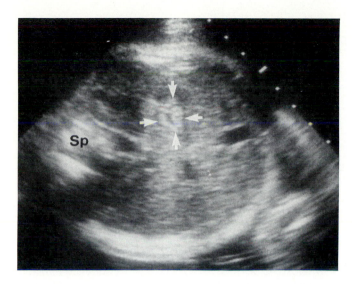

Figure 7–1. Transverse scan of the fetal abdomen in a fetus with esophageal atresia. A normal stomach is not visualized. The arrows point to the collapsed walls of the stomach. Sp, Spine.

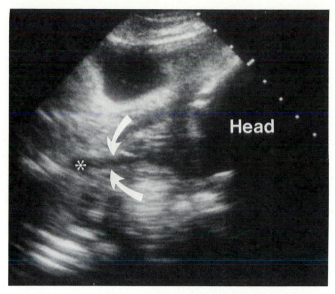

Figure 7–2. Coronal section of the neck in a fetus with esophageal atresia. Arrows point to the esophagus, which ends blindly (*).

cheoesophageal septum, forming the laryngotracheal tube and the esophagus. Development of the upper respiratory and gastrointestinal tracts takes place between the 21st day and the 5th week of gestation.[13] Given this common embryologic origin, it is not surprising that anomalies of the trachea and esophagus are often associated.

Pathology

There are different types of tracheoesophageal abnormalities. The five major varieties include (1) isolated esophageal atresia, (2) esophageal atresia with a fistula connecting the proximal portion of the esophagus with the trachea, (3) esophageal atresia with a fistula connecting the distal portion of the esophagus with the trachea, (4) esophageal atresia with a double fistula connecting both segments of the interrupted esophagus with the trachea, and (5) tracheoesophageal fistula without esophageal atresia. The most common variety is the third one, which accounts for more than 90 percent of all cases.[5]

Associated Anomalies

Cardiac, chromosomal (Down syndrome), gastrointestinal, and genitourinary anomalies are found in 58 percent of patients. The incidence of congenital heart disease varies between 15 and 39 percent.[4,10] Atrial and ventricular septal defects are the most common cardiac abnormalities.

Diagnosis

An esophageal atresia should be suspected in the presence of polyhydramnios. The increased amount of amniotic fluid is related to decreased turnover as a

consequence of the esophageal obstruction. The prenatal diagnosis of isolated esophageal atresia has been reported in a few cases.[3,8,14] Failure to visualize the stomach in serial ultrasound examinations allowed the diagnosis (Figs. 7–1, 7–2). It should be stressed that this diagnosis is only possible in 10 percent of patients. In the remaining patients, the gastric secretion or the occurrence of a tracheoesophageal fistula will allow visualization of some gastric distention.[2] Any time the stomach is not visualized, the fetal face should be examined to exclude otocephaly (see p. 110).

Prognosis

The prognosis of esophageal atresia with or without tracheoesophageal fistula depends on three factors: associated congenital anomalies, respiratory complications, and gestational age and weight at delivery. Infants born at term without anomalies or pneumonia survive in virtually all cases. Infants who weigh 1800 to 2500 g or have moderate respiratory complications or a non-life-threatening anomaly have a mortality rate ranging from 35 to 43 percent. The very small infants (<1800 g), those with severe respiratory complications, or those with severe associated congenital anomalies have a survival rate as low as 6 percent.[6] Unfortunately, 40 percent of children with esophageal atresia uncomplicated by any other major anomaly are below the 10th percentile of weight for gestational age, and 36 percent weigh less than 2500 g.[9]

These figures are based on postnatal series. There are limited data on the outcome of prenatally diagnosed cases. However, prognosis is expected to be more favorable, since intrauterine recognition will allow optimal neonatal management.

Ring et al.[12] have reported 16 cases of surgical treatment with jejunal interposition in 4 infants with isolated esophageal atresia and 12 with tracheoesophageal fistulas. The mean follow-up was 27 years, and no deaths occurred. There was excellent function of the anastomosis, and only 2 patients reported some dysphagia.

Obstetrical Management

A careful search for associated congenital anomalies is indicated. Fetal karyotyping and echocardiography should be included. Before viability, parents may opt for pregnancy termination. After viability, isolated esophageal atresia or tracheoesophageal fistula without associated congenital anomalies should not change obstetrical management.

In some instances, severe polyhydramnios is found, and this could lead to premature labor. Therefore, serial sonographic monitoring is indicated. If preterm labor occurs, tocolytic agents should be used. Amniotic fluid drainage can also be considered.

REFERENCES

1. Belsey RHR, Donnison CP: Congenital atresia of the oesophagus. Br Med J 2:324, 1950.
2. Bovicelli L, Rizzo N, Orsini LF, et al.: Prenatal diagnosis and management of fetal gastrointestinal abnormalities. Semin Perinatol 7:109, 1983.
3. Farrant P: The antenatal diagnosis of oesophageal atresia by ultrasound. Br J Radiol 53:1202, 1980.
4. Greenwood RD, Rosenthal A: Cardiovascular malformations associated with tracheoesophageal fistula and esophageal atresia. Pediatrics 57:87, 1976.
5. Gross RE: The Surgery of Infancy and Childhood: Its Principles and Techniques. Philadelphia, Saunders, 1953.
6. Grybowski J, Walker WA: Gastrointestinal Problems in the Infant, 2d ed. Philadelphia, Saunders, 1983, pp 165–172.
7. Ingalls TH, Prindle RA: Esophageal atresia with tracheoesophageal fistula; epidemiologic and teratologic implications. N Engl J Med 240:987, 1949.
8. Jassani MN, Gauderer MWL, Faranoff AA, et al.: A perinatal approach to the diagnosis and management of gastrointestinal malformations. Obstet Gynecol 59:33, 1982.
9. Jolleys A: An examination of the birthweights of babies with some abnormalities of the alimentary tract. J Pediatr Surg 16:160, 1981.
10. Landing BH: Syndromes of congenital heart disease with tracheobronchial anomalies. AJR 123:679, 1975.
11. Ravitch MM, Barton BA: The need for pediatric surgeons as determined by the volume of work and the mode of delivery of surgical care. Surgery 76:754, 1974.
12. Ring WS, Varco RL, L'Heureux PR, et al.: Esophageal replacement with jejunum in children. J Thorac Cardiovasc Surg 83:918, 1982.
13. Smith EI: The early development of the trachea and esophagus in relation to atresia of the esophagus and tracheoesophageal fistula. Contr Embryol, Carnegie Institute, Washington, DC, 36(no. 245):41, 1957.
14. Zemlyn S: Prenatal detection of esophageal atresia. J Clin Ultrasound 9:453, 1981.

Duodenal Atresia

Epidemiology

Duodenal atresia is the most common type of congenital small bowel obstruction. Its incidence is approximately 1 in 10,000 live births.[7]

Embryology

During the 5th week of embryonic life, the epithelium of the primitive duodenum proliferates and obliterates the lumen. By the 11th week, vacuolization leads to restoration of luminal patency. Defective vacuolization results in segmental obstruction or stenosis. The association of duodenal atresia with chromosomal abnormalities and other anomalies supports the view that the lesion is due to an early embryonic insult. Exposure to thalidomide between the 30th and 40th day of gestation has resulted in duodenal atresia in the human fetus, suggesting that this is the critical period of time for the development of the lesion.[9]

Most duodenal atresias result from failure of canalization of the primitive bowel by the 11th week. On rare occasions, duodenal atresia may also result from a vascular accident causing infarction of a segment of fetal bowel and subsequent atrophy and absorption.[11] In this case, the extent of the obstruction is greater and may involve the duodenum, jejunum, and ileum. Duodenal atresia has been reported after intrauterine midgut strangulation in a fetus with an omphalocele.[24]

Etiology

In many cases, the etiology of duodenal atresia is unknown. Most cases are sporadic, but a genetic component is suggested by the report of familial cases of pyloroduodenal atresia with an autosomal recessive pattern of inheritance.[19] Furthermore, duodenal atresia can be a feature of the autosomal recessive type of multiple bowel atresias.[15] A teratogenic origin is implicated in the cases of duodenal atresia reported in infants exposed to thalidomide.[9]

Pathology

Intestinal atresias can be classified into four types. Type I is characterized by one or more transverse diaphragms. In type II, the blind-ending loops are connected by a fibrous string. In type III, there is complete separation of the blind-ending loops. Type IV corresponds to the so-called apple-peel atresia of the small bowel, with absence of a large portion of the small bowel and typical apple-peel configuration of the small bowel along the mesenteric artery.[11]

The most frequent form of duodenal atresia (type I) results from the presence of a membrane or a diaphragm (web). In about 20 percent of patients, duodenal obstructions are associated with an annular pancreas, that is, a ring of pancreatic tissue encircling the distal portion of the duodenum.[17] One theory claims that the duodenal obstruction results from the extrinsic compression of the anomalous pancreas,[7,11,16] and another theory suggests that the annular pancreas does not have a role in the genesis of the lesion but rather is a consequence of a common development field defect.[18] Duodenal atresia can be part of an apple-peel or Christmas tree form of intestinal atresia, which probably results from prenatal occlusion of a branch of the superior mesenteric artery, either the right colic or marginal. This type of intestinal atresia is characterized by extensive small bowel atresia that may involve the distal duodenum, entire jejunum, and proximal ileum.

Associated Anomalies

Duodenal atresia is an isolated anomaly in only 30 to 52 percent of patients.[8,27] Vertebral anomalies are found in 37 percent of patients and include anomalous rib number, sacral agenesis, bilateral talipes equinovarus, presence of a sixth lumbar vertebra, bilateral absence of thumbs, sacral hemivertebrae, bilateral cervical ribs, and fusion of the cervical spine.[1] Other gastrointestinal anomalies occur in 26 percent of patients, including malrotation, esophageal atresia, imperforate anus, ileal atresia, transposed liver, duodenal duplication, and Meckel's diverticulum. Eight to 20 percent of patients will have congenital heart disease, mainly endocardial cushion defects and ventricular septal defects.[1,7] Renal anomalies have been identified in 8 percent of patients.[1]

Approximately one third of cases of duodenal atresias are associated with trisomy 21.[1,2,7,8] The le-

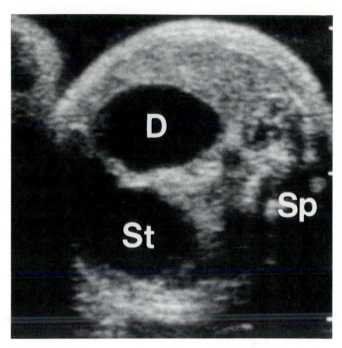

Figure 7–3. Transverse scan of the upper abdomen in an infant with duodenal atresia. The typical double bubble is seen. St, stomach; D, dilated duodenal bulb; Sp, spine.

sion has also occurred with interstitial deletion of the long arm of chromosome 9.[26]

Diagnosis

Diagnosis relies on the demonstration of the double bubble sign, which is due to the simultaneous distention of the stomach and the first portion of the duodenum (Figs. 7–3, 7–4, 7–5).[3] A connection between the two cystic structures can be demonstrated. We have noted that these infants frequently have increased peristaltic waves. Polyhydramnios is a constant feature in all intestinal atresias. On the other hand, intestinal atresias have been reported in 6 to 9 percent of patients with polyhydramnios.[6]

A critical issue relates to the time in gestation when the diagnosis can be made. Although some reports suggest that the diagnosis may not be possible before the third trimester,[23] we have recently made this diagnosis in four fetuses before 24 weeks of gestation and in one fetus as early as 19 weeks.

A potential pitfall in diagnosis of this condition is the visualization of a double bubble in a coronal plane of the fetal trunk as a consequence of a prominent incisura angularis of the stomach. The double bubble image is caused by the bidissection of an otherwise normal fetal stomach. This error can be easily overcome by scanning the abdomen in a transverse plane.[10] A choledochal cyst has been confused with duodenal atresia, since a double bubble image can occur also in this condition. One bubble corresponds

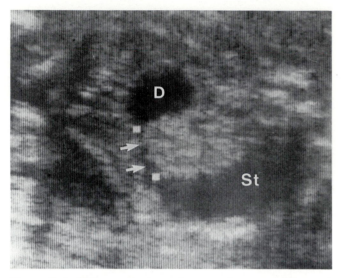

Figure 7–4. Oblique scan shows the stomach connected (*arrows*) with a dilated duodenal bulb through the pylorus. D, duodenum; St, stomach.

to the normal stomach and the other to the chole-dochal cyst. However, a communication between the two cystic masses cannot be demonstrated in cases of choledochal cysts. It may also be possible to demonstrate dilated biliary ducts entering the cyst.[5]

Attempts at a biochemical diagnosis of intestinal obstruction have been made by measuring the amniotic fluid levels of pancreatic lipase, bile acids, or bilirubin. A high concentration of these substances has been demonstrated in fetuses with duodenal obstruction distal to the ampulla of Vater.[4,13,20] However, the location of atresia or stenosis is postampullary in 20 to 50 percent of patients, limiting the value

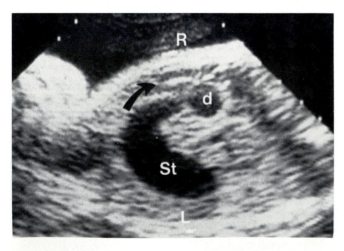

Figure 7–5. Oblique coronal scan in a fetus with duodenal atresia. A striking deviation of the duodenal bulb (d) upward and toward the right suggests an extrinsic lesion. The infant had a right diaphragmatic hernia. Upward rotation is indicated by black arrow. St, stomach; L, left; R, right.

of these markers.[7,11] Levels of intestinal enzymes, such as disaccharidases, are low in intestinal obstruction.[21] The role of these studies in the prenatal diagnosis of bowel atresia has not been clearly defined. An elevation of alpha-fetoprotein concentrations in amniotic fluid in the presence of a duodenal obstruction has been reported.[25]

In cases of associated duodenal and esophageal atresia without tracheoesophageal fistula, the sonographic picture is very similar to that of duodenal atresia, except that the distention of the two bubbles is far greater.[6,12] In these patients, the amniotic fluid concentration of bile acids should be normal.[4]

Distention of the stomach without a typical double bubble appearance has been found in congenital pyloric stenosis.[22,28] The reliability of ultrasound in making this diagnosis has not been established.

Prognosis

The prognostic factors for neonatally diagnosed duodenal atresia are gestational age at delivery, associated anomalies, and diagnostic delay. The morbidity associated with diagnostic delay includes vomiting, aspiration pneumonia, electrolyte imbalance, dehydration, and even stomach perforation. We have recently found that prenatal diagnosis reduces the morbidity associated with diagnostic delay in duodenal atresia. The main causes of death are associated congenital anomalies. Prematurity is thought to be related to polyhydramnios causing preterm labor. In one report, 40 percent of the babies with duodenal atresia uncomplicated by any other major anomaly weighed below the 10th percentile.[14] Surgical repair of duodenal atresia is performed during the neonatal period.

Obstetrical Management

The critical issue in the management of fetuses with duodenal atresia is the presence or absence of associated anomalies. Fetal karyotyping, echocardiography, and a careful examination of the anatomy are indicated. In some fetuses, the diagnosis will be made at an age close to the legal limit for pregnancy termination, and fetal blood sampling for rapid chromosomal analysis can be offered. Further management decisions depend on the results of these studies.

The option of pregnancy termination should be offered before viability. In continuing pregnancies and in those cases diagnosed after viability, the recognition of duodenal atresia does not alter standard obstetrical management. Delivery in a tertiary care center is desirable to expedite surgical repair.

Polyhydramnios may contribute to the onset of premature labor. Tocolytic agents are indicated in these patients. Amniotic fluid drainage may also be considered.

REFERENCES

1. Atwell JD, Klidjian AM: Vertebral anomalies and duodenal atresia. J Pediatr Surgery 17:237, 1982.
2. Aubrespy P, Derlon S, Seriat-Gautier B: Congenital duodenal obstruction: A review of 82 cases. Prog Pediatr Surg 11:109, 1978.
3. Balcar I, Grant D, Miller WA, et al.: Antenatal detection of Down syndrome by sonography. AJR 143:29, 1984.
4. Deleze G, Sidiropoulos D, Paumgartner G: Determination of bile acid concentration in human amniotic fluid for prenatal diagnosis of intestinal obstructions. Pediatrics 59:647, 1977.
5. Dewbury KC, Aluwihare APR, Birch SJ, et al.: Prenatal ultrasound demonstration of a choledochal cyst. Br J Radiol 53:906, 1980.
6. Duenhoelter JH, Santos-Ramos R, Rosenfeld CR, et al.: Prenatal diagnosis of gastrointestinal tract obstruction. Obstet Gynecol 47:618, 1976.
7. Fonkalsrud EW: Duodenal atresia or stenosis. In: Bergsma D: Birth Defects Compendium, 2d ed. New York, Alan R. Liss, 1979, p 350.
8. Fonkalsrud EW, de Lorimer AA, Hayes DM: Congenital atresia and stenosis of the duodenum. A review compiled from the members of the surgical section of the American Academy of Pediatrics. Pediatrics 43:79, 1969.
9. Gourevitch A: Duodenal atresia in the newborn. Ann R Coll Surg Engl 48:141, 1971.
10. Gross BH, Filly RA: Potential for a normal fetal stomach to simulate the sonographic "double bubble" sign. J Can Assoc Radiol 33:39, 1982.
11. Grybowski J, Walker WA: Gastrointestinal Problems in the Infant, 2d ed. Philadelphia, Saunders, 1983, pp 427–485.
12. Hayden CK, Schwartz MZ, Davis M, et al.: Combined esophageal and duodenal atresia: Sonographic findings. AJR 140:225, 1983.
13. Hisanaga S, Shimokawa H, Kurokawa T, et al.: Relation of the site of congenital upper gastrointestinal obstruction to amniotic fluid bilirubin concentration. Asia-Oceania J Obstet Gynecol 9:435, 1983.
14. Jolleys A: An examination of the birth weights of babies with some abnormalities of the alimentary tract. J Pediatr Surg 16:160, 1981.
15. Kao KJ, Fleischer R, Bradford WD, et al.: Multiple congenital septal atresias of the intestine: Histomorphologic and pathogenetic implications. Pediatr Pathol 1:443, 1983.
16. Kirillova IA, Kulazhenko VP, Kulazhenko LG, et al.: Pancreas annulare in human embryos. Acta Anat 118:214, 1984.
17. Lundquist G: Annular pancreas: Pathogenesis, clinical features, and treatment, with a report of two operation cases. Acta Chir Scand 117:451, 1959.
18. Merrill JR, Raffensperger JG: Pediatric annular pancreas: Twenty years' experience. J Pediatr Surg 11:921, 1976.
19. Mishalany HG, Idriss ZA, Der Kaloustian VM: Pyloroduodenal atresia (diaphragm type): An autosomal recessive disease. Pediatrics 62:419, 1978.
20. Mohide PT, Hill RE: Amniotic fluid lipase in two cases of duodenal obstruction. Am J Obstet Gynecol 132:221, 1978.
21. Morin PR, Potir M, Dallaire L, et al.: Prenatal detection of intestinal obstruction: Deficient amniotic fluid disaccharidases in affected fetuses. Clin Genet 18:217, 1980.
22. Nabekura J, Shin T, Koyanagi T, et al.: Identification of affected sites in fetal gastroduodenal obstructions by real-time ultrasonic tomography. Asia-Oceania J Obstet Gynecol 9:427, 1983.
23. Nelson LH, Clark CE, Fishburne JI, et al.: Value of serial sonography in the in utero detection of duodenal atresia. Obstet Gynecol 59:657, 1982.
24. Shigemoto H, Horiya Y, Isomoto T, et al.: Duodenal atresia secondary to intrauterine midgut strangulation by an omphalocele. J Pediatr Surgery 17:420, 1982.
25. Weinberg AG, Milunsky A, Harrod MJ: Elevated amniotic-fluid alpha-fetoprotein and duodenal atresia. Lancet 2:496, 1975.
26. Ying KL, Curry CJR, Rajani KB, et al.: De novo interstitial deletion in the long arm of chromosome 9: A new chromosome syndrome. J Med Genet 19:68, 1982.
27. Young DG, Wilkinson AW: Abnormalities associated with neonatal duodenal obstruction. Surgery 63:832, 1968.
28. Zimmerman HB: Prenatal demonstration of gastric and duodenal obstruction by ultrasound. J Assoc Can Radiol 29:138, 1978.

Bowel Obstruction

Incidence

Atresias and stenoses of the small bowel occur in 1 in 5000 live births; atresia and stenosis of the colon are less common and are reported to occur in 1 in 20,000 live births; and figures for imperforate anus are in the range of 1 in 2500 to 1 in 3300 live births.[9,26] Meconium ileus is the presenting symptom in 10 to 15 percent of cases of cystic fibrosis.[10,28]

Etiology

Intestinal atresia is generally the result of a vascular accident, volvulus, or intussusception.[17] It has also been reported as a complication of amniocentesis.[27,30,31] In multiple intestinal atresia, familial cases inherited with an autosomal recessive pattern have been described.[12,14,20] The apple-peel variety of small bowel atresia typically has a familial tendency.[6] In the majority of cases, meconium ileus is associated with cystic fibrosis (an autosomal recessive disease).[28]

Pathogenesis

Most cases of bowel atresia do not result from a disorder of embryogenesis but rather from a vascular insult during fetal life. The role of vascular compromise was originally suspected because of the association of volvulus, intussusceptions, snaring of the umbilical ring, and kinking with intestinal atresia. Experimental evidence suggests that ligation of the vessels supplying the intestine results in lesions similar to that of intestinal atresia.[18] The observation of bile, planocellular epithelium, and lanugo distal to the site of obstruction suggests that the lesion occurs after organogenesis. Indeed, bile is not secreted before the 11th week, planocellular epithelium before the 12th week, and lanugo before the 6th to 7th month. It is, therefore, not surprising that associated extragastrointestinal anomalies are rare in intestinal obstructions. On the other hand, gastrointestinal anomalies are common. A defective mesenterium could lead to the development of malrotation, volvulus, and intussusceptions, which in turn would cause vascular obstruction. It should be noted that lesions that could account for the vascular accident (e.g., volvulus) are found in only 25 percent of cases of intestinal atresias.[4] Experimental evidence gathered in chicken embryos suggests that even a temporary obstruction of blood supply can result in intestinal atresia.[32]

Pathology

Intestinal atresias are more common than stenosis and are usually multiple. They are classified in different ways.[10,17,19] In the most commonly used classification, type I is characterized by one or more transverse diaphragms, in type II, the blind-ending loops are connected by a fibrous string, and in type III, there is a complete separation of the blind-ending loops. Type IV corresponds to the so-called apple-peel atresia of the small bowel.[10] Type IV is thought to result from prenatal occlusion of a branch of the superior mesenteric artery, either the right colic or marginal, and it is characterized by extensive small bowel atresia that may involve the distal duodenum, entire jejunum, and proximal ileum.[34] The most common sites of atresias are the proximal jejunum and distal ileum.[11] Meconium ileus is caused by viscid, thick meconium that accumulates and obstructs the distal ileum. All these conditions may lead to dilatation of the bowel proximal to the obstruction and to perforation, with the development of meconium peritonitis.

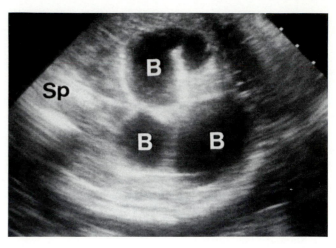

Figure 7–6. Transverse scan of the abdomen in a fetus with ileal atresia. Dilated loops of bowel (B) are visible. Sp, spine.

Associated Anomalies

The incidence of extragastrointestinal-associated anomalies is low.[23] However, gastrointestinal anomalies are present in approximately 45 percent of patients and include bowel malrotation (22.7 percent), intestinal duplications (3 percent), microcolon, and esophageal atresia (3 percent).[4,23]

Diagnosis

The diagnosis is made by demonstrating multiple distended bowel loops (Figs. 7–6, 7–7, 7–8). The differential diagnosis includes all conditions capable of producing intraabdominal anechoic images, such as duodenal atresia, hydronephrosis, ovarian cyst, and mesenteric cyst. Usually, the ultrasound appearance of distended bowel loops is striking because of the increased peristalsis and the presence of floating particulate matter (Fig. 7–8).[8,16] A careful examination of the visceral anatomy will reveal a normal urinary system and stomach. The presence of an increased echogenicity in the abdominal cavity can correspond to meconium ileus.[5,22] The earliest case was diagnosed in a 19-week fetus with cystic fibrosis.[22] However, the reader should be alerted that focal areas of increased echogenicity in the lower fetal abdomen can be a normal finding in the second trimester.[7] The development of ascites or of a highly echogenic mass is a sign of bowel perforation (see section on meconium peritonitis).

It should be stressed that there is considerable variability in the appearance of the bowel in the third trimester of pregnancy. In some cases, suspicion of an intestinal obstruction may arise. In our experience, this has occurred in fetuses who were normal at birth. Therefore, caution is recommended. Unless there is massive dilatation of intestinal loops, a definitive diagnosis is difficult. The index of suspicion should be raised when the inner diameter of the small bowel

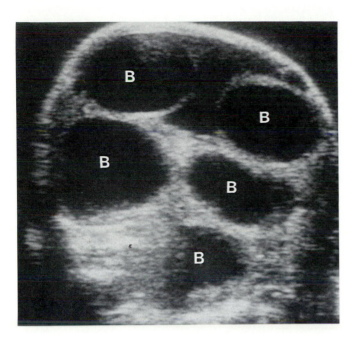

Figure 7–7. Transverse scan of the abdomen of a fetus with small bowel atresia. A volvulus was present. In real-time examination, increased peristalsis was seen. B, dilated bowel loops.

measures more than 7 mm (see Table 7–8, which shows the upper limit of the transverse diameter of the colon). Since obstruction of the small or large intestine results in greatly enlarged bowel loops, identification of the precise site of obstruction (small versus large intestine) may not be possible. Moreover, significant dilatation of the large bowel may not

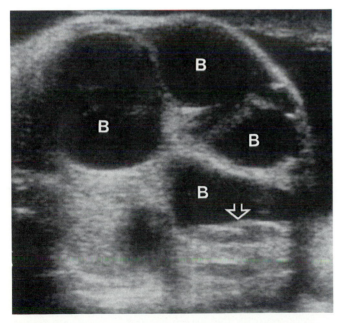

Figure 7–8. Transverse scan of the abdomen of a fetus with small bowel atresia. Dilated bowel loops (B) are clearly visible. Layering of meconium in one bowel loop is seen (*arrow*).

always be visible. This has been attributed to the fact that fluid is absorbed at this level by the colon mucosa, leading to little or no distention of the proximal bowel. However, a prenatal diagnosis of anal atresia has been reported.[1]

The sonographer should be aware that bowel distention can be associated with intestinal disorders that do not cause mechanical obstruction. Chronic chloride diarrhea is a condition inherited with an autosomal recessive pattern, found mainly in the northern European countries, and with a sonographic image similar to that of bowel obstruction.[15]

Polyhydramnios is a frequent feature in upper gastrointestinal obstructions, but it is rare in distal obstructions.[16]

Attempts at a biochemical diagnosis of intestinal obstruction have been made by measuring the amniotic fluid levels of pancreatic lipase and bile acids. These compounds are secreted into the bowel at the level of the ampulla of Vater. An intestinal obstruction distal to this point could lead to vomiting of the gastric contents and elevation of the amniotic fluid levels of these substances. Elevation of amniotic fluid bile acids has been reported in infants with ileal atresia.[3] Amniotic fluid levels of bilirubin can also increase in the presence of a high gastrointestinal obstruction.[13,33] This concept should be kept in mind when interpreting the results of spectrophotometric analysis of amniotic fluid in a sensitized pregnancy complicated by gastrointestinal obstruction. Under these circumstances, the difference in optical density (ΔOD) at 450 nm may not be an accurate indicator of hemolysis. Sonography and fetal blood sampling are the instruments of choice when evaluating such a fetus.

Another biochemical approach to the diagnosis of bowel obstruction involves measuring the level of intestinal enzymes in amniotic fluid. Disaccharidase activity in amniotic fluid has been shown to correlate with the activity of these enzymes in fetal jejunal mucosa between 16 and 21 weeks. This has been interpreted to indicate that the activity of disaccharidases in amniotic fluid reflects bowel discharge into the amniotic fluid.[25] Therefore, bowel obstruction would be associated with low disaccharidase activity.[21,24] A serious limitation of this approach is that the activity of dissacharidases normally decreases after the 22nd week of gestation, and their diagnostic value would be restricted to gestational ages between 14 and 21 weeks.

Prognosis

The prognosis depends on the site of the obstruction, the length of remaining bowel, birth weight, associated congenital anomalies, and the presence of meconium peritonitis. In general, the lower the obstruction, the better the outcome. Mortality rates of 50 percent and 35 percent have been reported in patients with jejunal atresia, depending on whether or not bowel resection is necessary.[10] Survival with distal atresias is virtually 100 percent if the infant is in good preoperative condition. Apple-peel atresia is associated with a high mortality rate due to the extent of the lesion.[6] Congenital volvulus has an extremely poor prognosis, with a mortality rate as high as 80 percent.[10] Intussusception is rarely a cause of congenital intestinal obstruction, but when present, it usually carries a good prognosis. The outcome of infants with meconium ileus is related to both the intestinal obstruction and the presence or absence of cystic fibrosis. Intestinal perforation worsens the prognosis. The overall mortality rate with meconium peritonitis is 62 percent.[2] A report shows that 61 percent of newborns with jejunal atresia weighed less than 2500 g and had a significantly higher mortality rate.[29]

Obstetrical Management

Even though there is a case report of prenatal diagnosis of meconium ileus in a midtrimester fetus at risk, it is unlikely that an intestinal obstruction could be reliably diagnosed with ultrasound before viability. The recognition of an intestinal obstruction should not change obstetrical management. These fetuses can be delivered vaginally at term, but it should be noted that polyhydramnios may lead to malpresentation. Delivery in a tertiary care center where a pediatric surgeon is available is recommended.

REFERENCES

1. Bean WJ, Calonje MA, Aprill CN, et al.: Anal atresia: A prenatal ultrasound diagnosis. JCU 6:111, 1978.
2. Bergmans MGM, Merkus JMWM, Baars AM: Obstetrical and neonatological aspects of a child with atresia of the small bowel. J Perinat Med 12:325, 1984.
3. Deleze G, Sidiropoulos D, Paumgartner G: Determination of bile acid concentration in human amniotic fluid for prenatal diagnosis of intestinal obstructions. Pediatrics 59:647, 1977.
4. De Lorimier AA, Fonkalsrud EW, Hays DM: Congenital atresia and stenosis of the jejunum and the ileum. Surgery 65:819, 1969.
5. Denholm TA, Crow HC, Edwards WH, et al.: Prenatal sonographic appearance of meconium ileus in twins. AJR 143:371, 1984.
6. Dickson JAS: Apple peel small bowel: An uncommon variant of duodenal and jejunal atresia. J Pediatr Surg 5:595, 1970.
7. Fakhry J, Reiser M, Shapiro LR, et al.: Increased echogenicity in the lower fetal abdomen: A common normal variant in the second trimester. J Ultrasound Med 5:489, 1986.

8. Fogel SR, Katragadda CS, Costin BS: New ultrasonographic findings in a case of fetal jejunal atresia. Tex Med 76:44, 1980.
9. Freeman NV: Congenital atresia and stenosis of the colon. Br J Surg 53:595, 1966.
10. Grybowski J, Walker WA: Gastrointestinal Problems in the Infant, 2d ed. Philadelphia, Saunders, 1983, pp 427–540.
11. Guttman FM, Braun P, Bensoussan AL, et al.: The pathogenesis of intestinal atresia. Surg Gynecol Obstet 141:203, 1975.
12. Guttman FM, Braun P, Garance PH, et al.: Multiple atresias and a new syndrome of hereditary multiple atresias involving the gastrointestinal tract from stomach to rectum. J Pediatr Surg 8:633, 1973.
13. Hisanaga S, Shimokawa H, Kurokawa T, et al.: Relation of the site of congenital upper gastrointestinal obstruction to amniotic fluid bilirubin concentration. Asia Oceania J Obstet Gynecol 9:435, 1983.
14. Kao KJ, Fleischer R, Bradford WD, et al.: Multiple congenital septal atresias of the intestine: Histomorphologic and pathogenetic implications. Pediatr Pathol 1:443, 1983.
15. Kirkinen P, Jouppila P: Prenatal ultrasonic findings in congenital chloride diarrhea. Prenat Diagn 4:457,1984.
16. Kjoller M, Holm-Nielsen G, Meiland H, et al.: Prenatal obstruction of the ileum diagnosed by ultrasound. Prenat Diagn 5:427, 1985.
17. Louw JH: Investigations into the etiology of congenital atresia of the colon. Dis Colon Rectum 7:471, 1964.
18. Louw JH, Barnard CN: Congenital intestinal atresia—Observations on its origin. Lancet 2:1065, 1955.
19. Martin LW, Zerella JT: Jejunoileal atresia: A proposed classification. J Pediatr Surg 11:399, 1976.
20. Mishalany HG, Der Kaloustian VM: Familial multiple-level intestinal atresias. Report of two siblings. J Pediatr 79:124, 1971.
21. Morin PR, Potier M, Dallaire L, et al.: Prenatal detection of intestinal obstruction: Deficient amniotic fluid disaccharidases in affected fetuses. Clin Genet 18:217, 1980.
22. Muller F, Frot JC, Aubry MC, et al.: Meconium ileus in cystic fibrosis fetuses. Lancet 1:223, 1984.
23. Nixon HH, Tawes R: Etiology and treatment of small intestinal atresia: Analysis of a series of 127 jejunoileal atresias and comparison with 62 duodenal atresia. Surgery 69:41, 1971.
24. Potier M, Dallaire L, Melancon SB: Prenatal detection of intestinal obstruction by disaccharidase assay in amniotic fluid. Lancet 2:982, 1977.
25. Potier M, Melancon SB, Dallaire L: Development patterns of intestinal disaccharidases in human amniotic fluid. Am J Obstet Gynecol 131:73, 1978.
26. Ravitch MM, Barton BA: The need for pediatric surgeons as determined by the volume of work and the mode of delivery of surgical care. Surgery 76:754, 1974.
27. Rickwood AMK: A case of ileal atresia and ileocutaneous fistula caused by amniocentesis. J Pediatr 91:312, 1977.
28. Rosenstein BJ, Langbaum TS: Incidence of meconium abnormalities in newborn infants with cystic fibrosis. Am J Dis Child 134:72, 1980.
29. Safra MJ, Oakley GP, Erickson D: Descriptive epidemi-

ology of small bowel atresia in metropolitan Atlanta. Teratology 14:143, 1976.

30. Swift PGF, Driscoll IB, Vowles KDJ: Neonatal small-bowel obstruction associated with amniocentesis. Br Med J 1:720, 1979.
31. Therkelsen AJ, Rehder H: Intestinal atresia caused by second trimester amniocentesis. Br J Obstet Gynecol 88:559, 1981.
32. Tibboel D, van Nie CJ, Molenaar JC: The effects of

temporary general hypoxia and local ischemia on the development of the intestines: An experimental study. J Pediatr Surg 15:57, 1980.
33. Wynn RJ, Schreiner RL: Spurious elevation of amniotic fluid bilirubin in acute hydramnios with fetal intestinal obstruction. Am J Obstet Gynecol 134:105, 1979.
34. Zivkovic SM, Milosevic VR: Duodenal and jejunal atresia with agenesis of the dorsal mesentery: "Apple peel" small bowel. Am J Surg 137:676, 1979.

Meconium Peritonitis

Definition
This term refers to the peritoneal inflammatory reaction seen in cases of intrauterine bowel perforation.

Incidence
Neonatal units see one case or more per year of meconium peritonitis occurring or developing during the neonatal period.[12] At least eight instances of prenatal diagnosis of meconium peritonitis have been reported.[1,5,9,11,14–17]

Etiopathogenesis and Pathology
Meconium peritonitis may occur after a bowel perforation associated with a bowel obstruction of any etiology (e.g., intestinal atresia, volvulus, meconium ileus). In 25 to 40 percent of all patients, it is secondary to meconium ileus due to cystic fibrosis.[4,10] Peritonitis can also occur with hydrometrocolpos.[8] In some cases, neither a bowel perforation nor an obstruction can be identified, and the etiology of the peritonitis remains unclear.

Two pathologic types have been described in fetuses: the fibroadhesive type and the cystic variety. The fibroadhesive type is characterized by an intense chemical reaction of the peritoneum, leading to formation of a dense mass with calcium deposits that eventually seals off the perforation. The second type is characterized by a cystic cavity formed by the fixation of the bowel loops surrounding the perforation site.[12,13] In this variety, the perforation is not sealed off, and meconium continues to escape into the cystic cavity, which is lined by a calcified peel. Since fetal meconium is sterile, perforation in the antenatal period does not lead to bacterial contamination.[7]

Diagnosis
The diagnosis of meconium peritonitis should be considered whenever a fetal intraabdominal hyperechogenic mass is detected.[7] A bright echogenic mass casting an acoustic shadow, especially if associated with ascites and polyhydramnios, is strongly indicative of meconium peritonitis (Figs. 7–9, 7–10, 7–11). Isolated ascites may also be a form of presentation of meconium peritonitis.[9a,11] The differential diagnosis includes intraabdominal teratomas and fetal gallstones. Intraabdominal teratomas generally are complex masses, and fetal gallstones can be recognized by their location inside the gallbladder.[3] Table 7–1 illustrates possible causes of fetal intraabdominal calcifications.

Polyhydramnios is not a typical feature in either of these conditions. The diagnosis should also be suspected in a fetus with a bowel obstruction that suddenly develops ascites or hydrops.[2] In one fetus, a confident diagnosis was made by a fetal paracentesis that demonstrated meconium-stained fluid with an intense inflammatory reaction rich in polymorphonuclear cells.[1]

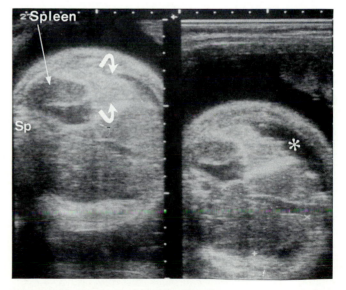

Figure 7–9. Meconium peritonitis in a 35-week fetus. Transverse scan of the abdomen showing a calcified mass (*arrows*) and ascites. Sp, spine. The right scan shows ascites (*).

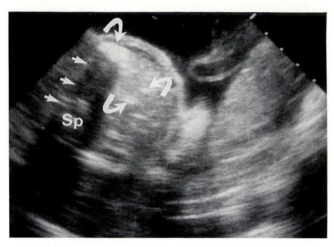

Figure 7–10. Transverse scan in a fetus with meconium peritonitis. Multiple intraabdominal calcifications are seen (*curved arrows*). The largest calcification casts an acoustic shadow (*arrowheads*). Sp, spine.

TABLE 7–1. DIFFERENTIAL DIAGNOSIS OF INTRAABDOMINAL CALCIFICATIONS

Peritoneal
  Meconium peritonitis
  Plastic peritonitis associated with hydrometrocolpos
Tumors
  Hemangioma
  Hemangioendothelioma
  Hepatoblastoma
  Metastatic neuroblastoma
  Teratoma
  Ovarian dermoid
Congenital infection
  Toxoplasmosis
  Cytomegalovirus infection

Prognosis

Meconium peritonitis is a serious condition. The mortality of treated infants in the neonatal period is as high as 62 percent.[4] Of the eight prenatally diagnosed fetuses reported in the literature, five survived, two died, and one pregnancy was electively terminated at 18 weeks. Deaths occurred in two premature infants weighing 610 and 1300 g.[1,5,9,11,14–17]

Obstetrical Management

There are scant data on which to base obstetrical management, since there are only a few prenatally diagnosed cases in the literature. We have made this diagnosis in the second trimester of pregnancy. At this point, the possibility of cystic fibrosis should be considered, and further investigation is recommended. Intestinal isoenzymes of alkaline phospha-

tase in amniotic fluid have been used recently for prenatal diagnosis of this condition.[6] In the future, prenatal diagnosis of cystic fibrosis probably will rely on the application of microbiologic techniques. Before viability, the option of pregnancy termination can be offered to the parents.

Our approach to the management of this condition after viability is dependent on the evolution of the disease. If there is a localized lesion that does not change over time and there is no associated ascites, intervention does not seem warranted. On the other hand, in the face of the rapid development and worsening of ascites, preterm delivery can be considered to avoid further damage to the bowel loops. The antenatal administration of steroids in cases of lung immaturity is indicated. There is no evidence that an elective cesarean section will improve the outcome for these infants. If severe abdominal distention and ascites are present, a fetal paracentesis before the induction of labor should be considered.[1] Delivery in a tertiary center is recommended, since these infants will require immediate surgical care.

REFERENCES

1. Baxi LV, Yeh MN, Blanc WA, et al.: Antepartum diagnosis and management of in utero intestinal volvulus with perforation. N Engl J Med 308:25, 1983.
2. Beischer NA, Fortune DW, Macafee J: Nonimmunologic hydrops fetalis and congenital abnormalities. Obstet Gynecol 38:86, 1971.
3. Beretsky I, Lankin DH: Diagnosis of fetal cholelithisis using real-time high-resolution imaging employing digital detection. J Ultrasound Med 2:381, 1983.
4. Bergsmans MGM, Merkus JMW, Baars AM: Obstetrical and neonatal aspects of a child with atresia of the small bowel. J Perinat Med 12:325, 1984.
5. Blumenthal DH, Rushovich AM, Williams RK, et al.: Prenatal sonographic findings of meconium peritonitis with pathologic correlation. J Clin Ultrasound 10:350, 1982.

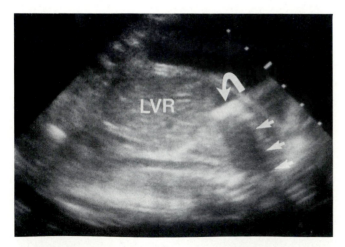

Figure 7–11. Longitudinal scan of the fetus shown in Figure 7–10. The intraabdominal calcification (*curved arrow*) is adjacent to the liver (LVR). Note the acoustic shadow (*arrowheads*).

6. Brock DJH, Bedgood D, Barron L, et al.: Prospective prenatal diagnosis of cystic fibrosis. Lancet 1:1175, 1985.

7. Brugman SM, Bjelland JJ, Thomasson JE, et al.: Sonographic findings with radiologic correlation in meconium peritonitis. J Clin Ultrasound 7:305, 1979.

8. Ceballos R, Hicks GM: Plastic peritonitis due to neonatal hydrometrocolpos: Radiologic and pathologic observations. J Pediatr Surg 5:63, 1970.

9. Clair MR, Rosenberg ER, Ram PC, et al.: Prenatal sonographic diagnosis of meconium peritonitis. Prenat Diagn 3:65, 1983.

9a. Dillard JP, Edwards DK, Leopold GR: Meconium peritonitis masquerading as fetal hydrops. J Ultrasound Med 6:49, 1987.

10. Finkel LI, Solvis TL: Meconium peritonitis, intraperitoneal calcifications and cystic fibrosis. Pediatr Radiol 12:92, 1982.

11. Garb M, Rad FF, Riseborough J: Meconium peritonitis presenting as fetal ascites on ultrasound. Br J Radiol 53:602, 1980.

12. Grybowski J, Walker WA: Gastrointestinal Problems in the Infant, 2d ed. Philadelphia, Saunders, 1983, p 260.

13. Kolawole TM, Bankole MA, Olurin EO, et al.: Meconium peritonitis presenting as giant cysts in neonates. Br J Radiol 46:964, 1973.

14. Lauer JD, Cradock TV: Meconium pseudocyst: Prenatal sonographic and antenatal radiologic correlation. J Ultrasound Med 1:333, 1982.

15. McGahan JP, Hanson F: Meconium peritonitis with accompanying pseudocyst: Prenatal sonographic diagnosis. Radiology 148:125, 1983.

16. Nancarrow PA, Mattrey RF, Edwards DK, et al.: Fibroadhesive meconium peritonitis: In utero sonographic diagnosis. J Ultrasound Med 4:213, 1985.

17. Schwimer SR, Vanley GT, Reinke RT: Prenatal diagnosis of cystic meconium peritonitis. J Clin Ultrasound 12:37, 1984.

Hirschsprung's Disease

Synonyms
Congenital intestinal aganglionosis, aganglionic megacolon, and anal aganglionosis.

Definition
Hirschsprung's disease is characterized by absence of the intramural myenteric parasympathetic ganglia in a segment of colon extending proximally from the anus to varying distances.

Incidence
This condition occurs in 1 in 8000 live births.[6] Males are affected more frequently than females.[3]

Embryology
The neuroblasts derived from the neural crest normally migrate to populate the stomach by the 6th week, the small bowel by the 7th week, the colon by the 8th week, and the rectum by the 12th week of development.[5] Neuroblasts continue to mature after birth up to 5 years of age. Hirschsprung's disease is thought to result from interrupted migration of the neuroblasts at different times of development before the 12th week or from failure of these cells to populate the full length of the gut. Alternatively, Hirschsprung's disease could be due to degeneration of normally migrated neuroblasts during prenatal or postnatal life.[4]

Etiology
In most cases, Hirschsprung's disease is a sporadic disorder. Four percent of the cases are familial, with a sex-modified multifactorial type of inheritance with a lower threshold in males. Families with the short segment of intestine variety (the rectum and sigmoid or rectum alone) have a higher incidence of affected males, whereas this sexual difference disappears in families with long segment involvement.[1] The recurrence risk for siblings of a proband is 10 percent in the long segment variety.[1,4] The possibility of an autosomal dominant variety with variable penetrance has been suggested in some cases.[4]

Pathology
The hallmark of the disease is the absence of the ganglion cells of the myenteric plexus. The involved area is usually limited to a segment of sigmoid or rectum. When involvement extends to the cecum, the condition is termed "long segment intestine variety" and is rare, accounting for only 6 to 21 percent of all cases.[3] In more rare instances, involvement is segmental, affecting the colon and sparing the rectum (skip aganglionosis). The term "total agangliosis coli" is used when the condition involves all the colon and a variable segment of small bowel; it accounts for 8 percent of all cases of Hirschsprung's disease.[3]

The symptoms of Hirschsprung's disease are due to a functional obstruction, since the aganglionic segment is unable to transmit the peristaltic wave.

Dilatation of the bowel proximal to the site of the obstruction will occur. Affected infants have a delay in the passage of meconium. Symptoms of the disease are constipation and abdominal distention. Rectal and colonic distention may cause obstructive uropathy.

Associated Anomalies

Two percent of patients have a chromosomal anomaly (frequently trisomy 21).[4] In a few infants, there is colonic atresia or imperforate anus.[7] Hirschsprung's disease has also been reported in association with neural tumors, such as neuroblastomas and pheochromocytomas, suggesting an embryologic disorder in the development of the neural crest or in the migration of neuroblasts from the neural crest.[2]

Diagnosis

Antenatal recognition of a bowel obstruction that ultimately proved to be Hirschsprung's disease has been made in one fetus.[9] The image was similar to that of intestinal obstruction. In another report, polyhydramnios and cystic areas thought to correspond to slightly dilated loops of bowel were seen.[8] Diagnostic considerations included Hirschsprung's disease, imperforate anus, and colonic atresia. The newborn underwent barium enema, which was inconclusive. Two months later, the infant had constipation and abdominal distention, and the diagnosis of Hirschsprung's disease was made on biopsy of the colon and rectum. Diagnosis with enzymatic analysis of amniotic fluid was attempted in one fetus,[4] but neither ultrasound nor disaccharidase activity in midtrimester amniotic fluid was helpful. Difficulties in prenatal diagnosis with enzymatic analysis may be due to lack of expression of the disease in the midtrimester. Indeed, only 70 to 80 percent of cases are diagnosed in the neonatal period.

Prognosis

In utero identification of a bowel obstruction later identified as caused by Hirschsprung's disease should avoid the complications of delayed diagnosis. These complications include enterocolitis, cecal per-foration, obstructive uropathy, malnutrition, and volvulus. The reported mortality is around 20 percent in infancy,[6] although this figure probably does not include those cases diagnosed during the neonatal period. The treatment consists of removal of the aganglionic segment of intestine. This may require a colostomy, with a deferred final repair.

Obstetrical Management

Hirschsprung's disease has not been diagnosed before viability. The diagnosis of bowel obstruction is an indication for serial examinations to exclude bowel perforation and meconium peritonitis. A precise diagnosis of Hirschsprung's disease seems difficult in the absence of a significant family history. Changes in standard obstetrical management are not indicated.

REFERENCES

1. Bodian M, Carter CO: A family study of Hirschsprung's disease. Ann Hum Genet 26:261, 1963.
2. Bower RJ, Adkins JC: Ondine's curse and neurocristopathy. Clin Pediatr 19:665, 1980.
3. Grybowski J, Walker WA: The gastrointestinal problems in the infant. Philadelphia, Saunders, 1983, pp 498–508.
4. Jarmas AL, Weaver DD, Padilla LM, et al.: Hirschsprung's disease: Etiologic implications of unsuccessful prenatal diagnosis. Am J Med Genet 16:163, 1983.
5. Okamoto E, Ueda T: Embryogenesis of intramural ganglia of the gut and its relation to Hirschsprung's disease. J Pediatr Surg 2:437, 1967.
6. Touloukian RJ: Colon aganglionosis. In: Bergsma D (ed): Birth Defects Compendium. New York, Alan R. Liss, 1979, pp 240–241.
7. Vanhoutte JV: Primary aganglionosis associated with imperforate anus: Review of the literature pertinent to one observation. J Pediatr Surg 4:468, 1969.
8. Vermesch M, Mayden KL, Confino E, et al.: Prenatal sonographic diagnosis of Hirschsprung's disease. J Ultrasound Med 5:37, 1986.
9. Wrobleski D, Wesselhoeft C: Ultrasonic diagnosis of prenatal intestinal obstruction. J Pediatr Surg 14:598, 1979.

Splenomegaly

The fetal spleen can be visualized in transverse scans of the fetal abdomen as a solid structure located behind the fetal stomach and lateral and cranial to the left kidney (Fig. 7–12). The echogenic texture of the spleen is similar to that of the kidney and is generally homogeneous. Nomograms are available for assessing the fetal spleen size. The longitudinal diameter (L) is measured in a transverse scan from the portion

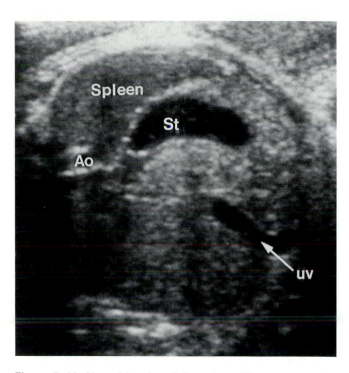

Figure 7–12. Normal location of the spleen. The organs can be visualized in a transverse scan as a structure posterior to the fetal stomach (st). Its echogenic texture is similar to that of the kidney. Ao, aorta; uv, umbilical vein.

of the organ closest to the anterior abdominal wall to the portion of the organ closest to the spine. The transverse diameter (T) is measured in the same plane, perpendicularly to the longitudinal diameter. The vertical diameter (V) is measured in a coronal plane. Spleen volume has been estimated by using the formula of the ellipsoid:

$$0.5233 \times L \times V \times T$$

Spleen perimeter is estimated using the formula of the ellipsoid:

$$\text{Spleen perimeter} = (\text{longitudinal} + \text{transverse}) \times 1.57$$

Nomograms for the assessment of splenomegaly have been derived and are displayed in Table 7–2.

Splenomegaly is suspected when the size of the spleen is above the 95th percentile. The correlation coefficient between spleen perimeter and gestational age is better than that between splenic volume and age (Figs. 7–13, 7–14).[3] Therefore, splenomegaly should probably be defined on the basis of spleen perimeter. The antenatal detection of splenomegaly has been reported once in the literature in a fetus with cytomegalovirus infection.[1] We have seen one case of spleno-

TABLE 7–2. FETAL SPLEEN DIAMETERS AND THE CALCULATED VOLUME AND PERIMETER

Gestational Age (weeks)	No. of Patients	Diameters (mm)									Volume (cm³)			Perimeter (mm)		
		Longitudinal			Vertical			Transverse								
		5th	Mean	95th	5th	Mean	95th	5th	Mean	95th	5th	Mean	95th	5th	Mean	95th
18	2	0.7	1.4	2.1	0.3	0.8	1.1	0.4	0.9	1.3	—	0.7	0.73	2.3	3.5	4.7
19	3	1.2	1.6	2.3	0.4	0.8	1.2	0.4	0.9	1.4	0.4	0.9	1.4	2.7	3.9	5.1
20	3	1.1	1.8	2.6	0.5	0.8	1.2	0.5	1.0	1.5	0.5	1.0	1.5	3.3	4.5	5.7
21	2	1.2	2.0	2.7	0.5	0.9	1.3	0.6	1.1	1.6	0.8	1.3	1.8	3.5	4.7	5.9
22	3	1.5	2.2	2.9	0.6	1.0	1.3	0.7	1.2	1.6	1.2	1.7	2.2	4.1	5.3	6.5
23	4	1.6	2.3	3.1	0.7	1.0	1.4	0.8	1.2	1.7	1.4	2.0	2.5	4.5	5.7	6.9
24	3	1.9	2.5	3.2	0.7	1.1	1.5	0.8	1.3	1.8	1.6	2.2	2.8	4.9	6.1	7.2
25	3	1.9	2.6	3.3	0.7	1.1	1.5	0.9	1.4	1.9	1.9	2.5	3.1	5.3	6.4	7.7
26	3	2.0	2.7	3.4	0.8	1.2	1.5	1.0	1.5	1.9	2.1	2.8	3.5	5.5	6.7	7.9
27	5	2.2	2.9	3.7	0.9	1.3	1.7	1.0	1.5	2.0	2.0	3.0	4.1	5.9	7.1	8.3
28	3	2.4	3.1	3.8	1.0	1.3	1.7	1.1	1.6	2.1	2.2	3.4	4.6	6.2	7.4	8.6
29	3	2.5	3.3	4.0	1.0	1.4	1.8	1.2	1.7	2.1	2.4	3.8	5.3	6.5	7.7	8.9
30	4	2.7	3.4	4.1	1.1	1.5	1.9	1.3	1.7	2.2	2.6	4.3	6.1	6.9	8.1	9.3
31	4	3.0	3.6	4.3	1.2	1.5	1.9	1.3	1.8	2.3	2.9	5.0	7.0	7.3	8.5	9.7
32	3	3.1	3.8	4.5	1.2	1.6	2.0	1.4	1.9	2.4	3.3	5.7	8.1	7.7	8.9	10.1
33	3	3.3	4.0	4.7	1.3	1.6	2.0	1.5	2.0	2.4	3.8	6.6	9.2	8.1	9.3	10.5
34	4	3.5	4.3	5.0	1.3	1.7	2.1	1.6	2.0	2.5	4.5	7.6	10.7	8.6	9.8	11.0
35	4	3.8	4.5	5.2	1.4	1.8	2.2	1.6	2.1	2.6	5.2	8.8	12.3	9.1	10.3	11.5
36	5	4.1	4.8	5.5	1.5	1.9	2.2	1.7	2.2	2.7	6.1	10.1	14.1	9.7	10.9	12.1
37	6	4.4	5.1	5.8	1.5	1.9	2.3	1.8	2.3	2.7	7.3	11.8	16.2	10.4	11.6	12.8
38	3	4.7	5.4	6.2	1.6	2.0	2.3	1.8	2.3	2.8	8.6	13.6	18.6	11.1	12.3	13.4
39	3	5.1	5.8	6.5	1.7	2.0	2.4	1.9	2.4	2.9	10.1	15.6	21.1	11.8	13.0	14.2
40	3	5.5	6.2	7.0	1.7	2.1	2.5	2.0	2.5	2.9	11.8	17.9	24.1	12.7	13.8	15.1

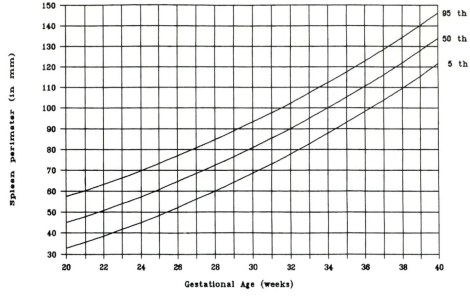

Figure 7–13. Growth of spleen perimeter with gestational age. *(Reproduced with permission from Schmidt et al.: J Ultrasound Med 4:667, 1985.)*

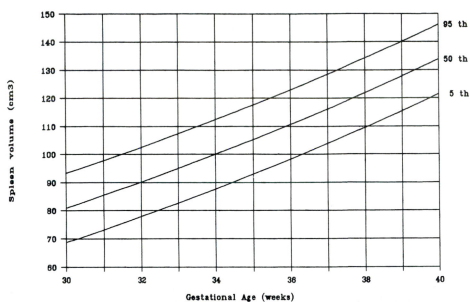

Figure 7–14. Growth of spleen volume with gestational age. *(Reproduced with permission from Schmidt et al.: J Ultrasound Med 4:667, 1985.)*

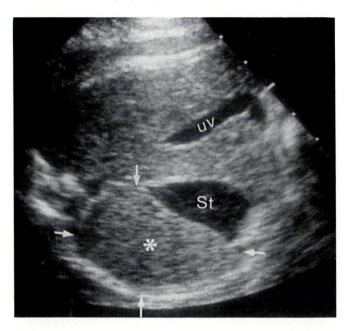

Figure 7–15. An enlarged spleen (∗) is visualized. The neonate had congenital syphilis. St, stomach; uv, umbilical vein.

TABLE 7–3. CAUSES OF SPLENOMEGALY IN NEONATAL PERIOD

Infection	Congestive heart failure
Bacterial	Neoplastic disorders
Viral (cytomegalovirus, rubella)	Leukemia
Syphilis	Lymphoma
Toxoplasmosis	Hamartoma
Hepatitis	Cysts
Hematologic conditions	Metabolic disorders
Isoimmunization	Other
Anemia	Beckwith-Wiedemann syndrome

megaly in an infant with congenital syphilis (Fig. 7–15). The differential diagnosis of splenomegaly in the newborn comprises a large number of entities, many of which are not amenable to prenatal diagnosis. In most cases, the cause of splenomegaly is infection (Table 7–3).[2,4] However, we have recently identified hepatosplenomegaly in a fetus diagnosed to have pyruvate kinase deficiency. More observations are required to formulate a coherent approach to the evaluation of these fetuses. Amniocentesis and percutaneous umbilical cord puncture are techniques that could be used for the prenatal diagnosis of some of these conditions.

REFERENCES

1. Eliezer S, Ester F, Ehund W, et al.: Fetal splenomegaly, ultrasound diagnosis of cytomegalovirus infection: A case report. J Clin Ultrasound 12:520, 1984.
2. Green M: Pediatric Diagnosis. Philadelphia, Saunders, 1986, pp 92–93.
3. Schmidt W, Yarkoni S, Jeanty P, et al.: Sonographic measurements of the fetal spleen: Clinical implications. J Ultrasound Med 4:667, 1985.
4. Tunnessen WW: Signs and Symptoms in Pediatrics. Philadelphia, Lippincott, 1983, pp 340–347.

Hepatomegaly

Isolated enlargement of the liver in the fetus is a rare finding. A nomogram for the evaluation of fetal liver size during the second half of pregnancy is available (Table 7–4).[15] The fetal liver length is measured in a paramedian section passing through the right liver lobe. The liver length is measured from the right hemidiaphragm to the tip of the right lobe (Fig. 7–16).

Isolated hepatomegaly is a rare finding. Liver enlargement is frequently associated with splenomegaly. Table 7–5 indicates the most common causes of hepatomegaly in the neonatal period.

Hemolytic anemias can be diagnosed either by umbilical cord puncture or analysis of the bilirubin content of amniotic fluid. Congenital infections can be ruled out by appropriate tests in maternal serum (VDRL, or serum titers for infectious agents) or fetal blood (e.g., IgM, liver function tests, specific rubella IgM). Microcephaly or hydrocephaly may be present in congenital rubella, toxoplasmosis, cytomegalovirus infection, or congenital syphilis.

Other syndromes, such as the Beckwith-Wiedemann syndrome, can be diagnosed prenatally with ultrasound (see p. 220). Zellweger syndrome has been diagnosed prenatally by culture of amniotic fluid cells and demonstration of the accumulation of very long chain fatty acids or of deficiency of both acyl-CoA-dihydroxyacetone phosphate acyltransferase and alkyl dihydroacetone phosphate synthase. These enzymes are crucial to the synthesis of plasmalogens.[13]

Liver tumors can cause hepatic enlargement or simply a change in the sonographic appearance of this organ. Hepatic hemangioma is a benign tumor that often appears as a large lesion with a hypoechogenic sonographic appearance.[1] It frequently results in arteriovenous shunting, leading to congestive heart failure and eventually to neonatal death.[2] In other circumstances, the tumor may rupture, causing shock and finally death.[5] A hemangioma has been detected prenatally in a 32-week-old infant as a well-circumscribed mass with a homogeneous appearance. Vessels were seen within the mass, and there were no signs of fetal hydrops.[12] After birth, the baby did well, and surgery was not required. In another antenatal visualization of this condition, high-output cardiac failure led to death in utero at 31 weeks' gestation (Fig. 7–17).[11]

Hepatoblastoma is the most frequent hepatic malignancy in fetal life. Its sonographic appearance is predominantly echogenic and may show areas of calcifications.[5] Alpha-fetoprotein levels are raised in 80 to 90 percent of cases.[10] Hepatoblastoma usually affects one lobe but is bilateral 30 percent of the time.[6]

TABLE 7–4. ULTRASOUND MEASUREMENTS OF THE FETAL LIVER

Gestational Age (weeks)	Liver Length (mm)		
	−2 SD	Mean	+2 SD
20	20.9	27.3	33.7
21	26.5	28.0	29.5
22	23.9	30.6	37.3
23	26.4	30.9	35.4
24	26.2	32.9	39.6
25	28.3	33.6	38.9
26	29.4	35.7	42.0
27	33.3	36.6	39.9
28	34.4	38.4	42.4
29	34.1	39.1	44.1
30	33.7	38.7	43.7
31	33.9	39.6	45.3
32	35.2	42.7	50.2
33	37.2	43.8	50.4
34	37.7	44.8	51.9
35	38.7	47.8	56.9
36	41.4	49.0	57.4
37	45.2	52.0	58.8
38	48.7	52.9	57.1
39	48.7	55.4	62.1
40	*	59.0	*

* Measurement obtained from only one fetus.
Modified with permission from Vintzileos et al.: Obstet Gynecol 66:477, 1985.

TABLE 7–5. COMMON CAUSES OF HEPATOMEGALY

Infectious causes
  Hepatitis
  Cytomegalovirus infection
  Rubella
  Toxoplasmosis
  Syphilis
  Varicella
  Coxsackievirus infection
Congenital anemia
  Congenital hemolytic anemias, such as spherocytosis
  Isoimmunization
Congestive heart failure
Hepatic tumors
  Mesenchymal hamartoma
  Hemangioma
  Metastatic neuroblastoma
  Hepatoblastoma
  Hemangiopericytoma
Metabolic disorders
  Galactosemia (AR)*
  Tyrosinemia (probably AR)
  Alpha$_1$-antitrypsin deficiency (AR)
  Disorders of the urea cycle (AR)
  Methylmalonic acidemia (probably AR)
  Infantile sialidosis (AR)
Genetic disorders
  Beckwith-Wiedemann syndrome (sporadic, some familial cases)
  Zellweger syndrome (AR)
Hepatic cysts
  Adult polycystic disease of liver and kidneys
  Solitary cyst

* Autosomal recessive.

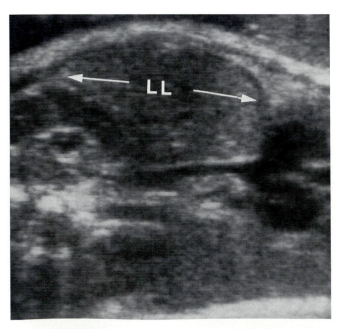

Figure 7–16. Longitudinal scan of fetal liver showing measurement of liver length (LL).

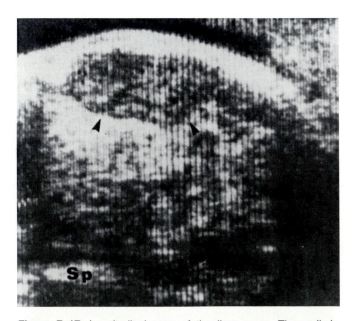

Figure 7–17. Longitudinal scan of the liver mass. The well-circumscribed borders and the homogeneity of the mass can be seen. Vessels were seen within the mass. Sp, spine. (Reproduced with permission from Platt et al.: J Ultrasound Med 2:521, 1983.)

Treatment is aimed at surgical excision, which carries a mortality of 20 to 25 percent.[10] At a 5-year follow-up, survival rate was 36 percent.[7] The tumor may lead to death from rupture, presumably during delivery.[5]

Mesenchymal hamartoma of the liver is a developmental abnormality rather than a true neoplasm. It generally appears as an irregular mass with cystic components that may fill the entire abdomen. Most hamartomas are detected in the first year of life. Histologically, hepatic hamartoma is characterized by an admixture of vascular and epithelial components. Overlapping between the histologic picture of a hamartoma and that of a hemangioma can occur. Calcifications may also be present.[1] Prenatal identification of this lesion was reported in a 33-week-old fetus whose fetal abdomen showed several hypoechoic masses that replaced the liver parenchyma. The infant was stillborn.[8] The available literature on hamartomas is based on infants diagnosed after birth. Most infants die from complications of surgery or events unrelated to the hamartoma.[8]

Hepatic calcifications can occur with fetal tumors, such as hepatoblastomas, and intrauterine infections.[14] We have seen cases of hepatic calcification without any demonstrable pathologic significance. Other authors have reported a similar finding.[4]

Asymptomatic hepatic cysts are found in about 30 percent of patients with adult polycystic disease of the kidney (APDK).[9] In these patients, renal involvement is usually minimal. Less frequently, cysts are found also in the pancreas, spleen, lung, ovary, and other organs.[9] The frequency of hepatic involvement in patients with an early onset of APDK in the fetal or neonatal period is unknown.

A solitary unilocular hepatic cyst has been detected antenatally at the 27th week of gestation.[3] It was shown to grow in subsequent ultrasonic examinations, and by the end of gestation, it measured 11 × 10 cm. At surgery, the cyst was noted to replace the entire left lobe of the liver. Postoperatively, the newborn did well.

REFERENCES

1. Abramson SJ, Lack EE, Teele RL: Benign vascular tumors of the liver in infants: Sonographic appearance. AJR 138:629, 1982.
2. Berdon WE, Baker DH: Giant hepatic hemangioma with cardiac failure in the newborn infant. Radiology 92:1523, 1969.
3. Chung WM: Antenatal detection of hepatic cyst. J Clin Ultrasound 14:217, 1986.
4. Corson VL, Sanders RC, Johnson TRB, et al.: Midtrimester fetal ultrasound: Diagnostic dilemmas. Prenat Diagn 3:47, 1983.
5. Cremin BJ, Nuss D: Calcified hepatoblastoma in a newborn. J Pediatr Surg 9:913, 1974.
6. Exelby PR, Filler RM, Grosfeld JL: Liver tumors in children in the particular reference to hepatoblastoma and hepatocellular carcinoma. American Academy of Pediatrics Surgical Section Survey—1974. J Pediatr Surg 10:329, 1975.
7. Foster JH, Berman MM: Major Problems in Clinic Surgery. Solid Liver Tumors. Philadelphia, Saunders, 1977, Vol. 22.
8. Foucar E, Williamson RA, Yiu-Chiu V, et al.: Mesenchymal hamartoma of the liver identified by fetal sonography. AJR 140:970, 1983.
9. Hartnett M, Bennett W: Extrarenal manifestations of cystic kidney disease. In: Gardner KD Jr (ed): Cystic Diseases of the Kidney. New York, Wiley, 1976, pp 201–219.
10. Murray-Lyon IM: Primary and secondary cancer of the liver. In: Gazet JC (ed): Carcinoma of the Liver, Biliary Tract and Pancreas. London, Arnold, 1983, pp 57–59.
11. Nakamoto SK, Dreilinger A, Dattel B, et al.: The sonographic appearance of hepatic hemangioma in utero. J Ultrasound Med 2:239, 1983.
12. Platt LD, Devore GR, Benner P, et al.: Antenatal diagnosis of a fetal liver mass. J Ultrasound Med 2:521, 1983.
13. Schutgens RBH, Schrakamp G, Wanders RJA, et al.: The cerebro-hepatorenal (Zellweger) syndrome: Prenatal detection based on impaired biosynthesis of plasmalogens. Prenat Diagn 5:337, 1985.
14. Shackelford GD, Kirks DR: Neonatal hepatic calcification secondary to transplacental infection. Pediatr Radiol 122:753, 1977.
15. Vintzileos AM, Neckles S, Campbell WA, et al.: Fetal liver ultrasound measurements during normal pregnancy. Obstet Gynecol 66:477, 1985.

Choledochal Cyst

Synonym
Cystic dilatation of the common bile duct.

Definition
Presence of a single cyst or, in rare instances, multiple cysts along the normal bile ducts, usually found in the common bile duct (ductus choledochus; hence, the name).

Etiology
Unknown. Sporadic occurrence is the rule. No famil-

TABLE 7–6. CLASSIFICATION OF ANOMALIES OF THE BILIARY TREE

I. Common
    A. Choledochal cyst
    B. Segmental dilatation
    C. Diffuse dilatation
II. Diverticulum type in the entire extrahepatic duct
III. Choledochocele
IV. Multiple cysts
    A. In intrahepatic and extrahepatic ducts
    B. In extrahepatic ducts
V. Intrahepatic cysts

ial cases have been reported. In twin pregnancies, only one twin is affected.[4]

Incidence

It is a rare disorder in the western world. Two thirds of the cases are reported in Japan. The male to female ratio is 1:3.5.[6,9]

Embryology of the Bile Ducts

The bile ducts arise from diverticula of the gut. The proximal portions form the common bile duct, the cystic duct (whose terminal dilatation will eventually become the gallbladder), and the hepatic ducts. Further branching of the hepatic ducts give rise to the secretory tubules of the liver.

Etiology

The pathogenesis of choledochal cysts is controversial. A choledocal cyst can be due to (1) segmental weakness of the wall of the common bile duct, which leads to dilatation, (2) obstruction of the distal part of the common bile duct, with increased back pressure and secondary dilatation of the proximal portion of the duct, or (3) a combination of these two factors. The observations that cystic dilatations can occur in different locations and take different shapes (Table 7–6), and that obstruction is not always a feature suggest that different factors may play a role in the pathogenesis of the cyst.[7]

Pathology

The cysts can be single or multiple and can involve the intrahepatic or extrahepatic portions of the biliary tree. Various classifications have been proposed. A recent[8] classification is reported in Table 7–6. Type IA is the most common cyst of the biliary tract. This variety has been identified in all prenatal diagnoses (choledochal cyst). The gallbladder is usually not affected by the cyst, but hepatic biliary cirrhosis may develop.

Diagnosis

A handful of cases of antenatal visualization of a choledochal cyst are reported in the English literature.[1–3,5] The cyst appeared as an echo-free,

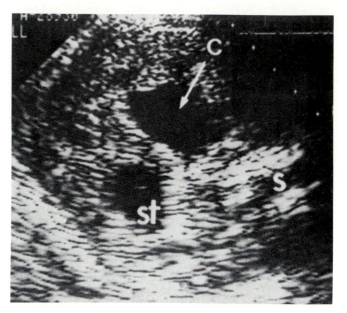

Figure 7–18. Transverse scan demonstrating the relationship of the choledochal cyst (c) to the stomach (st) and fetal spine (s). *(Reproduced with permission from Elrad et al.: J Ultrasound Med 4:553, 1985.)*

nonpulsatile mass in the right side of the fetal abdomen, near the portal vein. A correct diagnosis has been made in two patients[2,5] based on visualization of dilated hepatic ducts adjacent or leading to the cyst. The cyst did not measure more than 3 × 3 cm. The earliest visualization was at 25 weeks gestation.[3]

Differential diagnosis includes primarily duodenal atresia. Cysts in other organs, such as ovaries, mesentery, liver, pancreas, and omentum, should also be considered. In these cases, a normal fetal stomach, gallbladder, and kidneys can be identified, thus excluding these organs as the origin of the cyst (Fig. 7–18). The absence of polyhydramnios, of peristalsis inside the mass, and of any connection between the cyst and the stomach, which is not dilated, help in excluding duodenal atresia. A definite diagnosis relies on the finding of tubular structures arising from the cyst into the hepatic parenchyma (Fig. 7–19).

Prognosis

If the diagnosis of choledochal cysts is confirmed in the postnatal period, the neonate will require an operation.[5,6,9] Untreated choledochal cysts generally lead to progressive biliary cirrhosis and portal hypertension.[4] The size of the cyst and the presence of biliary obstruction are prognostic factors that determine the timing and severity of the clinical manifestations.[4] Obstruction accelerates the onset of symptoms.[9] Other complications of choledocal cysts include the development of calculi (8 percent), cyst rupture (1.8 percent), and development of adenocarcinoma (3.2 percent).[9]

Most fetuses diagnosed prenatally have been

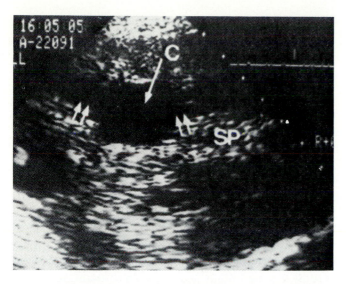

Figure 7–19. Transverse scan showing tubular structures (*arrows*) at both ends of the cystic mass (C). SP, spine. *(Reproduced with permission from Elrad et al.: J Ultrasound Med 4:553, 1985.)*

operated on during the neonatal period. The rationale has been to prevent biliary complications, since even in cases without obstruction, oral feedings stimulate bile production, leading to recurrent bouts of cholangitis and hepatic fibrosis.[5] In one infant in whom the obstruction occurred distal to the cyst, liver biliary cirrhosis was already present at 10 days after birth.[1] The reported operative mortality rate in the latest studies is about 10 percent.[9]

Obstetrical Management
Choledochal cysts are generally diagnosed in the late second–early third trimester.[5] The observation that some infants with choledochal cysts have meconium

in the bowel would support the view that the cysts developed relatively late in gestation. Furthermore, in one patient, the cyst appeared at the 31st week and had not been detected in previous examinations, confirming late development.[5]

There does not seem to be a need to change standard obstetrical management when the diagnosis is made after viability.

REFERENCES

1. Dewbury KC, Aluwihare APR, Chir M, et al.: Case reports. Prenatal ultrasound demonstration of a choledochal cyst. Br J Radiol 53:906, 1980.
2. Elrad H, Mayden KL, Ahart S, et al.: Prenatal ultrasound diagnosis of choledochal cyst. J Ultrasound Med 4:553, 1985.
3. Frank JL, Hill MC, Chirathivat S, et al.: Antenatal observation of a choledochal cyst by sonography. AJR 137:166, 1981.
4. Grybowski J, Walker WA: Gastrointestinal Problems in the Infant, 2d ed. Philadelphia, Saunders, 1983, pp 309–312.
5. Howell CG, Templeton JM, Weiner S, et al.: Antenatal diagnosis and early surgery for choledochal cyst. J Pediatr Surg 18:387, 1983.
6. Saito S: Choledochal cyst in infants. Am J Dis Child 126:533, 1973.
7. Saito S, Ishida M: Congenital choledochal cyst (cystic dilatation of the common bile duct). Prog Pediatr Surg 6:63, 1974.
8. Todani T, Watanabe Y, Narusue M, et al.: Congenital bile duct cysts: Classification, operative procedures and review of 37 cases, including cancer arising from choledochal cyst. Am J Surg 134:263, 1977.
9. Yamaguchi M: Congenital choledochal cyst. Analysis of 1,433 patients in the Japanese literature. Am J Surg 140: 653, 1980.

Mesenteric, Omental, and Retroperitoneal Cysts

Definition
These cysts may be located in the small or large bowel mesentery (mesenteric cysts), in the omentum (omental cysts), or in the retroperitoneal space (retroperitoneal cysts). They contain a clear amber fluid, with a serous or chylous appearance.[1]

Incidence
Rare. Only about 700 cases of mesenteric cysts and 150 cases of omental cysts have been reported in the world literature.[1,4] Retroperitonal cysts are even more rare.

Etiology
The cause of congenital mesenteric, omental, or-retroperitoneal cysts is unknown. They could be secondary to an obstruction of lymphatic vessels or ectopic lymphatic tissue. Since no obstruction of lymphatic vessels has ever been demonstrated on lymphangiography, these cysts are generally considered lymphatic hamartomas.[4]

Pathology
The cysts are most often single and multilocular[1] and may vary in size up to several centimeters. They are

lined by mesothelial cells, and the fluid may be serous, chylous, or occasionally, hemorrhagic. The most common location of mesenteric cysts is in the small bowel mesentery (78 percent of cases).[2] Most of the omental cysts are contained within the omentum, but on occasion they may be pedunculated.[1]

Diagnosis

Mesenteric or omental cysts should be considered in the differential diagnosis of an intraabdominal cystic lesion. Other conditions that should be considered include ovarian, pancreatic, choledochal, and hepatic cysts and lesions, such as duodenal atresia. In a female infant, the most common cause of a hypoechogenic intraabdominal lesion is an ovarian cyst. A choledochal cyst should be suspected when ducts corresponding to the biliary tree are seen on both sides of the hypoechogenic mass. Hepatic cysts are generally surrounded by liver parenchyma. In duodenal atresia, communication between the two bubbles can be demonstrated. A precise diagnosis of mesenteric cyst may be impossible. Omental cysts tend to be mobile.

Prognosis

These cysts are frequently asymptomatic and may be an incidental finding at surgery. Clinical manifestation of omental, retroperitoneal, and mesenteric cysts are related to the size and location of the lesion. Omental cysts may occur as a progressive abdominal enlargement or may twist, rupture, bleed, or lead to intestinal obstruction.[3] Surgery is the definitive treatment.

In mesenteric cysts, as in omental cysts, the symptoms may be acute or chronic. Malignant degeneration in adulthood has been described[2] and may lead to death. In half of the patients, surgical enucleation of the cyst cannot be accomplished, and bowel resections may be required.[2]

Retroperitoneal cysts have a high tendency to recur (22 percent in Kurtz' series) because their proximity to major blood vessels makes total excision difficult.[2] Unless intraabdominal cysts are giant and there is fear of rupture, their presence probably should not alter standard obstetrical management.

REFERENCES

1. Grybowski J, Walker WA: Gastrointestinal problems in the infant, 2d ed. Philadelphia, Saunders, 1983, pp 271–274.
2. Kurtz RJ, Heimann TM, Beck AR, et al.: Mesenteric and retroperitoneal cysts. Ann Surg 203:109, 1986.
3. Oliver GA: The omental cyst: A rare cause of acute abdominal crisis. Surgery 56:588, 1964.
4. Vanek VW, Phillips AK: Retroperitoneal, mesenteric and omental cysts. Arch Surg 119:838, 1984.

TABLE 7–7. MEASUREMENTS OF THE DIAMETERS OF THE FETAL STOMACH

Gestational Age (wk)	N	Anteroposterior (cm)	Transverse (cm)	Longitudinal (cm)
13–15	15	0.4 ± 0.1	0.6 ± 0.2	0.9 ± 0.3
16–18	29	0.6 ± 0.2	0.8 ± 0.2	1.3 ± 0.4
19–21	17	0.8 ± 0.2	0.9 ± 0.2	1.6 ± 0.5
22–24	11	0.9 ± 0.3	1.8 ± 0.3	1.9 ± 0.6
25–27	14	1.0 ± 0.5	1.9 ± 0.5	2.3 ± 1.0
28–30	17	1.2 ± 0.3	1.6 ± 0.4	2.3 ± 0.5
31–33	18	1.4 ± 0.3	1.6 ± 0.4	2.8 ± 0.9
34–36	15	1.4 ± 0.4	1.6 ± 0.4	2.8 ± 0.9
37–39	16	1.6 ± 0.4	2.0 ± 0.4	3.2 ± 0.9

Data are presented as mean ± 2SD.
Reproduced with permission from Goldstein, Reece, Yarkoni, et al.: Growth of the fetal stomach in normal pregnancies. Obstet Gynecol 70: (in press), 1987.

TABLE 7–8. TRANSVERSE COLONIC DIAMETER ACROSS GESTATIONAL AGE

Gestational Age (wk)	Percentile (cm)		
	10th	50th	90th
26	0.1	0.5	0.9
27	0.2	0.5	0.9
28	0.3	0.6	1.0
29	0.4	0.7	1.1
30	0.4	0.8	1.1
31	0.5	0.8	1.2
32	0.6	0.9	1.3
33	0.6	1.0	1.3
34	0.7	1.1	1.4
35	0.8	1.1	1.5
36	0.9	1.2	1.6
37	1.0	1.3	1.7
38	1.1	1.4	1.8
39	1.2	1.5	1.9
40	1.3	1.6	2.0
41	1.4	1.7	2.1
42	1.5	1.9	2.2

Reproduced with permission from Goldstein, Lockwood, Hobbins: Ultrasound assessment of fetal intestinal development in the evaluation of gestational age. Obstet Gynecol (in press), 1987.

8

The Urinary Tract and Adrenal Glands

Normal Anatomy of the Urinary Tract

Embryology

The three embryonic kidneys are the pronephros, mesonephros, and metanephros. The first two degenerate during fetal life but are important inducers of the development of the third. The ureteral bud, derived from the wolffian duct, grows toward the metanephros and induces differentiation of the nephrogenic blastema into renal parenchyma. The actively growing part of the ureteral bud, the ampulla, undergoes multiple divisions, induces the development of nephrons, and establishes communications with them. This activity continues throughout gestation until the 32d to 36th weeks. The ureteral bud gives rise to the renal pelvis, calyces, papillae, and collecting tubules, whereas the metanephric blastema gives origin to the nephron (glomeruli, proximal and distal convoluted tubules, and Henle's loop). The differentiation, elongation, and maturation of the components of the nephron continue even after birth.[6]

The metanephros is originally located in the fetal pelvis. Rapid growth of the caudal portion of the embryo results in displacement of the kidneys cephalad until they reach their normal position in the lumbar fossae. Abnormalities in this process result in ectopic kidneys. The renal pelves are initially directed anteriorly. They rotate so that the hilum of the kidney and calyces are directed medially at the end of

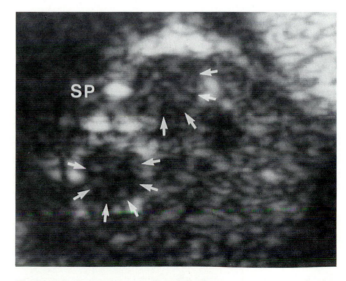

Figure 8–1. Transverse section of the fetal abdomen at 16 weeks. Arrows delineate kidneys. Sp, spine.

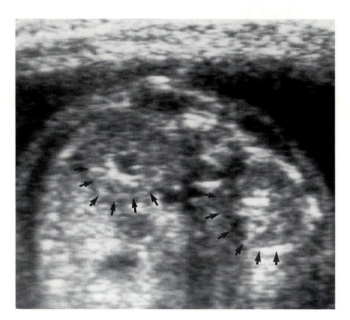

Figure 8–2. Transverse scan of a 27-week fetus. Arrows delineate the two kidneys. The pelvocaliceal system and capsule are visible.

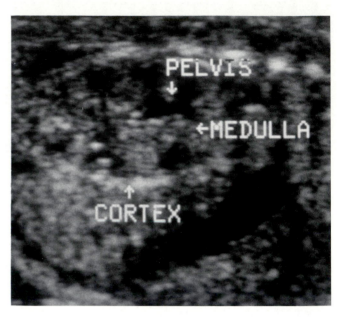

Figure 8–3. Longitudinal scan of a fetal kidney in late third trimester.

TABLE 8–1. NORMAL SIZE VALUES OF KIDNEY DIMENSIONS

Age (weeks)	Kidney Thickness (mm)			Kidney Width (mm)			Kidney Length (mm)			Kidney Volume (cm³)		
	5th	50th	95th	5th	50th	95th	5th	50th	95th	5th	50th	95th
16	2	6	10	6	10	13	7	13	18	—	0.4	2.6
17	3	7	11	6	10	14	10	15	20	—	0.6	2.8
18	4	8	12	6	10	14	12	17	22	—	0.7	2.9
19	5	9	13	7	10	14	14	19	24	—	0.9	3.1
20	6	10	13	7	11	15	15	21	26	—	1.1	3.3
21	6	10	14	8	12	15	17	22	28	—	1.4	3.6
22	7	11	15	8	12	16	19	24	29	—	1.7	3.9
23	8	12	16	9	13	17	21	26	31	—	2.1	4.3
24	9	13	17	10	14	18	22	28	33	0.3	2.5	4.7
25	10	14	18	11	15	19	24	29	34	0.8	3.0	5.2
26	11	15	19	12	16	19	25	31	36	1.3	3.5	5.7
27	11	15	19	12	16	20	27	32	37	1.9	4.1	6.3
28	12	16	20	13	17	21	28	33	38	2.5	4.7	6.9
29	13	17	21	14	18	22	29	35	40	3.2	5.4	7.6
30	14	18	22	15	19	23	31	36	41	3.9	6.1	8.3
31	14	18	22	16	20	24	32	37	42	4.6	6.8	9.0
32	15	19	23	17	20	24	33	38	43	5.4	7.5	9.7
33	16	20	23	17	21	25	34	39	44	6.1	8.3	10.5
34	16	20	24	18	22	26	35	40	45	6.8	9.0	11.2
35	17	21	25	18	22	26	35	41	46	7.4	9.6	11.8
36	17	21	25	19	23	27	36	41	47	8.1	10.2	12.4
37	18	22	26	19	23	27	37	42	47	8.6	10.8	13.0
38	18	22	26	19	23	27	37	43	48	9.0	11.2	13.4
39	19	23	27	19	23	27	38	43	48	9.4	11.6	13.8
40	19	23	27	19	23	27	38	44	49	9.6	11.8	14.0

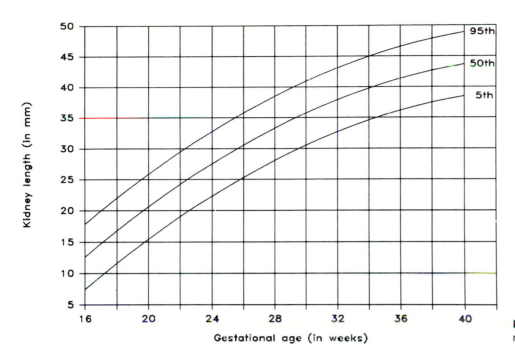

Figure 8–4. Relationship between kidney length and gestational age.

embryogenesis. Fusion of the kidneys to form a horseshoe kidney often occurs at the level of the lower pole.

The pathogenesis of renal congenital anomalies is poorly understood. The timing of the insult is responsible for the type of anomaly. For example, if the insult occurs within 5 weeks after conception, failure of communication between the ureteral bud and the metanephric blastema results in renal agenesis. Disturbances occurring immediately after union of these two structures would result in dysplastic cystic kidneys. If the insult takes place after most of the structural development of the kidney has occurred, a milder form of cystic kidney disease (Potter syndrome type IV) or hydronephrosis will ensue.

Sonographic Anatomy

The kidneys can be imaged as early as $9\frac{1}{2}$ weeks into gestation.[5] In early pregnancy, the kidneys appear as hypoechogenic, oval structures in the posterior midabdomen (Fig. 8–1). As the kidney matures, the pelvocaliceal system appears as an echo-poor structure (Fig. 8–2). The capsule becomes more visible,

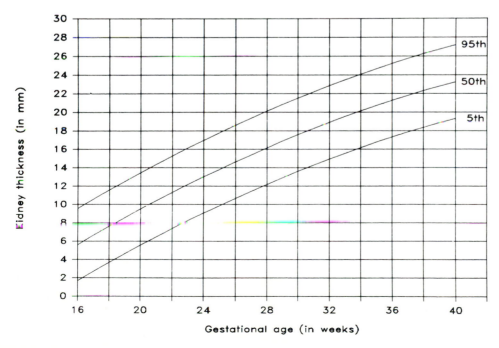

Figure 8–5. Relationship between kidney thickness and gestational age.

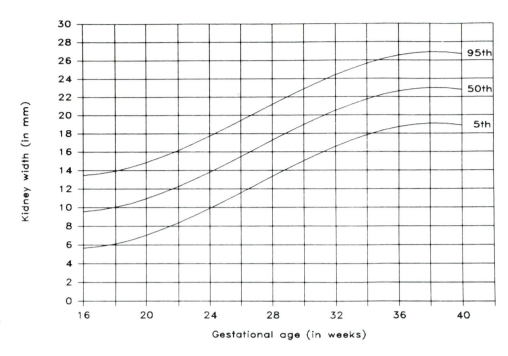

Figure 8–6. Relationship between kidney width and gestational age.

and the distinction between the pyramids and the cortex becomes apparent during the third trimester (Fig. 8–3). With high-resolution equipment, the arcuate arteries can be seen as little, bright echoes that are parallel to the cortex.

Renal biometry can be assessed quite readily.[1,3,4] The renal length is measured from the upper pole to the lower pole of the kidney in a longitudinal section of the fetus in a scan that is parallel to the long axis of the aorta. It is important to avoid using an oblique cut through the kidney. A practical hint is to keep the aorta in the same scan. The thickness, width, and

perimeter of the kidney are measured in a transverse section of the kidney. This section is obtained at the level of the renal pelvis, if visible; otherwise, it is obtained at the level where the renal section is the largest. Normal biometry is shown in Table 8–1 (Figs. 8–4 through 8–7). Caliper positioning can be difficult because of the low contrast between the renal parenchyma and the surrounding tissues. Respiratory movements, when present, are extremely helpful in defining the cleavage plane between the kidney and the adrenal glands, spleen, liver, and bowel.

The ratio of the kidney perimeter to the abdominal

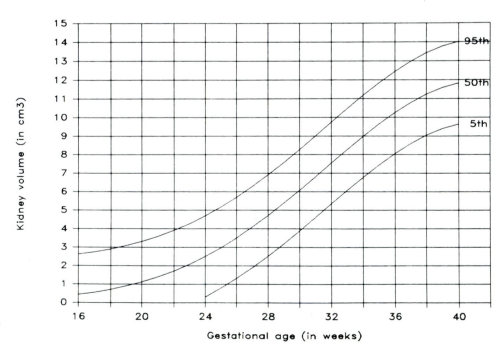

Figure 8–7. Growth of kidney volume through gestational age.

TABLE 8–2. KIDNEY PERIMETER TO ABDOMINAL PERIMETER RATIO

Gestational Age (weeks)	Ratio (%)	Percentile 5th	Percentile 95th
<17	28	24	32
17–20	30	24	36
21–25	30	26	34
26–30	29	24	33
31–35	28	22	34
36–40	27	19	35

Reproduced with permission from Jeanty, Romero: Obstetrical Ultrasound. New York, McGraw-Hill, 1983, p 146.

perimeter is a simple screening procedure for renal anomalies.[3] The ratio can be either computed or measured with a digitizer or a map reader.

The computed kidney perimeter to abdominal perimeter ratio is calculated as follows:

$$\text{Ratio} = \frac{(\text{kidney width} + \text{kidney thickness})}{(\text{anteroposterior abdominal diameter} + \text{transverse abdominal diameter})}$$

The normal values for the kidney perimeter to abdominal perimeter ratio are shown in Table 8–2.

The normal fetal bladder can be visualized as early as the 13th week of gestation. Changes in the size of this organ are generally apparent during the course of a sonographic examination because the fetus empties its bladder every 30 to 45 minutes. A technique for the calculation of fetal bladder volume has been proposed by Campbell et al.[2,7] They obtained three bladder diameters and use the formula:

$$\frac{\text{Bladder}}{\text{volume}} = \frac{4/3 \times \pi \times \text{diameter } a/2 \times}{\text{diameter } b/2 \times \text{diameter } c/2}$$

Diameter a is obtained from the bladder fundus to the bladder neck, diameter b is the maximum transverse diameter, and diameter c is the maximum anteroposterior diameter. Hourly urinary output was calculated

by doing serial examinations at 15 to 30 minute intervals. The urinary output increased with progressive gestational age from a mean of 12.2 ml/hr at 32 weeks to 28 ml/hr at 40 weeks.[7] The bladder walls are normally thin but in the presence of obstruction, they may undergo hypertrophy.

This chapter focuses on the most common renal abnormalities and tumors of the kidney. Bilateral renal agenesis, cystic diseases of the kidney, obstructive uropathies, and tumors will be discussed. Recently, Hill et al. have shown that ultrasound can identify pelvic kidneys in the fetus. Ectopic kidneys are found in 1:1200 autopsies but the frequency reported in clinical studies is 1:10,000. This suggests that they are frequently asymptomatic. Ectopic kidneys should be suspected when both kidneys are not seen in their normal position in a transverse scan of the fetal trunk. They may be associated with an increased incidence of hydronephrosis and other congenital anomalies involving the cardiovascular, skeletal, and gastrointestinal tracts.[3a]

REFERENCES
1. Bertagnoli L, Lalatta F, Gallicchio R, et al.: Quantitative characterization of the growth of the fetal kidney. J Clin Ultrasound 11:349, 1983.
2. Campbell S, Wladimiroff JW, Dewhurst CJ: The antenatal measurement of fetal urine production. J Obstet Gynaecol Br Commonw 80:680, 1973.
3. Grannum P, Bracken M, Silverman R, et al.: Assessment of fetal kidney size in normal gestation by comparison of ratio of kidney circumference to abdominal circumference. Am J Obstet Gynecol 136:249, 1980.
3a. Hill LM, Peterson CS: Antenatal diagnosis of fetal pelvic kidneys. J Ultrasound Med 6:393, 1987.
4. Jeanty P, Dramaix-Wilmet M, Elkhazen N, et al: Measurement of fetal kidney growth on ultrasound. Radiology 144:159, 1982.
5. Mahony BS, Filly RA: The genitourinary system in utero. Clin Diagn Ultrasound 18:1, 1986.
6. Potter EL: Normal and Abnormal Development of the Kidney. Chicago, Year Book, 1972.
7. Wladimiroff JW, Campbell S: Fetal urine-production rates in normal and complicated pregnancy. Lancet 1:151, 1974.

Bilateral Renal Agenesis

Definition
Bilateral absence of kidneys.

Epidemiology
The incidence of bilateral renal agenesis (BRA) varies between 0.1 and 0.3 per 1000 births.[11,16,45,57,60,74] The male to female ratio is 2.5:1.[17,57,58,74]

Etiology
BRA can be an isolated finding, or less frequently, it can be part of a syndrome. Syndromic BRA can occur in conjunction with the following disorders:

Chromosomal Disorders
1. Familial marker chromosome[24] involves the pres-

ence of an abnormal, small, extra chromosome, possibly a segment of chromosome 22.

2. Cat's eye syndrome[23] is characterized by iris coloboma, anal atresia, preauricular tags, and renal anomalies. It is probably due to a small, extra acrocentric autosome.

3. 4p-Syndrome[49] is characterized by multiple heterotopies of cells (in adrenals, brain, pancreas, and skin) and BRA. Cardiac, facial, and genital anomalies have been reported as well.

Autosomal Recessive Disorders

1. Fraser syndrome consists of cryptophthalmos (partial or complete absence of eyelid), syndactyly, auditory canal atresia, cleft palate, and malformation of the external genitalia. BRA and laryngeal atresia are less constant findings of the syndrome.[10,17,19,47,51]

2. Cerebro-oculo-facio-skeletal syndrome is a complex syndrome with some of the following abnormalities: microcephaly, microphthalmia, narrow palpebral fissures, high nasal bridge, large ears, micrognathia, kyphosis, scoliosis, flexion contraction of the extremities, and rocker-bottom foot. The prognosis is poor, and most infants die within the first 3 years of life.[59]

3. Acro-renal-mandibular syndrome[33] is characterized by severe split-hand/split-foot anomaly, renal and genital malformation: bilateral renal agenesis with lens prolapse and cataracts,[8] and syndrome of renal, genital, and middle ear abnormalities.[76]

Autosomal Dominant Disorders

1. Branchio-oto-renal syndrome[14] consists of preauricular pits, branchial fistulas, and renal anomalies.

2. Müllerian duct anomalies and renal agenesis.[7,6]

Nonmendelian Disorders. Other associations with BRA have been described suggesting a genetic basis. They include agnathia, tracheoesophageal fistula, duodenal atresia and renal agenesis,[65] VATER (vertebral defects, anal atresia, tracheoesophageal fistula, radial and renal dysplasia) association,[20,72] congenital cystic adenomatous malformation,[43] renal agenesis with cardiovascular and skeletal abnormalities,[38] and hypothalamic–hamartoma syndrome.[34]

Sporadic Syndromes. Some teratogenic conditions, such as diabetes mellitus, have been associated with BRA.[30,44,55]

Nonsyndromic BRA. Several patterns of inheritance have been proposed for familial cases of BRA, including autosomal recessive,[12,31,42,61,67,73] X-linked recessive,[54] and multifactorial.[9] In the largest available

series, the risk of a second affected sibling when recognized syndromes are excluded, ranges from 3.5 to 5.9 percent.[4,17,63] This frequency is too high to be explained purely on the basis of a multifactorial inheritance pattern. An alternative explanation is heterogeneity of cases included in the reported series. Indeed, they may have included cases of BRA as isolated malformation sequence inherited with a multifactorial pattern as well as BRA associated with mendelian syndromes (i.e., in families in which individuals have other renal anomalies).[25,66,74,79] In these cases, BRA may be a severe manifestation of an autosomal dominant gene with reduced penetrance and variable expressivity, milder in females and more severe in males.[9,20,52,75]

Risk of Recurrence

The etiology of BRA is not clear. In the presence of chromosomal defects, the risk of recurrence depends on the parents' karyotypes. Autosomal recessive and autosomal dominant syndromes have a 25 and 50 percent risk of recurrence, respectively.

In nonsyndromic cases, parents can be counseled with the following information:

1. The first relatives of a patient with BRA have an increased risk (13 percent) of having silent unilateral renal agenesis. In parents with two affected infants, the risk of silent renal anomalies increases to 30 percent.[63] Therefore, screening parents with ultrasound is indicated.

2. The risk of having another affected child is increased to 3 percent. This risk is higher if either parent has unilateral renal agenesis.[15] When BRA is part of a multiple malformation syndrome, the rate of malformed infants is 12.5 percent, and the risk of BRA is lower.[4] The high frequency of birth defects in this group suggests an autosomal recessive syndrome.

3. Infants of affected families are at risk not only for BRA but also for unilateral renal agenesis and renal dysplasia.[26] The risk for sirenomelia or caudal regression is probably not increased, since these represent a different genetic defect.[26,52]

Embryology

The three embryonic kidneys are the pronephros, mesonephros, and metanephros. The first two degenerate during fetal life but are important inducers of the development of the third. The ureteral bud, derived from the wolffian duct, grows toward the metanephros and induces differentiation of the nephrogenic blastema into renal parenchyma.

Renal agenesis might result from interruption in the normal embryologic sequence from pronephros to metanephros. Alternatively, failure of development of the ureteral bud or lack of stimulation of nephron formation in the metanephric blastema can also result in renal agenesis.

DuBois[22] has proposed the following classification of the various embryonic defects:

1. Normal ureteric bud growth but defective differentiation of the metanephric blastema results in renal aplasia, in which there is a nubbing of nonfunctional tissue.
2. Failure of the ureteric duct to reach the nephrogenic blastema results in the ureters ending blindly.
3. Failure of both the ureteral bud and the metanephric blastema results in absence of both kidneys and ureters.
4. Lack of development of the wolffian duct leads to both BRA and severe lower urogenital malformations.

Pathology

Potter[57] has suggested that the term BRA be reserved for those patients in whom both kidneys and ureters are absent (Fig. 8–8). Renal aplasia refers to the presence of ureters and rudimentary fragments of tissue that may have identifiable tubular structures. BRA may change the shape of the adrenal glands, which usually take a discoid configuration, since there is no upward pressure to give them their characteristic shape. This concept is important, since these organs have been confused with kidneys during prenatal[21] and postnatal[69] sonography.

BRA is associated with other anomalies in what has been termed the "Potter sequence," "Potter syndrome," or "oligohydramnios sequence." These anomalies include:

1. Pulmonary hypoplasia. Lungs often weigh less than one-half that expected from the total fetal weight.[1,46] There is a reduction in the number of alveoli and also of conducting airways. This suggests that the responsible insult occurs before the 16th conceptional week.[36]
2. Typical facies. Low set ears, redundant skin, prominent fold arising at inner canthus of each eye, parrot-beak nose, and receding chin.
3. Aberrant hand and foot positioning, bowed legs, clubbed feet, hip dislocation.

Severe oligohydramnios is thought to be responsible for this phenotype. Supporting evidence is that infants with severe oligohydramnios secondary to premature rupture of membranes or intrauterine growth retardation show the same spectrum of anomalies.[56] Furthermore, infants with BRA but without significant oligohydramnios and with other anomalies that impair amniotic fluid dynamics (e.g., intestinal obstruction) do not show the elements of the Potter sequence.[71] However, not all the anomalies of the

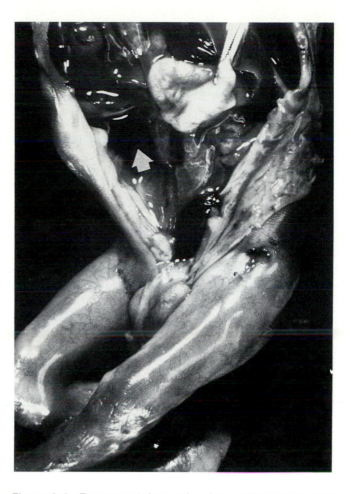

Figure 8–8. Empty renal fossa of a fetus with bilateral renal agenesis. White arrow points toward renal fossa.

Potter sequence are due to oligohydramnios. A relationship between low set ears and oligohydramnios has not been established.

Amniotic fluid is primarily produced as a dialysate of fetal blood.[53] The fetal kidney begins to produce urine at the 10th conceptional week of gestation. Oligohydramnios in the presence of BRA has been observed as early as the 14th week of gestation.[68]

Associated Anomalies

These vary in frequency in the different reports. Buchta et al.[9] suggest that anomalies due to oligohydramnios, such as facial anomalies, anomalies of the extremities, pulmonary hypoplasia, and intrauterine growth retardation, should not be classified as associated anomalies but simply as part of the sequence.

Associated anomalies can be divided into two categories[9,58]: (1) anomalies involving adjacent structures, ranging from mild forms of associated genital malformations to sirenomelia, and (2) multiple unrelated anomalies involving heart, CNS, face, and others. In two studies, anomalies involving adjacent structures occurred in 9 of 16 patients (56 percent)[63]

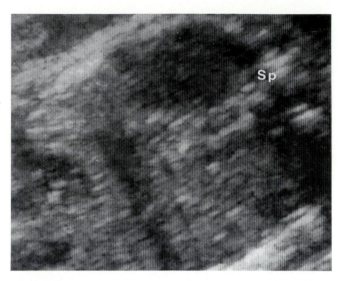

Figure 8–9. Typical sonographic image of a fetus with bilateral renal agenesis. The renal fossa is empty. Note the presence of severe oligohydramnios. Sp, spine.

and 89 of 134 (66 percent).[4] Anomalies of nonadjacent structures occurred in 7 of 16 patients (44 percent)[63] and 45 of 134 (34 percent).[4]

Various organ systems can be involved. Cardiovascular malformations (14 percent)[74] include tetralogy of Fallot, ventricular septal defect, atrial septal defect, hypoplastic left ventricle, coarctation of the aorta, dextrocardia, single ventricle, transposition of the great vessels, total anomalous pulmonary venous drainage, tricuspid atresia, and hypoplastic aorta.

Musculoskeletal malformations (40 percent)[74] include absent radius and fibula, digital anomalies, lumbar hemivertebrae, cleft palate, sacral agenesis, and diaphragmatic hernia.

Central nervous system malformations (11 percent)[74] include hydrocephaly, microcephaly, meningocele, cephaloceles, holoprosencephaly, and iniencephaly.

Gastrointestinal malformations (19 percent)[74] include duodenal atresia, imperforate anus, tracheoesophageal fistula, malrotation, absent stomach or gallbladder, and omphalocele.

Other anomalies include microphthalmia, single umbilical artery, and amnion nodosum.

Diagnosis

Prenatal diagnosis of BRA has been reported several times in the literature.[13,32,37,40,41,50,62] Criteria for a positive diagnosis include the following:

Absence of a Fetal Bladder. The bladder can be seen as early as $10\frac{1}{2}$ weeks of gestation but is not consistently imaged until 13 weeks. It is believed that it is never completely empty, with a normal fetus voiding at least once an hour.[13,77] In those cases in which there is poor visualization of this organ, serial exam-

inations at 30-minute intervals should reveal the presence of the bladder. Visualization of the bladder is difficult when the fetus is in breech presentation. The administration of furosemide has been used to induce fetal diuresis.[78] The furosemide test is performed by administering a single intravenous dose of 20 to 60 mg of furosemide to the mother and then monitoring filling of the fetal bladder during the next 2 hours. A distended bladder would obviously indicate the presence of functioning kidneys.

Several authors have reported failure of the furosemide test to reliably identify BRA from other causes of intrauterine renal failure.[35,64] Indeed, a case has been reported in which an infant with severe oligohydramnios that failed to respond to furosemide was found after delivery to have renal failure requiring peritoneal dialysis.[27]

Experimental data in an ovine model suggest that administration of furosemide to the mother at doses of 1 to 2 mg/kg body weight does not induce fetal diuresis.[18] Perhaps this observation can be explained by the poor transplacental passage of furosemide in the ovine model. Indeed, Chamberlain et al. did not find furosemide in the fetal venous plasma using an assay with a sensitivity of 100 ng/ml.[18] Furthermore, direct administration of furosemide to the fetus at doses of > 3 mg/kg body weight were required to induce diuresis in an inconsistent manner.[18] The value of these interesting observations to human pregnancy remains to be established because there are data to support the view that furosemide crosses the human placenta. Beerman et al. have reported cord levels of 330 to 340 µg/ml between 8.5 and 9.5 hours after maternal oral ingestion.[6] In our opinion, a negative test cannot be used to diagnose renal agenesis.

The diagnostic value of other imaging techniques, such as nuclear magnetic resonance, comput-

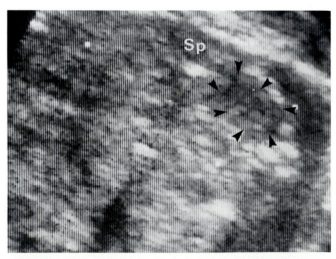

Figure 8–10. Fetus with severe oligohydramnios and bilateral renal agenesis. The shadow (*arrowheads*) in the renal fossa was confused with kidneys. It corresponded to an adrenal gland.

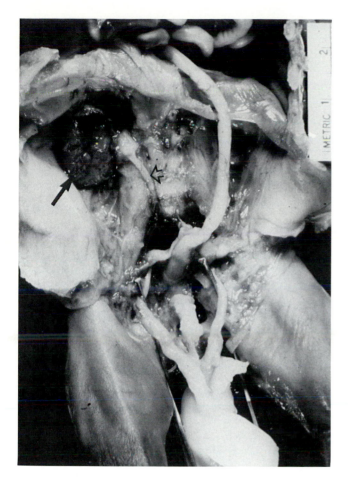

Figure 8–11. Autopsy specimen of an infant with bilateral renal agenesis. This photograph was shown in a pathologic conference. The adrenal gland (*black arrow*) was thought to be a kidney, and the structure indicated by the empty arrow was confused with a ureter but was an aberrant blood vessel.

erized tomography, intravenous pyelography,[40,50] and Doppler waveform analysis, of both maternal and fetal circulation has not been established.

Intravenous pyelography has been used to confirm the diagnosis. In this method, contrast medium is administered to the mother, and her abdomen is radiographed at 3 minutes and again 20 minutes later. This approach was originally proposed as a test for the detection of fetal life. Its overall accuracy was 47 percent.[70] Eighteen of 34 normal infants did not demonstrate kidneys in the pyelogram. The limitations of this approach are obvious.

Bilateral Absence of the Fetal Kidneys. The fetal kidneys can be visualized by the 10th menstrual week of gestation,[9] but it is only after the 12th week that they can be visualized in all fetuses. Since the adrenal glands are often enlarged during the second trimester, they can be confused with fetal kidneys (Figs. 8–9 through 8–12).[21,28,39,62,69] The differential diagnosis is based on visualization of a well-defined renal capsule and renal pelvis. In some cases, it is impossible to

differentiate between kidneys and adrenals. A method that could be used to improve visualization of the renal fossae is the instillation of warm saline (37C) into the amniotic cavity.

Oligohydramnios. The most severe examples of oligohydramnios are seen in BRA. This important finding may be present in BRA even early in the second trimester.[68] Less severe forms of oligohydramnios can be seen in cases associated with impaired dynamics of amniotic fluid exchange (e.g., esophageal atresia, pulmonary congenital cystic adenomatoid malformation).[43] The lack of amniotic fluid together with the fetal flexion often hampers clear visualization of the renal area.

The differential diagnosis should include the other renal malformations that can give rise to oligohydramnios and nonvisualization of the bladder (polycystic kidneys, multicystic kidneys, etc.).

An accurate diagnosis of BRA in all cases does not seem possible with ultrasound at this time. It is extremely difficult to establish the differential diagnosis between BRA and a functional cause of in utero renal failure.[35,64]

Some cases of BRA have come to the attention of the sonographer because of an elevated maternal serum AFP. The explanation for this observation is not known.[3,40]

Prognosis

BRA is invariably fatal. The infants are either stillborn or die in the first days of life due to pulmonary hypoplasia. Between 24 and 38 percent of infants with BRA are stillbirths.[57,60,74] The cause of intrauterine death is unknown. Neither pulmonary hypoplasia nor bilateral renal agenesis per se should cause fetal death, since the vital function of these organs in utero is executed by the placenta.

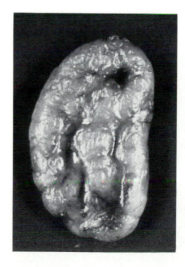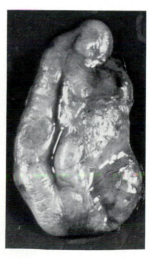

Figure 8–12. Discoid appearance of the adrenal glands of a fetus with bilateral renal agenesis.

Intrauterine growth retardation (IUGR) and associated congenital anomalies have been suggested as potential causes of death. As many as 47 percent of infants with BRA are growth retarded.[60] The incidence of IUGR seems to be higher after the 34th week of gestation.[2,57] Sixty percent of infants with BRA are born before the 37th week of gestation.[60]

Obstetrical Management

Identification of the sonographic signs associated with BRA conveys a poor prognosis to the pregnancy even if a specific diagnosis of BRA cannot be confidently made. Barss et al.[5] recently reported that all eight patients with severe oligohydramnios (largest amniotic fluid pocket <1 cm in any vertical plane) before 26 weeks of gestation died in utero or in the early neonatal period. Mercer et al.[48] reported 24 percent survivors in 33 patients with severe oligohydramnios before 26 weeks' gestation, with 18 percent having a good neonatal outcome. The option of pregnancy termination should be offered before viability. After 24 weeks of gestation, management depends on the certainty of the diagnosis. If a definitive diagnosis can be made, BRA would fulfill the criteria for offering pregnancy termination even in the third trimester (certain prenatal diagnosis and uniformly fatal disease). In the case of uncertainty secondary to difficulties in renal fossa visualization, expectant management is advised. A difficult problem involves the management of fetal distress in infants suspected of having BRA. This difficult clinical and ethical problem must await more data before firm guidelines can be offered. We advise our patients that severe oligohydramnios from early pregnancy seems to be associated with pulmonary hypoplasia and a poor outcome even if BRA is not present. Preliminary evidence suggests that the absence of fetal breathing in fetuses with oligohydramnios due to rupture of membranes in the second trimester is associated with poor prognosis.[8a]

REFERENCES

1. Alcorn D, Adamson TM, Lambert TF, et al.: Morphological effects of chronic tracheal ligation and drainage in the fetal lamb lung. J Anat 123:649, 1977.
2. Bain AD, Scott JS: Renal agenesis and severe urinary tract dysplasia. A review of 50 cases, with particular reference to the associated anomalies. Br Med J 1:841, 1960.
3. Balfour RP, Laurence KM: Raised serum AFP levels and fetal renal agenesis. Lancet 1:317, 1980.
4. Bankier A, De Campo M, Newell R, et al.: A pedigree study of perinatally lethal renal disease. J Med Genet 22:104, 1985.

5. Barss VA, Benacerraf BR, Frigoletto FD: Second trimester oligohydramnios, a predictor of poor fetal outcome. Obstet Gynecol 64:608, 1984.
6. Beermann B, Groschinsky-Grind M, Fahraeus L: Placental transfer of furosemide. Clin Pharmacol Ther 24:560, 1978.
7. Biedel CW, Pagon RA, Zapata JO: Müllerian anomalies and renal agenesis: Autosomal dominant urogenital adysplasia. J Pediatr 104:861, 1984.
8. Biedner B: Potter's syndrome with ocular anomalies. J Pediatr Ophthalmol Strabismus 17:172, 1980.
8a. Blott M, Greenough A, Nicolaides KH, et al.: Fetal breathing movements as predictor of favourable pregnancy outcome after oligohydramnios due to membrane rupture in second trimester. Lancet 2:129,1987.
9. Buchta RM, Viseskul C, Gilbert EF, et al.: Familial bilateral renal agenesis and hereditary renal adysplasia. Z Kinderheilk 115:111, 1973.
10. Burn J, Marwood RP: Fraser syndrome presenting as bilateral renal agenesis in three sibs. J Med Genet 19:360, 1982.
11. Butler N, Alberman E: Perinatal Problems. The Second Report of the British Perinatal Mortality Survey. London, Livingston, 1969.
12. Cain DR, Griggs D, Lackey DA, et al.: Familial renal agenesis and total dysplasia. Am J Dis Child 128:377, 1974.
13. Campbell S: The antenatal detection of fetal abnormality by ultrasonic diagnosis. In: Birth Defects Proceedings. Vienna, IV International Conference, 1973.
14. Carmi R, Binshtock M, Abeliovich D, et al.: The branchio-oto-renal (BOR) syndrome: Report of bilateral renal agenesis in three sibs. Am J Med Genet 14:625, 1983.
15. Carter CO: The genetics of urinary tract malformations. J Genet Hum 32:23, 1984.
16. Carter CO, Evans K: Birth frequency of bilateral renal agenesis. J Med Genet 18:158, 1981.
17. Carter CO, Evans K, Pescia G: A family study of renal agenesis. J Med Genet 16:176, 1979.
18. Chamberlain PF, Cumming M, Torchia MG, et al.: Ovine fetal urine production following maternal intravenous furosemide administration. Am J Obstet Gynecol 151:815, 1985.
19. Codere F, Brownstein S, Chen MF: Cryptophthalmos syndrome with bilateral renal agenesis. Am J Ophthalmol 91:737, 1981.
20. Curry CJR, Jensen K, Holland J, et al.: The Potter sequence: A clinical analysis of 80 cases. Am J Med Genet 19:679, 1984.
21. Dubbins PA, Kurtz AB, Wapner RJ, et al.: Renal agenesis: Spectrum of in utero findings. J Clin Ultrasound 9:189, 1981.
22. DuBois AM: The embryonic kidney. In: Rouiller C, Muller AF (eds): The Kidney: Morphology, Biochemistry, Physiology. New York, Academic Press, 1969, pp 1–50.
23. Egli F, Stalder G: Malformations of kidney and urinary tract in common chromosomal aberrations. Hum Genet 18:1, 1973.
24. Ferrandez A, Schmid W: Potter-syndrom (Nierenage-

nesie) mit chromosomaler aberration beim patient und mosaik beim vater. Helv Pediatr Acta 26:210, 1971.

25. Fitch N, Srolovitz H: Severe renal dysgenesis produced by a dominant gene. Am J Dis Child 130:1356, 1976.

26. Gilbert EF, Opitz JM: Renal involvement in genetic-hereditary malformation syndromes. In: Hamburger J, Crosnier J, Grunfeld JP (eds): Nephrology. New York, Wiley-Flammarion, 1979, pp 909–944.

27. Goldenberg RL, Davis RO, Brumfield CG: Transient fetal anuria of unknown etiology: A case report. Am J Obstet Gynecol 149:87, 1984.

28. Grannum P, Venus IH, Hobbins JC: Fetal urinary tract anomalies: Diagnosis and management. Clin Diagn Ultrasound 19:53, 1986.

29. Grannum P, Bracken M, Silverman R, et al.: Assessment of fetal kidney size in normal gestation by comparison of ratio of kidney circumference to abdominal circumference. Am J Obstet Gynecol 136:249, 1980.

30. Grix A Jr, Curry C, Hall BD: Patterns of multiple malformations in infants of diabetic mothers. Birth Defects 18:55, 1982.

31. Hack M, Jaffe J, Blankstein J, et al.: Familial aggregation in bilateral renal agenesis. Clin Genet 5:173, 1974.

32. Hadlock FP, Deter RL, Carpenter R, et al.: Review. Sonography of fetal urinary tract anomalies. AJR 137:261, 1981.

33. Halal F, Desgranges MF, Leduc B, et al.: Acro-renal-mandibular syndrome. Am J Med Genet 5:277, 1980.

34. Hall JG, Pallister PD, Clarren SK, et al.: Congenital hypothalamic hamartoblastoma, hypopituitarism, imperforate anus and postaxial polydactyly — A new syndrome? Part I: Clinical, causal and pathogenetic considerations. Am J Med Genet 7:47, 1980.

35. Harman CR: Maternal furosemide may not provoke urine production in the compromised fetus. Am J Obstet Gynecol 150:322, 1984.

36. Hislop A, Hey E, Reid L: The lungs in congenital bilateral renal agenesis and dysplasia. Arch Dis Child 54:32, 1979.

37. Hobbins JC, Grannum PAT, Berkowitz RL, et al.: Ultrasound in the diagnosis of congenital anomalies. Am J Obstet Gynecol 134:331, 1979.

38. Holzgreve W, Wagner H, Rehder H: Bilateral renal agenesis with Potter phenotype, cleft palate, anomalies of the cardiovascular system, skeletal anomalies including hexadactyly and bifid metacarpal. A new syndrome? Am J Med Genet 18:177, 1984.

39. Jeanty P, Chervenak F, Grannum P, et al.: Normal ultrasonic size and characteristics of the fetal adrenal glands. Prenat Diagn 4:21, 1984.

40. Kaffe S, Godmilow L, Walker BA, et al.: Prenatal diagnosis of bilateral renal agenesis. Obstet Gynecol 49:478, 1977.

41. Keirse MJNC, Meerman RH: Antenatal diagnosis of Potter syndrome. Obstet Gynecol 52:64S, 1978.

42. Kohn G, Borns PF: The association of bilateral and unilateral renal aplasia in the same family. J Pediatr 83:95, 1973.

43. Krous HF, Harper PE, Perlman M: Congenital cystic adenomatoid malformation in bilateral renal agenesis. Arch Pathol Lab Med 104:368, 1980.

44. Kucera J: Rate and type of congenital anomalies among offspring of diabetic women. J Reprod Med 7:61, 1971.

45. Leck I, Record RG, McKeown T, et al.: The incidence of malformations in Birmingham, England, 1950–1959. Teratology 1:263, 1968.

46. Leonidas JC, Bhan I, Beatty EC: Radiographic chest contour and pulmonary air leaks in oligohydramnios-related pulmonary hypoplasia (Potter's syndrome). Invest Radiol 17:6, 1982.

47. Lurie IW, Cherstvoy ED: Renal agenesis as a diagnostic feature of the crypthophthalmos–syndactyly syndrome. Clin Genet 25:528, 1984.

48. Mercer LJ, Brown LG: Fetal outcome with oligohydramnios in the second trimester. Obstet Gynecol 67:840, 1986.

49. Mikelsaar AVN, Lazjuk GL, Lurie JW, et al.: A 4p-syndrome: A case report. Hum Genet 19:345, 1973.

50. Miskin M: Prenatal diagnosis of renal agenesis by ultrasonography and maternal pyelography. AJR 132:1025, 1979.

51. Mortimer G, McEwan HP, Yates JRW: Fraser syndrome presenting as monozygotic twins with bilateral renal agenesis. J Med Genet 22:76, 1985.

52. Opitz JM, Gilbert EF: Editorial comment on the papers by Wilson and Hayden and Wilson and Baird on renal agenesis. Am J Med Genet 21:167, 1985.

53. Parmley TH, Seeds AE: Fetal skin permeability to isotopic water (THO) in early pregnancy. Am J Obstet Gynecol 108:128, 1970.

54. Pashayan H, Dowd T, Nigro AV: Bilateral absence of the kidneys and ureters. Three cases reported in one family. J Med Genet 14:205, 1977.

55. Passarge E, Lenz W: Syndrome of caudal regression in infants of diabetic mothers: Observations of further cases. Pediatrics 37:672, 1966.

56. Perlman M, Levin M: Fetal pulmonary hypoplasia, anuria, and oligohydramnios: Clinicopathologic observations and review of the literature. Am J Obstet Gynecol 118:1119, 1974.

57. Potter EL: Bilateral absence of ureters and kidneys. A report of 50 cases. Obstet Gynecol 25:3, 1965.

58. Potter EL: Normal and abnormal development of the kidney. Chicago, Year Book, 1972.

59. Preus M, Kaplan P, Kirkham T: Renal anomalies and oligohydramnios in the cerebro-oculo-facio-skeletal syndrome. Am J Dis Child 131:62, 1977.

60. Ratten GJ, Beischer NA, Fortune DW: Obstetric complications when the fetus has Potter's syndrome. I. Clinical considerations. Am J Obstet Gynecol 115:890, 1973.

61. Rizza JM, Downing SE: Bilateral renal agenesis in two female siblings. Am J Dis Child 121:60, 1971.

62. Romero R, Cullen M, Grannum P, et al.: Antenatal diagnosis of renal anomalies with ultrasound. III. Bilateral renal agenesis. Am J Obstet Gynecol 151:38, 1985.

63. Roodhooft AM, Birnholz JC, Holmes LB: Familial nature of congenital absence and severe dysgenesis of both kidneys. N Engl J Med 310:1341, 1984.

64. Rosenberg ER, Bowie JD: Failure of furosemide to induce diuresis in a growth-retarded fetus. AJR 142:485, 1984.

65. Saito R, Takata N, Matsumoto N, et al.: Anomalies of the auditory organ in Potter's syndrome. Arch Otolaryngol 108:484, 1982.
66. Schimke RN, King CR: Hereditary urogenital adysplasia. Clin Genet 18:417, 1980.
67. Schinzel A, Homberger C, Sigrist T: Bilateral renal agenesis in two male sibs born to consanguineous parents. J Med Genet 15:314, 1978.
68. Schmidt W, Kubli F: Early diagnosis of severe congenital malformations by ultrasonography. J Perinat Med 10:233, 1982.
69. Silverman PM, Carroll BA, Moskowitz PS: Adrenal sonography in renal agenesis and dysplasia. AJR 134:600, 1980.
70. Thomas CR, Lang EK, Lloyd FP: Fetal pyelography — A method for detecting fetal life. Obstet Gynecol 22:335, 1963.
71. Thomas IT, Smith DW: Oligohydramnios, cause of the nonrenal features of Potter's syndrome, including pulmonary hypoplasia. J Pediatr 84:811, 1974.
72. Uehling DT, Gilbert E, Chesney R: Urologic implications of the VATER association. J Urol 129:352, 1983.
73. Whitehouse W, Mountrose U: Renal agenesis in nontwin siblings. Am J Obstet Gynecol 116:880, 1973.
74. Wilson RD, Baird PA: Renal agenesis in British Columbia. Am J Med Genet 21:153, 1985.
75. Wilson RD, Hayden MR: Brief clinical report: Bilateral renal agenesis in twins. Am J Med Genet 21:147, 1985.
76. Winter JSD, Kohn G, Mellman WJ, et al.: A familial syndrome of renal, genital, and middle ear anomalies. J Pediatr 72:88, 1968.
77. Wladimiroff JW, Campbell S: Fetal urine-production rates in normal and complicated pregnancy. Lancet 1:151, 1974.
78. Wladimiroff JW: Effect of frusemide on fetal urine production. Br J Obstet Gynaecol 82:221, 1975.
79. Zonana J, Rimoin DL: Hollister DW, et al.: Renal agenesis—A genetic disorder. Pediatr Res 10:420 (Abstr), 1976.

Infantile Polycystic Kidney Disease

Synonyms

Polycystic kidney disease type I, infantile polycystic disease of the liver and kidney, renal tubular ectasia, microcystic kidney disease, and autosomal recessive polycystic kidney disease.

Definition

Infantile polycystic kidney disease (IPKD) is an autosomal recessive disorder characterized by bilateral and symmetrical enlargement of the kidneys. Normal parenchyma is replaced by dilated collecting tubules. There is no increased amount of connective tissue.

Incidence

Potter reported 2 cases in 110,000 infants.[10]

Etiology

The disease is inherited with an autosomal recessive pattern. Therefore, there is a 25 percent recurrence risk. The possibility of the dominantly inherited adult form of polycystic kidneys must be ruled out by a thorough examination of the parents and of the family history before genetic counseling.

Pathogenesis and Pathology

A primary defect of the collecting ducts appears to be responsible for the disease. Since the renal pelvis, calyces, and papilla are normal, a defect in the ureteral buds is unlikely. The normal number of nephrons and their intact development, except for the collecting ducts, suggest that the insult does not occur early in gestation and that the lesion is not due to defective metanephric blastema. Cysts are not a result of obstruction.[9]

The disease is always bilateral. The kidneys are grossly enlarged but retain their reniform configuration (Fig. 8–13). Enlargement may be so massive as to cause soft tissue dystocia.[5,6] The bladder, renal pelvis, and ureters are normal. Cystic lesions measuring 1 to 2 mm can be visualized on the surface of the kidney. Histologically, the parenchyma is occupied by large cystic structures lined by cuboidal cells. An important feature is the absence of marked proliferation of connective tissue as seen with dysplastic kidneys.

The disease has been classified into four groups according to the patient's age at the time of clinical presentation[1]:

1. Perinatal. Onset of renal failure occurs in utero or at birth. The kidneys are massively dilated, with 90 percent involvement, and there is rapid neonatal death.
2. Neonatal. Onset occurs within the first month after birth. This group has smaller kidney size, with 60 percent involvement, and there is mild hepatic fibrosis. Death occurs within one year.
3. Infantile. The disease appears by 3 to 6 months of age, with 20 percent renal involvement, moderate hepatic fibrosis, and hepatosplenomegaly. It

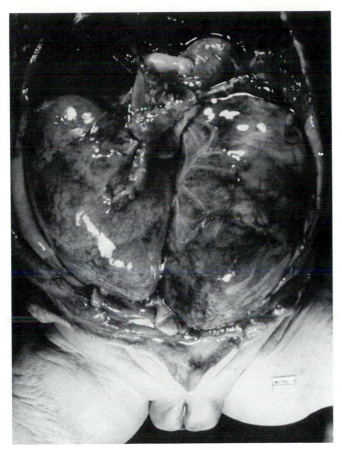

Figure 8–13. Bilaterally enlarged kidneys fill the abdomen of a fetus with infantile polycystic kidney disease.

progresses to chronic renal failure, hypertension, and portal hypertension.

4. Juvenile. The disease appears at 1 to 5 years of age. There is less renal involvement. The course of the disease is similar to that of the infantile group.

The most common clinical presentation is the perinatal variety.[2] Multiple allelism has been proposed as an explanation for the variable age at onset of the disease.[18] Recurrences tend to be group-specific,[1] although this observation has been challenged.[4,12]

Associated Anomalies

Infants with IPKD do not have an increased incidence of associated malformations when compared to the normal population.[12,15]

Cystic changes are also present in the liver. Portal and interlobular fibrosis accompanied by biliary duct hyperplasia and dilatation of the biliary tree may lead to portal hypertension. Hepatocytes are not affected.

Diagnosis

The criteria for diagnosis are (1) bilaterally enlarged kidneys, (2) oligohydramnios, and (3) absent fetal bladder. The typical hyperechogenic texture is attributed to

sound enhancement by the microscopic cystic structures present in the renal parenchyma (Fig. 8–14). Kidney enlargement can be assessed by using the kidney perimeter to abdominal perimeter ratio. An enlarged kidney should not be used as the sole diagnostic criterion, since nephromegaly has been reported without any demonstrable pathologic significance.[13,16]

Since there is a broad spectrum of renal compromise with IPKD, in utero diagnosis may be limited to the severe forms in which the signs can often be identified before the 24th week of gestation.[7,8,11] In some fetuses, prenatal diagnosis may not be possible until the third trimester[14] or not at all.[13] Our data, based on serial renal measurements, suggest that progressive enlargement of the kidneys occurs in utero and that kidney size may be normal in early stages of the disease.

Although some authors have claimed that a differential diagnosis with adult polycystic kidney disease cannot be made easily by ultrasound,[17] we believe that the massive enlargement of the kidneys (Figs. 8–13, 8–14) is rarely seen in adult polycystic kidney disease. Examination of the parents and other members of the family may be helpful as adult polycystic kidney disease is an autosomal dominant disorder.

Prognosis

The prognosis depends on the clinical variety of IPKD. The severe renal involvement typical of the perinatal type can lead to stillbirth[9,15] or neonatal death secondary to pulmonary hypoplasia. Death later in life is often the result of renal failure. In the juvenile form, renal involvement is less severe and may permit survival into later childhood or even into adult life.[3,11] It has been claimed that prognosis

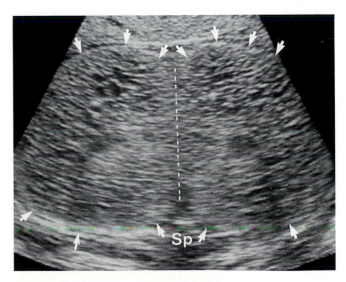

Figure 8–14. Transverse scan of a fetus with infantile polycystic kidney disease. Multiple small cysts are visualized. The kidneys fill the entire abdominal cavity. The abdominal circumference is 40 cm. At the time of delivery, severe soft tissue dystocia occurred because the kidneys were nonreducible.

correlates better with the intravenous pyelogram pattern than with the age of presentation.[4]

Obstetrical Management

When the diagnosis is made before viability, the option of pregnancy termination should be offered to the parents. In a fetus at risk, a severe variant diagnosed after viability (with severe oligohydramnios and nonvisualization of fetal bladder) is a condition for which termination of pregnancy in the third trimester may also be offered, since this condition is uniformly fatal. Massively enlarged kidneys may cause a soft tissue dystocia at delivery.

REFERENCES

1. Blyth H, Ockenden BG: Polycystic disease of kidneys and liver presenting in childhood. J Med Genet 8:257, 1971.
2. Bosniak MA, Ambos MA: Polycystic kidney disease. Semin Roentgenol 10:133, 1975.
3. Case records of the Massachusetts General Hospital. N Engl J Med 290:676, 1974.
4. Chilton SJ, Cremin BJ: The spectrum of polycystic disease in children. Pediatr Radiol 11:9, 1981.
5. Dalgaard OZ: Bilateral polycystic disease of the kidneys: A follow-up of two hundred eighty-four patients and their families. Acta Med Scand [Suppl] 328, 1957.
6. Greenberg LA, Altman DH, Litt RE: Cystic enlargement of the kidney in infancy. Radiology 89:850, 1967.
7. Habif DV, Berdon WE, Yeh MN: Infantile polycystic kidney disease: In utero sonographic diagnosis. Radiology 142:475, 1982.
8. Jung JH, Luthy DA, Hirsch JH, et al.: Serial ultrasound of a pregnancy at risk for infantile polycystic kidney disease (IPKD). Birth Defects 18:173, 1982.
9. Madewell JE, Hartman DS, Lichtenstein JE: Radiologic–pathologic correlations in cystic disease of the kidney. Radiol Clin North Am 17:261, 1979.
10. Potter EL: Type I cystic kidney: Tubular gigantism. In: Normal and Abnormal Development of the Kidney. Chicago, Year Book, 1972, pp 141–153.
11. Reilly KB, Rubin SP, Blanke BG, et al.: Infantile polycystic kidney disease: A difficult antenatal diagnosis. Am J Obstet Gynecol 133:580, 1979.
12. Resnik J, Vernier RL: Cystic disease of the kidney in the newborn infant. Clin Perinatol 8:375, 1981.
13. Romero R, Cullen M, Jeanty P, et al.: The diagnosis of congenital renal anomalies with ultrasound. II. Infantile polycystic kidney disease. Am J Obstet Gynecol 150:259, 1984.
14. Simpson JL, Sabbagha RE, Elias S, et al.: Failure to detect polycystic kidneys in utero by second trimester ultrasonography. Hum Genet 60:295, 1982.
15. Spence HM, Singleton R: Cysts and cystic disorders of the kidney: Types, diagnosis, treatment. Urol Surv 22:131, 1972.
16. Stapleton FB, Hilton S, Wilcox J: Transient nephromegaly simulating infantile polycystic disease of the kidneys. Pediatrics 67:554, 1981.
17. Sumner TE, Volberg FM, Martin JF: Real-time sonography of congenital cystic kidney disease. Urology 20:97, 1982.
18. Zerres K, Volpel MC, Weiss H: Cystic kidneys. Genetics, pathologic anatomy, clinical picture, and prenatal diagnosis. Hum Genet 68:104, 1984.

Adult Polycystic Kidney Disease

Synonyms

Autosomal dominant polycystic kidney disease and adult hepatorenal polycystic disease.

Definition

Adult polycystic kidney disease (APKD) is an autosomal dominant disease characterized by replacement of renal parenchyma with multiple cysts of variable size due to dilatation of the collecting tubules and other tubular segments of the nephrons.

Etiology

Unknown. The disorder is inherited as an autosomal dominant trait, and the recurrence risk is 50 percent. The genetic locus for this disorder is located on chromosome 16.

Incidence

One in 1000 people carries the mutant gene. APKD is one of the most common genetic disorders and the third most prevalent cause of chronic renal failure.[12] The penetrance of the gene is virtually 100 percent.[17] However, the expressivity of the gene may vary, ranging from severe forms that result in neonatal death to asymptomatic forms detected only at autopsy.[3] The disease is usually clinically manifested in the fourth decade of life, but infantile and neonatal cases have been reported.[1,4,5,7,9,11,16]

Pathogenesis and Pathology

APKD is one of the entities that can produce Potter's type III polycystic kidney. In Potter's type III kidneys, the defect seems to be at the level of the ampulla (distal end of the ureter bud), similar to that found in type II. However, the involvement is not universal, and some ampullae are normal. The result is the presence of cysts coexisting with normal renal tissue. The cysts correspond to both dilated collecting ducts and other tubular portions of the nephron.

There is considerable variation in the degree of renal involvement in patients of the same age, suggesting variability in the expressivity of the gene. Cysts are visible in nephrons and in collecting tubules, and there is a mixture of normal and abnormal elements.[14] Macroscopically, the kidneys are almost always bilaterally affected and often enlarged. Unilateral involvement may be the first manifestation of the disease.[17] The size of the cysts may vary, and some cysts may reach several centimeters.[10] Involvement of the liver is less prominent than in IPKD. The lesions consist of periportal fibrosis;[13] they may be focal and detected only by chance.[1]

Associated Anomalies

Clinically overt APKD has been associated with cystic lesions in other organs, including liver, pancreas, spleen, lungs, testes, ovaries, and epididymis.[3] An association between APKD and liver cysts has been clearly demonstrated.[19] Whether cysts in other organs are due to random occurrence, an actual increased incidence, or the consequence of a detailed autopsy in patients with a known anomaly has not been established.

It should be stressed that type III polycystic kidney disease is a common morphologic expression of a group of disorders other than APKD. Meckel syndrome (autosomal recessive), tuberous sclerosis (autosomal dominant), and Von-Hippel Lindau (autosomal dominant) are mendelian disorders associated with this type of renal disease.[19]

Diagnosis

There are several documented cases of prenatal diagnosis of this condition.[11,12a,18,20] The sonographic appearance has been described as similar to that of IPKD: enlarged kidneys with increased parenchymal echogenicity or multiple cysts (Fig. 8–15). The amount of amniotic fluid has been normal or decreased. The earliest diagnosis has been made at $23\frac{1}{2}$ weeks. In some fetuses where serial examinations were performed, the dimensions and appearance of the kidneys were normal in the midtrimester, and abnormalities were first detected at 30 and 36 weeks.[11] In some cases, the gross lesions may be more prominent in one kidney.[10,11] Therefore, unilateral involvement does not exclude diagnosis in the fetus. In one reported fetus, ascites was noted,[18] and in another, nonimmune hydrops was identified.[20]

APKD in the fetus should be suspected when cystic enlarged kidneys are detected in association with a normal amount of fluid. This condition is a late

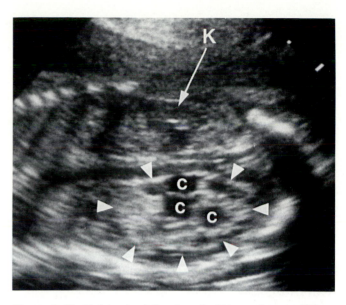

Figure 8–15. Unilateral adult polycystic kidney disease. This a coronal longitudinal section demonstrating both kidneys. The upper kidney (K) is normal. The lower kidney is polycystic and shows multiple cystic structures (C) and thickened renal parenchyma.

cause of renal failure, but the gross lesions may be present in fetuses and newborns.[1,4,6,7,9,15,19]

The diagnosis of APKD in a newborn or a fetus should prompt investigation of both parents. The prenatal diagnosis of APKD has been made by chronic villous sampling using a highly polymorphic DNA probe genetically linked to the locus of the mutant gene.[14]

Prognosis

Pretorius et al. have recently reviewed the follow-up of seven cases diagnosed in utero. One pregnancy was electively terminated at $23\frac{1}{2}$ weeks. One infant died in the neonatal period. Of the five remaining infants, four had normal renal function, and all infants but one had normal blood pressure (follow-up 2 months to 4 years and 10 months).[13a] Since this information is based upon a limited experience, parents may be informed about the natural history of the disease with data on APKD from postnatal series. APKD is a chronic disease that may become symptomatic over a wide range of ages from the newborn period to adulthood. Sometimes, the disease can be completely asymptomatic and will be detected at autopsy. The mean age of onset of symptoms is 35 years, and the mean age of diagnosis is 43 years.[19] The symptoms are loin pain, renal enlargement, renal insufficiency, and uremia. Hypertension can be observed in 50 to 70 percent of patients. Berry aneurysms are demonstrated in 10 to 30 percent of patients, and their rupture is a cause of death in 10 percent of patients with APKD. There are not sufficient data to formulate adequate prognostic guidelines for patients diagnosed in utero or in the immediate neonatal period. Stillbirth and early neonatal death have been reported by Potter.[13,16]

Obstetrical Management

Parents at risk should be counseled about the possibility of first trimester prenatal diagnosis. If the diagnosis is made before viability, the option of pregnancy termination should be offered to the parents. After viability, the diagnosis of APKD probably should not alter standard obstetrical management. Any time enlarged hyperechogenic kidneys are diagnosed in a fetus, members of the family should be screened with renal sonography. There are no data in which to base the management of fetuses with evidence of in utero renal failure.

REFERENCES

1. Blyth H, Ockenden BG: Polycystic disease of kidneys and liver presenting in childhood. J Med Genet 8:257, 1971.
2. Chilton SJ, Cremin BJ: The spectrum of polycystic disease in children. Pediatr Radiol 11:9, 1981.
3. Dalgaard OZ: Bilateral polycystic disease of the kidney: A follow-up of two hundred eighty-four patients and their families. Acta Med Scand [Suppl] 328, 1957.
4. Eulderink F, Hogewind BL: Renal cysts in premature children. Arch Pathol Lab Med 102:592, 1978.
5. Fellows RA, Leonidas JC, Beatty EC Jr: Radiologic features of "adult type" polycystic kidney disease in the neonate. Pediat Radiol 4:87, 1976.
6. Fryns JP, Van Den Berghe H: "Adult" form of polycystic kidney disease in neonates. Clin Genet 15:205, 1979.
7. Kaye C, Lewy PR: Congenital appearance of adult-type (autosomal dominant) polycystic kidney disease. J Pediatr 85:807, 1974.
8. Kissane JM: Congenital malformations. In: Heptinstall RH (ed): Pathology of the Kidney, 3d ed. Boston, Little, Brown, 1983, p 109.
9. Loh JP, Haller JO, Kassner EG, et al.: Dominantly

inherited polycystic kidneys in infants: Association with hypertrophic pyloric stenosis. Pediatr Radiol 6:27, 1977.
10. Madewell JE, Hartman DS, Lichtenstein JE: Radiologic–pathologic correlations in cystic disease of the kidney. Radiol Clin North Am 17:261, 1979.
11. Main D, Mennuti MT, Cornfeld D, et al.: Prenatal diagnosis of adult polycystic kidney disease. Lancet 2:337, 1983.
12. Milutinovic J, Fialkow PJ, Phillips LA, et al.: Autosomal dominant polycystic kidney disease: Early diagnosis and data for genetic counselling. Lancet 1:1203, 1980.
13. Potter EL: Type III cystic kidney: Combined ampullary and interstitial abnormality. In: Normal and Abnormal Development of the Kidney. Chicago, Year Book, 1972, pp 182–208.
13a. Pretorius DH, Lee ME, Manco-Johnson ML, et al.: Diagnosis of autosomal dominant polycystic kidney disease in utero and in the young infant. J Ultrasound Med 6:249, 1987.
14. Reeders ST, Zerres K, Ga IA, et al: Prenatal diagnosis of autosomal dominant polycystic kidney disease with a DNA probe. Lancet 2:6, 1986.
15. Ross DG, Travers H: Infantile presentation of adult-type polycystic kidney disease in a large kindred. J Pediatr 87:760, 1975.
16. Shokeir MHK: Expression of "adult" polycystic renal disease in the fetus and newborn. Clin Genet 14:61, 1978.
17. Spence HM, Baird SS, Ware EW: Cystic disorders of the kidney: Classification, diagnosis, treatment. JAMA 163:1466, 1957.
18. Zerres K, Weiss H, Bulla M: Prenatal diagnosis of an early manifestation of autosomal dominant adult-type polycystic kidney disease. Lancet 2:988, 1982.
19. Zerres K, Volpel MC, Weiss H: Cystic kidneys. Genetics, pathologic anatomy, clinical picture, and prenatal diagnosis. Hum Genet 68:104, 1984.
20. Zerres K, Hansmann M, Knopfle G, et al.: Clinical case reports. Prenatal diagnosis of genetically determined early manifestation of autosomal dominant polycystic kidney disease. Hum Genet 71:368, 1985.

Multicystic Kidney Disease

Synonyms

Potter's type II cystic kidney disease, multicystic dysplastic kidneys, polycystic kidney disease type II, and dysplastic kidney disease.

Definition

Multicystic kidney disease is a congenital renal disorder characterized by cystic lesions that correspond primarily to dilated collecting tubules. The disorder can be bilateral, unilateral, or segmental.

Etiology

MKD is generally a sporadic condition,[27] and familial occurrence is rare.[35] On occasion, MKD has been reported with maternal diabetes.

Potter's type II cystic kidney disease can occur within the spectrum of syndrome, usually as a secondary manifestation.[38]

Autosomal Recessive Syndromes. Meckel, Dandy-Walker, short-rib polydactyly type I or Saldino-

Noonan and type II or Majewsky, Zellweger (cerebrohepatorenal syndrome), retina–renal dysplasia, Ivemark (dysplasia of kidney, liver, and pancreas), Roberts, Fryns, Smith-Lemli-Opitz.

Autosomal Dominant Syndromes. Apert syndrome.

Chromosomal Defects. Trisomy C, del (15) (q22) (q24).

Incidence

The incidence of bilateral MKD is estimated to be 1 in 10,000.[29] This figure may represent an underestimation of the real incidence of the disease, since not all perinatal deaths are followed by autopsy. The male to female ratio is 2:1 in unilateral MKD.[28]

Pathogenesis

The pathogenesis of multicystic kidney disease (MKD) is unknown. The current understanding of this disease suggests that it is a complex abnormality that may be the result of two types of insults: (1) developmental failure of the mesonephric blastema to form nephrons or (2) an early obstructive uropathy.

The normal development of nephrons requires differentiation of the mesonephric blastema. This process is induced by the ampulla, which is the distal growing end of the ureteral duct. Failure of induction because of an abnormal response of the metanephric blastema or because of a defective ampulla results in disorganized differentiation of the metanephric blastema, giving rise to renal dysplasia. This term refers to a histologic picture characterized by structures generally not represented in normal morphogenesis, including (1) focally dilated tubules that are frequently surrounded by muscle, (2) small ducts with hyperchromatic epithelium, and (3) heterotopic mesodermic structures, such as cartilage. The mechanism by which the collecting tubules are transformed into cysts is unknown. This pathogenetic hypothesis is supported by the frequent association of ureteral malformations and renal dysplasia.

Some cases of multicystic kidney disease occur in association with obstructive uropathy.[10] Some renal function can persist.[37] The obstructive process must take place early in embryogenesis. Otherwise, the renal lesion would correspond to cystic kidney disease type IV, in which the cystic dilatation is limited to the terminal portion of the collecting tubules and to nephrons developed in the latter part of gestation.

The defective metanephric blastema hypothesis can explain those cases of multicystic kidney associated with a hypoplastic or a malformed ureteral bud. However, some cases of unilateral absence of the ureter on the affected side would challenge this view. The explanation that regression of the ureter has

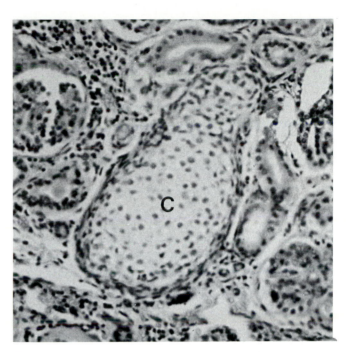

Figure 8–16. Histologic section of a multicystic kidney. C, cartilage.

occurred is not uniformly valid because, in some cases, there is agenesis of the hemitrigone. The pathogenesis in these cases cannot be attributed to a defective ampulla, and a plausible explanation is not available.

Pathology

MKD can be bilateral, unilateral, or limited to a localized portion of a kidney. The segmental variety of multicystic kidney disease is almost always unilateral and is frequently referred to as a "multilocular cyst." Potter[27] suggested that the disease be classified into IIA, characterized by normal or enlarged kidneys (multicystic–multilocular cyst group), and IIB, with small dysgenetic or aplastic kidneys. Recently, the cystic variety of MKD has been subdivided into two major categories: pelvicoinfundibular atresia[13] and the hydronephrotic variety,[10] according to the presence or absence of atresia of the ureter.

Macroscopically, multicystic kidneys may be enlarged (IIA), small (IIB), or of normal size. Enlarged kidneys may weigh several hundred grams and distend the abdomen. When the disease is type IIB, the kidneys may weigh as little as 1 g. Anytime there is involvement of an entire kidney, the ureter is virtually always affected with obstructive or developmental lesions. The renal artery is small or absent in most cases. Cartilage may be found in one third of affected kidneys (Fig. 8–16).

Cysts are usually terminal portions of collecting tubules, often located in the center of the kidney, and

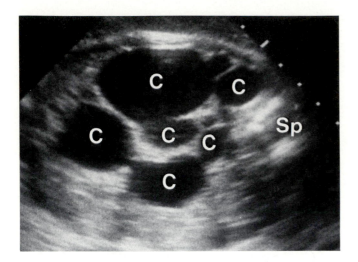

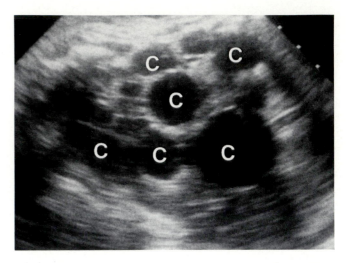

Figure 8–17. Transverse scan of a fetus with multicystic kidney disease. Note the multiple cystic structures (C). Sp, spine.

Figure 8–18. Coronal view of the same fetus shown in Figure 8–17. Cysts (C) do not communicate.

may be surrounded by zones of connective or myxomatous tissue.[38]

Unilateral MKD is often asymptomatic. In these patients, the contralateral urinary tract shows minor abnormalities in 30 to 50 percent of patients, including malrotation, ureteropelvic junction obstruction, horseshoe kidney, and other ureteral anomalies.[12,20,23,25,32] In some cases, the sonographic finding of contralateral hydronephrosis has been attributed to a compensatory overload on the functioning kidney.[4,29]

Associated Malformations

Besides the anomalies belonging to the Potter sequence or oligohydramnios sequence (p. 261), bilateral MKD may be associated with cardiovascular malformations, CNS abnormalities (anencephaly, hydrocephalus, iniencephaly, spina bifida, occipital meningocele), diaphragmatic hernia, cleft palate, microphthalmia, duodenal stenosis and imperforate anus,[27] tracheoesophageal fistula, and bilateral absence of radius and thumb.[8] In contradistinction to Potter type I or III, Potter II exhibits no cystic changes in the liver, pancreas, or other parenchymatous organs.[35]

An increased frequency of associated congenital anomalies is also found with unilateral multicystic kidneys.[3,12] They include hydrocephaly, anencephaly, spina bifida, myelomeningocele, esophageal atresia, imperforate anus, duodenal bands, tracheoesophageal fistula, ventricular septal defect, talipes equinovarus, hypospadias, vesical diverticulum, and patent urachus. Chromosomal anomalies can also occur.

Diagnosis

Multicystic kidneys have a typical appearance on ultrasound, and antenatal diagnosis of both the unilateral and the bilateral forms has been report-

ed on numerous occasions in the literature.[1,2,4,9,11,16,21,24,26,30] Ultrasound criteria for the diagnosis of bilateral multicystic kidney include:

1. Cystic kidneys. The cysts are multiple, peripheral, round, and of variable size. In most instances, the kidneys are enlarged (type IIA), but in some cases they are small and atrophic. The enlarged kidneys may fill a significant portion of the abdomen and may have a lobulated shape. In type IIa, the kidney may look like a cluster of grapes (Figs. 8–17, 8–18). The renal sinus cannot be identified (Fig. 8–17).
2. Failure to visualize the fetal bladder, even after furosemide administration. Limitations, interpretation, and technique of this test are discussed in the section on bilateral renal agenesis (p. 262).
3. Oligohydramnios. If amniotic fluid is present in association with a typical image of multicystic kidney, consideration should be given to the possibility of a unilateral MKD and incomplete or late obstruction of the contralateral kidney.

The differential diagnosis includes IPKD and ureteropelvic junction obstruction (UPJ). The differential diagnosis between UPJ obstruction and MKD is difficult,[28a] even in the neonatal period, using intravenous pyelography and scintillography.[5,29,33,36] Some criteria have been suggested for differential diagnosis in the newborn.[34] UPJ obstruction is suggested by:

1. Visible renal parenchyma
2. Cystic lesions nonspherical in shape and radiating from the renal pelvis
3. A dilated ureter or a single large cyst (multicystic kidney can occur as a single cyst as well) (Fig. 8–19).
4. Visualization of cysts that communicate with the renal pelvis

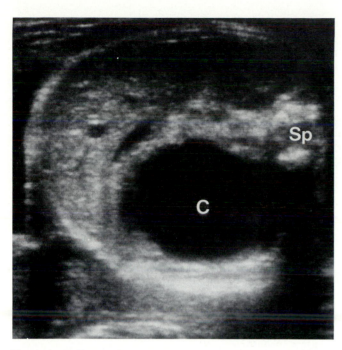

Figure 8-19. Fetus with unilateral multicystic kidney disease with a single cyst (C). This image stresses the difficult differential diagnosis between a UPJ obstruction and multicyctic kidney disease. The latter could occur as either multiple or single cystic structure. Sp, Spine.

Multilocular cysts should be differentiated from Wilms' tumor and hamartoma that has undergone necrosis.

In unilateral MKD, the only signs are renal in origin. The bladder and contralateral kidney may be completely normal. This type would be diagnosed only when focusing onto the size and morphology of kidneys in routine scans.

It must be stressed that the appearance of the kidney in MKD is related to the time of the insult. When this occurs early (between the 8th and 11th week of conception), the kidney adopts the classic morphology of MKD (there are 10 to 20 noncommunicating cysts, and the organ loses its reniform appearance). The renal pelvis and calyces are atretic or extremely small. If the insult occurs later, the morphology of the kidney depends on the duration of the obstruction. At an earlier stage, a typical hydronephrotic image is observed. Later, the typical image of the large multicystic kidney appears. Most characteristically, there are at least two cysts and a recognizable pelvis, which often communicates with the cysts. Some renal function can be demonstrated.[34]

Prognosis
Bilateral MKD is a fatal condition.[12] Cole et al.[7] reported one infant who was doing well at 41 months of age, but since an IVP showed "prompt visualization of distorted calyces," we think the diagnosis of bilateral MKD is doubtful.

There is a paucity of data concerning the prog-

nosis of unilateral MKD. One risk is the development of hypertension.[6,18] Generally, urologists advocate follow-up of the patient rather than prophylactic nephrectomy.[29]

Obstetrical Management
When the diagnosis of bilateral MKD is made early in gestation, the option of termination of pregnancy should be offered to the patient. Fetal karyotype should be considered. If the diagnosis is made after viability, aggressive intervention for fetal distress would seem unwarranted, since the disease is uniformly fatal. Unilateral MKD with a normal contralateral kidney, normal karyotype, and no associated anomalies should not influence obstetrical management. If an obstructive uropathy is diagnosed on the opposite side, delivery should be accomplished when pulmonic maturity is documented. Evaluation in the neonatal period will be required. Delivery in a tertiary care center is recommended.

REFERENCES

1. Bartley JA, Golbus MS, Filly RA, et al.: Prenatal diagnosis of dysplastic kidney disease. Clin Genet 11:375, 1977.
2. Bateman BG, Brenbridge ANAG, Buschi AJ: In utero diagnosis of multicystic kidney disease by sonography. J Reprod Med 25:256, 1980.
3. Bearman SB, Hine PL, Sanders RC: Multicystic kidney: A sonographic pattern. Radiology 118:685, 1976.
4. Beretsky I, Lankin DH, Rusoff JH: Sonographic differentiation between the multicystic dysplastic kidney and the ureteropelvic junction obstruction in utero using high resolution real-time scanners employing digital detection. J Clin Ultrasound 12:429, 1984.
5. Bloom DA, Brosman S: The multicystic kidney. J Urol 120:211, 1978.
6. Chen YH, Stapleton FB, Roy S, et al.: Neonatal hypertension from a unilateral multicystic, dysplastic kidney. J Urol 133:664, 1985.
7. Cole BR, Kaufman RL, McAlister WH, et al.: Bilateral renal dysplasia in three siblings: Report of a survivor. Clin Nephrol 5:83, 1976.
8. D'Alton M, Romero R, Grannum P, et al.: Antenatal diagnosis of renal anomalies with ultrasound. IV. Bilateral multicystic kidney disease. Am J Obstet Gynecol 54:532, 1986.
9. Dunne MG, Johnson ML: The ultrasonic demonstration of fetal abnormalities in utero. J Reprod Med 23:195, 1979.
10. Felson B, Cussen LJ: The hydronephrotic type of unilateral congenital multicystic disease of the kidney. Semin Roentgenol 10:113, 1975.
11. Friedberg JE, Mitnick JS, Davis DA: Antepartum ultrasonic detection of multicystic kidney. Radiology 131:198, 1979.
12. Greene LF, Feinzaig W, Dahlin DC: Multicystic

dysplasia of the kidney: With special reference to the contralateral kidney. J Urol 103:482, 1971.

13. Griscom NT, Vawter GF, Fellers FX: Pelvoinfundibular Atresia: The usual form of multicystic kidney: 44 unilateral and two bilateral cases. Semin Roentgenol 10:125, 1975.

14. Grote W, Weisner D, Janig U, et al.: Prenatal diagnosis of a short-rib polydactylia syndrome type Saldino-Noonan at 17 weeks' gestation. Eur J Pediatr 140:63, 1983.

15. Harcke HT, Williams JL, Popky GL, et al.: Abdominal masses in the neonate: A multiple modality approach to diagnosis. Radiographics 2:69, 1982.

16. Henderson SC, Van Kolken RJ, Rahatzad M: Multicystic kidney with hydramnios. J Clin Ultrasound 8:249, 1980.

17. Hobbins JC, Grannum P, Berkowitz RL, et al.: Ultrasound in the diagnosis of congenital anomalies. Am J Obstet Gynecol 134:331, 1979.

18. Javadpour N, Chelouhy E, Moncada L: Hypertension in a child caused by a multicystic kidney. J Urol 104:918, 1970.

19. Johannessen JV, Haneberg B, Moe PJ: Bilateral multicystic dysplasia of the kidneys. Beitr Pathol Bd 148:290, 1973.

20. Kyaw MM: Roentgenologic triad of congenital multicystic kidney. Am J Roentgenol 119:710, 1973.

21. Lee TG, Blake S: Prenatal fetal abdominal ultrasonography and diagnosis. Radiology 124:475, 1977.

22. Legarth J, Verder H, Gronvall S: Prenatal diagnosis of multicystic kidney by ultrasound. Acta Obstet Gynecol Scand 60:523, 1981.

23. Madewell JE, Hartman DS, Lichtenstein JE: Radiologic–pathologic correlations in cystic disease of the kidney. Radiol Clin North Am 17:261, 1979.

24. Mendoza SA, Griswold WR, Leopold GR, et al.: Intrauterine diagnosis of renal anomalies by ultrasonography. Am J Dis Child 133:1042, 1979.

25. Newman L, Simms K, Kissane J, et al.: Unilateral total renal dysplasia in children. AJR 116:778, 1972.

26. Older RA, Hinman CG, Crane LM, et al.: In utero diagnosis of multicystic kidney by gray scale ultrasonography. AJR 133:130, 1979.

27. Potter EL: Type II cystic kidney: Early ampullary inhibition. In: Normal and Abnormal Development of the Kidney. Chicago, Year Book, 1972, pp 154–181.

28. Resnick J, Vernier RL: Cystic disease of the kidney in the newborn infant. Clin Perinatol 8:375, 1981.

28a. Rizzo N, Gabrielli S, Pilu G, et al.: Prenatal diagnosis and obstetrical management of multicystic dysplastic kidney disease. Prenat Diagn 7:109, 1987.

29. Sanders RC, Hartman DS: The sonographic distinction between neonatal multicystic kidney and hydronephrosis. Radiology 151:621, 1984.

30. Santos-Ramos R, Duenhoelter JH: Diagnosis of congenital fetal abnormalities by sonography. Obstet Gynecol 45:279, 1975.

31. Saxton HM, Golding SJ, Chantler C, et al.: Diagnostic puncture in renal cystic dysplasia (multicystic kidney). Evidence on the aetiology of the cysts. Br J Radiol 54:555, 1981.

32. Scheible W, Leopold GR: High-resolution real-time ultrasonography of neonatal kidneys. J Ultrasound Med 1:133, 1982.

33. Siddiqui AR, Cohen M, Mitchell ME: Multicystic dysplastic kidneys suggesting hydronephrosis during Tc-DTPA imaging. J Nucl Med 23:892, 1982.

34. Stuck KJ, Koff SA, Silver TM: Ultrasonic features of multicystic dysplastic kidney: Expanded diagnostic criteria. Radiology 143:217, 1982.

35. Warkany J: Congenital Cystic Disease of the Kidney. Chicago, Year Book, 1981, pp 1044–1045.

36. Wood BP, Goske M, Rabinowitz R: Multicystic renal dysplasia masquerading as ureteropelvic junction obstruction. J Urol 132:972, 1984.

37. Young LW, Wood BP, Spohr C: Delayed excretory urographic opacification, a puddling effect in multicystic renal dysplasia. Ann Radiol (Paris) 17:391, 1974.

38. Zerres K, Volpel MC, Weiss H: Cystic kidneys. Genetics, pathologic anatomy, clinical picture, and prenatal diagnosis. Hum Genet 68:104–135, 1984.

Ureteropelvic Junction Obstruction

Definition
Obstruction of the urinary tract at the junction of the renal pelvis and the ureter.

Incidence
The incidence of ureteropelvic junction (UPJ) obstruction in utero is not known. In the cases diagnosed postnatally, it occurs more commonly in males than in females, with a sex ratio of 5:1.[1,16]

Etiology and Pathology
UPJ obstruction is essentially a sporadic phenomenon, although familial cases have been reported.[4,20]

In the family reported by Raffle, all affected patients were females, but males were not screened.[20] A dominant pattern of inheritance with incomplete penetrance and variable expression has been suggested for some cases of unilateral UPJ obstruction.[7] This could explain the occurrence of hydronephrosis in twins.[12]

The ureteropelvic junction is a frequent site of obstruction of the urinary tract. Anatomic causes responsible for UPJ obstruction include fibrous adhesions, bands, kinks, ureteral valves, aberrant lower pole vessels, abnormal ureteral insertion, and unusual shapes of the pyeloureteral outlet.[10] How-

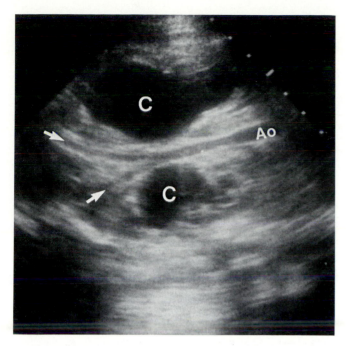

Figure 8–20. Coronal view of a fetus with bilateral ureteropelvic junction obstruction. Note the asymmetrical involvement of the kidneys. C, cystic dilatation of the renal pelvis; Ao; aorta; arrows point to bifurcation of the aorta.

ever, any of these anatomic causes for UPJ obstruction are seen in only a fraction of patients. Since in most instances of UPJ obstruction the junction is anatomically patent to the passage of a probe, the problem seems to be of functional nature.[2] The ureteropelvic junction is important in the formation and propulsion of the bolus of urine. The normal interwoven pattern of the muscularis of the ureter is considered critical for this function. Abnormal development of the musculature would impair bolus formation and propulsion. In one study, 69 percent of patients with UPJ obstruction had an abnormal muscular arrangement in which the circular layer was present but the longitudinal layer was not.[2]

The condition occurs bilaterally in 30 percent of cases usually with an asymmetrical involvement of the kidneys. When the obstruction is unilateral, it occurs more frequently on the left side.[8,16,17,21] Infants with UPJ obstruction frequently have other associated anomalies of the urinary tract,[16] including vesicoureteric reflux, bilateral ureteral duplication, bilateral obstructed megaureter, contralateral nonfunctioning kidney, contralateral renal agenesis, meatal stenosis, and hypospadias.[1,8,16] In a recent series, the incidence of such anomalies was 27 percent.[8]

Associated Anomalies

Anomalies in extraurinary systems occurs in up to 19 percent of cases.[18] UPJ obstruction has been described in association with Hirschsprung's disease, cardiovascular abnormalities, neural tube defects, sagittal synostosis, mandibular hypoplasia, esophageal atresia and distal fistula, imperforate anus, syndactyly, congenital hip dislocation, and adrenogenital syndrome.[2,18]

Diagnosis

The diagnosis depends on the demonstration of a dilated renal pelvis (Figs. 8–20 through 8–24). The two problems with the diagnosis of UPJ obstruction are (1) the criteria used to classify a renal pelvis as

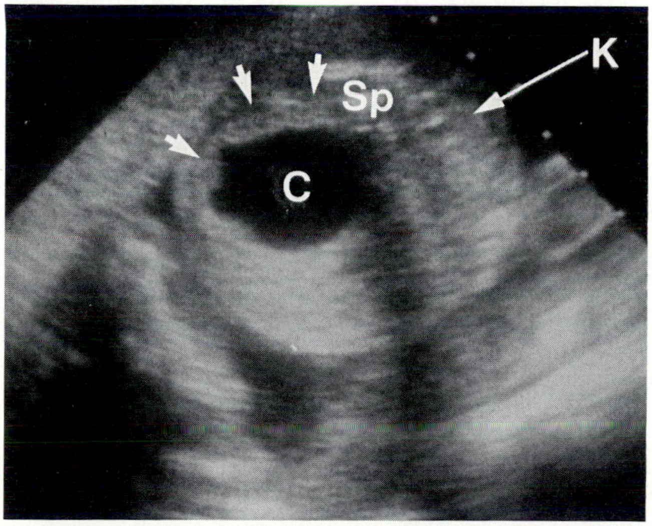

Figure 8–21. Transverse scan at the level of the renal fossa in a fetus with unilateral ureteropelvic junction obstruction. The cystic structure (C) corresponds to a dilated renal pelvis. The arrows point to the renal parenchyma. Sp, spine; K, contralateral normal kidney.

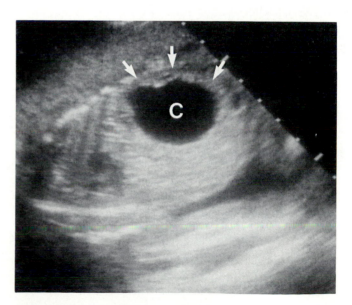

Figure 8–22. Longitudinal scan of the fetus shown in Figure 8–21. There is dilatation of the renal pelvis. Arrows point to the renal parenchyma. C, renal pelvis.

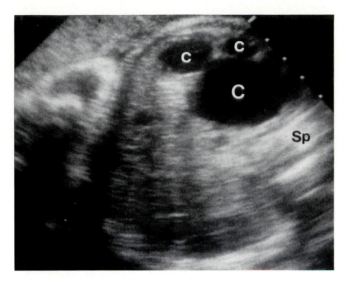

Figure 8–23. Transverse scan of a fetus with hydronephrosis. The largest cystic structures (C) correspond to the renal pelvis, and the other cystic structures (c) correspond to distended calyces. Sp, spine.

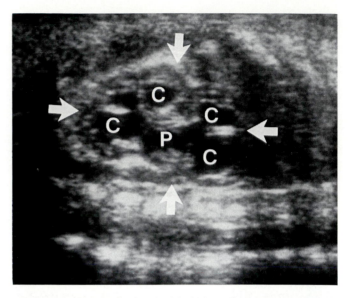

Figure 8–24. Longitudinal scan of the kidney of a fetus with unilateral hydronephrosis. An important clue in the differential diagnosis with multicystic kidney disease is that the cystic structures communicate with the renal pelvis. P, renal pelvis; C, dilated renal calyces.

dilated and (2) the natural history of the disease in utero.

At this time, there is no available nomogram of renal pelvis size and gestational age. Two criteria of renal pelvis measurements have been proposed[3]:

1. Anteroposterior diameter. Renal pelvises of less than 5 mm are normal, whereas those between 5 and 10 mm are normal in most instances but may require follow-up. In a recent study of eight fetuses with a ≥10 mm renal pelvis diameter, seven had an anatomic abnormality at postnatal examination.[14]
2. The ratio between the maximum transverse pelvic diameter and the renal diameter at the same level. Ratios above 50 percent would suggest hydronephrosis. However, diagnostic indices with this criterion are not available.

Harrison et al. have suggested a semiquantitative estimate of hydronephrosis.[11] Mild dilatation would show enlarged renal pelvis, branching infundibula, and calices. Severe dilatation would be characterized by only a large, unilocular fluid collection.[11]

Several patients have been reported in whom a diagnosis of hydronephrosis, either unilateral or bilateral, was initially made in utero, but follow-up scans in utero and postnatally failed to confirm the finding.[5,6,22] Interpreting these reports of transitory hydronephrosis is difficult because authors have not described the dimensions of the renal pelvis. However, this indicates that serial ultrasound scans are needed to predict trends in amniotic fluid volume and in hydronephrosis severity.

It has been suggested that the fetal renal pelvis may vary in size according to the volume state of the mother.[19] Some authors have recommended that patients be reexamined after 12 hours of water and fluid restriction. However, a study of the effect of this protocol on renal pelvis size failed to demonstrate a significant effect in 76.5 percent of cases.[14] Therefore, the phenomenon of transient hydronephrosis cannot be explained by changes in the hydration of the mother.

Most UPJ obstructions are unilateral, and the amount of amniotic fluid as well as bladder dynamics should be normal. In cases of unilateral UPJ obstructions, the presence of severe oligohydramnios should raise the suspicion of contralateral renal agenesis or dysplasia.

In those patients with bilateral dilatation of the renal pelvis, the amount of amniotic fluid can provide information about the severity of the obstruction. If the amount of fluid is normal and the bladder is visible, the obstruction is either of recent onset or incomplete.[5,15] A normal to increased amount of amniotic fluid may coexist with a bilateral poor renal function in cases of associated anomalies that lead to polyhydramnios, such as diaphragmatic hernia, congestive heart failure, and gastrointestinal atresia.[11,22]

The differential diagnosis includes multicystic dysplastic kidneys (Figs. 8–16 through 8–19, 8–24) and perinephric urinoma secondary to rupture of the severely dilated renal pelvis (see p. 272). A precise diagnosis is often impossible and would not change the dismal prognosis for that kidney.[6,11]

Prognosis

The overall prognosis for unilateral UPJ obstructions is good, and intervention is not urgent even after birth.

In one follow-up study of children who underwent surgery for unilateral or bilateral hydronephrosis secondary to UPJ obstruction within 6 months of age, there were no postoperative deaths. Although the calyceal dilatation did not improve and in some cases showed a deterioration on the excretory urogram, the clinical results in regard to symptomatology and renal function were good. Serum creatinine and urea were normal even in patients with bilateral disease.[1,21]

Obstetrical Management

Unilateral UPJ obstruction should not alter standard obstetrical management as long as the contralateral kidney looks normal. There are no data to support an early delivery for correction of the UPJ obstruction. Indeed, the only study available has shown no advantage to immediate surgical repair in cases of unilateral involvement diagnosed in utero versus those diagnosed postnatally after the onset of symptoms.[23] This report only presents data on short-term follow-up (mean follow-up 2 years) and, in our opinion, should not be used to unnecessarily delay the surgical correction of an obstructed kidney.

The management of bilateral UPJ obstruction is based on gestational age, the amount of amniotic fluid, and functional renal reserve. The management issues are similar to those of posterior urethral valves (see p. 286). In cases of bilateral involvement, the amount of amniotic fluid may provide an index of renal function[13] and it usually correlates with the severity of neonatal pulmonary hypoplasia. A better estimate of residual renal function can be provided by chemical analysis of a fetal urine sample.[9] This is necessary whenever a surgical correction is planned because in some cases even early (20 weeks) fetal intervention may be too late to prevent gross renal damage.[11] A careful search for associated anomalies is always indicated, and a fetal karyotype should be performed whenever an intervention in utero is considered.

REFERENCES

1. Ahmed S, Savage JP: Surgery of pelviureteric obstruction in the first year of life. Aust NZ J Surg 55:253, 1985.
2. Antonakopoulos GN, Fuggle WJ, Newman J, et al.: Idiopathic hydronephrosis. Arch Pathol Lab Med 109:1097, 1985.
3. Arger PH, Coleman BG, Mintz MC, et al.: Routine fetal genitourinary tract screening. Radiology 156:485, 1985.
4. Atwell JD: Familial pelviureteric junction hydronephrosis and its association with a duplex pelvicaliceal system and vesicoureteric reflux. A family study. Br J Urol 57:365, 1985.
5. Baker ME, Rosenberg ER, Bowie JD: Transient in utero hydronephrosis. J Ultrasound Med 4:51, 1985.
6. Blane CE, Koff SA, Bowerman RA, et al.: Nonobstructive fetal hydronephrosis: Sonographic recognition and therapeutic implications. Radiology 147:95, 1983.
7. Buscemi M, Shanske A, Mallet E, et al.: Dominantly inherited ureteropelvic junction obstruction. Urology 26:568, 1985.
8. Drake DP, Stevens PS, Eckstein HB: Hydronephrosis secondary to ureteropelvic obstruction in children: A review of 14 years of experience. J Urol 119:649, 1978.
9. Glick PL, Harrison MR, Golbus MS, et al.: Management of the fetus with congenital hydronephrosis. II: Prognostic criteria and selection for treatment. J Pediatr Surg 20:376, 1985.
10. Hanna MK, Jeffs RD, Sturgess JM, et al.: Ureteral structure and ultrastructure. Part II. Congenital ureteropelvic junction obstruction and primary obstructive megaureter. J Urol 116:725, 1976.
11. Harrison MR, Golbus MS, Filly RA: The Unborn Patient. Prenatal Diagnosis and Treatment. Orlando, FL, Grune & Stratton, 1984, pp 97–101, 304–348.
12. Hately W, Nicholls B: The ultrasonic diagnosis of bilateral hydronephrosis in twins during pregnancy. Br J Radiol 52:989, 1979.
13. Hellstrom WJG, Kogan BA, Jeffrey RB, et al.: The natural history of prenatal hydronephrosis with normal amounts of amniotic fluid. J Urol 132:947, 1984.
14. Hoddick WK, Fily RA, Mahony BS, et al.: Minimal fetal renal pyelectasis. J Ultrasound Med 4:85, 1985.
15. Hoffer FA, Lebowitz RL: Intermittent hydronephrosis: A unique feature of ureteropelvic junction obstruction caused by a crossing renal vessel. Radiology 156:655, 1985.
16. Johnston JH, Evans JP, Glassberg KI, et al.: Pelvic hydronephrosis in children: A review of 219 personal cases. J Urol 117:97, 1977.
17. Kelalis PP, Culp OS, Stickler GB, et al.: Ureteropelvic obstruction in children: Experiences with 109 cases. J Urol 106:418, 1971.
18. Lebowitz RL, Griscom NT: Neonatal hydronephrosis: 146 cases. Radiol Clin North Am 15:49, 1977.
19. Morin ME, Baker DA: The influence of hydration and bladder distension on the sonographic diagnosis of hydronephrosis. J Clin Ultrasound 7:192, 1979.
20. Raffle RB: Familial hydronephrosis. Br Med J 1:580, 1955.
21. Robson WJ, Rudy SM, Johnston JH: Pelviureteric obstruction in infancy. J Pediatr Surg 11:57, 1976.
22. Sanders R, Graham D: Twelve cases of hydronephrosis in utero diagnosed by ultrasonography. J Ultrasound Med 1:341, 1982.
23. Thorup J, Mortensen T, Diemer H, et al.: The prognosis of surgically treated congenital hydronephrosis after diagnosis in utero. J Urol 134:914, 1985.

Megaureter

Definition

Megaureter is a dilated ureter with or without dilatation of the renal pelvis and calyces.

Incidence

Ninety-two percent of in utero urinary tract obstructions are associated with megaureters. However, most of these obstructive uropathies are due to an obstacle to the passage of urine at the level of the bladder outlet associated with megaureters.[7] The disorder is more common in male than in female children.[5,25]

Etiology

Megaureter is a sporadic disease. For some specific causes of megaureter, such as primary vesicoureteral reflux, familial cases have been described.[11,12,17] Reflux has been found in 26 to 34 percent of asymptomatic siblings of patients with vesicoureteral reflux.[3,8]

Pathogenesis and Pathology

Ureteral enlargement may be caused by obstruction to the flow of urine, vesicoureteral reflux, or conditions in which neither obstruction nor reflux is present.[9,10,22] Distinction among these different conditions is important, since treatment varies. Obstructive or refluxing hydroureter requires sur-

gical correction, whereas nonrefluxing, nonobstructive megaureters can be managed expectantly. Figure 8–25 outlines the international classification of megaureter.[16]

The term "primary" refers to a ureteral defect, whereas "secondary" refers to a pathologic process in another organ leading to dilatation of the ureter. In primary obstructive megaureter, the obstruction is at or just above the ureterovesical junction. The obstacle may be caused by stenosis of the ureteral valves, but the most common cause is the presence of a narrow juxtavesical ureteral segment that does not dilate or transmit the peristaltic wave.[4,20,21] The pathologic basis for the obstruction may be segmental fibrosis or a localized absence of muscle. Developmental failure of the longitudinal muscle results in inability of the organ to propagate the peristaltic wave. In secondary obstructive megaureter, ureterectasis is due to an extrinsic pressure, such as by a vessel or tumor.

Primary refluxing megaureter is due to an abnormality of the ureterovesical junction, leading to failure of the antireflux mechanism at the level of the ureterovesical junction. Secondary refluxing megaureter is due to reflux associated with a coexistent abnormality (e.g., neurogenic bladder or posterior urethral valves). Primary nonrefluxing nonobstructive megaureter is an idiopathic dilatation of the ureter above the vesical junction, and secondary

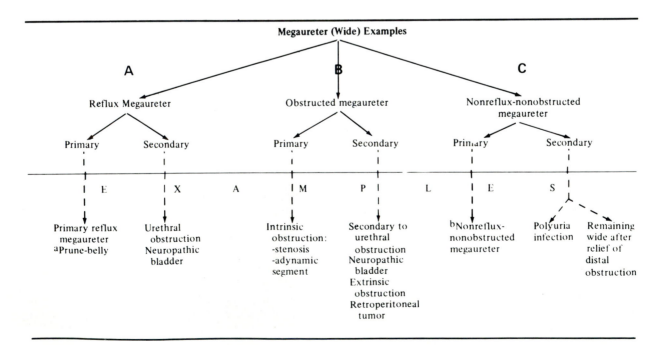

Figure 8–25. International classification of megaureter. *(Reprinted with permission from Smith et al.: Birth Defects 8(5):3, 1976.)*

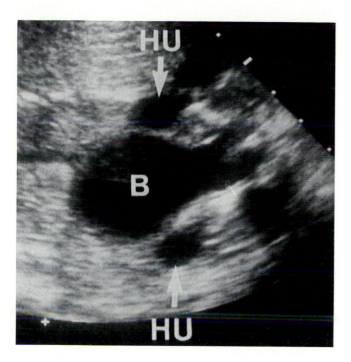

Figure 8–26. Coronal section of the fetal pelvis, showing bilateral dilatation of the ureters. This is a secondary obstructive megaureter. HU, hydroureter; B, bladder.

nonrefluxing nonobstructive megaureter is found with high rates of urine formation, such as in diabetes insipidus or infection, and in ureters that remain wide after spontaneous cessation of vesicoureteric reflux.

This chapter will only be concerned with primary megaureters, as secondary megaureters are discussed in other chapters.

Associated Anomalies

Megaureter may be associated with unilateral renal agenesis, complete or incomplete duplex system, ectopic kidney, contralateral cystic dysplastic kidney, horseshoe kidney, or Hirschsprung's disease.[15,19,25]

Diagnosis

Pathologic studies have shown that at 30 weeks the diameter of the middle portion of the fetal ureter is 1.5 mm, and, therefore, normal ureters are rarely visible with ultrasound in the human fetus. Megaureters are seen as hypoechogenic intraabdominal structures that can be traced back to the renal pelvis.

The diagnosis of a lower urinary tract obstruction is excluded by demonstrating a normal sized bladder. If an enlarged bladder is seen, the most likely diagnosis is a lower urinary tract obstruction (Fig. 8–26). However, exceptions to this have been reported. Megacystis and hydroureters associated with bilateral vesicoureteral reflux have been documented in the human fetus in the absence of any bladder outflow

obstruction.[14] The association of megaureter and megacystis has also been recognized in the absence of demonstrable obstruction or reflux (see p. 291).[18]

The renal pelvis may or may not be dilated (Fig. 8–27). In primary nonobstructive nonrefluxing megaureter, the renal pelvis is much smaller than one would expect from the ureteral dimensions, and the ureter has a straight course rather than the tortuous appearance seen in secondary refluxing hydroureter.[2] Ultrasound has been used to differentiate ureterovesical obstruction and megaureter in the neonatal period.[25]

The presence of a normal amount of amniotic fluid would suggest satisfactory renal function. However, megaureter may be associated with other malformations that lead to polyhydramnios (congestive heart failure, gastrointestinal tract abnormality). In these cases, therefore, the degree of renal deterioration is difficult to assess.[14]

Megaureter may be differentiated from mesenteric and adnexal masses because the shape of these cystic structures is not tubular but usually round. In bowel obstructions, there is usually polyhydramnios but no hydronephrosis. The dilated loops demonstrate peristalsis, and particulate matter may be seen in the lumen.

Prognosis

Whitaker and Witherow have shown that dilatations of the ureters are harmful to the kidney only if they are secondary to increased pressures within the urinary system.[23,24] At a 5-year follow-up, it was shown that when the pressure was elevated and operation was performed, improvement in the upper tract function was achieved. When the pressure was ele-

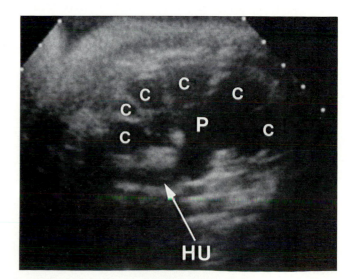

Figure 8–27. Coronal scan of a fetus with hydroureter (HU). Note the mild dilatation of the renal pelvis (P) and calices (C).

vated and operation was delayed, deterioration occurred. When the pressure was low, renal function did not worsen without operation, even though the intravenous urography appearance was unchanged. Attempts at surgical repair may worsen the prognosis by producing obstruction in at least 10 percent of patients.[1,23] Therefore, operation in these patients seems unnecessary.[24]

Obstetrical Management

Unilateral megaureter does not require a change in standard obstetrical management. Early delivery to preserve renal function may lead to respiratory distress and death of the infant.[13]

Bilateral involvement, with a normal amount of amniotic fluid, requires no intervention. There are no precedents for the management of bilateral megaureters (in the absence of lower urinary tract obstruction) associated with severe oligohydramnios.

REFERENCES

1. Belman AB: Megaureter. Classification, etiology, and management. Urol Clin North Am 1:497, 1974.
2. Deter RL, Hadlock FP, Gonzales ET, et al.: Prenatal detection of primary megaureter using dynamic image ultrasonography. Obstet Gynecol 56:759, 1980.
3. Dwoskin JY: Sibling uropathology. J Urol 115:726, 1976.
4. Gosling JA, Dixon JS: Functional obstruction of the ureter and renal pelvis. A histological and electron microscopic study. Br J Urol 50:145, 1978.
5. Hanna MK, Jeffs RD: Primary obstructive megaureter in children. Urology 6:419, 1975.
6. Harrison MR, Golbus MS, Filly RA: The Unborn Patient. Prenatal Diagnosis and Treatment. Orlando, FL, Grune & Stratton, 1984, pp 277–348.
7. Hobbins JC, Romero R, Grannum P, et al.: Antenatal diagnosis of renal anomalies with ultrasound. I. Obstructive uropathy. Am J Obstet Gynecol 148:868, 1984.
8. Jerkins GR, Noe HN: Familial vesicoureteral reflux: A prospective study. J Urol 128:774, 1982.
9. King LR: Ureter and ureterovesical junction. In: Kelalis PP, King LR, Belman AB (eds): Clinical Pediatric Urology, 2d ed. Philadelphia, Saunders, 1985, p 486.
10. King LR, Levitt SB: Vesicoureteral reflux, megaureter, and ureteral reimplantation. In: Walsh PC (ed): Campbell's Urology, 5th ed. Philadelphia, Saunders, 1986 , p 2031.
11. Mebust WK, Forest JD: Vesicoureteral reflux in identical twins. J Urol 108:635, 1972.
12. Mogg RA: Familial and adult reflux. Birth Defects 8(5):365, 1977.
13. Montana MA, Cyr DR, Lenke RR, et al.: Sonographic detection of fetal ureteral obstruction. AJR 145:595, 1985.
14. Philipson EH, Wolfson RN, Kedia KR: Fetal hydronephrosis and polyhydramnios associated with vesicoureteral reflux. J Clin Ultrasound 12:585, 1984.
15. Sant GR, Barbalias GA, Klauber GT: Congenital ureteral valves — An abnormality of ureteral embryogenesis. J Urol 133:427, 1985.
16. Smith ED, Cussen LJ, Glenn J, et al.: Report of Working Party to Establish an International Nomenclature for the Large Ureter. Birth Defects 8(5):3, 1977.
17. Stephens FD, Joske RA, Simmons RT: Megaureter with vesicoureteric reflux in twins. Aust NZ J Surg 24:192, 1955.
18. Swenson O, Fisher JH: The relation of megacolon and megaloureter. N Engl J Med 253:1147, 1955.
19. Swenson O, MacMahon E, Jaques WE, et al.: A new concept of the etiology of megaloureters. N Engl J Med 246:41, 1952.
20. Tokunaka S, Koyanagi T: Morphologic study of primary nonreflux megaureters with particular emphasis on the role of ureteral sheath and ureteral dysplasia. J Urol 128:399, 1982.
21. Tokunaka S, Koyanagi T, Tsuji I: Two infantile cases of primary megaloureter with uncommon pathological findings: Ultrastructural study and its clinical implication. J Urol 123:214, 1980.
22. Tokunaka S, Koyanagi T, Matsuno T, et al.: Paraureteral diverticula: Clinical experience with 17 cases with associated renal dysmorphism. J Urol 124:791, 1980.
23. Whitaker RH: Methods of assessing obstruction in dilated ureters. Br J Urol 45:15, 1973.
24. Witherow RON, Whitaker RH: The predictive accuracy of antegrade pressure flow studies in equivocal upper tract obstruction. Br J Urol 53:496, 1981.
25. Wood BP, Ben-Ami T, Teele RL, et al.: Ureterovesical obstruction and megaloureter: Diagnosis by real-time ultrasound. Radiology 156:79, 1985.

Posterior Urethral Valves

Definition

Lower urinary tract obstruction caused by a membranelike structure in the posterior urethra. It affects male fetuses almost exclusively.

Etiology

The disorder is usually sporadic. However, some cases of posterior urethral valves (PUV) have been reported in twins[7,20,31,32,38] and in siblings,[9,11,24,31] suggesting a genetic basis in some instances.

Embryology

Between 4 and 6 weeks of development, the primitive cloaca of a normal embryo is divided by the urorectal septum into the urinary and rectal compartments. The wolffian (mesonephric) ducts, which enter the

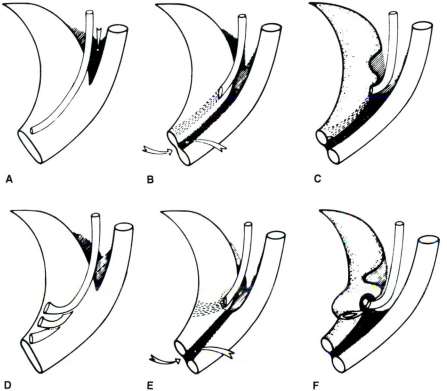

A   B   C

D   E   F

Figure 8–28. Development of type I valves. **A, B, C.** Normally, the orifices of the wolffian ducts migrate from their anterolateral position to the level of verumontanum, on the posterior wall of the urorectal septum. Normal remnants of this migration are the longitudinally oriented plicae colliculi. **D, E, F.** Abnormal anterior insertion of the wolffian duct orifices and consequent abnormal migration of the terminal ends of the ducts, resulting in circumferential obliquely oriented ridges. (*Reproduced with permission from King: In: Kelalis, King, Belman (eds): Clinical Pediatric Urology, 2d ed. Philadelphia, Saunders, 1985, Vol 1, pp 527–558.*)

anterior wall of the cloaca, recede to the level of the verumontanum (an elevation of the posterior wall of the prostatic urethra where the seminal ducts enter) in the posterior wall of the urinary compartment of the newly divided cloaca. Hence, the posterior wall of the urethra has two normal folds, called the "urethrovaginal folds" or "plicae colliculi." They are considered remnants of the cephalad migration of the wolffian ducts (Fig. 8–28). They extend longitudinally from Müller's tubercule (a prominence located between the entrance of the two müllerian ducts in the

urogenital sinus) to the origin of the Cowper or Bartholin glands.

Urethral valves are of heterogeneous embryologic origin.[29] Some valves (Young type I) seem to result from an exaggerated development of the urethrovaginal folds with an abnormal insertion of the distal end of the wolffian ducts. Other valves (Young type III) develop because of abnormal canalization of the urogenital membrane. This explanation is consistent with the morphology of type III valves (Fig. 8–29).

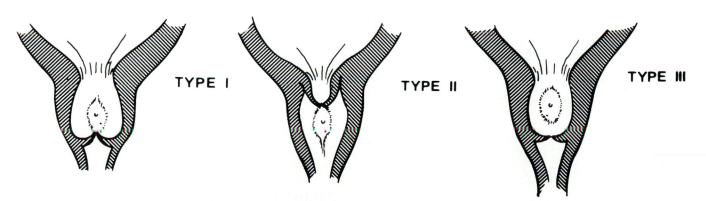

TYPE I   TYPE II   TYPE III

Figure 8–29. Young's classification of posterior urethral valves into three types. (*Reproduced with permission from King: In: Kelalis, King, Belman (eds): Clinical Pediatric Urology, 2d ed. Philadelphia, Saunders, 1985, Vol 1, pp 527–558.*)

Pathology

The classification of urethral valves is that proposed by Young et al. in 1919 and is simply based on the gross anatomic characteristic of the valves.[47] Type I valves are folds distal to the verumontanum that insert into the lateral wall of the urethra (Fig. 8–29). Type II valves are folds arising in the verumontanum, passing proximally to the bladder neck where they divide into fingerlike membranes. Type III valves consist of a diaphragmlike structure with a small perforation and are located distal to the verumontanum but not attached to it. In practice, type II valves do not cause obstruction, and only types I and III have clinical relevance.[14,36] Type I valves are much more common than are type III. The valves may be extremely thin and covered purely by their transitional epithelium or may contain variable amounts of connective tissue, which in extreme cases gives them a fleshy appearance.

Obstruction of the urinary flow due to the urethral valves results in compensatory hypertrophy of the detrusor. The portion of the detrusor within the

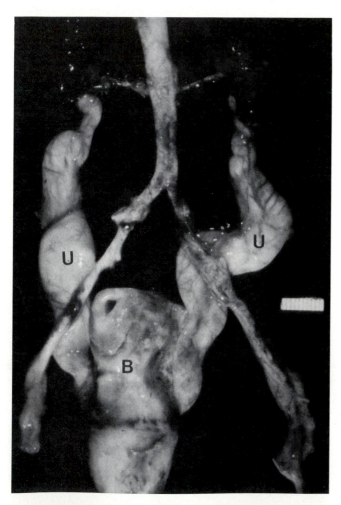

Figure 8–30. Anatomic specimen of a fetus born with posterior urethral valves. Note the distended bladder (B), tortuous ureters (U), and atrophic kidneys.

bladder neck also undergoes hypertrophy and may give the appearance of a bladder neck contracture in voiding cystourethrograms. The bladder neck may, in itself, obstruct the urine outflow.

Distention of the bladder (megacyst) eventually leads to vesicoureteral reflux and hydronephrosis (Fig. 8–30). The vesicoureteral reflux is thought to be produced by the shortening of the intravesical portion of the ureters when there is bladder distention. The portion of the ureter contained in the bladder wall is crucial for the prevention of reflux, since it acts as a valve preventing retrograde flow of urine into the ureter when intravesical pressure increases. Bilateral reflux, though not necessarily symmetrical, has a higher mortality rate and is usually present in PUV cases detected in utero. In neonatal series, reflux is generally unilateral.[28,37,46] In these patients, reflux is mainly on the left side,[21,28] the corresponding kidney is severely affected, and the contralateral kidney is usually spared, leading to a favorable prognosis.

Experimental and clinical evidence suggests that urinary obstruction severe enough to lead to hydronephrosis can cause renal dysplasia. This phenomenon is critically dependent on the time at which the obstruction occurs.[15] Observations in human and animal fetuses indicate that early obstruction leads to renal dysplasia, whereas late obstruction does not. Beck[3] demonstrated that ureteral obstruction in the fetal lamb before 70 days of gestation (term, 147 to 150 days) resulted in a renal picture similar to that of renal dysplasia (large amounts of undifferentiated mesenchymal stroma, parenchymal disorganization, cystic dilatation of the Bowman spaces, and marked fibrosis). Ligature of the ureters after 80 days of gestation resulted in hydronephrosis, but renal dysplasia did not occur. More recently, Harrison's group reported similar findings[18] and demonstrated that early in utero decompression may prevent the development of renal dysplasia.[17]

According to Potter's classification, the type of cystic kidney associated with obstructive uropathy varies depending on the timing of the obstruction. Type II dysplastic kidneys result from early obstruction. (See section on multicystic kidney disease for further details about the pathology of this condition.) If the obstruction occurs late in intrauterine life, a type IV cystic kidney results. With this variety of cystic disease, all structures are normal except for the terminal portion of the collecting tubes and the nephrons derived from them, which are dilated. There is no proliferation of connective tissue, and renal dysplasia does not occur.[25,43]

Associated Anomalies

PUV are associated in sequence with other abnormalities of the urinary tract, depending on the severity of

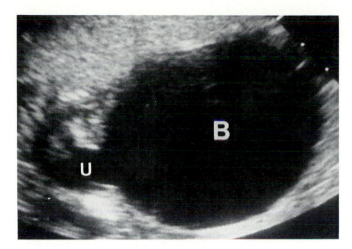

Figure 8–31. A markedly dilated bladder (B) suggests an outlet obstruction. The proximal portion of the urethra (U) is dilated.

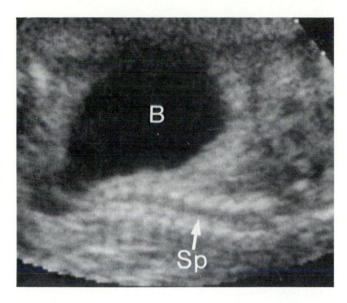

Figure 8–32. A dilated bladder (B) and proximal urethra in a fetus with posterior urethral valves. Sp; spine.

the obstruction: megacystis, megaureter, hydrone-phrosis, paraureteral diverticula, and dilatation of proximal urethra. The pathogenesis of these abnor-malities is obviously related to the increased up-stream pressure.[36]

Other anomalies of the genitourinary tract that are associated with PUV include duplication of the urethra,[12,39] megalourethra,[33] cryptorchidism,[34] and hypospadias.[37]

Reported extraurinary anomalies include tra-cheal hypoplasia, patent ductus arteriosus, total anomalous pulmonary vein drainage, mitral stenosis, scoliosis, skeletal anomalies in lower extremities, imperforate anus.[16,37] Chromosomal abnormalities, including trisomies 18 and 13, del 2q, and 69 XXY have been reported in 9 of 38 cases with documented obstructive uropathy.[41]

Diagnosis

Visualization of the urethral valves is not possible with ultrasound because of their small size. A diag-nosis of PUV should be suspected in the presence of sonographic signs of lower urinary tract obstruction (dilated bladder, hydroureter, and hydronephrosis) in a male infant (Figs. 8–31, 8–32, 8–33). Sex determi-nation is important, since PUV do not occur in female infants. Causes of lower urinary tract obstruction in females include agenesis of the urethra, megacystis–microcolon–intestinal hypoperistalsis syndrome, and variants of the caudal regression syndrome. Some-times it is possible to demonstrate the dilated poste-rior urethra proximal to the valves (Figs. 8–31, 8–32).

Another sign of PUV is bladder wall hyper-trophy, which is visible after relief of the obstruction (Fig. 8–34). The ureters are characteristically dilated and tortuous, and in severe cases their entrance into the bladder can be observed.

The degree of dilatation of the renal pelvis is variable. In some patients, there may be severe obstruction and renal dysplasia in the absence of marked distention of the renal pelvis. This can be explained by one of the following reasons: (1) renal dysplasia has decreased urinary production, (2) rup-ture at the level of the bladder or any other point along the urinary tract has resulted in decompression of the renal pelvis, or (3) there is pelviureteric atresia.

The most important consideration in regard to the kidney involves the prenatal detection of renal dysplasia.[40] Renal dysplasia can occur with both small and enlarged kidneys. The most important sonographic signs of renal dysplasia are multiple

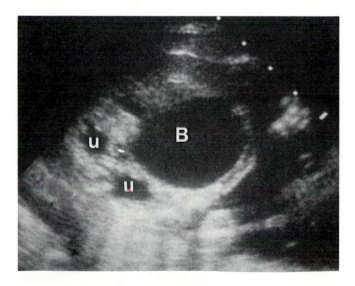

Figure 8–33. Dilated bladder (B) and bilateral hydroureters (u).

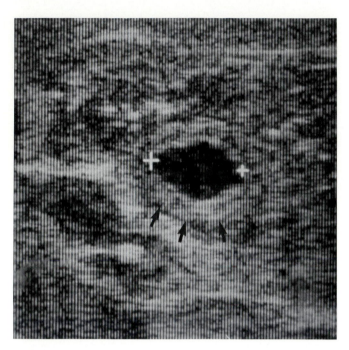

Figure 8–34. A fetus who had posterior urethral valves and experienced resolution of the obstructive process in utero after shunting. A thickened bladder wall is visible. Arrows point to the outer bladder wall.

cysts and the hyperechogenicity of the renal parenchyma. Table 8–3 shows the diagnostic indices of renal dysplasia. The detection of renal cysts is relatively insensitive, but their presence indicates dysplastic kidneys (Fig. 8–35). Renal echogenicity is more sensitive but also less specific (Fig. 8–36). Hydronephrosis is the weakest of the renal signs in the prediction of renal dysplasia.

Urine can extravasate into the peritoneal cavity (ascites) or the perirenal space.[1,15,22] The mechanisms responsible for urine extravasation are often unknown. Rupture of the bladder can account for some cases, but the rest are attributed to transudation of urine into the peritoneal cavity. The degree of ascites is variable and can reach extreme proportions, leading to atrophy of the abdominal wall muscles (the prune-belly sequence). On occasion, there is no free-floating ascites, but an isolated perirenal urinoma persists.

Oligohydramnios is not an invariable finding and is related to the severity and duration of the obstruction. The presence of severe oligohydramnios is considered a poor prognostic sign; conversely, a normal amount of amniotic fluid is a good prognostic sign.[8,13]

In utero intravenous pyelograms have been used to confirm the diagnosis.[19] After the placement of a needle in the urinary tract, dye (2.5 ml of renographin 69) was injected to procure better visualization. The

indications for this diagnostic maneuver decrease as experience with ultrasound increases.

Some fetuses with PUV have come to the attention of the sonographer because of an elevated amniotic fluid and maternal serum AFP.[8]

The differential diagnosis includes other obstructive uropathies, such as ureteropelvic junction (UPJ) obstruction, ureterovesical junction (UVJ) obstruction, primary megaureter, and massive vesicoureteral reflux.[42] In both UPJ and UVJ obstructions, the bladder should not be dilated. The differential diagnosis between PUV and other causes of low urinary tract obstruction, such as absence of the urethra or detrusor hypertrophy, may not be possible in all cases.[27] Megacystic–microcolon–intestinal hypoperistalsis syndrome (MMIHS) is a rapidly fatal triad that affects females in 91 percent of cases and is characterized by a massively dilated, thick-walled bladder, normal to increased amniotic fluid, dilatation of the stomach with little peristaltic activity, bilateral hydronephrosis with no signs of renal damage, and no hydroureters (see p. 291).

A critical aspect of evaluation of the fetus with obstructive uropathy is the assessment of renal reserve. Infants with bilateral dysplastic kidneys have a uniformly poor prognosis. Although sonographic detection of cortical cystic changes has excellent specificity in the prenatal diagnosis of renal dysplasia, its sensitivity is relatively poor. Therefore, infants with normal kidneys on ultrasound can still be born with nonfunctioning kidneys. Management decisions, such as pregnancy termination and in utero surgery, rely on assessment of renal reserve. For example, a diagnosis of renal dysfunction even in the absence of sonographic findings would render in utero shunting useless.

Attempts at evaluating renal reserve have been undertaken with (1) single drainage of the fetal bladder and documentation of reaccumulation of urine, (2) furosemide stimulation of urine production, and (3) electrolyte determination in fetal urine. The first two methods have proven to be unreliable and, therefore, have been abandoned in favor of the third option.

TABLE 8–3. DIAGNOSTIC INDICES OF DIFFERENT SONOGRAPHIC CRITERIA FOR THE IDENTIFICATION OF RENAL DYSPLASIA IN OBSTRUCTIVE UROPATHY

	Sensitivity (%)	Specificity (%)	PPV (%)	NPV (%)
Renal cysts	44	100	100	44
Hyperechogenic renal parenchyma	73	80	89	57
Hydronephrosis	41	73	78	35

Reproduced with permission from Mahony, Filly, Callen, et al.: Radiology 152:143, 1984.

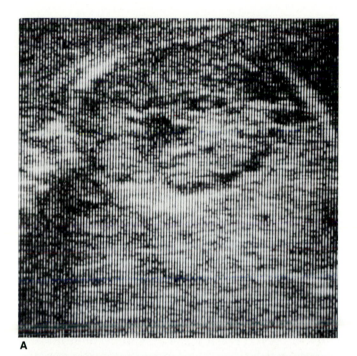

A

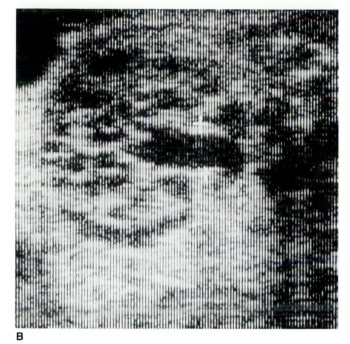

B

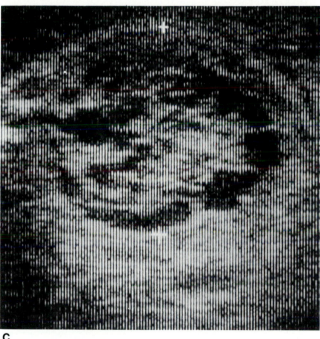

C

Figure 8–35. This sequence of images demonstrates the in utero development of cystic dysplasia of the kidneys. **A**. There is enlargement of the kidney and formation of cystic structures close to the cortex. **B**. Further enlargement of the kidney and cystic structures. **C**. Severe cystic dysplastic kidney.

Studies have been accomplished by puncturing the bladder and assaying electrolytes and osmolarity in the first urine sample obtained.[16] In addition, fetal urinary output has been measured by placing a balloon-tipped catheter (4F Model JC-211, Critikon Inc, Tampa, FL) into the dilated fetal bladder. The concentrations of sodium, chloride, and osmolarity correlated with renal function at birth. Poor function was defined as the presence of severe renal dysplasia and pulmonary hypoplasia at autopsy or biopsy, or renal and pulmonary insufficiency at birth. Good function was based on nondysplastic kidneys at autopsy or biopsy or normal renal and pulmonary function at birth. Table 8–4 illustrates the prognostic criteria for fetuses with bilateral obstructive uropathy. The fetus with renal damage acts as a salt loser, and, therefore, the concentration of electrolytes and osmolarity in the urine are elevated. With the exception of urinary output per hour, information about these prognostic criteria can be obtained by a single puncture of the fetal bladder and a sonographic examination. It is unclear if quantitation of fetal

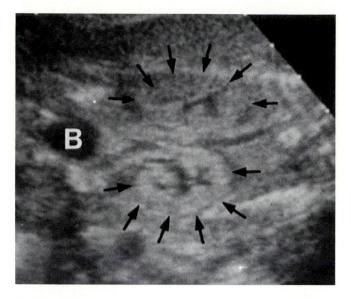

Figure 8–36. Coronal scan showing increased echogenicity of the renal parenchyma of a fetus with posterior urethral valves. There is oligohydramnios, and a normal-sized bladder (B). The infant was born with cystic dysplastic kidneys. Arrows point to the renal parenchyma.

diuresis provides valuable information. Furthermore, infectious complications have occurred during exteriorization of the fetal bladder, leading to death in 3 of 9 fetuses. Therefore, this invasive procedure does not seem justified.

Prognosis

The only data on long-term prognosis have been gathered from cases diagnosed after birth. Caution is advised in extrapolating these figures to infants diagnosed in utero, since the natural history of the disease may be different. The timing of the occurrence of urinary obstruction is a critical factor in determining the extent and severity of renal damage. When the condition is diagnosed in utero, the prognosis seems much worse. Affected neonates are at high risk (32 to 50 percent) for death,[10,44] as a result of pneumomediastinum and pneumothorax related to pulmonary hypoplasia, associated congenital anomalies, renal failure, and surgical complications after decompressive surgery.[37] Survivors have a higher incidence of growth retardation, expressed as a lower percentile of height and weight for a given age. Catch-up growth occurs after corrective surgery.[35] Improvement in renal function is demonstrated in most patients after surgery. However, chronic parenchymal deterioration can continue despite treatment. Renal hypoplasia and dysplasia and chronic pyelonephritis are thought to play a role, but the precise mechanisms for progressive renal failure despite correction of the obstruction are unknown. The development of end-stage renal disease may be delayed for 9 to 10 years.[45]

The incidence of chronic renal failure in infants diagnosed in the first 3 months of life is 39 percent.[1] The most important prognostic factor for the prediction of good renal function seems to be the postoperative nadir of serum creatinine during the first year. Levels of 0.8 mg/ml or less are associated with good prognosis, and levels of 1 mg/ml or less are associated with long-term normal growth.[46]

The outcome of infants who have undergone vesicoamniotic shunt is available from the International Fetal Surgery Registry. Of a total of 73 treated patients, 11 elected to terminate the pregnancy after shunt placement. The reasons for termination were an abnormal karyotype ($n = 6$) or the development of sonographic signs of renal dysplasia. The survival for the remaining 62 patients was 48 percent. Survival could not be related to fetal age at the time of diagnosis or treatment but was related to fetal sex and to the etiology of the obstruction. Male infants did better (survival = 51 percent) than female infants (survival = 20 percent). There were 3 stillbirths and 29 postnatal deaths. Pulmonary hypoplasia was the most common cause of neonatal death.

Obstetrical Management

Once the diagnosis of the lower urinary tract obstruction is made, management depends on the detection of other life-threatening anomalies, gestational age at diagnosis, and status of renal function.

A search for associated anomalies is important, but sonographic evaluation is frequently hampered by the associated oligohydramnios. The instillation of fluid into the amniotic cavity may be required to improve visualization. This can be accomplished by the injection of a solution warmed to 37C. Chromosomal analysis should be undertaken when feasible by either amniocentesis or fetal blood sampling. A recent study indicated that 23 percent of infants with obstructive uropathy had chromosomal abnormalities.[41] If a chromosomal or anatomic anomaly incompatible with life is detected (e.g., trisomy 18 or holoprosencephaly), the option of preg-

TABLE 8–4. PROGNOSTIC CRITERIA FOR FETUSES WITH BILATERAL OBSTRUCTIVE UROPATHY

Poor Prognostic Signs	Good Prognostic Signs
Severe oligohydramnios	Normal amniotic fluid
Cystic kidneys	Normal kidneys
Na > 100 mEq/ml	Na < 100 mEq/ml
Cl > 90 mEq/ml	Cl < 90 mEq/ml
Osmolarity > 210 mOsm	Osmolarity < 210 mOsm
Urinary output of < 2 ml/hr*	Urinary output > 2 ml/hr

* Urinary output was measured by exteriorizing the fetal bladder with an indwelling catheter for several hours.
Reproduced with permission from Glick, Harrison, Golbus, et al.: J Pediatr Surg 20:376, 1985.

nancy termination at any stage of gestation can be considered.

The next step in the evaluation process is assessing the renal reserve by referring to the criteria outlined in Table 8–4. Of particular importance is the amniotic fluid volume, since infants with normal amniotic fluid seem to have an excellent prognosis.

With good prognostic criteria, there are little data to advise parents about the long-term risks to the infant. Theoretical risks would include worsening of the condition in utero, requirement of in utero surgery or premature delivery, development of pulmonary hypoplasia, or some long-term impairment of renal function.

If prognosis is poor based on the criteria outlined in Table 8–4, alternatives include pregnancy termination or nonintervention. If the prognosis is good, further management decisions are based on the gestational age. If the diagnosis is made at a gestational age when pulmonic maturity is likely, an L:S ratio determination is indicated. In the presence of lung maturity, the patient should be delivered in a tertiary care center where urologic evaluation can be performed after birth. The mode of delivery should not be affected by the diagnosis.

When the diagnosis has been made after viability but before lung maturity, weekly serial examinations are required. The options are (1) preventive utero decompression or (2) expectant management and intervention only when the amniotic fluid volume decreases. The optimal management between these options has not been established. Harrison's group[23] at the University of California, San Francisco, favors the second option.

Choice of Intrauterine Surgery. Two different procedures can be performed for decompression of obstructive uropathy in utero: placement of a shunt and suprapubic vesicostomy. Indwelling catheters frequently become dislodged or occluded, and, therefore, they are most effective when used in circumstances that require short-term decompression (urinary obstructions detected in late pregnancy while awaiting fetal lung maturity). Harrison's group[23] has performed two suprapubic vesicostomies in early pregnancy. This procedure seems more efficient in the treatment of an obstruction, since the likelihood of reobstruction is small. However, it requires a hysterotomy, and the risks of this operation are yet to be established.

Technique for Catheter Placement. The procedure requires sedation of both fetus and mother. This can be accomplished by the parenteral administration of diazepam or morphine. In the presence of severe oligohydramnios, the instillation of fluid into the amniotic cavity is necessary to create a space in which the amniotic coil can be placed.

Several catheters have been employed to create a vesicoamniotic shunt. We have used a 6.5 Fr polyethylene instrument constructed from an angiographic catheter.[5] Harrison's group uses a kit that contains a Harrison fetal bladder stent, 8 Fr (Model 03408-1, VPI, Inc., Spencer, IN).[23] The catheters have a double pigtail. One end is destined to coil into the bladder and the other into the amniotic cavity. The catheters are constructed from material that maintains the curved shape and will not disappear even when the catheter is mounted onto a straight needle for insertion. This property is referred to as the "memory" of the shunt. Several lateral sideholes are made along both coils. The straight portion of the catheter should not contain any holes; otherwise, leakage of urine into the fetal peritoneal cavity will occur.

The needle is 19 gauge and 29 cm long. A pusher made of the same material as the catheter is required and should be long enough to permit advancement of the catheter. The other instrument required is a sterile ruler to intraoperatively assess the amount of catheter that has been advanced. The catheter is specifically designed for each patient, taking measurements of the fetal bladder and of the fetal abdominal wall into account.

The procedure can be conducted in three major steps:

1. Introduction of the catheter into the fetal bladder. A small incision in the maternal abdominal wall and rectus sheath is performed with a scalpel. Local anesthesia is required. Once the needle is in the fetal bladder, the catheter is advanced the length of the distal pigtail. The last orifice of the pigtail should be inside the fetal bladder. Ultrasound can demonstrate the coiled catheter within this organ.

2. Withdrawal of a segment of the needle until its tip is in the amniotic cavity. The length of needle to be removed corresponds to the straight portion of the catheter. During this maneuver, the pusher must not be moved. It is important that a pocket of fluid be created at the beginning of the procedure if one was not already present. Otherwise, the creation of the second coil becomes extremely difficult.

3. Advancement of the pusher until the second coil is created inside the amniotic cavity. This is the most difficult part of the procedure. If calculations have not been correct, the distal end of the catheter may end up in the uterine or maternal abdominal wall. Another technique of inserting the catheter through an introducer needle is now being evaluated. Initial results are encouraging.

REFERENCES

1. Adzick NS, Harrison MR, Flake AW, et al.: Urinary extravasation in the fetus with obstructive uropathy. J Pediatr Surg 20:608, 1985.
2. Atwell JD: Posterior urethral valves in the British Isles: A multicenter B.A.P.S. review. J Pediatr Surg 18:70, 1983.
3. Beck AD: The effect of intra-uterine urinary obstruction upon the development of the fetal kidney. J Urol 105:784, 1971.
4. Bellinger MF, Comstock CH, Grosso D, et al.: Fetal posterior urethral valves and renal dysplasia at 15 weeks gestational age. J Urol 129:1238, 1983.
5. Berkowitz RL, Glickman MG, Smith GJW, et al.: Fetal urinary tract obstruction: What is the role of surgical intervention in utero? Am J Obstet Gynecol 144:367, 1982.
6. Cass AS, Khan AU, Smith S: Neonatal perirenal urinary extravasation with posterior urethral valves. Urology 18:258, 1981.
7. Davidsohn I, Newberger C: Congenital valves of the posterior urethra in twins. Arch Pathol 16:57, 1933.
8. Dean WM, Bourdeau EJ: Amniotic fluid alpha-fetoprotein in fetal obstructive uropathy. Pediatrics 60:537, 1980.
9. Doraiswamy NV, Al Badr MSK: Posterior urethral valves in siblings. Br J Urol 55:448, 1983.
10. Egami K, Smith ED: A study of the sequelae of posterior urethral valve. J Urol 127:84, 1982.
11. Farkas A, Skinner DG: Posterior urethral valves in siblings. Br J Urol 48:76, 1976.
12. Fernbach SK, Maizels M: Posterior urethral valves causing urinary retention in an infant with duplication of the urethra. J Urol 132:353, 1984.
13. Garrett WJ, Kossoff G, Osborn RA: The diagnosis of fetal hydronephrosis, megaureter and urethral obstruction by ultrasonic echography. Br J Obstet Gynaecol 82:115, 1975.
14. Glassberg KI: Current issues regarding posterior urethral valves. Urol Clin North Am 12:175, 1985.
15. Glazer GM, Filly RA, Callen PW: The varied sonographic appearance of the urinary tract in the fetus and newborn with urethral obstruction. Radiology 144:563, 1982.
16. Glick PL, Harrison MR, Golbus MS, et al.: Management of the fetus with congenital hydronephrosis. II. Prognostic criteria and selection for treatment. J Pediatr Surg 20:376, 1985.
17. Glick PL, Harrison MR, Adzick NS, et al.: Correction of congenital hydronephrosis in utero IV: In utero decompression prevents renal dysplasia. J Pediatr Surg 19:649, 1984.
18. Glick PL, Harrison MR, Noall RA, et at.: Correction of congenital hydronephrosis in utero III: Early mid-trimester ureteral obstruction produces renal dysplasia. J Pediatr Surg 18:681, 1983.
19. Gore RM, Callen PW, Filly RA, et al.: Prenatal percutaneous antegrade pyelography in posterior urethral valves: Sonographic guidance. AJR 139:994, 1982.
20. Grajewski RS, Glassberg KI: The variable effect of posterior urethral valves as illustrated in identical twins. J Urol 130:1188, 1983.
21. Greenfield SP, Hensle TW, Berdon WE: Urinary extravasation in the newborn male with posterior urethral valves. J Pediatr Surg 17:751, 1982.
22. Griscom NT, Colodny AH, Rosenberg HK et al.: Diagnostic aspects of neonatal ascites: Report of 27 cases. AJR 128:961, 1977.
23. Harrison MR, Golbus MS, Filly RA: The Unborn Patient. Prenatal Diagnosis and Treatment. New York, Grune & Stratton, 1984, pp 277–348.
24. Hasen HB, Song YS: Congenital valvular obstruction of the posterior urethra in two brothers. J Pediatr 47:207, 1955.
25. Henneberry MO, Stephens FD: Renal hypoplasia and dysplasia in infants with posterior urethral valves. J Urol 123:912, 1980.
26. Hobbins JC, Romero R, Grannum P, et al.: Antenatal diagnosis of renal anomalies with ultrasound. I. Obstructive uropathy. Am J Obstet Gynecol 148:868, 1984.
27. Hurwitz A, Yagel S, Rabinovitz R, et al.: Hydramnios caused by pure megacystis. J Clin Ultrasound 12:110, 1984.
28. Johnston JH: Vesicoureteric reflux with urethral valves. Br J Urol 51:100, 1979.
29. Kelalis PP, King LR, Belman AB: Posterior urethra. In: Kelalis PP, King LR, Belman AB (eds). Clinical Pediatric Urology, 2d ed. Philadelphia, Saunders, 1985, p 527.
30. King LR: Posterior urethral valves. In : Kelalis PP, King LR, Belman AB (eds). Clinical Pediatric Urology, 2d ed. Philadelphia, Saunders, 1985, Vol 1, pp 527–558.
31. Kjellberg SR, Ericsson NO, Rudhe U: Urethral valves. In: The Lower Urinary Tract in Childhood. Some Correlated Clinical and Roentgenologic Observations. Stockholm: Almqvist & Wiksell, 1957, pp 203–254.
32. Kroovand RL, Weinberg N, Emami A: Posterior urethral valves in identical twins. Pediatrics 60:748, 1977.
33. Krueger RP, Churchill BM: Megalourethra with posterior urethral valves. Urology 18:279, 1981.
34. Krueger RP, Hardy BE, Churchill BM: Cryptorchidism in boys with posterior urethral valves. J Urol 124:101, 1980.
35. Krueger RP, Hardy BE, Churchill BM: Growth in boys with posterior urethral valves. Primary valve resection vs upper tract diversion. Urol Clin North Am 7:265, 1980.
36. Kurth KH, Alleman RJ, Schroder FH: Major and minor complications of posterior urethral valves. J Urol 126:517, 1981.
37. Lebowitz RL, Griscom NT: Neonatal hydronephrosis: 146 Cases. Radiol Clin North Am 15:49, 1977.
38. Livne PM, Delaune J, Gonzales ET Jr: Genetic etiology of posterior urethral valves. J Urol 130:781, 1983.
39. Lorenzo RL, Turner WR, Bradford BF, et al.: Duplication of the male urethra with posterior urethral valves. Pediatr Radiol 11:39, 1981.
40. Mahony BS, Filly RA, Callen PW, et al.: Fetal renal dysplasia: Sonographic evaluation radiology. Radiology 152:143, 1984.

41. Nicolaides KH, Rodeck CH, Gosden CM: Rapid karyotyping in non-lethal fetal malformations. Lancet 1:283, 1986.
42. Reuter KL, Lebowitz RL: Massive vesicoureteral reflux mimicking posterior urethral valves in a fetus. J Clin Ultrasound 13:584, 1985.
43. Schwarz RD, Stephens FD, Cussen LJ: The pathogenesis of renal dysplasia. II. The significance of lateral and medial ectopy of the ureteric orifice. III. Complete and incomplete urinary obstruction. Invest Urol 19:97, 1981.
44. Tsingoglou S, Dickson JAS: Lower urinary obstruction in infancy. A review of lesions and symptoms in 165 cases. Arch Dis Child 47:215, 1972.
45. Warshaw BL, Edelbrock HH, Ettenger RB, et al.: Progression to end-stage renal disease in children with obstructive uropathy. J Pediatr 100:183, 1982.
46. Warshaw BL, Hymes LC, Trulock TS, et al.: Prognostic features in infants with obstructive uropathy due to posterior urethral valves. J Urol 133:240, 1985.
47. Young HH, Frontz WA, Baldwin JC: Congenital obstruction of the posterior urethra. J Urol 3:289, 1919.

Prune-Belly Syndrome

Synonyms

Triad syndrome (abdominal wall distention, urinary tract obstruction, and cryptorchidism) and Eagle-Barret syndrome.

Definition

Prune-belly syndrome describes the association of hypotonic abdominal wall, large hypotonic bladder with dilated ureters, and cryptorchidism. Prune-belly syndrome may be considered a malformation sequence due to intrauterine abdominal wall distention. Such distention is most frequently due to an obstructive uropathy, but other causes could lead to the morphologic features of the syndrome in the absence of urinary involvement.

Epidemiology

The incidence varies from 1 in 35,000 to 1 in 50,000 live births.[9] The overwhelming majority of affected infants are males. Fewer than 20 of more than 300 reported cases have been females.

Etiology

Genetic basis for prune-belly syndrome has not been established, although it has been documented in siblings.[2,8] The risk of recurrence of this condition is unknown, but parents should probably be told that this is a possibility. Cases associated with chromosomal anomalies (trisomy 13, 18, and 45XO) have been reported.[3,7,13]

There is an association between prune-belly syndrome and twinning. The incidence of twinning in the general population is 1:80, and in prune-belly syndrome, it is 1:23.[11] All reported cases in twins are discordant for the syndrome.

Pathogenesis

There are two theories to explain this syndrome. The mesodermal defect theory proposes that abdominal wall laxity is the result of an early embryologic insult affecting the mesoderm of the anterior abdominal wall and the urinary tract.[4,5] However, increasing evidence suggests that the pathogenesis of prune-belly syndrome can be explained by the urethral obstruction malformation complex.[15,17] According to this view, urethral obstruction leads to massive distention of the bladder and ureters, which in turn causes pressure atrophy of the abdominal wall muscles. Bladder distention also interferes with the descent of the testes and is responsible for cryptorchidism. The obstructive nature of the bladder distention explains the presence of muscular hypertrophy in the bladder wall, tortuous hydroureters, renal dysplasia, and a persistently open urachus. A distended bladder could also exert compression on the iliac vessels and lead to limb deficiencies. The urethral obstruction causes severe oligohydramnios and features of the oligohydramnios sequence, such as pulmonary hypoplasia, skeletal deformities, and Potter facies.

The major objection to this theory has been that not all newborns with prune-belly syndrome have a urethral obstruction at birth. However, it is possible for transient in utero urinary obstruction to cause the sequence responsible for the syndrome.[6] Prune-belly syndrome could be the result of an intraabdominal distention unrelated to obstruction of the urinary tract. For example, transient ascites,[12,19] intestinal duplication cysts,[16] and megacystis-microcolon syndrome also cause the malformation sequence.

Pathology

The deficiency in abdominal wall muscles ranges from a virtual agenesis to hypoplasia.[10] Poor abdominal wall musculature does not increase significantly the risk for postoperative hernias. The impaired support of the lower chest contributes to ineffective coughing, hence, the susceptibility of these infants to respiratory infections. Cryptorchidism is associated with impaired fertility probably due to abnormal spermatogenesis.[21] Hormonal production by the undescended testes is normal. Intraabdominal testes are at risk for malignant transformation.[23] The limb deformities have a wide spectrum, from those associated with oligohydramnios (equinovarus and dimple in the elbow and knee joint) to amputations. Most patients also have some intestinal malrotation, which has been attributed to a universal mesentery with unattached cecum.[22] Congenital heart disease has been reported in 10 percent of patients.[1]

Diagnosis

Prune-belly syndrome can be diagnosed in utero if spontaneous resolution of the intraabdominal distention responsible for the sequence occurs. Then, an abnormal tendency of the abdominal wall to depress when in contact with solid parts of the fetus (limbs) or to move by external percussion applied to the maternal abdomen can be documented.[14,19,20]

Prognosis

Prune-belly syndrome has a wide spectrum of severity. Some infants with severe oligohydramnios die in the neonatal period because of pulmonary hypoplasia or pneumothorax (type I prune-belly syndrome). Others survive the neonatal period and may develop renal insufficiency if urinary obstruction was the cause of the sequence (type II). The mild cases may have incomplete extrarenal features of the syndrome; the uropathy is less severe, and renal function is stable (type III).[22]

The abdomen offers a serious cosmetic problem. Several operations are available to assist in the correction of the abdominal wall reconstruction.[18] The other aspect of the rehabilitation of patients with prune-belly syndrome is the surgical treatment of the obstructive uropathy (see Posterior Urethral Valves, p. 280). Urologic evaluation is mandatory. Surgical correction of the large bladder, vesicoureteral reflux, and megaurethra may be required. Undescended testes are generally treated surgically.[23]

REFERENCES

1. Adebonojo FO: Dysplasia of the anterior abdominal musculature with multiple congenital anomalies: Prune-belly or triad syndrome. J Natl Med Assoc 65:327, 1973.
2. Adeyokunnu AA, Familusi JB: Prune belly syndrome in two siblings and a first cousin. Am J Dis Child 136:23, 1982.
3. Beckmann H, Rehder H, Rauskolb R: Letter to the Editor: Prune-belly sequence associated with trisomy 13. Am J Med Genet 19:603, 1984.
4. Burton BK, Dillard RG; Brief clinical report. Prune-belly syndrome: Observations supporting the hypothesis of abdominal overdistention. Am J Med Genet 17:669, 1984.
5. Bruton OC: Agenesis of abdominal musculature associated with genito-urinary and gastro-intestinal tract anomalies. J Urol 66:607, 1951.
6. Fitzsimons RB, Keohane C, Galvin J: Prune-belly syndrome with ultrasound demonstration of reduction of megacystis in utero. Br J Radiol 58:374, 1985.
7. Frydman M, Magenis RE, Mohandas TK, et al.: Chromosome abnormalities in infants with prune-belly anomaly: Association with trisomy 18. Am J Med Genet 15:145, 1983.
8. Gaboardi F, Sterpa A, Thiebat E, et al.: Prune-belly syndrome: Report of three siblings. Helv Paediatr Acta 37:283, 1982.
9. Garlinger P, Ott J: Prune-belly syndrome: Possible genetic implications. Birth Defects 10:173, 1974.
10. Geary DF, MacLusky IB, Churchill BM, et al.: A broader spectrum of abnormalities in the prune-belly syndrome. J Urology 135:324, 1986.
11. Ives E J: The abdominal muscle deficiency triad syndrome: Experience with 10 cases. Birth Defects 10:127, 1974.
12. Lubinsky M, Rapoport P: Transient fetal hydrops and "prune-belly" in one identical female twin. N Engl J Med 308:256, 1983.
13. Lubinsky M, Doyle K, Trunca C: The association of "prune-belly" with Turner's syndrome. Am J Dis Child 134:1171, 1980.
14. Meizner I, Bar-Ziv J, Katz M: Prenatal ultrasonic diagnosis of the extreme form of prune-belly syndrome. J Clin Ultrasound 13:581, 1985.
15. Moerman P, Fryns JP, Goddeeris P, et al.: Pathogenesis of the prune-belly syndrome: A functional urethral obstruction caused by prostatic hypoplasia. Pediatrics 73:470, 1984.
16. Nakayama DK, Harrison MR, Chinn DH, et al.: The pathogenesis of prune belly. Am J Dis Child 138:834, 1984.
17. Pagon RA, Smith DW, Shepard TH: Urethral obstruction malformation complex: A cause of abdominal muscle deficiency and the "prune belly." J Pediatr 94:900, 1979.
18. Randolph J, Cavett C, Eng G: Surgical correction and rehabilitation for children with "prune-belly" syndrome. Ann Surg 193:757, 1981.
19. Shapiro I, Sharf M: Spontaneous intrauterine remission of hydrops fetalis in one identical twin: Sonographic diagnosis. J Clin Ultrasound 13:427, 1985.
20. Shih WJ, Greenbaum LD, Baro C: In utero sonogram in prune-belly syndrome. Urology 20:102, 1982.
21. Uehling DT, Zadina SP, Gilbert E: Testicular histology in triad syndrome. Urology 23:364, 1984.
22. Woodard JR, Trulock TS: Prune-belly syndrome. In: Walsh PC (ed): Campbell's Urology, 5th ed. Philadelphia, Saunders, 1986, pp 2159–2178.
23. Woodhouse CRJ, Snyder HMC: Testicular and sexual function in adults with prune-belly syndrome. J Urol 133:607, 1985.

Megacystis–Microcolon–Intestinal Hypoperistalsis Syndrome

Synonym
Neonatal hollow visceral myopathy.[6]

Definition
Megacystis–microcolon–intestinal hypoperistalsis (MMIH) syndrome consists of the association of a distended unobstructed bladder, a dilated small bowel, and distal microcolon.

Incidence
This syndrome was first described in 1976,[2] and since then, 26 cases have been reported in the literature. The condition affects predominantly female infants. Of the 26 reported cases, only 3 have occurred in males.[4,9]

Etiology
Most cases are sporadic, although some familial cases have been reported.[2]

Pathology
There is a distended unobstructed bladder. Hydronephrosis is present in virtually all patients. Gastric and intestinal motility is impaired and leads to malnutrition. The small bowel is short, dilated, and malfixed, but no anatomic obstruction can be found in most patients. Microcolon (narrow rectum and sigmoid colon) is a transient feature of the syndrome, possibly related to the hypoperistalsis. Should the baby survive, all the segments of the colon become normal in size or dilated.[9] Histologically, there are normal ganglia.[1,3] Puri et al.[6] called attention to the similarity between MMIH syndrome and a smooth muscle disorder seen in adults, chronic idiopathic intestinal pseudoobstruction (CIIP). This syndrome is a familial condition characterized by bladder, intestinal, ureteral, and esophageal dysfunction. Electromicroscopic studies have shown vacuolar degeneration of smooth muscle similar to that reported by Puri et al. in MMIH. Therefore, it is possible that MMIH syndrome and CIIP represent expressions of the same disorder.

Diagnosis
In eight cases, antenatal visualization of this syndrome has been reported.[4–8] MMIH syndrome should be suspected in the presence of a distended bladder with a normal or increased amount of amniotic fluid in a female fetus. There may be hydronephrosis. The main differential diagnosis is obstructive uropathy due to posterior urethral valves. In a female fetus, a low urinary tract obstruction can be due to absence of the urethra, to variants of the caudal regression syndrome, or to the rare detrusor hypertrophy. In these conditions oligohydramnios is severe.

Prognosis
MMIH syndrome is a lethal condition in most cases. Of the 23 reported patients, 21 died in the immediate postoperative period or shortly thereafter. The cause of death is bowel renal dysfunction. Infants have died despite hyperalimentation. Sepsis is frequently noted in published reports as a final complication.

Obstetrical Management
In the absence of a positive family history, it is unclear if this diagnosis can be made with certainty. A massively dilated bladder has been a cause of soft tissue dystocia in one patient.[6] Therefore, consideration should be given to prenatal drainage of this organ. There does not seem to be any reason to induce preterm delivery of these infants.

REFERENCES

1. Amoury RA, Fellows RA, Goodwin CD, et al.: Megacystis–microcolon–intestinal hypoperistalsis syndrome: A cause of intestinal obstruction in the newborn period. J Pediatr Surg 12:1063, 1977.
2. Berdon WE, Baker DH, Blanc WA, et al.: Megacystis–microcolon–intestinal hypoperistalsis syndrome: A new cause of intestinal obstruction in the newborn. Report of radiologic findings in five newborn girls. AJR 126:957, 1976.
3. Jona JZ, Werlin SL: The megacystis microcolon intestinal hypoperistalsis syndrome: Report of a case. J Pediatr Surg 16:749, 1981.
4. Krook PM: Megacystis–microcolon–intestinal hypoperistalsis syndrome in a male infant. Radiology 136:649, 1980.
5. Manco LG, Osterdahl P: The antenatal sonographic features of megacystis–microcolon–intestinal hypoperistalsis syndrome. J Clin Ultrasound 12:595, 1984.
6. Puri P, Lake BD, Gorman F, et al.: Megacystis–microcolon–intestinal hypoperistalsis syndrome: A visceral myopathy. J Pediatr Surg 18:64, 1983.
7. Vezina WC, Morin FR, Winsberg F: Megacystis–microcolon–intestinal hypoperistalsis syndrome: Antenatal ultrasound appearance. AJR 133:749, 1979.
8. Vintzileos AM, Eisenfeld LI, Herson VC, et al.: Megacystis–microcolon–intestinal hypoperistalsis syndrome—Prenatal sonographic findings and review of the literature. Am J Perinatol 3:297, 1986.
9. Young LW, Yunis EJ, Girdany BR, et al.: Megacystis–microcolon–intestinal hypoperistalsis syndrome: Additional clinical, radiologic, surgical, and histopathologic aspects. AJR 137:749, 1981.

Congenital Mesoblastic Nephroma

Synonyms
Leiomyomatous hamartoma, fetal mesenchymal hamartoma, and fetal renal hamartoma.

Incidence
Congenital mesoblastic nephroma (CMN) is a rare renal tumor occurring in the neonatal period.[10] It affects males more frequently than females.[13]

Pathology
CMN is generally a solid tumor that is identified as a unilateral mass varying in weight from 35 to 450 g.[5] On several occasions, it has been confused with Wilms tumor,[7,16,17,19] from which it is indistinguishable by radiography and sonography.[7,11,15] However, prognosis and treatment of the two tumors are very different.

Macroscopically, CMN occurs most often as a solid, circumscribed mass resembling leiomyoma of the uterus, but the tumor may exhibit pseudocystic areas resulting from cavitation necrosis or hemorrhage.[4,10–12,18,20]

Histologically, it is composed of mesenchymal cells, regarded as smooth muscle cells, immature fibroblasts, or both,[2,5,7,22] with islands of glomeruli, tubules, vascular structures, and hematopoietic elements. The tumor is not encapsulated and may infiltrate the tissues located nearby. In rare instances, it may show a malignant pattern ("malignant mesenchymal nephroma of infancy") with irregularly shaped cells, a high nucleus:cytoplasm ratio, areas of necrosis, and more than 10 mitoses per 10 HPF (high power fields).[2,10,16]

Associated Anomalies
Of 51 children with CMN, 7 had congenital anomalies (14 percent), including polydactyly, gastrointestinal malformations, hydrocephalus, and genitourinary anomalies.[13]

Diagnosis
The antenatal visualization of mesoblastic nephroma has been reported on several occasions,[1,6,11,14,21,23] with the earliest diagnosis made at 26 weeks.[1] A specific diagnosis is not feasible with ultrasound. The condition can be detected by identification of a unilateral solid mass in one of the upper abdominal quadrants (Fig. 8–37). The mass usually arises from the renal fossa and compresses the involved kidney. The interface between the tumor and the normal parenchyma may give the sonographic appearance of a capsule surrounding the tumor. Polyhydramnios is always present although the reason for this association is unknown.[3]

Differential diagnosis should include Wilms tumor, other renal tumors, such as teratomas, and neuroblastomas of adrenal glands. IPKD can be excluded by the association of oligohydramnios and nonvisualization of the fetal bladder, with bilaterally enlarged kidneys.

Prognosis
All babies in whom the tumor was diagnosed in utero were operated on in the neonatal period and did well. Preterm labor or premature rupture of membranes complicated four of the pregnancies in which there was prenatal visualization of the tumor.[1,9,14,21] The mean weight of the patients diagnosed prenatally was 2140 g. In one report, 7 of 30 infants with CMN weighed less than 2275 g.[3] To date, the tumor has been reported in two stillborn infants.[19] The prognosis for this condition is generally good since it is unilateral and nearly always benign. However, reports in the literature have documented recurrences after incomplete surgical excision[7,13,16,20] in one infant[20] and metastases to the lung in another.[10] It would seem that infants diagnosed in the first 3 months of life usually have a benign variety of this tumor, with more aggressive behaviors appearing after 3 months of age.[10]

The treatment of choice is surgical removal (ne-

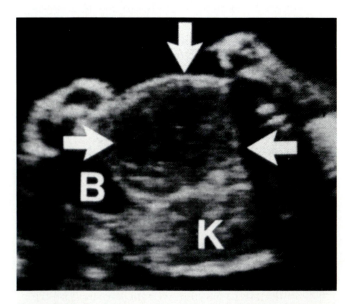

Figure 8–37. Transverse section of the fetal abdomen demonstrating a unilateral solid mass in the renal fossa adjacent to the fetal bladder (B). The contralateral kidney (K) is normal. *(Reproduced with permission from Giulian: Radiology 152:69, 1984.)*

phrectomy).[5,8,13] If the histologic status is worrisome or there is some residual tumor left behind following surgery, follow-up is indicated and postoperative chemotherapy or radiotherapy may be necessary.[2,10]

Obstetrical Management
The diagnosis of a renal tumor is an indication for serial sonography to monitor tumor growth and to check for associated anomalies.

REFERENCES

1. Apuzzio JJ, Unwin W, Adhate A, et al.: Prenatal diagnosis of fetal renal mesoblastic nephroma. Am J Obstet Gynecol 154:636, 1986.
2. Beckwith JB: Mesenchymal renal neoplasms of infancy revisited. J Pediatr Surg 9:803, 1974.
3. Blank E, Neerhout RC, Burry KA: Congenital mesoblastic nephroma and polyhydramnios. JAMA 240:1504, 1978.
4. Bogdan R, Taylor DEM, Mostofi FK: Leiomyomatous hamartoma of the kidney. A clinical and pathologic analysis of 20 cases from the Kidney Tumor Registry. Cancer 31:462, 1973.
5. Bolande RP, Brough AJ, Izant RJ Jr: Congenital mesoblastic nephroma of infancy. A report of eight cases and the relationship to Wilms' tumor. Pediatrics 40:272, 1967.
6. Ehman RL, Nicholson SF, Machin GA: Prenatal sonographic detection of congenital mesoblastic nephroma in a monozygotic twin pregnancy. J Ultrasound Med 2:555, 1983.
7. Fu YS, Kay S: Congenital mesoblastic nephroma and its recurrence. Arch Pathol 96:66, 1973.
8. Gerber A, Gold JH, Bustamante S, et al.: Cogenital mesoblastic nephroma. J Pediatr Surg 16:758, 1981.
9. Giulian BB: Prenatal ultrasonographic diagnosis of fetal renal tumors. Radiology 152:69, 1984.
10. Gonzalez-Crussi F, Sotelo-Avila C, Kidd JM: Mesenchymal renal tumors in infancy: A reappraisal. Hum Pathol 12:78, 1981.
11. Grider RD, Wolverson MK, Jagannadharao B, et al.: Congenital mesoblastic nephroma with cystic component. J Clin Ultrasound 9:43, 1981.
12. Hartman DS, Lesar MSL, Madewell JE: Mesoblastic nephroma: Radiologic–pathologic correlation of 20 cases. AJR 136:69, 1981.
13. Howell CG, Othersen HB, Kiviat NE, et al.: Therapy and outcome in 51 children with mesoblastic nephroma: A report of the national Wilms' tumor study. J Pediatr Surg 17:826, 1982.
14. Howey DD, Farrell EE, Scholl J, et al.: Congenital mesoblastic nephroma: Prenatal ultrasonic findings and surgical excision in a very-low-birth-weight infant. J Clin Ultrasound 13:506, 1985.
15. Jaffe MH, White SJ, Silver TM, et al.: Wilms tumor: Ultrasonic features, pathologic correlation and diagnostic pitfalls. Radiology 140:147, 1981.
16. Joshi VV, Kay S, Milsten R, et al.: Congenital mesoblastic nephroma of infancy: Report of a case with unusual clinical behavior. Am J Clin Pathol 60:811, 1973.
17. Kay S, Pratt CB, Salzberg AM: Hamartoma (leiomyomatous type) of the kidney. Cancer 19:1825, 1966.
18. Slasky BS, Penkrot RJ, Bron KM: Cystic mesoblastic nephroma. Urology 19:220, 1982.
19. Waisman J, Cooper PH: Renal neoplasms of the newborn. J Pediatr Surg 5:407, 1970.
20. Walker D, Richard GA: Fetal hamartoma of the kidney: Recurrence and death of patient. J Urol 110:352, 1973.
21. Walter JP, McGahan JP: Mesoblastic nephroma: Prenatal sonographic detection. J Clin Ultrasound 13:686, 1985.
22. Wigger HJ: Fetal mesenchymal hamartoma of kidney — A tumor of secondary mesenchyme. Cancer 36:1002, 1975.
23. Yambao TJ, Schwartz D, Henderson R, et al.: Prenatal diagnosis of congenital mesoblastic nephroma. A case report. J Reprod Med 31:257, 1986.

Wilms' Tumor

Synonym
Nephroblastoma.

Incidence
The random risk of developing Wilms' tumor has been estimated to be 1 in 10,000 live births.[17] The annual incidence has been estimated to be 7.8 per 1,000,000 children under the age of 15 years.[10,14] The precise incidence of this tumor in the neonatal period is unknown. The male to female ratio is nearly 1:1.[2,14]

Etiology
The tumor can occur sporadically or with a familial tendency. The pattern of inheritance has been suggested to be autosomal dominant with variable penetrance (the likelihood that an individual who inherits the gene will develop the disease) and expressivity (the clinical variability of the inherited disease). The

overall penetrance for inherited tumors is 63 percent. Bilateral tumors are more likely to be familial than unilateral tumors. The likelihood that a sibling will have the tumor after one affected sibling is less than 1 percent if the tumor is unilateral and 1 to 2 percent with bilateral tumors. The offspring of a patient with Wilms' tumor has a 5 percent risk of having the neoplasm if the tumor was unilateral and a 32 percent risk if the tumor was bilateral.[3]

Wilms' tumor can be part of Perlman syndrome, a condition inherited with an autosomal recessive trait, characterized by renal dysplasia, fetal gigantism, and hyperplasia of the endocrine pancreas.[12,13]

Pathology
The tumor possibly results from abnormal differentiation of metanephric blastema. Most cases are unilateral (95 percent). Spread occurs by local invasion and also by vascular and lymphatic dissemination. However, it can develop simultaneously and multifocally in both kidneys,[11] suggesting a coexisting malformation.[15] The tumor is solid, and growth can be exophytic or endophytic. The renal parenchyma is frequently replaced by the tumor.

Associated Anomalies
Similarly to mesoblastic nephroma, Wilms' tumor is associated with an increased incidence of congenital anomalies, with a reported incidence of 13.7 percent.[2]

Genitourinary abnormalities account for 28 percent of all anomalies seen in Wilms' tumor, and they are found in 3.9 percent of all patients.[2] External genital abnormalities seem to be 12 times more common in bilateral than in unilateral tumors.[1] Most of these anomalies cannot be detected antenatally. They include cryptorchidism, hypospadias, double collecting system, fused kidneys, and ambiguous genitalia.

Hemihypertrophy consists of total, segmental, or crossed hypertrophy of the body. This complication may not be present at the time of birth, and, therefore, it may not be diagnosable in utero. It is more common in association with bilateral Wilms' tumor, and the overall incidence of this complication is 2.47 percent. If the Beckwith-Wiedemann syndrome (exophthalmos. macroglosia, gigantism, and visceromegaly) is associated with hemihypertrophy, the likelihood of a neoplasm is 25 percent. This tumor could be an adrenocortical neoplasia, Wilms' tumor, hepatoblastoma, or gonadoblastoma.

An association of Wilms' tumor with deletion of 11p13 and aniridia has been reported. Other occasional chromosomal abnormalities reported with Wilms' tumor include trisomy 18, Turner syndrome, and a B-C chromosomal translocation.[7]

Diagnosis
The prenatal diagnosis of this tumor has not been reported as yet, but is seems feasible, since Wilms' tumor is known to occur in newborns[5,6,8,9,13,16] and in fetuses.[15] The condition should be considered in the presence of a solid mass in the fetal renal fossa, even though the most common tumor in the neonatal period is mesoblastic nephroma, which is not distinguishable sonographically from Wilms' tumor.[10] Careful examination of the opposite side is indicated.

Prognosis
The prognosis depends on the histologic type, lymph node invasion, and stage and size of the tumor at the time of the diagnosis. The treatment approach includes surgery (nephrectomy), with adjuvant therapy according to the stage and histologic type. Adjuvant therapy consists of chemotherapy or radiotherapy. The results of the second national Wilms' tumor study revealed over a 90 percent 2-year survival rate for patients with a favorable histology in stages I, II, and III, 60 percent in stage IV with a favorable histology, and 35 percent in stage IV with an unfavorable histology.[4]

REFERENCES

1. Beheshti M, Mancer JRK, Hardy BE, et al.: External genital abnormalities associated with Wilms' tumor. Urology 24:130–133, 1984.
2. Breslow NE, Beckwith JB: Epidemiological features of Wilms' tumor: Results of the National Wilms' Tumor Study. J Natl Cancer Inst 68:429, 1982.
3. Brodeur GM: Genetic and cytogenetic aspects of Wilms' tumor. In: Pochedly C, Baum, ES (eds): Wilms' Tumor: Clinical and Biological Manifestations. New York, Elsevier, 1984, pp 125–145.
4. D'Angio GJ, Evans A, Breslow N, et al.: The treatment of Wilms' tumor: Results of the Second National Wilms' Tumor Study. Cancer 47:2302, 1981.
5. Giangiacomo J, Kissane JM: Congenital Wilms' Tumor. In: Pochedly C, Baum ES, (eds): Wilms' Tumor. Clinical and Biological Manifestations. New York, Elsevier, 1984, pp 103–108.
6. Giangiacomo J, Penchansky L, Monteleone PL, et al.: Bilateral neonatal Wilms' tumor with B-C chromosomal translocation. J Pediatr 86:98, 1975.
7. Greenwood MF, Holland P: Clinical and biochemical manifestations of Wilms' tumor. In: Pochedly C, Baum ES (eds): Wilms' Tumor: Clinical and Biological Manifestations. New York, Elsevier, 1984, pp 9–30.
8. Jaffe MH, White SJ, Silver TM: Wilms' tumor: Ultrasonic features pathologic correlation, and diagnostic pitfalls. Radiology 140:147, 1981.
9. Kalousek DK, de Chadarevian JP, Bolande RP: Congenital Wilms' tumor with metastasis. Pediatr Radiol 4:124, 1976.

10. Kramer SA: Pediatric urologic oncology. Urol Clin North Am, 12:31, 1985.
11. Lago CM, Gonzalez FC, Lorenzo CG: Bilateral multifocal Wilms' tumor. J Pediatr Surg 20:552–553, 1985.
12. Neri G, Martini-Neri ME, Katz BE, et al.: The Perlman syndrome: Familial renal dysplasia with Wilms' tumor, fetal gigantism and multiple congenital anomalies. Am J Med Genet 19:195, 1984.
13. Perlman M, Levin M, Wittles B: Syndrome of fetal gigantism, renal hamartomas, and nephroblastomatosis with Wilms' tumor. Cancer 35:1212, 1975.
14. Third National Cancer Survey: Incidence data. In: Cutler SJ, Young JL Jr (eds). National Cancer Institute Monograph 41. Bethesda, MD, National Cancer Institute, 1975, p 420.
15. Warkany J: Wilms' tumor. In: Congenital Malformations. Chicago, Year Book, 1981, p 1061.
16. Wexler HA, Poole CA, Fojaco RM: Metastatic neonatal Wilms' tumor: A case report with review of the literature. Pediatr Radiol 3:179, 1975.
17. Young JL Jr, Miller RW: Incidence of malignant tumors in U.S. children. J Pediatr 86:254, 1975.

Normal Anatomy of the Adrenal Glands

The adrenal glands are relatively large organs in the fetus and the newborn (Fig. 8–38). Relative to body weight, their size is 10 to 20 times greater in the fetus than in the adult.[1]

The adrenal glands consist of two different endocrine organs: the medulla and the cortex. The medulla is of ectodermic origin, and the cortex is a mesodermal derivative. The large size of the fetal adrenal glands is due to the cortex, which decreases in size after birth.

The normal adrenal glands can be imaged with ultrasound as early as $9\frac{1}{2}$ weeks of gestation. They appear as bilateral midecho structures located immediately above the fetal kidneys (Figs. 8–39, 8–40).

During early gestation, they may appear as a hypoechogenic ring with a central hyperechogenic line. The thickness of the central hyperechogenic line gradually increases from one third to one half after 35 weeks. The large vessels can be used as two landmarks to define adrenal gland position; the inferior vena cava is close to the anterior part of the right adrenal gland, and the aorta is close to the left adrenal gland.[2,3]

Normal dimensions of the adrenal gland are given in Table 8–5. The thickness and width are measured in a transverse scan obtained by moving the transducer slowly cephalically to a transverse scan of the kidney. The longitudinal section is of

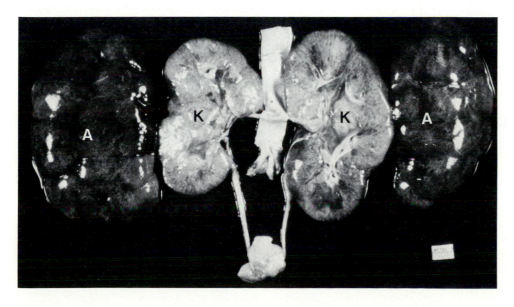

Figure 8–38. Pathologic specimen from a stillbirth. Note the relative large size of the adrenal glands (A) compared to the kidney (K).

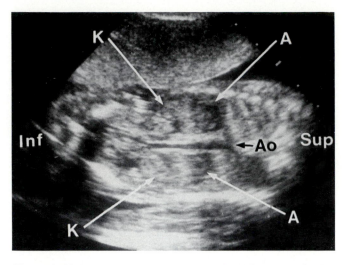

Figure 8–39. Longitudinal scan of a 21-week-old fetus showing the adrenal gland (A). The kidneys (K) can be demonstrated inferior to the adrenals. Ao, aorta; Sup, superior; Inf, inferior.

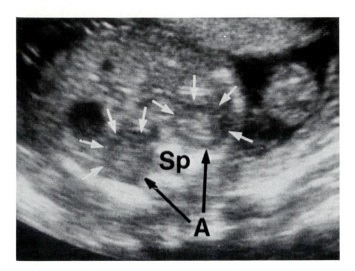

Figure 8–40. Transverse scan in a 22-week-old fetus. White arrows point to both adrenal glands (A). The hypoechogenic image anterior to the adrenal corresponds to the fetal stomach. Sp, Spine.

TABLE 8–5. SIZE OF THE FETAL ADRENALS

Gestational Age (weeks)	Mean Thickness (range) (mm)	Mean Width (range) (mm)
20–25	3 (2–5)	10 (7–12)
26–30	5 (2–8)	13 (12–17)
31–35	5 (3–7)	16 (14–18)
36–40	6 (4–9)	19 (16–24)

Reprinted with permission from Jeanty et al.: Prenat Diagn 4:21, 1984.

limited value because acoustic shadowing from the ribs often conceals the interface between the kidney and the adrenal gland.

The sonographer should be familiar with the image of the fetal adrenals to avoid confusing them with fetal kidneys. Furthermore, some pathologic conditions, such as adrenoblastomas, could be diagnosed with ultrasound. The value of fetal adrenal biometry in the prenatal diagnosis of congenital adrenal disorders is speculative at this time.

REFERENCES

1. Gardner LI: Development of the normal fetal and neonatal adrenal. In: Gardner LI (ed). Endocrine and Genetic Diseases of Childhood and Adolescence, 2d ed. Philadelphia, Saunders, 1975, pp 460–476.
2. Jeanty P, Chervenak F, Grannum P, et al.: Normal ultrasonic size and characteristics of the fetal adrenal glands. Prenat Diagn 4:21, 1984.
3. Lewis E, Kurtz AB, Dubbins PA, et al.: Real-time ultrasonographic evaluation of normal fetal adrenal glands. J Ultrasound Med 1:265, 1982.

Congenital Adrenal Neuroblastoma

Synonym
Adrenoblastoma.

Incidence
Congenital adrenal neuroblastoma is the most common abdominal tumor found in newborns, and it accounts for 12.3 percent of all perinatal neoplasms.[23] Its incidence has been estimated to vary from 1 in 10,000 to 1 in 7100 live births.[13,52] The neuroblastoma in situ is a histologic variant of malignant neuroblastoma characterized by its microscopic size and absence of metastases. Autopsy series show that incidental neuroblastomas in situ occur in 1 in 200 to 250 stillbirths and infants who have died under 3 months of age. This is 40 times greater than the incidence of clinically manifested neuroblastoma.[6,20,43] Therefore,

neuroblastoma in situ is either not a true tumor or has an extremely high rate of spontaneous regression.[22,27]

Embryology
The cortex and the medulla of the adrenal glands have different origins. The cortex develops during the 6th week of conceptional age by an aggregation of mesenchymal cells from the coelomic epithelium that lines the posterior abdominal wall between the dorsal mensentery and the developing gonad. The medulla originates from neuroectoderm. Neuroblasts migrate from the neural crest into the developing adrenal cortex to form the adrenal medulla.

Etiology
Adrenal neuroblastomas are considered a defect in neuroblast maturation. The presence of tumor-specific chromosome abnormalities in some neuroblastomas suggests a hereditary form.[32] Indeed, there are reports of neuroblastomas in monozygotic twins[30] and in families.[11,17,19,29,39] This, together with the tumor bilaterality and its occurrence in early life, suggests a familial tendency. It has been estimated that about 20 percent of neuroblastomas have a hereditary component.[28] Neuroblastoma has been associated with fetal hydantoin syndrome.[1,13]

Pathology
Neuroblastomas are almost always unilateral tumors. Fifty percent have metastases at birth.[42] They can invade the surrounding tissues (e.g., kidneys) or produce distant metastases. In the fetus, the most common sites for metastasis are liver (two thirds), and subcutaneous tissue (one third).[5,42] Placental involvement, both as tumor embolism and metastatic spread, has been described.[2,25,37,45,46,48]

Macroscopically, these tumors are soft, often with areas of hemorrhage, calcification, or necrosis. The histology may vary, ranging from the very malignant and poorly differentiated neuroblastoma through the ganglioneuroblastoma to the relatively benign and mature ganglioneuroma. Different patterns of malignancy can be found in the same tumor, and histologic type has not been found to be a reliable indicator of prognosis. Staging of the tumor is based on surgical findings. Stage I is a tumor limited to the adrenal gland, stage II consists of regional spreading that does not cross the midline, stage III refers to tumors extending over the midline, and stage IV includes patients with metastasis to distant lymph nodes, bone, brain, or lung. A special category is stage IV-S which includes patients with a small primary tumor and distant metastases limited to liver, skin, and bone marrow without radiologic

evidence of bony metastases.[15] In 75 to 90 percent of cases, neuroblastomas have hormonal activity with production of cathecolamines.[15,41] However, endocrine symptoms are rare, probably because the catecholamines are quickly converted into the inactive vanillylmandelic and homovanillic acids, which are excreted in the urine.[14]

Associated Anomalies
Neuroblastoma may be associated with other lesions resulting from maldevelopment of the neural crest, such as Hirschsprung's disease.[8,11] The possible association of neuroblastomas with other anomalies has been a matter of discussion. Most associated anomalies have been reported with neuroblastoma in situ. Since this entity is a relatively common finding in autopsy series and is thought to represent a normal variation of the morphogenesis of the adrenal glands,[6] such associations are not relevent to clinical neuroblastomas.[47] This view is supported by the report of Miller, who reviewed the records of 502 children with clinically apparent neuroblastoma and could not find an increased incidence of associated anomalies.[31] Furthermore, a case-controlled study of 157 children who died from neuroblastoma did not show an increased incidence of associated anomalies.[26]

Diagnosis
Prenatal visualization of neuroblastomas has been made in the third trimester.[4,18,24] The tumor appears as a mixed cystic and solid mass in the upper part of the kidney (Fig. 8–41), but its sonographic aspect varies considerably.[51] Calcifications may be present. A precise identification of the adrenal origin of the mass is difficult. The visualization of the kidneys separate from the mass would be helpful. These organs may be deformed by the tumor. In one patient, the primary tumor was not visualized, but cervical metastasis resulted in the visualization of solid masses in the region of the neck.[16] In some patients, congenital neuroblastoma is associated with hydrops fetalis.[2,16,25,33,34,38,46,48] No clear explanation has been proposed for this association.

About 75 to 90 percent of neuroblastomas release catecholamines. Transplacental passage of these hormones can lead to maternal symptoms and signs of catecholamine excess (nausea, vomiting, nervousness, sweating, headaches, hypertension).[34,49] The combination of maternal symptoms of cathecolamine excess and a suspected fetal mass is highly suggestive of fetal adrenoblastoma. Objective evidence of a cathecolamine excess can be gathered by demonstrating elevated vanillylmandelic and homovanillic acid in a 24-hour maternal urine specimen.

The differential diagnosis should include Wilms

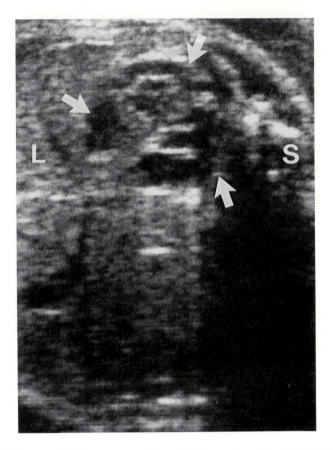

Figure 8–41. Oblique scan of the fetal abdomen shows a complex mass with mixed solid and cystic elements interposed between liver (L) and spine (S). *(Reproduced with permission from Giulian et al.: J Clin Ultrasound 14:225, 1986.)*

tumor, renal mesoblastic nephroma, multicystic kidney, liver diseases (hepatic hamartoma or hemangioma), and retroperitoneal teratoma. Sonographic differentiation is difficult also in children.[21,51] A definitive diagnosis is often possible only at laparotomy and after histologic examination. Nonetheless, a rapidly enlarging mass suggests a tumor.

Prognosis

Rare cases of stillborn infants with diffuse neuroblastoma have been reported in the literature.[2,3,7,40,46,48] After birth, the prognosis depends on age at diagnosis and stage.[12,36,41,44] The younger the infant at the time of diagnosis, the better the prognosis. The demonstration of catecholamine excretion does not seem to alter the prognosis.[41] Patients with a favorable prognosis are younger (under 2 years), have the tumor in an extraabdominal or midline location, and are in stages I, II, or IV-S.[35] The clinical course of neuroblastomas is unpredictable. Spontaneous regressions have been reported even in patients with metastasis.[10] The primary therapy is surgery, but this tumor is both radiosensitive and susceptible to chemotherapeutic agents.

Obstetrical Management

The detection of an enlarging adrenal mass should prompt repeated ultrasonic examinations to evaluate the speed of growth of the tumor. In one report, the tumor diameter doubled in 2 weeks.[24] The timing and method of delivery depend in part on the behavior of the tumor; explosive tumoral growth may require preterm delivery. Hemoperitoneum from rupture of the neuroblastoma has been reported following both nontraumatic and traumatic delivery.[9] Fetal hydrops or metastatic liver enlargement may cause dystocia.[46,48,50] A cesarean section may need to be considered.

REFERENCES

1. Allen RW, Ogden B, Bentley FL, et al.: Fetal hydantoin syndrome, neuroblastoma, and hemorrhagic disease in the neonate. JAMA 244:1464, 1980.
2. Anders D, Kindermann G, Pfeifer U: Metastasizing fetal neuroblastoma with involvement of the placenta simulating fetal erythroblastosis. Report of two cases. J Pediatr 82:50, 1973.
3. Andersen HJ, Hariri J: Congenital neuroblastoma in a fetus with multiple malformations. Virchows Arch [Pathol Anat] 400:219, 1983.
4. Atkinson GO, Zaatari GS, Lorenzo RL, et al.: Cystic neuroblastoma in infants: Radiographic and pathologic features. AJR 146:113, 1986.
5. Becker JM, Schneider KM, Krasna IH: Neonatal neuroblastoma. Prog Clin Cancer 4:382, 1970.
6. Beckwith JB, Perrin EV: In situ neuroblastomas: a contribution to the natural history of neural crest tumors. Am J Pathol 43:1089, 1963.
7. Birner WF: Neuroblastoma as a cause of antenatal death. Am J Obstet Gynecol 82:1388, 1961.
8. Bower RJ, Adkins JC: Ondine's curse and neurocristopathy. Clin Pediatr 19:665, 1980.
9. Brock CE, Ricketts RR: Hemoperitoneum from spontaneous rupture of neonatal neuroblastoma. Am J Dis Child, 136:370, 1982.
10. Cassady JR: A hypothesis to explain the enigmatic natural history of neuroblastoma. Med Pediatr Oncol 12:64, 1984.
11. Chatten J, Voorhess ML: Familial neuroblastoma. N Engl J Med 277:1230, 1967.
12. Coldman AJ, Fryer CJH, Elwood JM, et al.: Neuroblastoma: Influence of age at diagnosis, stage, tumor site, and sex on prognosis. Cancer 46:1896, 1980.
13. Ehrenbard LT, Chaganti RSK: Cancer in the fetal hydantoin syndrome. Lancet 2:97, 1981.
14. Evans AE, D'Angio GJ, Koop CE: Diagnosis and treatment of neuroblastoma. Pediatr Clin North Am 23:161, 1976.
15. Evans AE: Staging and treatment of neuroblastoma.

Cancer 45:1799, 1980.

16. Gadwood KA, Reynes CJ: Prenatal sonography of metastatic neuroblastoma. J Clin Ultrasound 11:512, 1983.

17. Gerson JM, Chatten J, Eisman S: Familial neuroblastoma. A follow-up. N Engl J Med 290:1487, 1974.

18. Giulian BB, Chang CNC, Yoss BS: Prenatal ultrasonographic diagnosis of fetal adrenal neuroblastoma. J Clin Ultrasound 14:225, 1986.

19. Griffin ME, Bolande RP: Familial neuroblastoma with regression and maturation to ganglioneurofibroma. Pediatrics 43:377, 1969.

20. Guin GH, Gilbert EF, Jones B: Incidental neuroblastoma in infants. Am J Clin Pathol 51:126, 1969.

21. Hendry GMA: Cystic neuroblastoma of the adrenal gland — A potential source of error in ultrasonic diagnosis. Pediatr Radiol 12:204, 1982.

22. Ikeda Y, Lister J, Bouton JM, et al.: Congenital neuroblastoma, neuroblastoma in situ and the normal fetal development of the adrenal. J Pediatr Surg 16:636, 1981.

23. Isaacs H Jr: Perinatal (congenital and neonatal) neoplasms: A report of 110 cases. Pediatr Pathol 3:165, 1985.

24. Janetschek G, Weitzel D, Stein W, et al.: Prenatal diagnosis of neuroblastoma by sonography. Urology 24:397, 1984.

25. Johnson AT Jr, Halbert D: Congenital neuroblastoma presenting as hydrops fetalis. NCMJ 35:289, 1974.

26. Johnson CC, Spitz MR: Neuroblastoma: Case-control analysis of birth characteristics. J Natl Cancer Inst 74:789, 1985.

27. Knudson AG, Meadows AT: Regressing of neuroblastoma IV-S: A genetic hypothesis. N Engl J Med 302:1254, 1980.

28. Knudson AG Jr, Strong LC: Mutation and cancer: Neuroblastoma and pheochromocytoma. Am J Hum Genet 24:514, 1972.

29. Leape LL, Lowman JT, Loveland GC: Multifocal nondisseminated neuroblastoma. J Pediatr 92:75, 1978.

30. Mancini AF, Rosito P, Faldella G, et al.: Neuroblastoma in a pair of identical twins. Med Pediatr Oncol 10:45, 1982.

31. Miller RW: Relation between cancer and congenital defects in man. N Engl J Med 275:87, 1966.

32. Moss RB, Blessing-Moore J, Bender SW, et al.: Cystic fibrosis and neuroblastoma. Pediatrics 76:814, 1985.

33. Moss TJ, Kaplan L: Association of hydrops fetalis with congenital neuroblastoma. Am J Obstet Gynecol 132:905, 1978.

34. Newton ER, Louis F, Dalton ME, et al: Fetal neuroblastoma and catecholamine-induced maternal hypertension. Obstet Gynecol 65:49s, 1985.

35. Nickerson HJ, Nesbit ME, Grosfeld JL, et al.: Comparison of stage IV and IV-S neuroblastoma in the first year of life. Med Pediatr Oncol 13:261, 1985.

36. O'Neill JA, Littman P, Blitzer P, et al.: The role of surgery in localized neuroblastoma. J Pediatr Surgery 20:708, 1985.

37. Perkins DG, Kopp CM, Haust MD: Placental infiltration in congenital neuroblastoma: A case study with ultrastructure. Histopathology 4:383, 1980.

38. Perlin BM, Pomerance JJ, Schifrin BS: Nonimmunologic hydrops fetalis. Obstet Gynecol 57:584, 1981.

39. Ploechl E, Kaeser H, Klein H: Excretion of catecholamines in relatives of patients with familial neuroblastoma. Cancer Res 36:10, 1976.

40. Potter EL, Parrish JM: Neuroblastoma, ganglioneuroma and fibroneuroma in a stillborn fetus. Am J Pathol 18:141, 1942.

41. Pritchard J, Kemshead J: Neuroblastoma: Recent developments in assessment and management. In: Duncan W (ed): Paediatric Oncology. New York, Springer-Verlag, 1983, pp 69–78.

42. Schneider KM, Becker JM, Krasna IH: Neonatal neuroblastoma. Pediatrics 36:359, 1965.

43. Shanklin DR, Sotelo-Avila C: In situ tumors in fetuses, newborns and young infants. Biol Neonatol 14:286, 1969.

44. Shimada H, Chatten J, Newton WA, et al.: Histopathologic prognostic factors in neuroblastic tumors: Definition of subtypes of ganglioneuroblastoma and an age-linked classification of neuroblastomas. J Natl Cancer Inst 73:405, 1984.

45. Smith CR, Chan HSL: Placental involvement in congenital neuroblastoma. J Clin Pathol 34:785, 1981.

46. Strauss L, Driscoll SG: Congenital neuroblastoma involving the placenta. Pediatrics 34:23, 1964.

47. Sy WM, Edmonson JH: The developmental defects associated with neuroblastoma—Etiologic implications. Cancer 22:234, 1968.

48. Van der Slikke JW, Balk AG: Hydramnios with hydrops fetalis an disseminated fetal neuroblastoma. Obstet Gynecol 55:250, 1980.

49. Voute PA Jr, Wadman SK, van Putten WJ: Congenital neuroblastoma: Symptoms in the mother during pregnancy. Clin Pediatr 9:206, 1970.

50. Weinberg T, Radman HM: Fetal dystocia due to neuroblastoma of the adrenals with metastases to the liver. Am J Obstet Gynecol 46:440, 1943.

51. White SJ, Stuck KJ, Blane CE, et al.: Sonography of neuroblastoma. AJR 141:465, 1983.

52. Young JL Jr, Miller RW: Incidence of malignant tumors in US children. J Pediatr 86:254, 1975.

9

The Genital Tract

Fetal Gender

Embryology

Before the 8th menstrual week, the genitalia are in an ambiguous state. Normal female external genitalia are formed in the absence of testosterone. This hormone induces differentiation of the external genitalia in a male pattern. This process occurs between the 8th and 10th weeks (menstrual age).

Diagnosis

The most informative scanning planes for examination of fetal genitalia are coronal (Figs. 9–1, 9–2) and tangential sections (Figs. 9–3, 9–4).

A male fetus can be identified by visualization of a penis or scrotum as early as the 15th week. Testicular descent can also be diagnosed in utero. Birnholz has reported that descent occurs in 62 percent of

infants by the 30th week and in 93 percent of infants by the 32d week.[1] The incidence of cryptorchidism based on the pediatric literature varies according to gestational age and weight. The incidence is only 0.7 percent for those infants weighing above 3500 g, but as high as 17 percent in infants weighing between 2000 and 2500 g.[4] A pitfall in identification of a penis is confusion with the umbilical cord or fetal fingers. An author has recently reported movement resembling fetal masturbation.[4a]

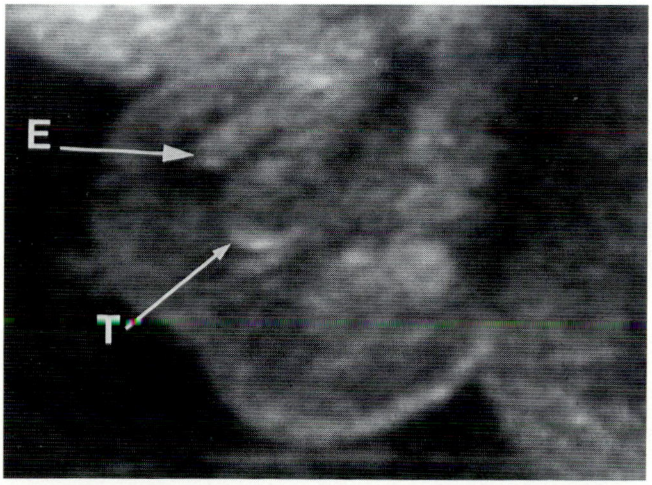

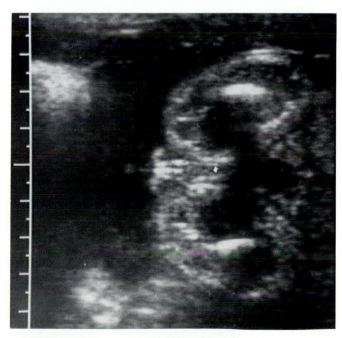

Figure 9–1. Coronal section of a third trimester male fetus. E, epididymis; T, testicle.

Figure 9–2. Coronal scan of a female fetus. Labia majora and minora are visible.

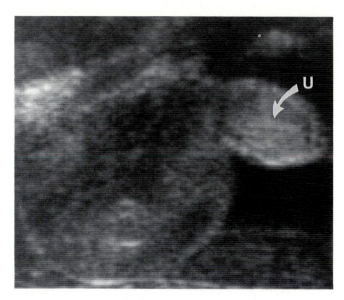

Figure 9–3. Male fetus scanned in a sagittal section. The scrotum and penis are visible. U, urethra.

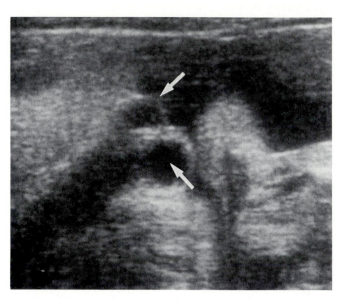

Figure 9–5. Edema of the labia majora. Arrows point to enlarged labia majora.

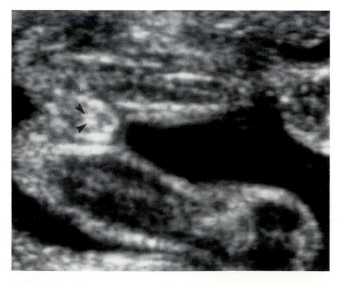

Figure 9–4. Scan of a female fetus. Arrowheads point to the labia minora.

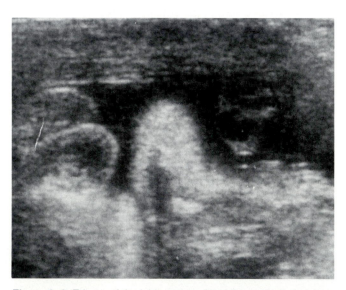

Figure 9–6. Edema of the labia majora. Note the similarity between the appearance of the swollen labia and the scrotum.

TABLE 9–1. REVIEW OF PRENATAL GENDER DIAGNOSIS WITH ULTRASOUND

Study	Weeks of Gestation
	13 14 15 16 17 18 19 20 21 22 23 24 25 26 27 28 29 30 31 32 33 34 35 36 37 38 39 40
1. Schorzman (1977)	V 75%* (25 →40) ; E 8%
2. Stocker (1977)	V 59% (30 →40) ; E 2.5%
4. Le Lann (1979)	V 57 (25 →31) 57 (31 →35) 34 (35 →) ; E NA
5. De La Fuente (1979)	(25 →40) ; E O
6. Sholly (1980)	V 64% (25 →40) ; E O
7. De Crespigny (1981)	V 55% (25 →28) 71% (28 →33) 74% (33 →36) 64% (36 →) ; E — 1% 1%
8. Shaley (1981)	V 91.6% (16 →18) V 95.1% (22 →) ; E 0% Male, E 16% Female
9. Plattner (1983)	V 56% (15 →19) 65% (19 →23) 85.5% (23 →) ; E 11.8% 4.3% 1.1%
10. Dunne (1983)	0% (13) V 15% (15 →18) V 70% (19 →22)
11. Birnholz (1983)	V 29% (15 →19) 66% (19 →23) 89% 90% 925 83.9 ; E 3.3% 0.44% ; V 40% / E 3% 16–24 weeks' gestation
12. Stephens (1983)	100% (15 →16) ; 0%
13. Elejalde (1985)	V 19% (15 →17) 39% (17 →20) 85% (21 →23) 86% (24 →28) 94% (29 →) ; E 3.8% 3.2% 1.1% 0% 0% ; V One examination 62% / Two examinations 78.3% Data of 13–24 weeks pooled ; E First examination 3.5% / Second examination 0%

* On top of each line is the number of fetuses visualized (V), and below the line is the number of errors (E). The distribution by weeks was taken from the original paper. Due to the variability periods chosen by the different authors, it was not possible to do a tabulation including all of them. For papers 11 and 13, an extra line has been added to pool the data between 13 and 24 weeks.

Reproduced with permission from Elejalde et al.: J Ultrasound Med 4:633, 1985.

The female genitalia can be identified by visualization of the labia majora. A separation between the labia minora also may be observed (Fig. 9–4).[7] In some cases, edema of the labia can be demonstrated (Figs. 9–5, 9–6). The sonographer should be aware of this condition to avoid a mistaken prenatal sex assignment (e.g., a male infant with hydrocele).

Medical indications for gender assessment include (1) patients with X-linked disorders (e.g., hemophilia), in which a female fetus would not be affected, but a male fetus would have a 50 percent chance of having the disease, (2) the assessment of dizygocity in twin gestation (discrepant sex = dizygocity), (3) exclusion of maternal cell contamination during amniocentesis when a mixed population of cells is observed at karyotyping, and (4) assistance in the prenatal diagnosis of some genetic conditions. The index of suspicion for campomelic syndrome is increased when there is a genotypic/phenotypic discrepancy in a fetus with a skeletal dysplasia (see p. 347).

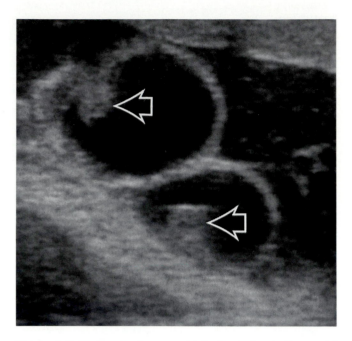

Figure 9–7. Hydrocele. Arrows point to the testes in the scrotal cavities.

Reliability of Prenatal Sex Determination. Published information about the accuracy of prenatal sex determination was reviewed recently by Elejalde et al. (Table 9–1).[3] The accuracy is dependent on gestational age and operator experience. Stephens and Sherman are the only authors who claim 100 percent accuracy of sex diagnosis from the 16th to the 18th week.[9] Elejalde et al. visualized fetal genitalia in 19 percent of infants between 15 and 18 weeks, with an error rate of 3.8 percent.[3] Because of the finite error rate, we prefer to rely on chromosomal analysis rather than ultrasound in assessing the risk of genetic disease in X-linked conditions.

Congenital Anomalies of External Genitalia

Hydrocele is the collection of fluid along the processus vaginalis. The processus vaginalis forms as an outpouching of peritoneum adjacent to the gubernaculum testis and progressively enlongates through the inguinal canal. During the seventh month of gestation, it extends into the scrotum, followed by the descent of the epididymis and testes. The condition has been classified as noncommunicating and communicating. In the noncommunicating variety, fluid accumulates in the scrotum during the normal descent of the testes through the processus vaginalis. The communicating variety may be associated with an inguinal hernia. A prenatal diagnosis of hydrocele has been made by demonstrating the presence of fluid within the scrotum (Fig. 9–7).[5,6] If the amount of fluid remains unchanged, the hydrocele is most likely of the noncommunicating variety. This condition requires no specific treatment and resolves spontaneously in most infants by 1 year of age. If the hydrocele enlarges throughout gestation, a communicating variety should be suspected. The neonatologist should look for an inguinal hernia.

Prenatal diagnosis of ambiguous genitalia by ultrasound has been reported by Cooper et al.[2] in a fetus at 34 weeks with extremely short limbs and ambiguous genitalia (Fig. 9–8). Chromosomal analysis showed a 46 XY karyotype with translocation from chromosome 9 to chromosome 3 (3q+ syndrome). Conditions that should be considered if ambiguous genitalia are diagnosed include adrenal hyperplasia, maternal androgen excess (due to ingestion in early pregnancy or to endogenous overproduction, such as an ovarian or adrenal tumor), and true hermaphroditism.

Figure 9–8. Ambiguous genitalia. Representative scan at 34 weeks showing ambiguous genitalia. Left sonogram shows a small midline cleft (*arrowhead*) separating two rounded structures (*arrows*), suggesting either labia majora or scrotal sac. A more cephalic scan (*right sonogram*) displays a small midline structure (*open arrow*) projecting between the two rounded structures (*closed arrows*). *(Reproduced with permission from Cooper et al.: J Ultrasound Med 4:433, 1985.)*

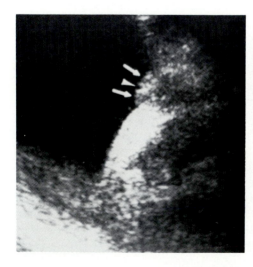
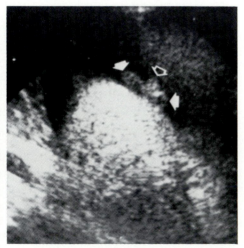

The most common cause of ambiguous genitalia in chromosomically XX fetuses is congenital adrenal hyperplasia. The frequency of the disorder in the United States and Europe is between 1 in 5000 and 1 in 15,000.[10] This common disorder is inherited as an autosomal recessive trait; its gene frequency is second only to that of cystic fibrosis. An early diagnosis is important because the condition may be life threatening during the newborn period due to electrolyte imbalance. The most common enzyme deficiency is 21-hydroxylase; 11-beta-hydroxylase deficiency also causes ambiguous genitalia. The metabolic abnormality results in deficient cortisol production, which increases the level of ACTH release with further steroid stimulation and an elevation of circulating androgens (see White et al.[11,12]). A prenatal diagnosis of 21-hydroxylase deficiency has been made in a fetus at risk by measuring amniotic fluid levels of 17-hydroxy-progesterone and delta$_4$-androstenedione,[10] and also by HLA typing of amniotic fluid cells. Although there are limitations to each method, a prenatal diagnosis is highly accurate when based on both techniques. Regrettably, amniocentesis is generally performed at 16 weeks; at this time, masculinization of affected females has already occurred. Diagnosis in the first trimester (chorionic villous sampling) may be possible in the future with the use of specific probes such as probes to the closely linked HLA class I and II genes.[12] Prenatal treatment with steroid administration to the mother from the 10th week may prevent ambiguous genitalia in female fetuses.[12] Testicular feminization syndrome has been diagnosed in an infant with an XY karyotype who had female genitalia.[8]

REFERENCES

1. Birnholz JC: Determination of fetal sex. N Engl J Med 309:942, 1983.
2. Cooper C, Mahony BS, Bowie JD: Prenatal ultrasound diagnosis of ambiguous genitalia. J Ultrasound Med 4:433, 1985.
3. Elejalde BR, de Elejalde MM, Heitman T: Visualization of the fetal genitalia by ultrasonography: A review of the literature and analysis of its accuracy and ethical implications. J Ultrasound Med 4:633, 1985.
4. Kogan SJ: Cryptorchidism. In: Kelalis PP, King LR, Belman AB (eds): Clinical Pediatric Urology, 2d ed. Philadelphia, Saunders, 1985, pp 864–887.
4a. Meizner I: Sonographic observation of in utero fetal "masturbation." J Ultrasound Med 6:111, 1987.
5. Meizner I, Katz M, Zmora E, et al.: In utero diagnosis of congenital hydrocele. J Clin Ultrasound 11:449, 1983.
6. Miller EI, Thomas RH: Fetal hydrocele detected in utero by ultrasound. Br J Radiol 52:624, 1979.
7. Schotten A, Giese C: The "female echo": Prenatal determination of the female fetus by ultrasound. Am J Obstet Gynecol 138:463, 1980.
8. Stephens JD: Prenatal diagnosis of testicular feminisation. Lancet 2:1038, 1984.
9. Stephens JD, Sherman S: Determination of fetal sex by ultrasound. N Engl J Med 309:984, 1983.
10. Warsos SL, Larsen JW, Kent SG, et al.: Prenatal diagnosis of congenital adrenal hyperplasia. Obstet Gynecol 55:751, 1980.
11. White PC, New MI, Dupont B: Congenital adrenal hyperplasia (first of two parts). N Engl J Med 316:1519, 1987.
12. White PC, New MI, Dupont B: Congenital adrenal hyperplasia (second of two parts). N Engl J Med 316:1580, 1987.

Hydrometrocolpos

Definition
Hydrometrocolpos is a distention of the uterus (metro) and vagina (colpos) caused by obstruction to the drainage of genital secretions.

Incidence
Less than 1 in 16,000 female births.[11]

Etiology
Most cases of hydrometrocolpos are sporadic. Twenty-five cases of McKusick-Kaufman syndrome have been reviewed by Robinow and Shaw.[9] This syndrome consists of the association of hydrometrocolpos, polydactyly, and heart defects and is inherited with an autosomal recessive pattern. In this condition, hydrometrocolpos is due to either cervical or vaginal atresia and not to an imperforate hymen. Polydactyly and polysyndactyly are only postaxial and can be the only manifestation of the condition in males. Congenital heart disease may be a ventricular septal defect or a single atrium. Anorectal anomalies, such as rectovaginal fistulas, anal atresia, and vaginal and uterine duplication, occur in some cases.[9]

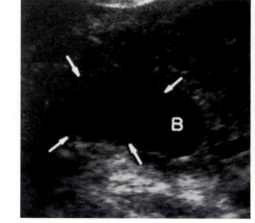
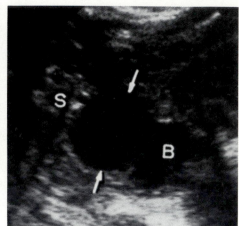

Figure 9–9. Sonogram of a hypo-echogenic, predominantly cystic, fetal pelvic mass (*arrows*). The left figure is a longitudinal scan, and the right is a transverse scan. B, bladder, S, spine. (*Reproduced with permission from Davis et al.: J Ultrasound Med 3:371, 1984.*)

Pathology

Obstruction to the flow of secretions from the genital tract is due to a membrane that is frequently referred to as an "imperforate hymen." However, Dewhurst pointed out that the membrane does not correspond to the hymen, which can usually be seen externally to the obstructing membrane.[4] Agenesis of the vagina or cervix can also be responsible for the obstruction.

The secretions that distend the uterus and vagina are produced by the uterine and cervical mucosas. These organs are under significant steroidal stimulation during fetal life.

The spectrum of hydrometrocolpos is broad, ranging from mild cases undetected until adolescence, when hematometrocolpos develops, to conditions occurring in the newborn as a huge pelviabdominal mass, with distention of the introitus and obstruction of the urinary tract. Sometimes, the con-

dition has been confused with an ovarian cyst. This diagnostic error has resulted in unnecessary hysterectomy.[4]

Associated Anomalies

If the obstruction is due to a membrane, associated anomalies are absent. However, if the hydrometrocolpos is due to cervical or vaginal atresia, other anomalies are common and include imperforate anus, persistent urogenital sinus, unilateral renal agenesis or hypoplasia, polycystic kidneys, duplication of vagina and uterus, esophageal atresia, and sacral hypoplasia.[5,7,8,11] Hydrometrocolpos has been described occasionally with Ellis-van Creveld syndrome.[1]

Diagnosis

Hydrometrocolpos has been identified in utero [3,6,10] The condition occurred as a retrovesical mass with a

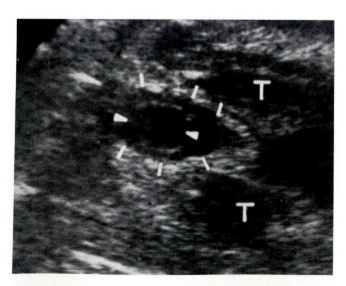

Figure 9–10. Transverse sonogram of the fetal perineum. Notice the hypoechogenic cystic space (*arrowheads*) spreading the labia majora (*lines*). T, thigh. (*Reproduced with permission from Davis et al.: J Ultrasound Med 3:371, 1984.*)

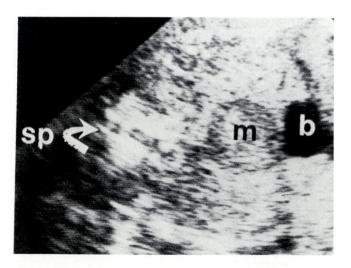

Figure 9–11. Tranverse scan through the fetal lower abdomen. A solid mass (m) is seen behind the bladder (b). sp, spine. (*Reproduced with permission from Hill, Hirsch: J Ultrasound Med 4:323, 1985.*)

sonographic appearance that in two patients was cystic[3,10] and in one patient had midlevel echoes.[6]

An elegant prenatal diagnosis has been made by Davis et al.,[3] who found a hypoechogenic pelvic mass posterior to the bladder and anterior to the spine (Fig. 9–9). The mass extended cephalically into the fetal abdomen and caudally into the vagina. A coronal scan of the perineum showed spreading of the labia majora and protrusion of the mass (Fig. 9–10). Hydrometrocolpos is part of the differential diagnosis of any cystic intraabdominal mass in a female fetus (ovarian and mesenteric cysts, cystic tumors, anterior meningoceles). A precise diagnosis is difficult. When present, visualization of the perineal findings should be quite specific.

When hydrometrocolpos occurs as a noncystic mass (Fig. 9–11), differential diagnosis should include solid ovarian tumors, sacral tumors, such as chordoma or chondroma, and distended rectum.[6] The solid sonographic image of some cases of fetal hydrometrocolpos is presumably due to the mucous nature of the secretion. To this extent, the term "hydrometrocolpos" would be a misnomer, and a more accurate term would be "mucometrocolpos."[6]

The pelvic mass frequently causes urinary tract obstruction, which may appear as hydronephrosis.[3,8,10] A rare complication described by Ceballos and Hicks is aseptic fibrous peritonitis after spillage of the genital secretions through the tubes into the peritoneal cavity.[2]

Prognosis

Hydrometrocolpos caused by a membrane can be treated easily by establishing vaginal patency. A more complex problem arises when the hydrometrocolpos is due to vaginal atresia or cervical atresia. An abdominal approach may be required. In the past, a mortality rate of up to 50 percent had been reported when infants underwent an exploratory laparotomy because of an undiagnosed hydrometrocolpos. There are no data concerning the future fertility of infants with hydrometrocolpos.

Obstetrical Management

After viability, obstetrical management is not altered by this diagnosis. Serial scans are recommended to monitor the lesion.

REFERENCES

1. Akoun R, Bagard M: La maladie d' Ellis-van Creveld. Algerie Med 60:769,1956
2. Ceballos R, Hicks GM: Plastic peritonitis due to neonatal hydrometrocolpos: Radiologic and pathologic observations. J Pediatr Surg 5:63, 1970.
3. Davis GH, Wapner RJ, Kurtz AB, et al.: Antenatal diagnosis of hydrometrocolpos by ultrasound examination. J Ultrasound Med 3:371, 1984.
4. Dewhurst J: Practical Pediatric and Adolescent Gynecology. New York, Marcell Dekker, 1980, pp 67–74.
5. Graivier L: Hydrocolpos. J Pediatr Surg 4:563, 1969.
6. Hill SJ, Hirsch JH: Sonographic detection of fetal hydrometrocolpos. J Ultrasound Med 4:323, 1985.
7. Lide TN, Coker WG: Congenital hydrometrocolpos. Review of the literature and report of a case with uterus duplex and incompletely septate vagina. Am J Obstet Gynecol 64:1275, 1952.
8. Reed MH, Griscom NT: Hydrometrocolpos in infancy. AJR 118:1, 1973.
9. Robinow M, Shaw A: The McKusick-Kaufman syndrome: Recessively inherited vaginal atresia, hydrometrocolpos, uterovaginal duplications, anorectal anomalies, postaxial polydactyly and congenital heart disease. J Pediatr 94:776, 1979.
10. Russ PD, Zavitz WR, Pretorius DH, et al. Hydrometrocolpos, uterus didelphys, and septate vagina: An antenatal sonographic diagnosis. J Ultrasound Med 5:211, 1986.
11. Westerhout FC, Hodgman JE, Anderson GV, et al.: Congenital hydrocolpos. Am J Obstet Gynecol 89:957, 1964.

Ovarian Cysts

Definition

An ovarian cyst is a fluid-filled ovarian tumor.

Incidence

Congenital ovarian cysts are rare. Less than 100 neonatal cases have been reported.

Etiology and Pathology

Unilateral cysts are more common than bilateral, and unilocular cysts are more common than septated cysts. Size varies and ranges from small cysts to structures filling the entire abdomen.

The majority are benign cysts of germinal or graafian origin, such as simple cysts, theca-lutein cysts, and corpus luteum cysts. Granulosa cell tumors, benign cystic teratomas, and mesonephromas have also been reported in the newborn period, but they are rare compared to the cysts of germinal origin.[2,7]

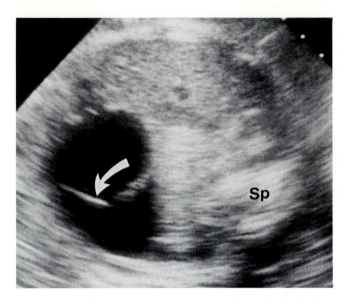

Figure 9–12. Transverse scan of the abdomen of a female fetus. A cystic lesion fills the anterior portion of the abdomen. A septum is indicated by the curved arrow. Sp, spine.

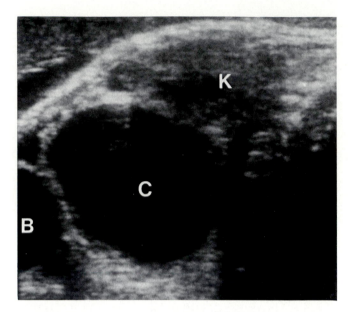

Figure 9–13. Oblique scan of a fetus with an ovarian cyst. The cystic lesion (C) is clearly seen. The bladder (B) is the hypoechogenic image below the cyst. The kidney (K) is posterior to it.

Associated Anomalies

Associated congenital hypertrophic pyloric stenosis was reported in one patient. Hydrocephalus and absence of corpus callosum and of the pyramidal system were detected in another patient.[13] Congenital hypothyroidism has been diagnosed in two patients.[5]

Diagnosis

An ovarian cyst should be suspected when a female fetus has a cystic intraabdominal mass, which is separated from the organs of the urinary and gastrointestinal tract (Figs. 9–12, 9–13).[3,10,12–14,16,17] Layering echoes may be present inside the cyst.[12]

Differential diagnoses include urachal and mesenteric cysts, enteric duplication, duodenal atresia, and dilated bowel. Urachal cysts are single and anterior, extending from the bladder to the umbilicus. Mesenteric cysts and enteric cysts may be indistinguishable from ovarian cysts. The shape of enteric bowel duplication is generally tubular, but this is not enough for a differential diagnosis. Duodenal atresia has a typical double bubble appearance. A communication between the two bubbles may be shown, and polyhydramnios is the rule. Bowel obstructions show multiple dilated bowel loops and increased peristalsis. Polyhydramnios has been reported in 10 percent of cases of fetal ovarian cysts and probably results from gastrointestinal obstruction.[14]

Prognosis

The prognosis for ovarian cysts is good, since most are benign. In the newborn, large cysts may cause ascites,[1] undergo torsion[8] and infarction,[9] lead to intestinal obstruction by membranous adhesions,[4] rupture,[15] or bleed.[11] Death may ensue because of massive hemoperitoneum. The frequency with which these accidents occur in utero is unknown.

Obstetrical Management

The detection of an intraabdominal hypoechogenic image compatible with an ovarian cyst does not alter standard obstetrical care. An exception to this is the extremely large cyst, which may cause dystocia or rupture during vaginal delivery. In one patient, this accident led to neonatal death.[7] If soft tissue dystocia is suspected, an elective cesarean section is a logical approach. An alternative would be to drain the cysts under ultrasound guidance. The theoretical risks of such an approach include spillage of an irritant (e.g., dermoid cysts) or a malignant tumor into the peritoneal cavity. The overwhelming majority of neonatal ovarian tumors are follicular or germinal in nature, and, therefore, the probability of this accident is low. Serial ultrasound examinations during pregnancy are recommended to monitor the growth of the cyst and possible complications. Torsion and bleeding of a pedunculated ovarian cyst can be suspected by the layering echoes inside the cyst[12] and by the transformation of a hypoechogenic mass into a hyperechogenic one. Newborns with ovarian cysts should probably be evaluated for hypothyroidism.[6]

REFERENCES

1. Ahmed S: Neonatal and childhood ovarian cysts. J Pediatr Surg 6:702, 1971.
2. Carlson DH, Griscom NT: Ovarian cysts in the newborn. AJR 116:664, 1972.
3. Crade M, Gillooly L, Taylor KJM: In utero demonstration of an ovarian cyst mass by ultrasound. J Clin Ultrasound 8:251, 1980.
4. Dieter RA Jr, Kindrachuk W, Muller RP: Neonatal intestinal obstruction due to torsion of an ovarian cyst. J Fam Pract 10:533, 1980.
5. Evers JL, Rolland R: Primary hypothyroidism and ovarian activity: Evidence for an overlap in the synthesis of pituitary glycoproteins. Case report. Br J Obstet Gynecol 88:195, 1981.
6. Jafri SZ, Bree RL, Silver TM, et al.: Fetal ovarian cysts: Sonographic detection and association with hypothyroidism. Radiology 150:809, 1984.
7. Jouppila P, Kirkinen P, Tuononen S: Ultrasonic detection of bilateral ovarian cysts in the fetus. Eur J Obstet Gynecol Reprod Biol 131:87, 1982.
8. Karrer FW, Swenson SA: Twisted ovarian cyst in a newborn infant: Report of a case. Arch Surg 83:921, 1961.
9. Marshall JR: Ovarian enlargements in the first year of life: Review of 45 cases. Ann Surg 161:372, 1965.
10. Mitsutake K, Abe I, Masumoto R, et al.: Prenatal diagnosis of fetal abdominal masses by real-time ultrasound. Kurume Med J 28:329, 1981.
11. Monson R, Rodgers BM, Nelson RM, et al.: Ruptured ovarian cyst in a newborn infant. J Pediatr 93:324, 1978.
12. Preziosi P, Fariello G, Maiorana A, et al.: Antenatal sonographic diagnosis of complicated ovarian cysts. J Clin Ultrasound 14:196, 1986.
13. Sandler MA, Smith SJ, Pope SG, et al.: Prenatal diagnosis of septated ovarian cysts. J Clin Ultrasound 13:55, 1985.
14. Tabsh KMA: Antenatal sonographic appearance of a fetal ovarian cyst. J Ultrasound Med 1:329, 1982.
15. Tietz KG, Davis JB: Ruptured ovarian cyst in a newborn infant. J Pediatr 51:564, 1957.
16. Touloukian RJ, Hobbins JC: Material ultrasonography in the antenatal diagnosis of surgically correctable fetal abnormalities. J Pediatr Surg 15:373, 1980.
17. Valenti C, Kassner EG, Yermakov V, et al.: Antenatal diagnosis of a fetal ovarian cyst. Am J Obstet Gynecol 123:216, 1975.

10

Skeletal Dysplasias

Normal Anatomy of the Fetal Skeleton

The skeleton is one of the earliest and easiest structures to image in the fetus. Details of the normal anatomy of the cranial, facial, and spinal components of the skeleton are discussed in Chapters 1 and 2. This chapter focuses specifically on the anatomy and biometry of the limbs and other bones not previously discussed.

The fetal skeleton becomes visible with ultrasound as soon as bones are calcified. Long bones have a primary ossification center in the diaphysis and secondary ossification centers in the epiphyses. The primary ossification center is developed in early pregnancy and is the first structure imaged with ultrasound. Secondary ossification centers develop in late pregnancy and the neonatal period, and therefore, they are not hyperechogenic structures during intrauterine life. However, the cartilages of the epiphyses can be demonstrated with ultrasound as hypoechogenic structures (e.g., head of femur and humerus).

The technique for measuring long bones is quite simple, and is described in basic texts on obstetrical ultrasound.[2] Measurements of the long bones include only the shaft. The distal and proximal epiphyses are not included. The femur is measured from the major trocanter to the distal end of the femoral shaft. For

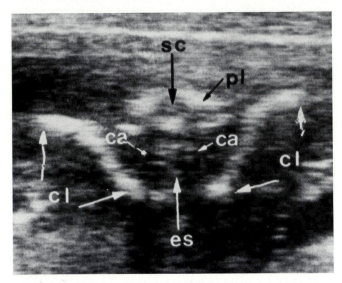

Figure 10–1. Transverse section at the level of the clavicles (cl). ca, carotid artery; es, esophagous; sc, spinal cord; pl, pedicle of thoracic vertebra. *(Reproduced with permission from Jeanty, Romero: Obstetrical Ultrasound. New York, McGraw-Hill, 1983.)*

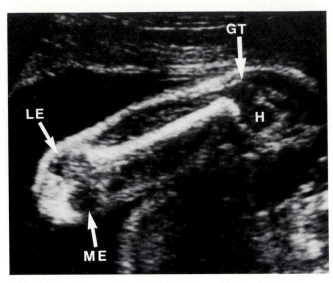

Figure 10–3. Longitudinal section of the humerus at 28 weeks' gestation. The cartilage of the humeral head (H) and greater tubercle (GT) can be seen proximally, while the cartilage of the lateral epicondyle (LE) and medial epicondyle (ME) are visible distally.

assessment of the fetus at risk for skeletal dysplasias, identification of each bone is extremely important, since there are disorders in which only a particular bone is hypoplastic (e.g., tibia, scapula). An easy task is to identify the bones of the forearm and leg. In a longitudinal scan of the forearm, the ulna extends farther into the elbow joint than the radius. In a transverse section of the leg, the tibia is the bone with the most central location, whereas the fibula is closest to the skin. In a longitudinal section, the tibia can be distinguished from the fibula by imaging its proximal

plate at the knee. Carpal bones become ossified after birth and, therefore, they are either not demonstrable or appear as hypoechogenic structures. Metacarpals and phalanges ossify in utero and are visible from the second trimester on. Talus and calcaneous begin calcifying at the 22d to 24th week of gestation. Metatarsal and phalanges of the toes are also calcified during the second trimester. The successive appearance of epiphyseal ossification centers of long bones has been used to date pregnancies. The distal femoral epiphysis appears at 32 to 35 weeks, and the proximal

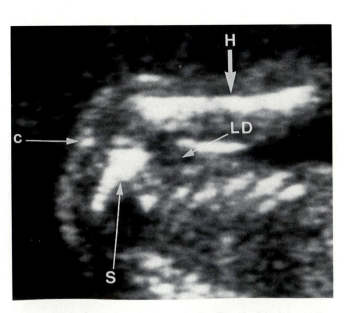

Figure 10–2. Section of the scapula (S). The clavicle (c) and the humerus (H) are visualized. LD, latissimus dorsi.

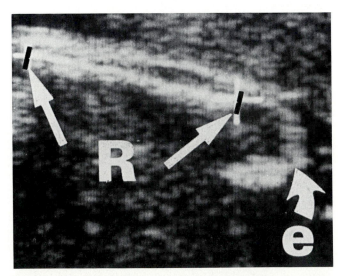

Figure 10–4. This longitudinal section of the forearm shows the radius (R), which is shorter than the ulna and does not extend as high as the ulna into the elbow joint. At the level of the wrist, both radius and ulna terminate at approximately the same level. e, elbow.

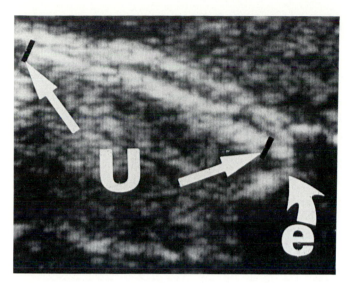

Figure 10–5. Longitudinal section of the forearm showing the ulna (u). e, elbow joint.

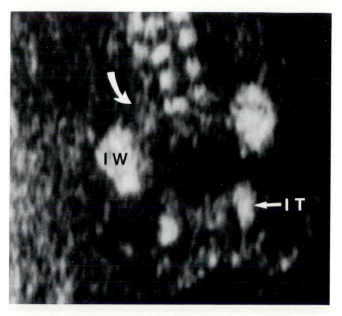

Figure 10–7. Coronal scan of a male fetal pelvis. The curved arrow points to the right iliopsoas muscle. IW, iliac wings; IT, ischial tuberosities.

tibial epiphysis calcifies 2 to 3 weeks later. Proximal humeral epiphysis is visualized at around 40 weeks. Nomograms for the assessment of the normal length of the long bones in the upper and lower extremities are displayed in Tables 10–3 and 10–4 (see pp. 323 and 324). Figures 10–1 to 10–10 show the normal anatomy of the appendicular skeleton.

BIRTH PREVALENCE AND CONTRIBUTION TO PERINATAL MORTALITY

Skeletal dysplasias are a heterogeneous group of bone growth disorders resulting in abnormal shape and size of the skeleton. The birth prevalence of skeletal dysplasias recognizable in the neonatal period has been estimated to be 2.4 per 10,000 births (95 percent confidence limits: 1.8 to 3.2 per 10,000 births).

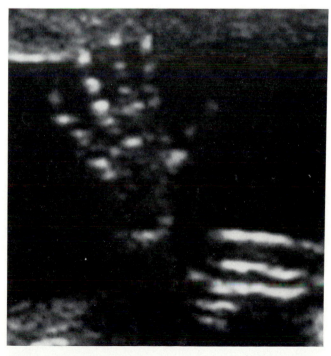

Figure 10–6. Fetal hand in the second trimester. Metacarpal bones and phalanges can be visualized. Carpal bones cannot be imaged because they are not ossified.

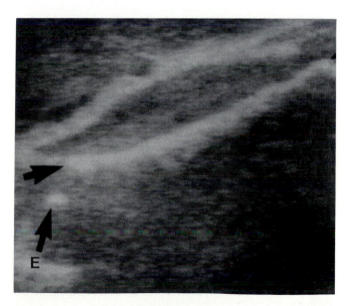

Figure 10–8. This figure illustrates a normal degree of femur bowing. The large black arrow points to the femur. E, distal femoral epiphysis.

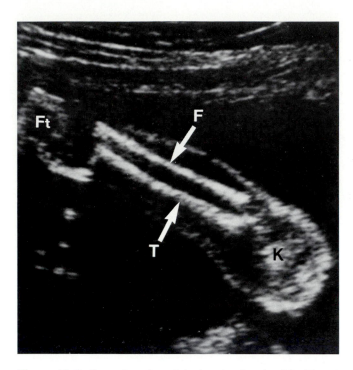

Figure 10–9. Coronal section of the leg showing the tibia (T) and fibula (F). The tibia is longer than the fibula and originates more proximally than the fibula at the knee (K). Ft, foot.

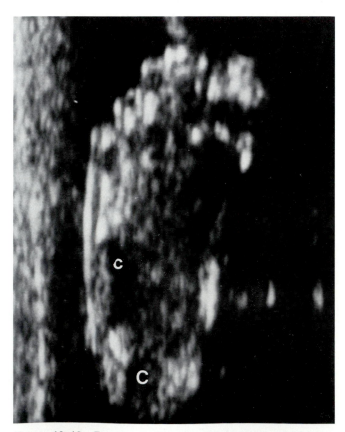

Figure 10–10. Fetal foot at 28 weeks. The five toes and the fourth and fifth metatarsal bones are clearly visible. Large C, cartilage of the calcaneal tuberosity; small c, cartilage of the cuboid bone.

TABLE 10–1. BIRTH PREVALENCE (PER 10,000 TOTAL BIRTHS) OF SKELETAL DYSPLASIAS

	Birth Prevalence (per 10,000)	Frequency among Perinatal Deaths
Thanatophoric dysplasia	0.69	1:246
Achondroplasia	0.37	—
Achondrogenesis	0.23	1:639
Osteogenesis imperfecta type II	0.18	1:799
Osteogenesis imperfecta, other types	0.18	—
Asphyxiating thoracic dysplasia	0.14	1:3196
Chondrodysplasia punctata	0.09	—
Campomelic dysplasia	0.05	1:3196
Chondroectodermal dysplasia	0.05	1:3196
Larsen syndrome	0.05	—
Mesomelic dysplasia (Langer's type)	0.05	—
Other	0.46	1:800
Total	2.44	1:110

Reproduced with permission from Camera, Mastroiacovo: In Papadatos, Bartsocas (eds): Skeletal Dysplasias. New York, Alan R. Liss, 1982, pp 441–449.

These data come from an Italian multicentric monitoring system for birth defects in which newborns (stillbirths and live births) with limb shortness or limb trunk disproportion, delivered in 90 hospitals, were radiographed and photographed.[1] Figures are based on 217,061 deliveries (215,392 live births and 1669 stillbirths). Among the 53 cases of skeletal dysplasias, 23 percent were stillbirths and 32 percent died during the first week of life. The overall frequency of skeletal dysplasias among perinatal deaths was 9.1 per 1000.

The birth prevalence of the different skeletal dysplasias and their relative frequency among perinatal deaths is shown in Table 10–1.[1] The four most common skeletal dysplasias were thanatophoric dysplasia, achondroplasia, osteogenesis imperfecta, and achondrogenesis. Thanatophoric dysplasia and achondrogenesis accounted for 62 percent of all lethal skeletal dysplasias.

CLASSIFICATION OF SKELETAL DYSPLASIAS

The existing nomenclature for skeletal dysplasias is complicated. There is a lack of uniformity about definition criteria. For example, they can be referred to by eponyms (e.g., Ellis-van Creveld syndrome, Larsen dysplasia), by Greek terms describing a salient feature of the disease (e.g., diastrophic = twisted; metatropic = changeable), or the presumed pathogenesis of the disease (e.g., osteogenesis imperfecta, achondrogenesis). The fundamental problem with any classification of skeletal dysplasias is that the patho-

TABLE 10–2. INTERNATIONAL CLASSIFICATION FOR DYSPLASIAS

Osteochondrodysplasias

Abnormalities of cartilage and/or bone growth and development

A. *Defects of growth of tubular bones and/or spine*

a. *Identifiable at birth*

α. Usually lethal before or shortly after birth

1. Achondrogenesis type I (Parenti-Fraccaro)	AR	**
2. Achondrogenesis type II (Langer-Saldino)		**
3. Hypochondrogenesis		*
4. Fibrochondrogenesis	AR	*
5. Thanatophoric dysplasia		***
6. Thanatophoric dysplasia with cloverleaf skull		**
7. Atelosteogenesis		*
8. Short rib syndrome (with or without polydactyly)		
a. Type I (Saldino-Noonan)	AR	**
b. Type II (Majewski)	AR	*
c. Type III (lethal thoracic dysplasia)	AR	*

β. Usually nonlethal dysplasia

9. Chondrodysplasia punctata		
a. Rhizomelic form autosomal recessive	AR	**
b. Dominant X-linked form; lethal in male	XLD	**
c. Common mild form (Sheffield)		
Exclude: symptomatic stippling (warfarin, chromosomal aberration)		***
10. Campomelic dysplasia		**
11. Kyphomelic dysplasia	AR	*
12. Achondroplasia	AD	****
13. Diastrophic dysplasia	AR	***
14. Metatropic dysplasia (several forms)	AR, AD	**
15. Chondroectodermal dysplasia (Ellis–Van Creveld)	AR	***
16. Asphyxiating thoracic dysplasia (Jeune)	AR	**
17. Spondyloepiphyseal dysplasia congenita		
a. Autosomal dominant form	AD	**
b. Autosomal recessive form	AR	**
18. Kniest dysplasia	AD	**
19. Dyssegmental dysplasia	AR	*
20. Mesomelic dysplasia		
a. Type Nievergelt	AD	*
b. Type Langer (probable homozygous dyschondrosteosis)	AR	*
c. Type Robinow		*
d. Type Rheinardt	AD	*
e. Others		***
21. Acromesomelic dysplasia	AR	**
22. Cleidocranial dysplasia	AD	****
23. Otopalatodigital syndrome		
a. Type I (Langer)	XLSD	**
b. Type II (André)	XLR	**
24. Larsen syndrome	AR, AD	**
25. Other multiple dislocation syndromes (Desbuquois)	AR	

b. *Identifiable in later life*

1. Hypochondroplasia	AD	***
2. Dyschondrosteosis	AD	***
3. Metaphyseal chondrodysplasia type Jansen	AD	*
4. Metaphyseal chondrodysplasia type Schmid	AD	**
5. Metaphyseal chondrodysplasia type McKusick	AR	**
6. Metaphyseal chondrodysplasia with exocrine pancreatic insufficiency and cyclic neutropenia	AR	**
7. Spondylometaphyseal dysplasia		
a. Type Kozlowski	AD	**
b. Other forms		***
8. Multiple epiphyseal dysplasia		
a. Type Fairbank	AD	****
b. Other forms		***
9. Multiple epiphyseal dysplasia with early diabetes (Wolcott-Rallisson)	AR	**
10. Arthro-ophthalmopathy (Stickler)	AR	***
11. Pseudoachondroplasia		
a. Dominant	AD	***
b. Recessive	AR	**
12. Spondyloepiphyseal dysplasia tarda (X-linked recessive)	XLR	**
13. Progressive pseudorheumatoid chondrodysplasia	AR	**
14. Spondyloepiphyseal dysplasia, other forms		***
15. Brachyolmia		
a. Autosomal recessive	AR	*
b. Autosomal dominant	AD	*
16. Dyggve-Melchior-Clausen dysplasia	AR	**
17. Spondyloepimetaphyseal dysplasia (several forms)		***
18. Spondyloepimetaphyseal dysplasia with joint laxity	AR	**
19. Otospondylomegaepiphyseal dysplasia (OSMED)	AR	*
20. Myotonic chondrodysplasia (Catel-Schwartz-Jampel)	AR	**
21. Parastremmatic dysplasia	AD	*
22. Trichorhinophalangeal dysplasia	AD	**
23. Acrodysplasia with retinitis pigmentosa and nephropathy (Saldino-Mainzer)	AR	**

B. *Disorganized development of cartilage and fibrous components of skeleton*

1. Dysplasia epiphyseal hemimelica		**
2. Multiple cartilaginous exostoses	AD	****
3. Acrodysplasia with exostoses (Giedion-Langer)		**
4. Enchondromatosis (Ollier)		***
5. Enchondromatosis with hemangioma (Maffucci)		**
6. Metachondromatosis	AD	**
7. Spondyloenchondroplasia	AR	*
8. Osteoglophonic dysplasia		*
9. Fibrous dysplasia (Jaffe-Lichtenstein)		***
10. Fibrous dysplasia with skin pigmentation and precocious puberty (McCune-Albright)		***
11. Cherubism (familial fibrous dysplasia of the jaws)	AD	**

C. *Abnormalities of density of cortical diaphyseal structure and/or metaphyseal modeling*

1. Osteogenesis imperfecta (several forms)	AR, AD	****

(continued)

TABLE 10–2. *(Continued)*

2. Juvenile idiopathic osteoporosis		**
3. Osteoporosis with pseudoglioma	AR	*
4. Osteopetrosis		
a. Autosomal recessive lethal	AR	**
b. Intermediate recessive	AR	**
c. Autosomal dominant	AD	***
d. Recessive with tubular acidosis	AR	**
5. Pycnodysostosis	AR	***
6. Dominant osteosclerosis type Stanescu	AD	**
7. Osteomesopycnosis	AD	**
8. Osteopoikilosis	AD	***
9. Osteopathia striata	AD	***
10. Osteopathia striata with cranial sclerosis	AD	**
11. Melorheostosis		***
12. Diaphyseal dysplasia (Camurati-Engelmann)	AD	***
13. Craniodiaphyseal dysplasia	AR	**
14. Endosteal hyperostosis		
a. Autosomal dominant (Worth)	AD	**
b. Autosomal recessive (Van Buchem)	AR	**
c. Autosomal recessive (sclerosteosis)	AR	**
15. Tubular stenosis (Kenny-Caffey)	AD	*
16. Pachydermoperiostosis	AD	**
17. Osteodysplasty (Melnick-Needles)	AD	**
18. Frontometaphyseal dysplasia	XLR	**
19. Craniometaphyseal dysplasia (several forms)	AD	***
20. Metaphyseal dysplasia (Pyle)	AR or AD	**
21. Dysosteosclerosis	AR or XLR	**
22. Osteo-ectasia with hyperphosphatasia	AR	**
23. Oculo-dento-osseous dysplasia		
a. Mild type	AD	***
b. Severe type	AR	*
24. Infantile cortical hyperostosis (Caffey disease, familial type)	AD	**

Dysostoses
Malformation of individual bones, singly or in combination

A. Dysostoses with cranial and facial involvement

1. Craniosynostosis (several forms)		***
2. Craniofacial dysostosis (Crouzon)		***
3. Acrocephalosyndactyly		
a. Type Apert	AD	***
b. Type Chotzen	AD	**
c. Type Pfeiffer	AD	**
d. Other types		***
4. Acrocephalopolysyndactyly (Carpenter and others)	AR	**
5. Cephalopolysyndactyly (Greig)	AD	*
6. First and second branchial arch syndromes		
a. Mandibulofacial dysostosis (Treacher-Collins, Franceschetti)	AD	***
b. Acrofacial dysostosis (Nager)		**
c. Oculo-auriculo-vertebral dysostosis (Goldenhar)	AR	***
d. Hemifacial microsomia		***
e. Others		***
(Probably parts of a large spectrum)		
7. Oculomandibulofacial syndrome (Haller-mann-Streiff-François)		**

B. Dysostoses with predominant axial involvement

1. Vertebral segmentation defects (including Klippel-Feil)		**
2. Cervico-oculo-acoustic syndrome (Wilder-vanck)		***
3. Sprengel anomaly		***
4. Spondylocostal dysostosis		
a. Dominant form	AD	**
b. Recessive forms	AR	**
5. Oculovertebral syndrome (Weyers)		*
6. Osteo-onychodysostosis	AD	***
7. Cerebrocostomandibular syndrome	AR	**

C. Dysostoses with predominant involvement of extremities

1. Acheiria		**
2. Apodia		**
3. Tetraphocomelia syndrome (Roberts) (SC pseudothalidomide syndrome)	AR	**
4. Ectrodactyly		
a. Isolated		***
b. Ectrodactyly–ectodermal dysplasia, cleft palate-syndrome	AD	**
c. Ectrodactyly with scalp defects	AD	**
5. Oro-acral syndrome (aglossia syndrome, Hanhart syndrome)		*
6. Familial radioulnar synostosis		**
7. Brachydactyly, types A, B, C, D, E (Bell's classification)	AD	****
8. Symphalangism	AD	***
9. Polydactyly (several forms)		****
10 Syndactyly (several forms)		****
11. Polysyndactyly (several forms)		***
12. Camptodactyly		****
13. Manzke syndrome		*
14. Poland syndrome		***
15. Rubinstein-Taybi syndrome		**
16. Coffin-Siris syndrome		**
17. Pancytopenia-dysmelia syndrome (Fanconi)	AR	***
18. Blackfan-Diamond anemia with thumb anomalies (Aase syndrome)	AR	**
19. Thrombocytopenia-radial-aplasia syndrome	AR	**
20. Orodigitofacial syndrome		
a. Type Papillon-Leage; lethal in males	XLD	**
b. Type Mohr	AR	**
21. Cardiomelic syndromes (Holt-Oram and others)	AD	***
22. Femoral focal deficiency (with or without facial anomalies)		**
23. Multiple synostoses (includes some forms of symphalangism)	AD	***
24. Scapulo-iliac dysostosis (Kosenow-Sinios)	AD	**
25. Hand–foot–genital syndrome	AD	**
26. Focal dermal hypoplasia (Goltz); lethal in males	XLD	**

Idiopathic Osteolyses

1. Phalangeal (several forms)		**
2. Tarsocarpal		
a. Including François form and others	AR	**
b. With nephropathy	AD	**
3. Multicentric		
a. Hajdu-Cheney form	AD	**
b. Winchester form	AR	*
c. Torg form	AR	*
d. Other forms		**

TABLE 10–2. (*Continued*)

Miscellaneous Disorders with Osseous Involvement		
1. Early acceleration of skeletal maturation		
a. Marshall-Smith syndrome		*
b. Weaver syndrome		*
c. Other types		*
2. Marfan syndrome	AD	****
3. Congenital contractural arachnodactyly	AD	**
4. Cerebrohepatorenal syndrome (Zellweger)		**
5. Coffin-Lowry syndrome	SLR	**
6. Cockayne syndrome	AR	**
7. Fibrodysplasia ossificans congenita	AD	***
8. Epidermal nervus syndrome (Solomon)		**
9. Nevoid basal cell carcinoma syndrome		**
10. Multiple hereditary fibromatosis		**
11. Neurofibromatosis	AD	****

Chromosomal Aberrations

Primary Metabolic Abnormalities

A. *Calcium and/or phosphorus*		
1. Hypophosphatemic rickets	XLD	****
2. Vitamin D dependency or pseudodeficiency rickets		
a. Type I with probable deficiency in 25-hydroxy vitamin D 1-α-hydroxylase	AR	**
b. Type II with target-organ resistancy	AR	**
3. Late rickets (McCance)		**
4. Idiopathic hypercalciuria		***
5. Hypophosphatasia (several forms)	AR	***
6. Pseudohypoparathyroidism (normo- and hypocalcemic forms, including acrodysostosis)	AD	***
B. *Complex carbohydrates*		
1. Mucopolysaccharidosis type I (α-L-iduronidase deficiency)		
a. Hurler form	AR	***
b. Scheie form	AR	**
c. Other forms	AR	**
2. Mucopolysaccharidosis type II—Hunter (sulfoiduronate sulfatase deficiency)	XLR	***
3. Mucopolysaccharidosis type III—Sanfilippo		***
a. Type III A (heparin sulfamidase deficiency)	AR	

b. Type III B (N-acetyl-α-glucosaminidase deficiency)	AR	
c. Type III C (α-glucosaminide-N-acetyl transferase deficiency)	AR	
d. Type III D (N-acetyl-glucosamine-6 sulfate sulfatase deficiency)	AR	
4. Mucopolysaccharidosis type IV		**
a. Type IV A—Morquio (N-acetyl-galactosamine-6 sulfate sulfatase deficiency)	AR	
b. Type IV B (β-galactosidase deficiency)	AR	
5. Mucopolysaccharidosis type VI—Maroteaux-Lamy (arylsulfatase B deficiency)	AR	
6. Mucopolysaccharidosis type VII (β-glucuronidase deficiency)	AR	**
7. Aspartyl glucosaminuria (aspartylglucosaminidase deficiency)	AR	**
8. Mannosidosis (α-mannosidase deficiency)	AR	**
9. Fucosidosis (α-fucosidase deficiency)	AR	**
10. GMI-Gangliosidosis (β-galactosidase deficiency) (several forms)	AR	**
11. Multiple sulfatases deficiency (Austin-Thieffry)	AR	**
12. Isolated neuraminidase deficiency, several forms including		**
a. Mucolipidosis I	AR	
b. Nephrosialidosis	AR	
c. Cherry red spot myoclonia syndrome	AR	
13. Phosphotransferase deficiency; several forms including		**
a. Mucolipidosis II (I cell disease)	AR	
b. Mucolipidosis III (pseudopolydystrophy)	AR	
14. Combined neuraminidase β-galactosidase deficiency	AR	*
15. Salla disease	AR	*
C. *Lipids*		
1. Niemann-Pick disease (sphingomyelinase deficiency) (several forms)	AR	***
2. Gaucher disease (β-glucosidase deficiency) (several types)	AR	****
3. Farber disease lipogranulomatosis (ceraminidase deficiency)	AR	**
D. *Nucleic acids*		
1. Adenosine-deaminase deficiency and others	AR	**
E. *Amino acids*		
1. Homocystinuria and others	AR	***
F. *Metals*		
1. Menkes syndrome (kinky hair syndrome and others)	AR	**

[a] Mode of transmission.
[b] Frequency.
AR, autosomal recessive
XLD, X-linked dominant
AD, autosomal dominant
XLR, X-linked recessive
SLR, sex-linked recessive
**** 1000 + cases.
*** 100–1000 cases.
** 20–100 cases.
* Fewer than 20 cases.

(Estimates of the relative frequency of these conditions are based on the compilers' experience and a review of the literature.)

Reproduced with permission from Kozlowski K, Beighton P: Gamut Index of Skeletal Dysplasias (An aid to radiodiagnosis). Berlin, Springer-Verlag, 1986.

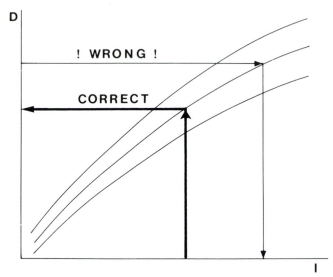

Figure 10–11. The statistical technique used to establish the relationship between gestational age and a biometric fetal parameter is regression analysis. This method uses an independent variable (I) to predict the value of a dependent variable (D). It is incorrect to use the dependent variable to predict the independent one. *(Reproduced with permission from Jeanty, Romero: Obstetrical Ultrasound. New York, McGraw-Hill, 1983.)*

genesis of these diseases is rarely known. Therefore, the current system relies on purely descriptive findings of either a clinical or radiologic nature.

In an attempt to develop a uniform terminology, a group of experts met in Paris in 1977 and proposed an International Nomenclature for Skeletal Dysplasias. This classification was subsequently revised in 1983 (Table 10–2). The system subdivides the diseases into five different groups: (1) osteocondro-dysplasias (abnormalities of cartilage or bone growth and development) (2) dysostoses (malformations of individual bones singly or in combination), (3) idiopathic osteolyses (disorders associated with multifocal resorption of bone), (4) skeletal disorders associated with chromosomal aberrations, and (5) primary metabolic disorders.

A comprehensive description of these diseases is beyond the scope of this book. This section focuses primarily on the osteochondrodysplasias that are recognizable at birth. Although more than 200 skeletal dysplasias have been described, only a few can be recognized with the use of sonography in the antepartum period. Most of these disorders result in short stature, and the term "dwarfism" has been used to refer to this clinical condition. Because this term carries a negative connotation, the term "dysplasia" has substituted it.

EMBRYOLOGY

The skeletal system develops from mesoderm. In most bones (e.g., the long bones), ossification is preceded by cartilage (endochondral ossification).

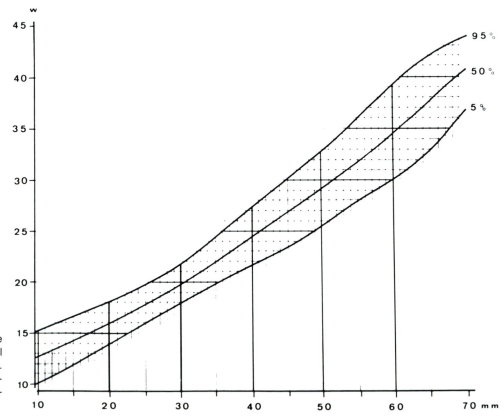

Figure 10–12. This figure shows the graph used to predict the gestational age from a given humeral length. Note that the humerus is on the horizontal axis, and age (dependent variable) is on the vertical axis.

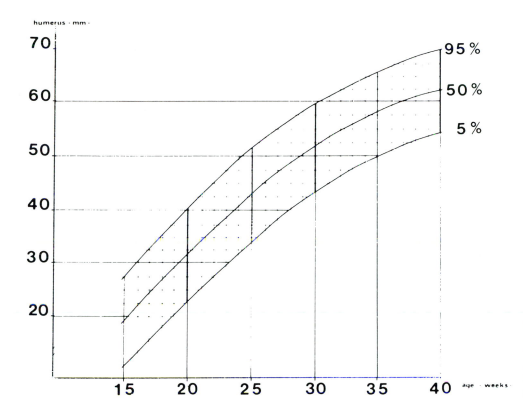

Figure 10–13. This figure represents an example of a correct graph required to assess the normality of a given biometric parameter. Note that the fetal age is the independent variable (horizontal axis).

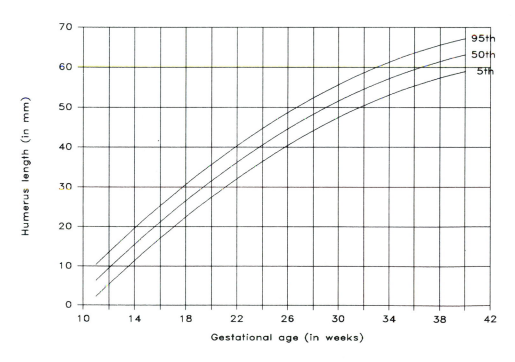

Figure 10–14. Growth of the humerus across gestational age.

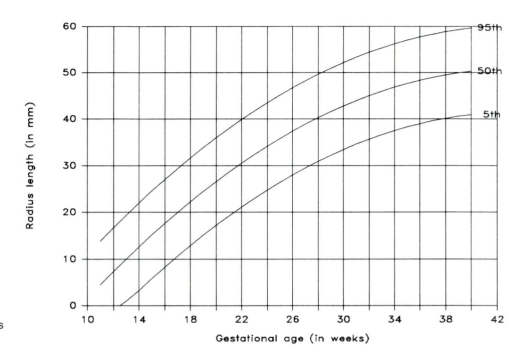

Figure 10–15. Growth of the radius across gestational age.

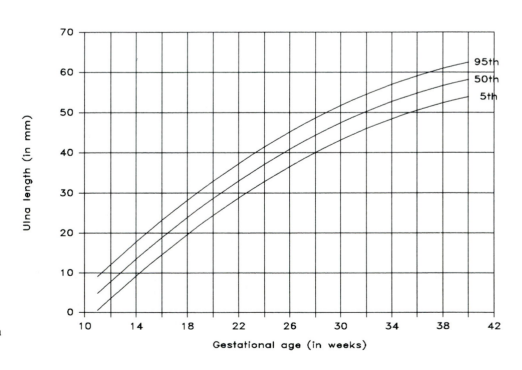

Figure 10–16. Growth of the ulna across gestational age.

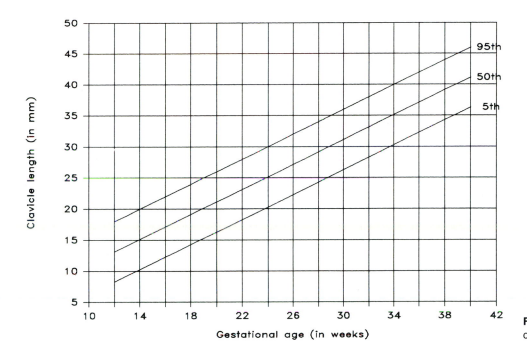

Figure 10–17. Growth of the clavicle across gestational age.

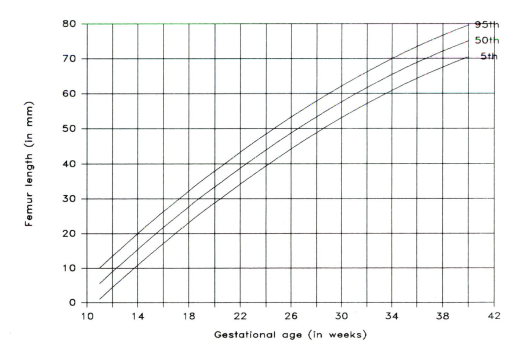

Figure 10–18 Growth of the femur across gestational age.

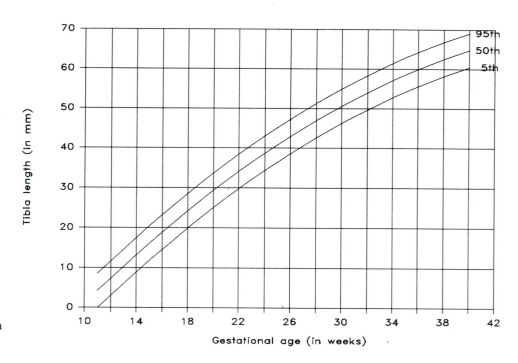

Figure 10–19. Growth of the tibia across gestational age.

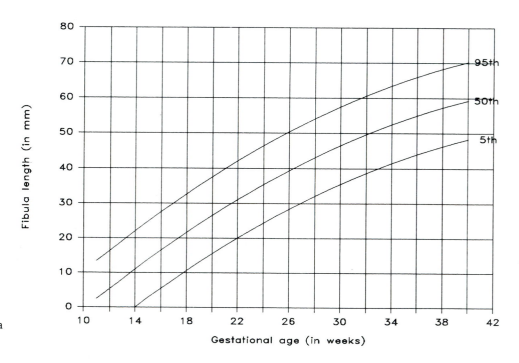

Figure 10–20. Growth of the fibula across gestational age.

TABLE 10–3. NORMAL VALUES FOR THE ARM

Age (weeks)	Humerus (mm) Percentile			Ulna (mm) Percentile			Radius (mm) Percentile		
	5th	50th	95th	5th	50th	95th	5th	50th	95th
12	—	9	—	—	7	—	—	7	—
13	6	11	16	5	10	15	6	10	14
14	9	14	19	8	13	18	8	13	17
15	12	17	22	11	16	21	11	15	20
16	15	20	25	13	18	23	13	18	22
17	18	22	27	16	21	26	14	20	26
18	20	25	30	19	24	29	15	22	29
19	23	28	33	21	26	31	20	24	29
20	25	30	35	24	29	34	22	27	32
21	28	33	38	26	31	36	24	29	33
22	30	35	40	28	33	38	27	31	34
23	33	38	42	31	36	41	26	32	39
24	35	40	45	33	38	43	26	34	42
25	37	42	47	35	40	45	31	36	41
26	39	44	49	37	42	47	32	37	43
27	41	46	51	39	44	49	33	39	45
28	43	48	53	41	46	51	33	40	48
29	45	50	55	43	48	53	36	42	47
30	47	51	56	44	49	54	36	43	49
31	48	53	58	46	51	56	38	44	50
32	50	55	60	48	53	58	37	45	53
33	51	56	61	49	54	59	41	46	51
34	53	58	63	51	56	61	40	47	53
35	54	59	64	52	57	62	41	48	54
36	56	61	65	53	58	63	39	48	57
37	57	62	67	55	60	65	45	49	53
38	59	63	68	56	61	66	45	49	54
39	60	65	70	57	62	67	45	50	54
40	61	66	71	58	63	68	46	50	55

Reprinted with permission from Jeanty, Romero: Obstetrical Ultrasound. New York, McGraw-Hill, 1983.

However, cartilage does not become bone but rather is destroyed and bone is formed in its place. In other cases, such as flat bones, ossification develops directly in the mesenchyme without cartilage formation (intramembranous ossification).

In long bones, ossification proceeds in an orderly fashion. It first begins in the shaft, or diaphysis, and extends from the middle toward both ends (epiphyses), where two areas of cartilage remain. During the last weeks of gestation and the first weeks of neonatal life, ossification centers appear in the epiphyses and lead to bone formation. The area of cartilage between the diaphysis and the epiphyses is called the metaphysis and represents the growing portion of the bone. Once adult size is achieved, this area ossifies, and the diaphysis joins permanently to the epiphyses.

BIOMETRY OF THE FETAL SKELETON IN THE DIAGNOSIS OF BONE DYSPLASIAS

Long bone biometry has been used extensively in the prediction of gestational age. Nomograms available for this purpose use the long bone as the independent variable and the estimated fetal age as the dependent variable (Figs. 10–11, 10–12). However, the type of nomogram required to assess the normality of bone dimensions uses the gestational age as the independent variable and the long bone as the dependent variable (Fig. 10–13). For the proper use of these nomograms the clinician must know accurately the gestational age of the fetus (Figs. 10–14 through 10–20, Tables 10–3, 10–4). Therefore, patients at risk for skeletal dysplasias should be advised to seek prenatal care early to assess all clinical estimators of gestational age. For those patients with uncertain gestational age, we have provided a set of nomograms that use the head perimeter as the independent variable (Figs. 10–21, 10–22). Other authors have used the biparietal diameter, but the head perimeter has the advantage of being shape independent. A limitation of this approach is the assumption that the cranium is not involved in the dysplastic process. The nomograms provide the mean, 5th, and 95th percentile for a given parameter. The 5th and 95th confidence limits are arbitrary statistical definitions of

TABLE 10–4. NORMAL VALUES FOR THE LEG

Age (weeks)	Tibia (mm) Percentile			Fibula (mm) Percentile			Femur (mm) Percentile		
	5th	*50th*	*95th*	*5th*	*50th*	*95th*	*5th*	*50th*	*95th*
12	—	7	—	—	6	—	4	8	13
13	—	10	—	—	9	—	6	11	16
14	7	12	17	6	12	19	9	14	18
15	9	15	20	9	15	21	12	17	21
16	12	17	22	13	18	23	15	20	24
17	15	20	25	13	21	28	18	23	27
18	17	22	27	15	23	31	21	25	30
19	20	25	30	19	26	33	24	28	33
20	22	27	33	21	28	36	26	31	36
21	25	30	35	24	31	37	29	34	38
22	27	32	38	27	33	39	32	36	41
23	30	35	40	28	35	42	35	39	44
24	32	37	42	29	37	45	37	42	46
25	34	40	45	34	40	45	40	44	49
26	37	42	47	36	42	47	42	47	51
27	39	44	49	37	44	50	45	49	54
28	41	46	51	38	45	53	47	52	56
29	43	48	53	41	47	54	50	54	59
30	45	50	55	43	49	56	52	56	61
31	47	52	57	42	51	59	54	59	63
32	48	54	59	42	52	63	56	61	65
33	50	55	60	46	54	62	58	63	67
34	52	57	62	46	55	65	60	65	69
35	53	58	64	51	57	62	62	67	71
36	55	60	65	54	58	63	64	68	73
37	56	61	67	54	59	65	65	70	74
38	58	63	68	56	61	65	67	71	76
39	59	64	69	56	62	67	68	73	77
40	61	66	71	59	63	67	70	74	79

Reprinted with permission from Jeanty, Romero: Obstetrical Ultrasound. New York, McGraw-Hill, 1983.

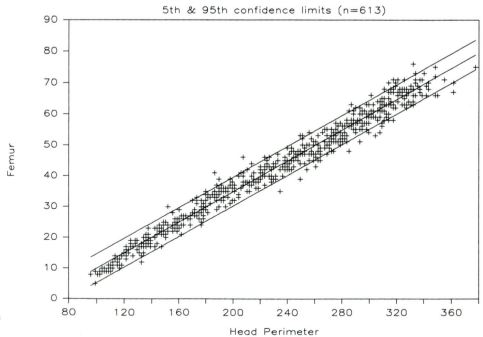

Figure 10–21. Relationship between the head perimeter and the femur.

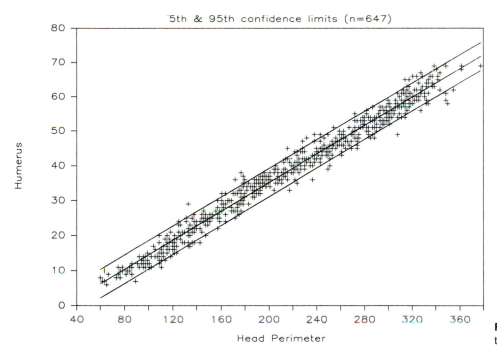

Figure 10–22. Relationship between the head perimeter and the humerus.

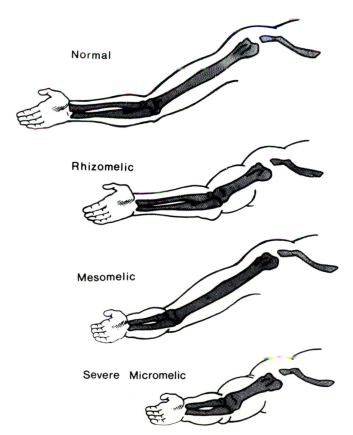

Figure 10–23. Varieties of short limb dysplasia according to the segment involved.

abnormality. A small proportion (2.5 percent) of the general population will have shortened long bones if these nomograms are employed. This point is illustrated in Figures 10–21, 10–22, 10–24, and 10–25. The crosses in these figures are measurements taken from fetuses subsequently born without short limb skeletal dysplasias. It may be better to use the 1st and 99th confidence limits because with this threshold, only 0.5 percent of the general population would be considered to have abnormally short bones. Larger studies are required for these boundaries to be established with accuracy. Our experience in the prenatal diagnosis of infants with skeletal dysplasias indicates that affected fetuses have dramatic deviations from the 5th and 95th confidence limits. An exception to this is heterozygous achondroplasia (see p. 359).

TERMINOLOGY FREQUENTLY USED IN DESCRIPTION OF BONE DYSPLASIAS

Shortening of the extremities can involve the entire limb (micromelia), the proximal segment (rhizomelia), the intermediate segment (mesomelia), or the distal segment (acromelia) (Fig. 10–23). The diagnosis of rhizomelia and mesomelia requires comparison between the bone dimensions of the leg and

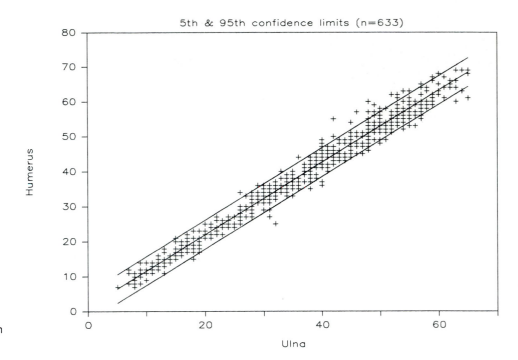

Figure 10–24. Relationship between the ulna and the humerus.

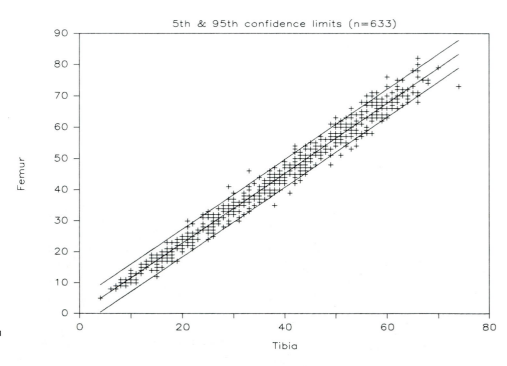

Figure 10–25. Relationship between the tibia and the femur.

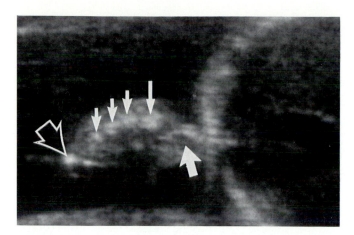

Figure 10–26. Polydactyly. A fetus with short rib–polydactyly syndrome showing six fingers. The large solid arrow points to the thumb. Small arrows indicate the next four fingers. The open arrow points to an extra digit. The presence of the extra digit on the ulnar side defines postaxial polydactyly.

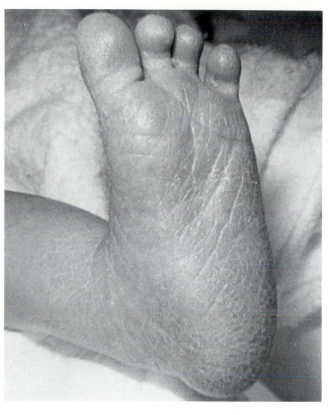

Figure 10–27. Syndactyly. There are only four digits on this foot.

forearm and of the thigh and arm. Figures 10–24 and 10–25 illustrate the relationship between these bones.

Several skeletal dysplasias feature alteration of hands and feet. Polydactyly refers to the presence of more than five digits (Fig. 10–26). It is classified as postaxial if the extra digits are on the ulnar or fibular side and preaxial if they are located on the radial or tibial side. Syndactyly refers to soft tissue or bony fusion of adjacent digits (Figs. 10–27, 10–28). Clinodactyly is a deviation of one or more fingers (Figs. 10–29, 10–30).

The most common spinal abnormality in skeletal dysplasias is platyspondyly, a flattening of the vertebral bodies. The antenatal detection of this abnormality has not been reported. Scoliosis can be identified in utero (Fig. 10–31).

CLINICAL PRESENTATION

The challenge of the antenatal diagnosis of skeletal dysplasias will generally occur in one of two ways: (1) a patient who has delivered an infant with a skeletal dysplasia and desires antenatal assessment of a subsequent pregnancy or (2) the incidental finding of a shortened, bowed, or anomalous extremity during a

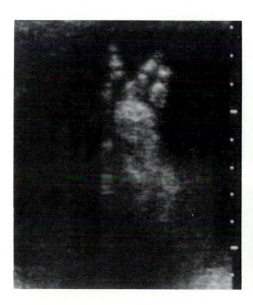

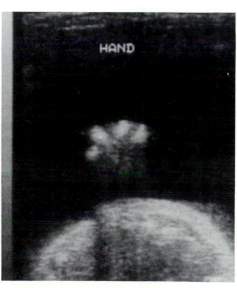

Figure 10–28. Syndactyly. Only four fingers are visualized. The left photograph shows a long axis view of the hand; the right photograph shows a transverse section of the hand. *(Courtesy of Dr. Carl Otto.)*

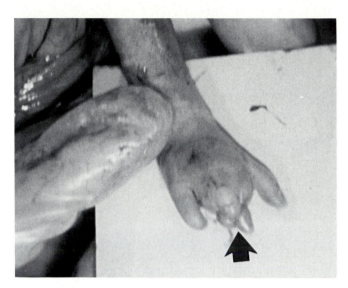

Figure 10–29. Clinodactyly. Note the overlapping fingers *(black arrow)* in this midtrimester fetus.

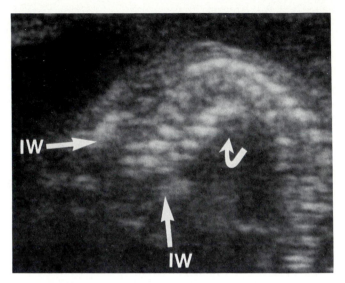

Figure 10–31. Coronal scan demonstrating severe scoliosis *(curved arrow)*. IW, iliac wings.

Figure 10–30. Sonogram of a fetus with clinodactyly. *(Reproduced with permission from Jeanty et al.: J Ultrasound Med 4:595, 1985.)*

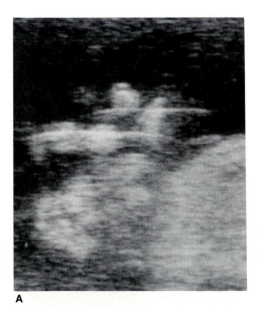

A

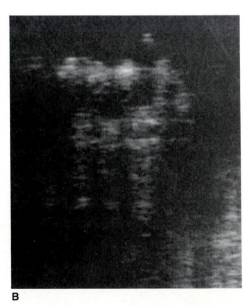

B

TABLE 10–5. LETHAL SKELETAL DYSPLASIAS

Achondrogenesis
Thanatophoric dysplasia
Short rib–polydactyly syndromes types I, II, and III
Fibrochondrogenesis
Atelosteogenesis
Homozygous achondroplasia
Osteogenesis imperfecta, perinatal type
Hypophosphatasia, perinatal type

routine sonographic examination. The task is easier when looking for a particular phenotype in a patient at risk. The inability to obtain reliable information about skeletal mineralization and the involvement of other systems (e.g., skin) with sonography is a limiting factor for an accurate diagnosis after identification of an incidental finding. Another limitation is the paucity of information about the in utero natural history of skeletal dysplasias.

Despite these difficulties and limitations there are good medical reasons for attempting an accurate prenatal diagnosis of skeletal dysplasias. A number of these disorders are uniformly lethal, and a confident antenatal diagnosis would allow options for the pregnancy termination to be considered. Table 10–5 lists such disorders.

APPROACH TO THE DIAGNOSIS OF SKELETAL DYSPLASIAS

Our approach to diagnosing skeletal dysplasias follows an organized examination of the fetal skeleton.

Long Bones

All long bones should be measured in all extremities. Comparisons with other segments should be made to establish if the limb shortening is predominantly

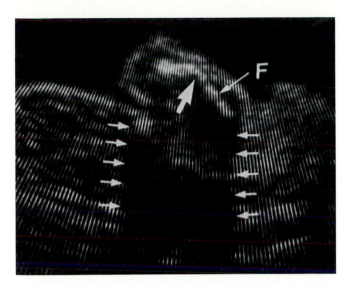

Figure 10–33. In utero fracture in a case of osteogenesis imperfecta. F, femur. The large arrow corresponds to the fracture site. The small arrows outline the decreased shadowing cast by the bone.

rhizomelic, mesomelic, or involves all segments. A detailed examination of each bone is necessary to exclude the absence or hypoplasia of individual bones (e.g., fibula or scapula).

An attempt should be made to assess the degree of mineralization by examining the acoustic shadow behind the bone and the echogenicity of the bone itself. However, there are limitations in the sonographic evaluation of mineralization. In our experience, the reflection of ultrasound waves at the interfacies between the skull and the amniotic fluid may lead to an overestimation of bone density. An

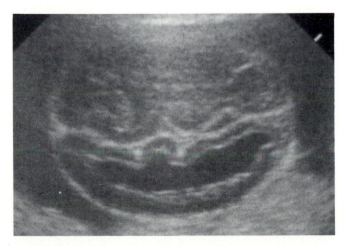

Figure 10–32. Demineralization of the skull in a case of congenital hypophosphatasia.

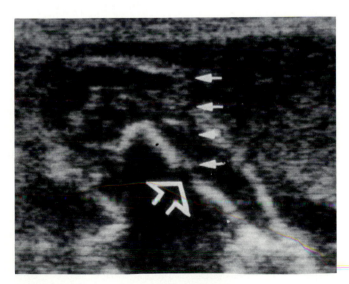

Figure 10–34. Potential pitfall. Shadowing from an upper extremity (*arrows*) creates the false image of a femur fracture (*open arrow).*

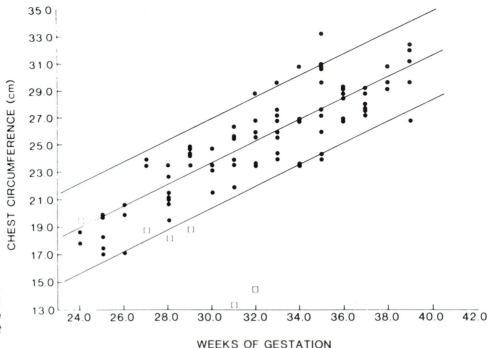

Figure 10–35. Relationship between thoracic circumference and gestational age. *(Reproduced with permission from Nimrod et al.: Obstet Gynecol 68:495, 1986.)*

example of skull demineralization is depicted in Figure 10–32. The pitfall is depicted in Fig. 10–65.

The degree of long bone curvature should be examined. At present, there is no objective means for this assessment; only by experience can an operator discern the boundary between normality and abnormality. Campomelia (excessive bowing) is characteristic of certain disorders (e.g., campomelic syndrome, osteogenesis imperfecta, etc.; see Table 10–6).

Finally, the possibility of fractures should be considered. They can be detected in conditions like osteogenesis imperfecta and hypophosphatasia. The fractures may be extremely subtle or may lead to angulation and separation of the segments of the affected bone (Figs. 10–33, 10–34).

Evaluation of Thoracic Dimensions

Several skeletal dysplasias are associated with a hypoplastic thorax (Table 10–6). Chest restriction may lead to pulmonary hypoplasia, a frequent cause of death in these conditions. Thoracic dimensions can be assessed by measuring the thoracic circumference at the level of the four chamber view of the heart. Figure 10–35 illustrates the relationship between the gestational age and thoracic circumference.

Evaluation of Hands and Feet

Hands and feet should be examined to exclude polydactyly and syndactyly, and extreme postural deformities as those seen in diastrophic dysplasia.

Evaluation of the Fetal Cranium

Several skeletal dysplasias are associated with defects of membranous ossification and, therefore, affect skull bones. Orbits should be measured to exclude hypertelorism. Other findings that should be investigated are micrognathia, short upper lip, abnormally shaped ear, frontal bossing, and cloverleaf skull deformity. Table 10–6 illustrates the conditions associated with these findings.

Postnatal Workup

Despite all efforts to establish an accurate prenatal diagnosis, a careful study of the newborn is required in all instances. The evaluation should include a detailed physical examination performed by a geneticist or an individual with experience in the field of skeletal dysplasias and radiograms of the skeleton. The latter should include anterior, posterior, lateral, and Towne views of the skull and anteroposterior views of the spine and extremities, with separate films of the hands and feet. Examination of the skeletal radiographs will permit precise diagnoses in the majority of cases, since the classification of skeletal dysplasias is largely based on radiographic findings. Histologic examination of the chondro-osseous tissue should be considered. Chromosomal studies should also be considered because there is a specific group of constitutional bone disorders associated with cytogenetic abnormalities. Biochemical studies are helpful in rare instances (e.g., hypophosphatasia). DNA studies and enzymatic activity assays should be considered in patients whose

TABLE 10–6. PARAMETERS FOR THE DIFFERENTIAL DIAGNOSIS OF SKELETAL DYSPLASIAS

Extreme micromelia
Achondrogenesis
Thanatophoric dysplasia
Fibrochondrogenesis
Atelosteogenesis
Short rib–polydactyly syndromes
Diastrophic dysplasia
Dyssegmental dysplasia
Roberts syndrome

Rhizomelia
Thanatophoric dysplasia
Atelosteogenesis
Chondrodysplasia punctata rhizomelic
    type
Diastrophic dysplasia
Congenital short femur

Mesomelia
Mesomelic dysplasia
COVESDEM association

Acromesomelia
Ellis-van Creveld syndrome

**Metaphyseal flaring (dumbbell-shaped
    bones)**
Metatropic dysplasia
Kniest syndrome
Dyssegmental dysplasia
Weissenbacher-Zweymuller syndrome
Fibrochondrogenesis
Short rib–polydactyly syndrome type III

Curved or bowed long bones
Campomelic syndrome
Osteogenesis imperfecta
Dyssegmental dysplasia
Otopalatodigital syndrome
Thanatophoric dysplasia (telephone
    receiver femur)
Roberts syndrome
Hypophosphatasia

Bone fractures
Osteogenesis imperfecta
Hypophosphatasia
Achondrogenesis

Hypoplastic or absent fibula
Fibrochondrogenesis
Atelosteogenesis
Mesomelic dysplasia, Langer's and Rein-
    hart's types
Otopalatodigital syndrome

Hypoplastic scapulae
Campomelic syndrome

Normal long bones
Larsen syndrome
Cleidocranial dysplasia
Craniosynostoses
Arthrogryposis multiplex congenita
Jarcho-Levin syndrome

Clubfoot deformity
Diastrophic dysplasia
Osteogenesis imperfecta
Kniest dysplasia
Spondiloepiphyseal congenita
Metatropic dysplasia
Mesomelic dysplasia, Nievergeit type
Chondrodysplasia punctata
Roberts syndrome
Pena-Shokeir syndrome
Arthrogryposis multiplex congenita
Larsen syndrome

Postaxial polydactyly
Chondroectodermal dysplasia
Short rib–polydactyly syndromes

Preaxial polydactyly
Chondroectodermal dysplasia
Short rib–polydactyly syndromes

Hitchhiker thumbs
Diastrophic dysplasia

Long, narrow thorax
Asphyxiating thoracic dysplasia
Chondroectodermal dysplasia
Metatropic dysplasia
Fibrochondrogenesis
Atelosteogenesis
Campomelic dysplasia
Jarcho-Levin syndrome
Achondrogenesis
Hypophosphatasia

Hypoplastic thorax
Short rib–polydactyly syndromes
Thanatophoric dysplasia
Homozygous achondroplasia

Congenital cardiac disease
Chondroectodermal dysplasia (atrial sep-
    tal defect, common atria)
Short rib–polydactyly syndrome type I
    (transposition of great vessels, double
    outlet right and left ventricle, ventricu-
    lar septal defect)
Short rib–polydactyly syndrome type II
    (transposition of great vessels)

Vertebral disorganization
Jarcho-Levin syndrome
Mesomelic dysplasia, Robinow type
Dyssegmental dysplasia
COVESDEM association
VACTERL association

Spine demineralization
Achondrogenesis

Large head
Achondroplasia
Thanatophoric dwarfism

Cloverleaf skull
Thanatophoric dysplasia
Campomelic syndrome

Hypertelorism
Mesomelic dysplasia, Robinow type
Larsen syndrome
Roberts syndrome
Otopalatodigital syndrome

Depressed nasal bridge
Atelosteogenesis
Thanatophoric dysplasia
Achondrogenesis
Achondroplasia
Campomelic dysplasia
Kniest syndrome
Larsen syndrome
Chondrodysplasia punctata nonrhizome-
    lic variety
Osteogenesis imperfecta type II

Cleft palate
Roberts syndrome
Larsen syndrome
Otopalatodigital syndrome
Kniest dysplasia
Diatrophic dysplasia
Spondyloepiphyseal dysplasia
Campomelic syndrome

Short upper lip
Chondroectodermal dysplasia

Micrognathia
Campomelic dysplasia
Diastrophic dysplasia
Weissenbacher-Zweymuller syndrome
Otopalatodigital syndrome
Achondrogenesis
Mesomelic dysplasia, Langer's type
Pena-Shokeir syndrome types I
    and II

Hypothonia
Pena-Shokeir syndrome

phenotype suggests a metabolic disorder, such as a mucopolysaccharidosis. Although a full discussion of such disorders is beyond the scope of this text, they are well-known causes of constitutional bone disease.

REFERENCES

1. Camera G, Mastroiacovo P: Birth prevalence of skeletal dysplasias in the italian multicentric monitoring system for birth defects. In: Papadatos CJ, Bartsocas CS (eds): Skeletal Dysplasias. New York, Alan R. Liss, 1982, pp 441–449.
2. Jeanty P, Romero R: Obstetrical Ultrasound. New York, McGraw-Hill, 1983, pp 183–194.
3. Jeanty P, Romero R, d'Alton M, et al.: In utero sonographic detection of hand and foot deformities. J Ultrasound Med 4:595, 1985.
4. Mahoney BS, Filly RA: High-resolution sonographic assessment of the fetal extremities, J Ultrasound Med 3:489, 1984.

Achondrogenesis

Synonym
Anosteogenesis.

Definition
Lethal chondrodystrophy characterized by extreme micromelia, short trunk, and a disproportionately large cranium (Fig. 10–36).

Incidence
This condition has been recognized only in the last 15 years, and not all of the 100 cases reported in the literature fit the diagnostic criteria for achondrogenesis. The birth prevalence is 0.23 in 10,000 births (see Table 10–1).

Etiology
The disease is inherited with an autosomal recessive pattern.

Pathology
Two types exist, with distinct histologic and radiologic features. Type I, Parenti-Fraccaro type, is a disorder of both endochondral and membranous ossification characterized by partial or complete lack of ossification of the calvarium and spine as well as extremely short long bones and, frequently, multiple rib fractures (Fig. 10–37). Type II, Langer-Saldino type, is a disorder of endochondral ossification only, is less severe than type I, and shows varied calcification of the calvarium and spine, as well as absence of rib fractures. Table 10–7 describes the main characteristics of the classic subdivision of achondrogenesis.[3] At least two different authors have proposed a subdivision of type II into different groups.[8,12] Whitley and Gorlin[12] have proposed a reclassification of the disease into four types. Table

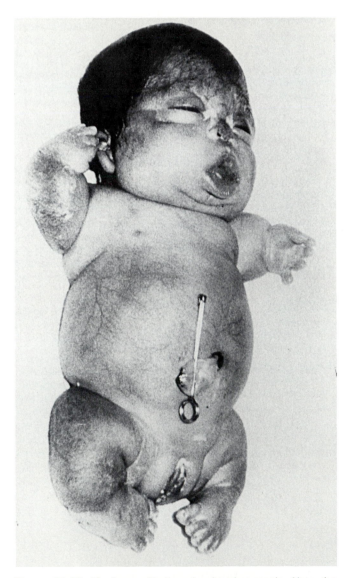

Figure 10–36. Newborn with type I achondrogenesis. Note the short limbs (micromelia), short trunk, and large head. There is redundancy of soft tissue, giving the image of hydrops fetalis. *(Reproduced with permission from Johnson et al.: J Ultrasound Med 3:223, 1984.)*

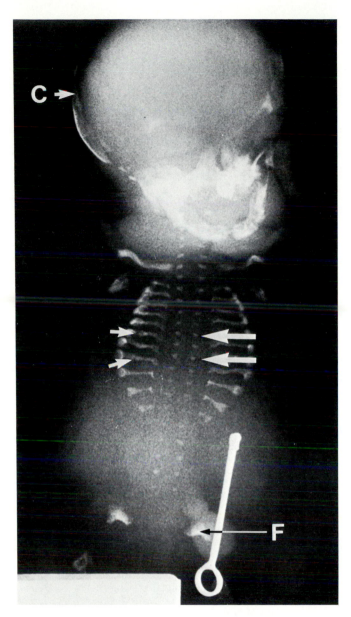

Figure 10–37. Radiograph of infant shown in Figure 10–36. Note the poor ossification of the calvarium (C) and spine (*large arrows*). Ribs are short, and fractures are visible (*small arrows*). Femurs (F) are extremely shortened. *(Reproduced with permission from Johnson et al.: J Ultrasound Med 3:223, 1984.)*

TABLE 10–7. MAJOR RADIOGRAPHIC FEATURES IN ACHONDROGENESIS

Site	Type	Features
Limbs	I	Gross shortening and irregularity, to extent of rudimentary ossicles
	II	Changes less gross, but severe shortening with metaphyseal widening and cupping present
Thorax	I	Thin ribs with flared anterior ends, possible fractures
	II	Ribs relatively short and stubby
Pelvis	I	Very poorly ossified iliac bones, sacrum and pubic bones absent
	II	Iliac bones small but moderately well ossified, deficient sacrum and pubic bones
Spine	I	Deficient ossification of vertebral bodies, from absence to small ossified center
	II	Nonossification of some vertebral bodies, especially in the lumbar region
Skull	I	Variable degree of vault underossification
	II	Good ossification of vault

Reproduced with permission from Cremin, Beighton: Bone Dysplasias of Infancy. A Radiological Atlas. Berlin, Springer-Verlag, 1978, pp 17–20.

dence to suggest that achondrogenesis tends to recur in a type-specific fashion.[12]

Histopathologically, achondrogenesis is characterized by a failure of cartilaginous matrix formation. At present, histologic studies have been described in the two classic types. In type I, there is increased cellular density in the resting cartilages with

10–8 illustrates the diagnostic criteria. In essence, type I remains unchanged, and the classic type II is subdivided into three prototypes that have the absence of rib fractures in common. There is progression from type II to IV toward a lesser involvement of the long bones. An index of endochondral bone growth, the femoral cylinder index, (CI femur) has been proposed for the classification (Fig. 10–38). It is calculated by dividing the femoral length by the femoral width and the midshaft in an anteroposterior projection. Whitley and Gorlin have presented evi-

TABLE 10–8. CRITERIA AND TABULATION OF ACHONDROGENESIS TYPES

Type	Descriptive Criteria	CI Femur*	Relative Frequency (%)
I	Multiple rib fractures, crenated ilia, stellate long bones	1.0–2.8	22
II	Unfractured ribs, crenated ilia, stellate long bones	1.0–2.8	18
III	Unfractured ribs, halberd ilia, mushroom-stem long bones	2.8–4.9	40
IV	Unfractured ribs, sculptured ilia, well-developed long bones	4.9–8.0	20

* CI femur, femoral cylinder index.
Reproduced with permission from Whitley, Gorlin: Radiology 148:693, 1983.

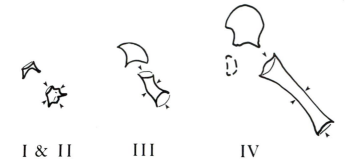

I & II   III   IV

Figure 10–38. Femoral cylinder index in achondrogenesis and a scheme of the four types of achondrogenesis. *(Reproduced with permission from Whitley, Gorlin: Radiology 148:693, 1983.)*

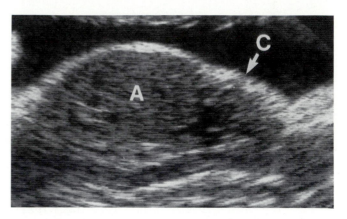

Figure 10–40. Sagittal scan demonstrating the narrow chest (C) and protruding abdomen (A). *(Reproduced with permission from Johnson et al.: J Ultrasound Med 3:223, 1984.)*

vacuolated PAS-positive inclusions inside the chondrocytes, as well as adequate cartilaginous matrix.[2] Large channels are visualized within the cartilage. Electron microscopy shows that the inclusion bodies correspond to an enlargement of the rough endoplasmic reticulum, which contains amorphous electron-opaque material.[10] In type II, the hypercellular cartilage is accompanied by a markedly deficient cartilaginous matrix and primitive mesenchymal chondrocytes with abundant, clear cytoplasm.[2] However, the distinction between the two entities is mainly based on radiologic criteria.[2]

Diagnosis

The prenatal diagnosis of this condition has been reported by several authors[1,4,5–7,9,11] and should be suspected by demonstration of the triad: (1) severe short limb dwarfism (Figs. 10–39, 10–40), (2) lack of vertebral ossification (Fig. 10–41), and (3) large head with normal to slightly decreased ossification of the calvarium. Although these findings are quite specific for achondrogenesis, the spectrum of the disease is broad (Table 10–8). Some patients will have vertebral ossification (mild forms of type II), and others will have calvarium demineralization (type I). Polyhydramnios and hydrops have been reported in association with achondrogenesis.[1,2] However, the association with hydrops has been questioned recently by the suggestion that these infants have a hydropic appearance because of an excess of soft tissue mass over a limited skeletal frame.[9] A definitive diagnosis is usually made radiographically, although a correct diagnosis has been made with prenatal sonography.[1,7,9]

Prognosis

The disease is uniformly lethal. Infants are either stillborn or die in the neonatal period.

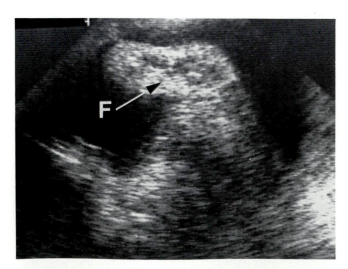

Figure 10–39. Intrauterine sonogram of fetus shown in Figures 10–36 and 10–37. Note the extremely short femur (F). *(Reproduced with permission from Johnson et al.: J Ultrasound Med 3:223, 1984.)*

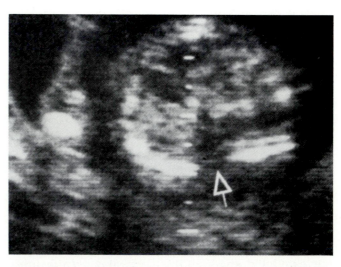

Figure 10–41. Transverse scan through the thorax showing absence of spinal echoes (*arrow*). *(Reproduced with permission from Mahony et al.: J Ultrasound Med 3:333, 1984.)*

Obstetrical Management

The option of pregnancy termination could be offered any time a definitive diagnosis is made (e.g., a pregnant patient carrying a fetus with a short limb dysplasia and who delivered an infant with achondrogenesis).

REFERENCES

1. Benacerraf B, Osathanondh R, Bieber FR: Achondrogenesis type I: Ultrasound diagnosis in utero. J. Clin Ultrasound 12:357, 1984.
2. Chen H, Liu CT, Yang SS: Achondrogenesis: A review with special consideration of achondrogenesis type II (Langer-Saldino). Am J Med Genet 10:379, 1981.
3. Cremin BJ, Beighton P: Bone Dysplasias of Infancy. A Radiological Atlas. Berlin, Springer-Verlag, 1978, pp 17–20.
4. Glenn LW, Teng SSK: In utero sonographic diagnosis of achondrogenesis. J Clin Ultrasound 13:195, 1985.
5. Golbus MS, Hall BD, Filly RA, et al.: Prenatal diagnosis of achondrogenesis. J Pediatr 91:464, 1977.
6. Graham D, Tracey J, Winn K, et al.: Early second trimester sonographic diagnosis of achondrogenesis. J Clin Ultrasound 11:336, 1983.
7. Johnson VP, Yiu-Chiu VS, Wierda DR, et al.: Midtrimester prenatal diagnosis of achondrogenesis. J Ultrasound Med 3:223, 1984.
8. Kozlowski K, Masel J, Morris L, et al.: Neonatal death dwarfism. Aust Radiol 21:164, 1977.
9. Mahony BS, Filly RA, Cooperberg PL: Antenatal sonographic diagnosis of achondrogenesis. J Ultrasound Med 3:333, 1984.
10. Molz G, Spycher MA: Achondrogenesis type I: Light and electron microscopic studies. Eur J Pediatr 134:69, 1980.
11. Smith WL, Breitweiser TD, Dinno N: In utero diagnosis of achondrogenesis type I. Clin Genet 19:51, 1981.
12. Whitley CB, Gorlin RJ: Achondrogenesis: New nosology with evidence of genetic heterogeneity. Radiology 148:693, 1983.

Thanatophoric Dysplasia

Synonym
Thanatophoric dwarfism.

Definition
Thanatophoric dysplasia is a lethal skeletal dysplasia characterized by extreme rhizomelia, bowed long bones, normal trunk length but narrow thorax, and a relatively large head (Fig. 10–42).

Incidence
0.69 per 10,000 births. It is the most common skeletal dysplasia (see Table 10–1).

Etiology
Unknown. Most cases of thanatophoric dysplasia are sporadic.[9] Some cases in the same sibship have been reported, and therefore an autosomal recessive pattern of inheritance has been suggested.[3,7,8,9,14] Alternatively, some authors have suggested a polygenic transmission with a 2 percent recurrence risk.[15] Familial cases of thanatophoric dysplasia may represent a separate type of lethal short limb dysplasia (i.e., fibrochondrogenesis).

Pathology
The limbs show rhizomelic shortening. The femurs are extremely short and bowed, and, in the most severe forms, may be shaped like a telephone receiver. The thorax is narrow in the anteroposterior dimension, with short ribs. However, the trunk is of normal length. The spine shows flattened vertebral bodies with wide intervertebral spaces giving a typical radiologic appearance similar to an "H" (Fig. 10–43). The cranium has a short base, and, frequently, the foramen magnum is decreased in size. The forehead is prominent, and hypertelorism and a saddle nose may be present. Hands and feet are normal, but the fingers are short and sausage-shaped.

Thanatophoric dysplasia is a disorder of endochondral ossification characterized by a very

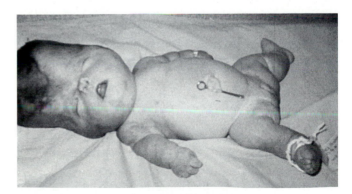

Figure 10–42. Infant with thanatophoric dysplasia. *(Reproduced with permission from Isaacson et al.: Am J Dis Child 137:896, 1983.)*

abnormal histology of the growth plate. There is decreased or absent proliferation and maturation of chondrocytes, which are not arranged in columns but distributed irregularly. The bony trabecula are oriented vertically and horizontally (under normal circumstances, the trabecula should be oriented only vertically). Metachromatic inclusions can be seen in the chondrocytes.

Associated Anomalies

Thanatophoric dysplasia is associated with a form of craniosynostosis called "cloverleaf skull" in 14 percent of cases.[10] The cloverleaf skull results from premature closure of the coronal and lambdoid sutures. If hydrocephaly occurs, the rostral expansion of the cortex and of the ventricular system results in an enlarged anterior fontanel and separation and depression of the temporal bones. The term "cloverleaf" refers to the three leaves formed by the prominent vertex of the calvarium in the middle and the two temporal bones on the sides. The mechanism responsible for this skull anomaly is poorly understood. A defect of endochondral ossification resulting in a short skull base and a defect of membranous ossification producing premature synostosis of some cranial sutures has been suggested as the pathogenesis.[10]

Horseshoe kidney, hydronephrosis,[7] atrial septal defect, defective tricuspid valve,[11] imperforate anus, and radioulnar synostosis have been described.[16]

Diagnosis

The sonographic antenatal diagnosis can be made in the presence of short-limbed dwarfism (Fig. 10–44), hypoplastic thorax (Fig. 10–45) and cloverleaf skull (Figs. 10–46, 10–47).[2,12] Frontal bossing can also be detected (Figs. 10–48, 10–49). Femur bowing, narrow thorax, large head size even without ventriculomegaly,[6] and redundant soft tissues are features that become more pronounced with advancing gestation, but may not be present in midtrimester.[1,2] In 71 percent of cases, thanatophoric dysplasia is associated with polyhydramnios, which may be massive and lead to premature labor.[17] Fetal movements do not seem to be affected by the disease,[1] but a decrease in motion during the third trimester has been reported.[2] A specific diagnosis of thanatophoric dysplasia seems possible only when severe micromelia is associated with cloverleaf skull.[12] On two occasions the temporal bulges of the cloverleaf skull were mistaken for encephalocele,[4,13] but an intact calvarium can be visualized.

In the absence of cloverleaf skull, the disease should be suspected when severe rhizomelic dwarfism and a narrow thorax are detected. The differential diagnosis should include Ellis–van Creveld syndrome

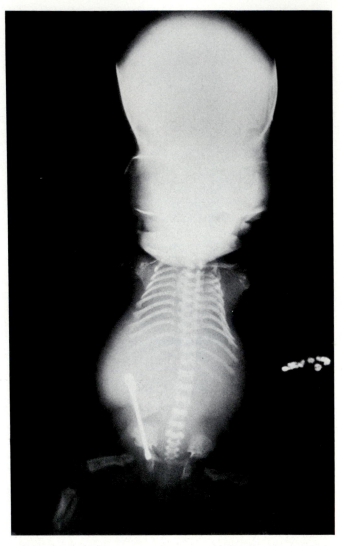

Figure 10–43. Radiograph of a newborn with thanatophoric dysplasia. *(Reproduced with permission from Isaacson et al.: Am J Dis Child 137:896, 1983.)*

(chondroectodermal dysplasia), asphyxiating thoracic dysplasia, short rib–polydactyly syndrome, and homozygous achondroplasia.

Homozygous achondroplasia may be differentiated because it is an autosomal dominant disease, and therefore, both parents must be affected. In the heterozygous form, the long bones are only mildly shortened and not bowed. Kurtz et al. have recently shown that none of seven fetuses affected with heterozygous achondroplasia had an abnormal short femur in the early second trimester. The relationship between femur and BPD became abnormal after the 21st and 27th weeks (see p. 359). On the other hand, the micromelia of thanatophoric dysplasia may be so severe that it can be observed in some cases even at the 19th week.

Asphyxiating thoracic dysplasia can be distin-

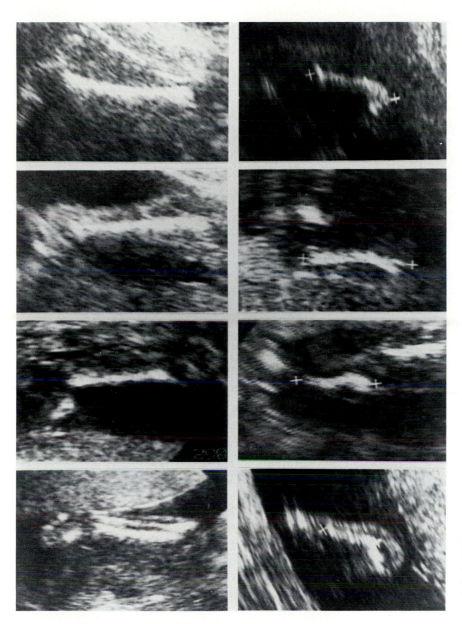

Figure 10–44. Sonographic comparison of long bones of a fetus affected with thanatophoric dysplasia (*right*) and a normal fetus of the same gestational age (*left*). Top to bottom, femur, humerus, tibia, and radius. *(Courtesy of Dr. Burrows.)*

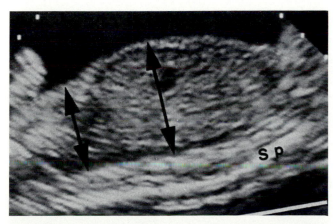

Figure 10–45. Longitudinal section of a fetus affected with thanatophoric dysplasia. Note the significant disproportion between the chest and the abdomen. Sp, spine. *(Reproduced with permission from Jeanty, Romero: Obstetrical Ultrasound. New York, McGraw-Hill, 1983.)*

guished because the bone shortening is less marked and the vertebrae are typically spared. It is conceivable that prenatal radiologic studies of the fetal spine may be helpful for diagnosis. Real-time ultrasound could be used to orient the radiographer so that a proper view of the spine can be obtained. Thanatophoric dysplasia is characterized by an H configuration to the vertebral bodies.

In chondroectodermal dysplasia, the presence of a well-formed postaxial extra digit is rather typical and the short limb dysplasia is acromesomelic (p. 349). Fibrochondrogenesis is characterized by dumbbell-shaped metaphyses (p. 339).

Prognosis
This disease is uniformly fatal shortly after birth. The cause of death is cardiorespiratory failure probably related to restrictive respiratory disease.

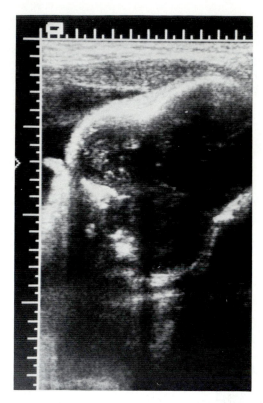

Figure 10–46. Coronal scan of the head of a fetus with thanatophoric dysplasia with cloverleaf skull.

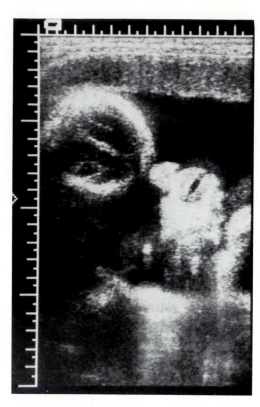

Figure 10–48. Frontal bossing in a fetus with cloverleaf skull. Note the prominent forehead. Under normal circumstances, the forehead is not visible in a scan that allows imaging of the mouth and nose.

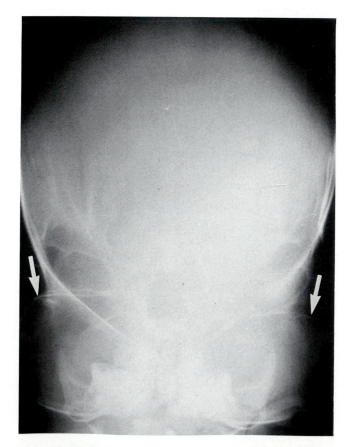

Figure 10–47. Radiograph of a newborn with thanatophoric dysplasia showing the lateral displacement of both temporal bones (cloverleaf skull) (*arrows* point to bulging temporal bones).

Obstetrical Management

When a confident diagnosis is made, the option of pregnancy termination can be offered at any time during gestation because the condition is uniformly fatal. The hydrocephaly associated with cloverleaf skull may result in significant macrocrania and lead to

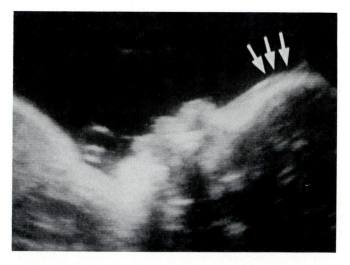

Figure 10–49. Frontal bossing in a sagittal scan. The arrows point to the prominent frontal bone.

cephalopelvic disproportion. In this case, cephalocentesis could be used to accomplish vaginal delivery.[4]

REFERENCES

1. Beetham FGT, Reeves JS: Early ultrasound diagnosis of thanatophoric dwarfism. J Clin Ultrasound 12:43, 1984.
2. Burrows PE, Stannard MW, Pearrow J, et al.: Early antenatal sonographic recognition of thanatophoric dysplasia with cloverleaf skull deformity. AJR 143:841, 1984.
3. Chemke J, Graff G, Lancet M: Familial thanatophoric dwarfism. Lancet 1:1358, 1971.
4. Chervenak FA, Blakemore KJ, Isaacson G, et al.: Antenatal sonographic findings of thanatophoric dysplasia with cloverleaf skull. Am J Obstet Gynecol 146:984, 1983.
5. Filly RA, Golbus MS, Carey JC, et al.: Short-limbed dwarfism: Ultrasonographic diagnosis by mensuration of fetal femoral length. Radiology 138:653, 1981.
6. Fink IJ, Filly RA, Callen PW, et al.: Sonographic diagnosis of thanatophoric dwarfism in utero. J. Ultrasound Med 1:337, 1982.
7. Graff G, Chemke J, Lancet M: Familial recurring thanatophoric dwarfism. Obstet Gynecol 39:515, 1971.
8. Harris R, Patton JT: Achondroplasia and thanatophoric dwarfism in the newborn. Clin Genet 2:61, 1971.
9. Horton WA, Harris DJ, Collins DL: Discordance for the kleeblattschaedel anomaly in monozygotic twins with thanatophoric dysplasia. Am J Med Genet 15:97, 1983.
10. Iannaccone G, Gerlini G: The so-called "cloverleaf skull syndrome": A report of three cases with a discussion of its relationships with thanatophoric dwarfism and craniostenosis. Pediatr Radiol 2:175, 1974.
11. Isaacson G, Blakemore KJ, Chervenak FA: Thanatophoric dysplasia with cloverleaf skull. Am J Dis Child 137:896, 1983.
12. Mahony BS, Filly RA, Callen PW, et al.: Thanatophoric dwarfism with the cloverleaf skull: A specific antenatal sonographic diagnosis. J Ultrasound Med 4:151, 1985.
13. Moore QS, Banik S: Ultrasound scanning in a case of thanatophoric dwarfism with clover-leaf skull. Br J Radiology 53:241, 1980.
14. Partington MW, Gonzales-Crussi F, Khakee SG, et al.: Cloverleaf skull and thanatophoric dwarfism. Report of four cases, two in the same sibship. Arch Dis Child 46:656, 1971.
15. Pena SDJ, Goodman HO: The genetics of thanatophoric dwarfism. Pediatrics 51:104, 1973.
16. Smith DW: Recognizable Patterns of Human Malformation. Genetic, Embryologic and Clinical Aspects, 3d ed. Philadelphia, Saunders, 1982, pp 242–243.
17. Thompson BH, Parmley TH: Obstetric features of thanatophoric dwarfism. Am J Obstet Gynecol 109:396, 1971.

Fibrochondrogenesis

Definition
Fibrochondrogenesis is a lethal short limb skeletal dysplasia inherited with an autosomal recessive pattern. The disorder is characterized by rhizomelic limb shortening, with broad, dumbbell-shaped metaphyses, pear-shaped vertebral bodies, and short and distally cupped ribs. Histopathologically, there is disorganization of the growth plate, with unique interwoven fibrous septae and fibroblastic dysplasia of chondrocytes.[3]

Incidence
A total of five cases have been reported in the literature.[1–3]

Etiology
Autosomal recessive.

Pathology
The condition was first described by LazzaroniFossati et al.[2] in an infant who manifested many of the same characteristics of thanatophoric dysplasia. However, marked methaphyseal flaring of long bones, clefting of the vertebral bodies, and a distinctive morphologic lesion of the growth plate distinguish fibrochondrogenesis from thanatophoric dysplasia.

Infants are afflicted with moderate to severe micromelia (shortening of all segments of an extremity). Tubular bones are short and broad, with wide metaphyses. The fibula may be disproportionately short. The ribs are short and cupped, vertebral bodies are flat and clefted, clavicles are long and thin, and pelvic bones are hypoplastic. Hand and foot contractures have also been observed.

The face is round and flat with protuberant eyes. Other features include frontal bossing, wide flat nasal bridge, small palpebral fissures with antimongoloid obliquity, low set abnormally formed ears, small mouth, cleft palate, and hypertelorism. An omphalocele has been described in one patient.[1] Light microscopy demonstrates a grossly disorganized growth plate. Chondrocytes are large and round, and the intercellular matrix shows interwoven fibrous septae. However, both diaphyseal and metaphyseal bone formations are normal.

Diagnosis

A specific prenatal diagnosis of fibrochondrogenesis has not been reported. However, in one fetus, severe micromelia was detected prenatally.[3] The differential diagnosis should include conditions associated with significant metaphyseal flaring, such as metatropic dysplasia, Kniest dysplasia, and spondyloepiphyseal dysplasia congenita. Thanatophoric dysplasia should also be considered.

Prognosis

All of the reported cases of fibrochondrogenesis either have been stillborn or have died shortly after birth. The longest survivor lived 3 weeks and required mechanical ventilation.

Obstetrical Management

A certain diagnosis of fibrochondrogenesis can be made if there has been a previously affected child.

The option of pregnancy termination should be offered to the parents before viability. As fibrochondrogenesis is considered a lethal disorder, the option of pregnancy termination after viability could be offered. Only five cases of this disorder have been reported in the literature, however.

REFERENCES

1. Eteson DJ, Adomian GE, Ornoy A, et al.: Fibrochondrogenesis: Radiologic and histologic studies. Am J Med Genet 19:277, 1984.
2. Lazzaroni-Fossati F, Stanescu V, Stanescu R, et al.: La fibrochondrogenese. Arch Fr Pediatr 35:1096, 1978.
3. Whitley CB, Langer LO, Ophoven J, et al.: Fibrochondrogenesis: Lethal, autosomal recessive chondrodysplasia with distinctive cartilage histopathology. Am J Med Genet 19:265, 1984.

Atelosteogenesis

Synonyms

Spondylohumerofemoral hypoplasia[5] and giant cell chondrodysplasia.

Definition

Atelosteogenesis is a lethal chondrodysplasia featuring deficient ossification of various bones, particularly the thoracic spine, humerus, femur, and hand bones, resulting clinically in a form of micromelic dwarfism. It is characterized by hypoplasia of the distal segment of the humerus and femur with enlargement of the proximal portion.

Incidence

Atelosteogenesis was first recognized as a distinct entity in 1983. The original report described six cases and identified four previous cases in the literature as fitting the description of the disease.[2,4] Subsequently, isolated cases have been reported.[1,5]

Etiology

Unknown. Neither parental consanguineity nor familial cases have been reported. Both sexes can be affected.

Pathology

The disorder is characterized by micromelia with severe shortening of the proximal segment of the extremities. Bowing of the long bones, dislocation of

the elbow or knee, clubfeet, and hyperlaxity of the ligaments may be present. There is no pathognomonic facies; however, a depressed nasal bridge, cleft palate and a frontal cephalocele have also been reported.[1]

The diagnosis is based primarily on the radiographic appearance of the spine, long bones, and hand. There is coronal clefting of the lumbar and lower thoracic vertebral bodies and hypoplasia of the upper thoracic bodies and ribs in that area. The humerus and femur are hypoplastic, with the distal segment thinned and the proximal portion enlarged, resulting in a club-shaped appearance. The ulna may be hypoplastic, and the fibulae are generally absent. Femoral and tibial epiphyses are not ossified, whereas the proximal humeral epiphysis may be prematurely ossified. There is a lack of ossification in some metacarpals and phalanges, although others may demonstrate near normal development.

Histologically, degenerating chondrocytes surrounded by fibrous material are found in degenerative areas of the matrix of the cartilage and growth plate.[3]

Diagnosis

The prenatal recognition of an affected infant with shortened long bones has been documented in one case.[1] The specific diagnosis of atelosteogenesis was not made until postmortem examination. Although the ultrasonic diagnosis of micromelia is easy, the specific diagnosis of atelosteogenesis is unlikely because of its sporadic occurrence. Differential diagnosis includes all disorders manifested by micromelic dwarfism such as achondrogenesis, thanatophoric dysplasia, and fibrochondrogenesis.

Prognosis

Atelosteogenesis is a lethal condition. Patients either have been stillborn or have died shortly after birth.

Obstetrical Management

Although the condition is lethal, it is doubtful that a precise prenatal diagnosis can be made.

REFERENCES

1. Chervenak FA, Isaacson G, Rosenberg JC, et al.: Antenatal diagnosis of frontal cephalocele in a fetus with atelosteogenesis. J Ultrasound Med 5:111, 1986.
2. Kozlowski K, Tsuruta T, Kameda Y, et al.: New forms of neonatal death dwarfism. Report of three cases. Pediatr Radiol 10:155, 1981.
3. Maroteaux P, Spranger J, Stanescu V, et al.: Atelosteogenesis. Am J Med Genet 13:15, 1982.
4. Rimoin DL, Sillence DO, Lachman RS, et al.: Giant cell chondrodysplasia: a second case of a rare lethal newborn skeletal dysplasia. Am J Hum Genet 32:125A, 1980.
5. Sillence DO, Lachman RS, Jenkins T, et al.: Spondylohumerofemoral hypoplasia (giant cell chondrodysplasia): A neonatally lethal short limb skeletal dysplasia. Am J Med Genet 13:7, 1982.

SKELETAL DYSPLASIAS ASSOCIATED WITH A SMALL THORAX

A group of skeletal dysplasias is characterized by a narrow thorax, which may lead to respiratory failure and death in the newborn period or shortly thereafter (Fig. 10–50). These conditions include asphyxiating thoracic dysplasia, the short rib–polydactyly syndromes, campomelic dysplasia, and chondroectodermal dysplasia. Prenatal diagnoses of these conditions have been reported. A precise diagnosis of the specific entity responsible for the narrow chest is extremely difficult even after neonatal examination and radiography. A specific identification of a disease entity in a relative makes diagnosis much simpler, since all these conditions are inherited with an autosomal recessive pattern. In the absence of this family history, the sonographer's task is to recognize the small thorax and the most commonly associated anomalies, with the realization that a specific antenatal diagnosis is extremely difficult. A specific prenatal diagnosis is probably not critical, since severe thoracic constriction seems to be associated with an extremely poor prognosis. Table 10–9 illustrates the criteria used by Cremin and Beighton for the differential diagnosis of some of these conditions. The radiologic features are not always discernible in utero with ultrasound. It should be stressed that other skeletal dysplasias may feature a hypoplastic thorax, but this finding is not the main characteristic of the disease (e.g., thanatophoric dysplasia (p. 335), atelosteogenesis (p. 340), fibrochondrogenesis (p. 339), achondrogenesis (p. 332), and Jarcho-Levin syndrome (p. 382).

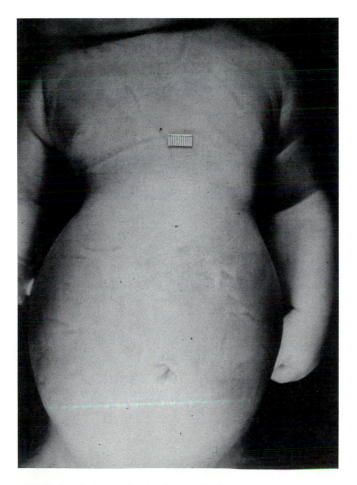

Figure 10–50. Marked thoracic hypoplasia in an infant with short rib–polydactyly syndrome.

TABLE 10–9. DISORDERS WITH THORACIC DYSPLASIA AND POLYDACTYLY

	Asphyxiating Thoracic Dysplasia (Jeune)	Chondroectodermal Dysplasia (Ellis–van Creveld)	Short Rib–Polydactyly Syndrome Type I (Saldino-Noonan)	Short Rib–Polydactyly Syndrome Type II (Majewski)	Short Rib Syndrome Type III (Naumoff)
Relative prevalence	Common	Uncommon	Common	Extremely rare	Rare
Clinical Features					
Thoracic constriction	+ +	+	+ + +	+ + +	+ + +
Polydactyly	+	+ +	+ +	+ +	+ +
Limb shortening	+	+	+ + +	+	+ +
Congenital heart disease	–	+ +	+ +	+ +	–
Other abnormalities	Renal disease	Ectodermal dysplasia	Genitourinary and gastrointestinal anomalies	Cleft lip and palate	Renal abnormalities
Radiographic features					
Tubular bone shortening	+	+	+ + +	+ +	+ + +
Distinctive features in femora	–	–	Pointed ends	–	Marginal spurs
Short, horizontal ribs	+ +	+ +	+ + +	+ + +	+ + +
Vertical shortening of ilia and flat acetabula	+ +	+ +	+ +	–	+ +
Defective ossification of vertebral bodies	–	–	+ +	–	+
Shortening of skull base	–	–	–	–	+

Reproduced with permission from Cremin, Beighton: Bone Dysplasias of Infancy: A Radiological Atlas. Berlin, Springer-Verlag, 1978.

Asphyxiating Thoracic Dysplasia

Synonyms
Jeune syndrome, Jeune thoracic dystrophy syndrome, infantile thoracic dystrophy, and thoraco-pelvic–phalangeal dystrophy.

Incidence
Rare. Approximately 100 cases of asphyxiating thoracic dysplasia (ATD) have been reported in the literature.[2]

Etiology
It is accepted that the disorder is transmitted in an autosomal recessive pattern. Minor manifestations have been recognized in parents of affected children, and, therefore, the possibility of a heterozygous expression has been suggested.[1,17]

Pathology
The most prominent feature is a narrow and bell-shaped thorax, with short and horizontal ribs. The clavicles may be inverted, with a high handlebar appearance. Tubular bones are either normal or mildly shortened and not bowed. The ilia are small and flattened.

The disease has a wide spectrum of manifestations. A dramatic reduction in chest dimensions leads to pulmonary hypoplasia and respiratory insufficiency.[2] In very rare instances, the disease is diagnosed because of an incidental chest x-ray that demonstrates the typical findings.[10]

Associated Anomalies
Visceral abnormalities include involvement of kidneys (tubular dysplasia, cystic dilatation of the collecting ducts, periglomerula fibrosis),[2,3,6,7,17] liver (polycystic liver disease, periportal fibrosis, hyperplasia of the bile ducts),[2,17] and pancreas (interstitial fibrosis).[2] Dental and nail defects,[13] polydactyly,[16,18] and cleft lip and palate[9] have been reported in some patients. However, these anomalies are more common in Ellis–van Creveld syndrome or chondroectodermal dysplasia (p. 349).

Diagnosis
Several prenatal diagnoses have been made.[4,11,15,16] One was made at 18 weeks in a fetus at risk because of an affected sibling.[4] In this case, serial scans performed before the 18th week failed to demonstrate the abnormality, and the condition was diagnosed by the presence of a narrow thorax and long bones in the third percentile for gestational age.

The most important diagnostic criterion is a hypoplastic thorax (Fig. 10–51). In most reports, recognition of a hypoplastic chest was based on the sonographer's subjective impression, since these cases predated the availability of thoracic fetal

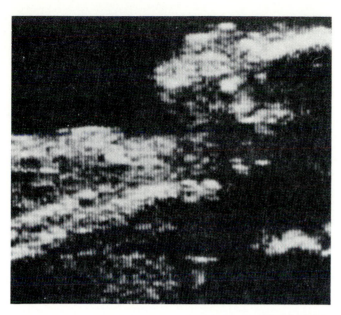

Figure 10–51. Longitudinal scan of a fetus with asphyxiating thoracic dysplasia. Note the reduced anteroposterior dimension of the chest. *(Reproduced with permission from Schinzel et al.: Radiology 154:777, 1985.)*

biometric nomograms.[4,15] In one case, the chest was narrow only in the anteroposterior diameter, whereas the transverse diameter was normal.[16] In all cases prenatally diagnosed with ultrasound, there was short limb dwarfism, with long bones that were two standard deviations below the mean for gestational age. This probably represents ascertainment biases, since this condition may be present with only mild limb shortening. The differential diagnosis between ATD and Ellis–van Creveld syndrome is impossible in atypical cases. Typically, ATD lacks polydactyly, ectodermal abnormalities, and congenital heart disease. Polyhydramnios has been associated frequently with this condition.

Prognosis
Eighty percent of affected infants die in the neonatal period from respiratory failure and infections.[4,8] Long-term survivors have been reported, but they seem to have the milder form of the disease.[5,10,13] However, with time, visceral involvement may lead to renal failure or hepatic cirrhosis. Of the four cases prenatally diagnosed (three with ultrasound and one with radiography), three underwent termination of pregnancy before viability, and one survived. The survivor developed hepatomegaly and mild jaundice.[13]

Obstetrical Management
The option of pregnancy termination should be offered if the diagnosis is made in the second trimester. There is a paucity of data on which to base the management of cases diagnosed in the third trimes-

ter. Until the predictive value of sonographically diagnosed thoracic hypoplasia for neonatal death is established, it seems that traditional obstetrical management should not be altered.

REFERENCES
1. Barnes ND, Hull D, Milner AD, Waterston DJ: Chest reconstruction in thoracic dystrophy. Arch Dis Child 46:833, 1971.
2. Beckwitt-Turkel S, Diehl EJ, Richmond JA: Necropsy findings in neonatal asphyxiating thoracic dystrophy. J Med Genet 22:112, 1985.
3. Bernstein J, Brough AJ, McAdams AJ: The renal lesions in syndromes of multiple congenital malformations; cerebrohepatorenal syndrome; Jeune asphyxiating thoracic dystrophy; tuberous sclerosis, Meckel syndrome. Birth Defects 10:35, 1974.
4. Elejalde BR, de Elejalde MM, Pansch D: Prenatal diagnosis of Jeune syndrome. Am J Med Genet 21:433, 1985.
5. Friedman JM, Kaplan HG, Hall JG: The Jeune syndrome (asphyxiating thoracic dystrophy) in an adult. Am J Med 59:857, 1975.
6. Gruskin AB, Baluarte HJ, Cote ML, et al.: The renal disease of thoracic asphyxiant dystrophy. Birth Defects 10:44, 1974.
7. Herdman RC, Langer LO: The thoracic asphyxiant dystrophy and renal disease. Am J Dis Chil 116:309, 1968.
8. Kaufman HJ, Kirkpatrick JA: Jeune thoracic dysplasia — A spectrum of disorders? Birth Defects 10:101, 1974.
9. Kohler E, Babbitt DP: Dystrophic thoraces and infantile asphyxia. Radiology 94:55, 1970.
10. Kozlowski K, Masel J: Asphyxiating thoracic dystrophy without respiratory distress. Report of 2 cases of the latent form. Pediatr Radiol 5:30, 1976.
11. Lipson M, Waskey J, Rice J, et al.: Prenatal diagnosis of asphyxiating thoracic dysplasia. Am J Med Genet 18:273, 1984.
12. Ozonoff MB: Asphyxiating thoracic dysplasia as a complication of metaphyseal chondrodysplasia (Jansen type). Birth Defects 10:72, 1974.
13. Penido R, Carrell R, Chialastri AJ: Case review: asphyxiating thoracic dystrophy in a teenager. J Pediatr 2:338, 1978.
14. Resnik R: Amniotic fluid. In: Creasy RK, Resnik R (ed): Maternal–Fetal Medicine. Principles and Practice. Philadelphia, Saunders, 1984, pp 135–139.
15. Russell JGB, Chouksey SK: Asphyxiating thoracic dystrophy. Br J Radiol 43:814, 1970.
16. Schinzel A, Savoldelli G, Briner J, et al: Prenatal sonographic diagnosis of Jeune syndrome. Radiology 154:777, 1985.
17. Shokeir MHK, Houston CS, Awen CF: Asphyxiating thoracic chondrodystrophy. Association with renal disease and evidence for possible heterozygous expression. J Med Genet 8:107, 1971.
18. Tahernia AC, Stamps P: Jeune syndrome (asphyxiating thoracic dystrophy): Report of a case, a review of the literature, and an editor's commentary. Clin Pediatr 16:903, 1977.

Short Rib–Polydactyly Syndromes

Short rib–polydactyly syndromes (SRPS) are a group of lethal disorders characterized by short limb dysplasia, constricted thorax, and postaxial polydactyly. Classically, three different types have been described, but some other variants have been recognized subsequently. It is likely that SRPS types I and III represent different manifestations of a single entity.[3,4] Varying expressivity could be due to different alleles at a single locus.[2] Although SRPS are ascertained on the basis of the skeletal abnormality, it is becoming clearer that generalized abnormalities of other organ systems are present. Therefore, the disorder may represent a fundamental defect of cellular differentiation during early embryogenesis. The different phenotypes could be the result of interaction with other intrauterine factors. For example, hydrops may be due to associated cardiovascular defects. The differential diagnosis of the three classic forms of SRPS with asphyxiating thoracic dysplasia and Ellis–van Creveld syndrome is outlined in Table 10–9.

The view that SRPS require the presence of polydactyly has been challenged by a number of authors who have reported cases that fit the morphologic description of SRPS but without polydactyly.[1,5] The term "short rib syndrome" has, therefore, been proposed to refer to entities in which this bone abnormality is responsible for a narrow thorax. Confusion results from the fact that there are no specific biochemical or histopathologic markers for these diseases. Also, the small number of cases reported in the literature precludes a rigorous statistical analysis of the different phenotypic variants.

An interesting feature of SRPS is the female sex preponderance. Recent data indicate that such preponderance may be artifactual and that failure of development of secondary sexual characteristics can occur. Indeed, in some cases, although the chromosomal constitution is XY, and the gonads are testes, the phenotype is female or ambiguous.[2] The other skeletal dysplasia in which this type of sex discrepancy has been documented is campomelic syndrome.

REFERENCES

1. Beemer FA, Langer LO, Klep-de Pater JM, et al.: A new short rib syndrome: Report of two cases. Am J Med Genet 14:115, 1983.
2. Bernstein R, Isdale J, Pinto M, et al.: Short rib–polydactyly syndrome: A single or heterogeneous entity: A re-evaluation prompted by four new cases. J Med Genet 22:46, 1985.
3. Cherstvoy ED, Lurie IW, Shved IA, et al.: Difficulties in classification of the short rib–polydactyly syndromes. Eur J Pediatr 133:57, 1980.
4. Sillence DO: Invited editorial comment: Non-Majewski short rib–polydactyly syndrome. Am J Med Genet 7:223, 1980.
5. Wladimiroff JW, Niermeijer MF, Laar J, et al.: Prenatal diagnosis of skeletal dysplasia by real-time ultrasound. Obstet Gynecol 63:360, 1984.

TYPE I OR SALDINO-NOONAN SYNDROME

Etiology
Autosomal recessive.

Pathology
There is severe micromelia with hypoplastic tubular bones. The femurs are typically pointed at both ends. The thorax is narrowed, and the ribs are extremely short. Vertebral bodies are distorted, with deficient ossification and incomplete coronal clefts.

Associated Anomalies
Associated anomalies of the heart (transposition of the great vessels, double outlet right ventricle, endocardial cushion defect), gastrointestinal tract (imperforate anus, agenesis of the gallbladder, intes-

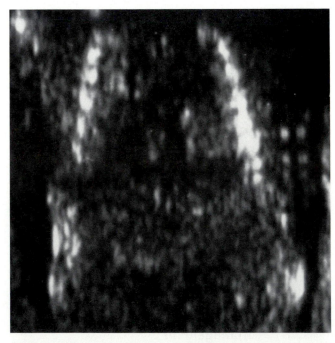

Figure 10–52. Coronal section of a fetus with short rib–polydactyly syndrome. Note the disproportion between the thoracic and abdominal cavities.

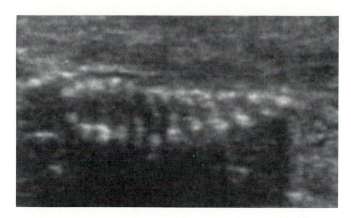

Figure 10–53. Longitudinal section of a fetus with short rib–polydactyly syndrome showing the very short ribs.

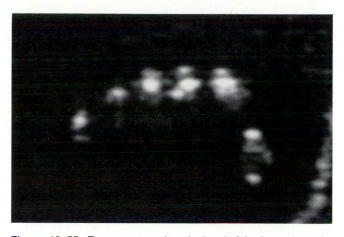

Figure 10–55. Transverse section of a hand of the fetus shown in Figures 10–53 and 10–54. Postaxial polydactyly is present. Six digits are easily identified.

tinal atresia), and genitourinary system (hypoplastic or polycystic kidneys) have been reported.[1,3,5,6]

Diagnosis
This condition has been identified antenatally with ultrasound in fetuses at risk.[2,4] The first fetus was identified with the combination of radiography and ultrasound. In the second fetus, oligohydramnios prevented the evaluation of the fetal long bones. The condition was suspected because of ascites in a fetus at risk. Figures 10–52 through 10–55 illustrate the sonographic findings in this condition in one of our prenatally diagnosed cases.

In the absence of a positive family history, a specific diagnosis of type I SRPS seems impossible. It should be suspected in fetuses with short limb dysplasia, narrow thorax, and polydactyly.

Prognosis
The disease is uniformly fatal.

Obstetrical Management
The option of pregnancy termination could be offered any time the diagnosis is made during gestation in a pregnancy at risk.

REFERENCES

1. Cherstvoy ED, Lurie IW, Shved IA, et al.: Difficulties in classification of the short rib–polydactyly syndromes. Eur J Pediatr 133:57, 1980.
2. Grote W, Weisner D, Jaenig U, et al.: Prenatal diagnosis of a short rib–polydactylia syndrome type Saldino-Noonan at 17 weeks gestation. Eur J Pediatr 140:63, 1983.
3. Kaibara N, Eguchi M, Shibata K, et al.: Short rib–polydactyly syndrome type I, Saldino-Noonan. Eur J Pediatr 133:63, 1980.
4. Richardson MM, Beaudet AL, Wagner ML, et al.: Prenatal diagnosis of recurrence of Saldino-Noonan dwarfism. J Pediatr 91:467, 1977.
5. Saldino RM, Noonan CD: Severe thoracic dystrophy with striking micromelia, abnormal osseous development, including the spine and multiple visceral abnormalities. AJR 114:257, 1972.
6. Spranger J, Grimm B, Weller M, et al.: Short rib–polydactyly (SRP) syndromes, types Majewski and Saldino-Noonan. Z Kinderheilk 116:73, 1974.

TYPE II OR MAJEWSKI TYPE

Etiology
Autosomal recessive.

Pathology
Distinctive features of this type of SRPS are less severe micromelia, cleft lip or palate, markedly short tibia with an ovoid shape, and normal pelvis and spine.

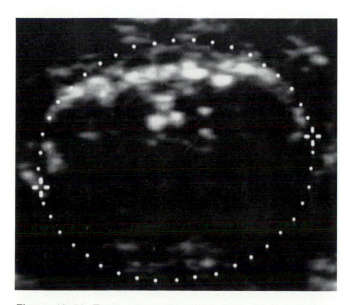

Figure 10–54. Transverse section of the chest of the fetus shown in Figure 10–53. Note the short ribs.

Associated Anomalies

Associated anomalies include hypoplasia of the epiglottis, larynx, ambiguous genitalia, polycystic kidneys, pancreatic fibrosis, and cardiovascular and gastrointestinal (malrotation) anomalies.[1–3,5,6]

Diagnosis

The prenatal diagnosis has been made in fetuses at risk by identification of short tibia, polydactyly, and cleft lip at fetoscopy,[7] or severe micromelia, short ribs with narrow thorax, and polydactyly at ultrasound.[4,6] The earliest diagnosis has been made at the 16th week of gestation.[4]

Cases resembling the Majewski type of SRPS but without polydactyly and with bowing of the long bones[8] are more consistent with a newly described short rib syndrome.

The diagnosis should be suspected whenever a hypoplastic thorax, polydactyly, short limb dysplasia (with short tibia), and cleft lip or palate are visualized. The differential diagnosis with other conditions is outlined in Table 10–9. In the absence of a positive family history, a specific differential diagnosis is difficult even after birth.

Prognosis

The disease is uniformly fatal.

Obstetrical Management

The option of pregnancy termination can be offered any time the diagnosis is made during gestation in a pregnancy at risk.

REFERENCES

1. Bernstein R, Isdale J, Pinto M, et al: Short rib–polydactyly syndrome: A single or heterogeneous entity? A re-evaluation prompted by four new cases. J Med Genet 22:46, 1985.
2. Chen H, Yang SS, Gonzalez E, et al.: Short rib–polydactyly syndrome, Majewski type. Am J Med Genet 7:215, 1980.
3. Cooper CP, Hall CM: Lethal short rib–polydactyly syndrome of the Majewski type: A report of three cases. Ped Radiology 144:513, 1982.
4. Gembruch U, Hansmann M, Foedisch HJ: Early prenatal diagnosis of short rib–polydactyly (SRP) syndrome type I (Majewski) by ultrasound in a case at risk. Prenat Diagn 5:357, 1985.
5. Spranger J, Grimm B, Weller M, et al.: Short rib–polydactyly (SRP) syndromes, types Majewski and Saldino-Noonan. Z Kinderheilk 116:73, 1974.
6. Thomson GSM, Reynolds CP, Cruickshank J: Antenatal detection of recurrence of Majewski dwarf (short rib–polydactyly syndrome type II Majewski). Clin Radiol 33:509, 1982.
7. Toftager-Larsen K, Benzie RJ: Fetoscopy in prenatal diagnosis of the Majewski and the Saldino-Noonan types of the short rib–polydactyly syndromes. Clin Genet 26:56, 1984.
8. Wladimiroff JW, Niermeijer MF, Laar J, et al.: Prenatal diagnosis of skeletal dysplasia by real-time ultrasound. Obstet Gynecol 63:360, 1984.

TYPE III OR NAUMOFF TYPE

Although originally considered a different entity, growing evidence supports the view that type I and type III are similar disorders.[1]

Etiology

Autosomal recessive.

Pathology

This type is characterized by vertebral hypoplasia, long bones with widened metaphyses and marginal spurs, short base of the skull, bulging forehead, and depressed nasal bridge. Urogenital abnormalities are frequently associated.[2,3,5]

Diagnosis

The diagnosis of this variety has been described in a fetus scanned because of the clinical suspicion of polyhydramnios. The fetus showed hydrops, a narrow chest, short limbs, polydactyly, hypoplastic vertebrae, and widened metaphyses of the femurs.[2]

It has been proposed that the differential diagnosis between type I and type III SRPS can be made on the basis of the appearance of the extremities of the long bones. Sharp ends are seen in type I, whereas widened metaphyses are seen in type III.[5] As stated before, it is possible that types I and III SRPS be different expressions of the same disorder.[1] Some authors have suggested the name "non-Majewski SRPS" for these two conditions.[4]

Prognosis

The disease is uniformly fatal.

Obstetrical Management

The option of pregnancy termination can be offered any time the diagnosis is made during gestation in a pregnancy at risk.

1. Bernstein R, Isdale J, Pinto M, et al.: Short rib–polydactyly syndrome: A single or heterogeneous entity? A reevaluation prompted by four new cases. J Med Genet 22:46, 1985.
2. Meizner I, Bar-Ziv J: Prenatal ultrasonic diagnosis of short rib–polydactyly syndrome (SRPS) type III: A case report and a proposed approach to the diagnosis of SRPS and related conditions. J. Clin Ultrasound 13:284, 1985.

3. Naumoff P, Young LW, Mazer J, et al.: Short rib–poly-dactyly syndrome type III. Ped Radiology 122:443, 1977.
4. Sillence DO: Invited editorial comment: Non-Majewski shortrib–polydactylysyndrome.AmJMedGenet7:223,1980.

5. Yang SS, Lin CS, Al Saadi A, et al.: Short rib-polydactyly syndrome, type III with chondrocytic inclusions. Report of a case and review of the literature. Am J Med Genet 7:205, 1980.

Campomelic Dysplasia

Synonyms
Campomelic dwarfism and campomelic syndrome.

Definition
Campomelic dysplasia (*campomelic* means bent limb) is a condition characterized by bowing of the long bones (particularly lower extremities), hypoplastic scapulae, and a wide variety of associated abnormalities, including hydrocephalus, congenital heart disease, and hydronephrosis. In a significant number of cases the phenotype is female, but the chromosomal constitution is XY and the gonads are testes.[2]

Incidence
Campomelic dysplasia has been reported in 0.05 per 10,000 births (see Table 10–1).

Etiology
Although the pattern of inheritance is not clearly defined, the frequency of parental consanguineity suggests an autosomal recessive transmission.[3,5,11,12] Many cases are sporadic.[8]

Pathology
The most prominent and invariable feature is bowing of the tibiae and femurs. Tubular bones are either normal in length or shortened.[8] Craniofacial anomalies, such as macrocephaly, cleft palate, and micrognathia, are seen in 90 to 99 percent of cases. Hypoplastic scapulae have been reported in 92 percent of patients.[2] The chest is narrow and bell-shaped. The vertebral bodies are frequently hypoplastic, and the pedicles are nonmineralized. The iliac wings are vertically narrow in 98 percent of patients, and hip dislocation is a frequent finding.

The association of hypoplastic scapulae, nonmineralized thoracic pedicles, and vertically narrowed iliac bones is quite unique for campomelic syndrome.[5]

Khajavi et al.[8] have suggested that the campomelic syndrome is a heterogeneous group of disorders that include two forms: (1) long-limbed campomelic syndrome with bent bones of normal width, only slightly shortened, and rarely involving the upper limbs and (2) short-limbed campomelic syndrome, in which the bent bones are short and

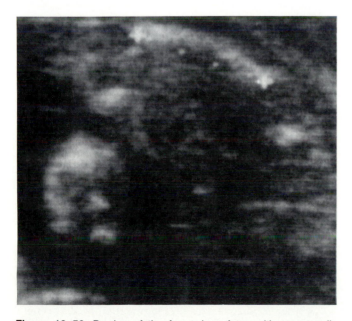

Figure 10–56. Bowing of the femur in a fetus with campomelic syndrome.

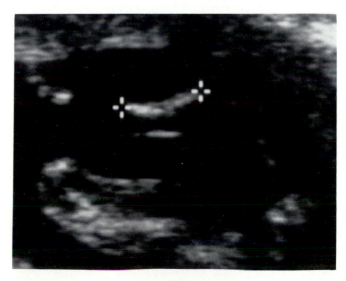

Figure 10–57. Bowing of a long bone in a fetus with campomelic syndrome.

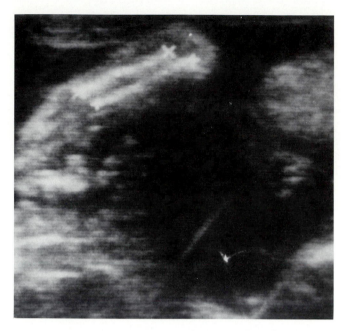

Figure 10–58. Leg of a fetus with campomelic syndrome. Note that bowing is absent.

wide. This variety can be classified into a craniosynostotic type with cloverleaf skull and a normocephalic type.

Associated Anomalies

Hydrocephalus has been reported in 23 percent of patients, congenital heart disease (VSD, ASD, Tetralogy of Fallot, aortic stenosis) in 30 percent, and hydronephrosis, frequently unilateral, in 30 percent. Fifty percent of the affected females have an XY chromosomal constitution.[2]

Diagnosis

Prenatal diagnosis of this condition has been reported in patients at risk.[4,6,7,13] In two reports, the condition was visualized antenatally, but a correct diagnosis was made only in the newborn.[1,10] The condition should be suspected any time there is a skeletal dysplasia with bowing of long bones, particularly if it is associated with other anomalies, such as congenital heart disease or hydronephrosis.

Some physiologic bowing can be seen in normal fetuses. There are no objective means available to differentiate pathologic from physiologic bowing. Experience is needed to make this assessment. All the patients we have seen had marked bowing (Figs. 10–56, 10–57); however it is not specific for campomelic syndrome. Other skeletal dysplasias associated with this finding include osteogenesis imperfecta, hypophosphatasia, thanatophoric dysplasia, and mesomelic dysplasia Reinhart variety. In addition, congenital bowing of the long bones could be a benign condition with no

other metabolic disorder. Long bone curvilinear deformation in campomelic syndrome may be limited to the proximal segment of the limbs (Fig. 10–58).

Prognosis

Beluffi and Fraccaro reviewed all the reported cases of campomelic dysplasia.[2] They found that of 92 infants for whom follow-up was available, 89 died within the first 10 months of life. At the time of their report, the age of the three survivors was 7 months, 19 months, and 17 years. The main cause of death was respiratory failure. Despite this gloomy overall prognosis, some patients may have reasonably normal psychomotor development. Long-term survivors can develop hearing loss and severe kyphosis.[9]

Obstetrical Management

The option of pregnancy termination should be offered before viability. After viability, standard obstetrical management is not altered.

REFERENCES

1. Balcar I, Bieber FR: Sonographic and radiologic findings in campomelic dysplasia. AJR 141:481, 1983.
2. Beluffi G, Fraccaro M: Genetical and clinical aspects of campomelic dysplasia. Prog Clin Biol Res 104:53, 1982.
3. Cremin BJ, Orsmond G, Beighton P: Autosomal recessive inheritance in campomelic dwarfism (letter). Lancet 1:488, 1973.
4. Fryns JP, van der Berghe K, van Assche A, et al.: Prenatal diagnosis of campomelic dwarfism. Clin Genet 19:199, 1981.
5. Hall BD, Spranger JW: Campomelic dysplasia. Further elucidation of a distinct entity. Am J Dis Child 134:289, 1980.
6. Hobbins JC, Bracken MB, Mahoney MJ: Diagnosis of fetal skeletal dysplasias with ultrasound. Am J Obstet Gynecol 142:306, 1982.
7. Hobbins JC, Grannum PAT, Berkowitz RL, et al.: Ultrasound in the diagnosis of congenital abnormalities. Am J Obstet Gynecol 134:331, 1979.
8. Khajavi A, Lachman R, Rimoin D, et al.: Heterogeneity in the campomelic syndromes: Long- and short- bone varieties. Radiology 120:641, 1976.
9. Opitz JM: Comment to: Genetical and clinical aspects of campomelic dysplasia. Beluffi G, Fraccaro M. Progr Clin Biol Res 104:66, 1982.
10. Pretorius DH, Rumack CM, Manco-Johnson ML, et al.: Specific skeletal dysplasias in utero: Sonographic diagnosis. Radiology 159:237, 1986.
11. Stuve A, Wiedemann HR: Congenital bowing of the long bones in two sisters (letter). Lancet 2:495, 1971.
12. Thurmon TF, DeFraites EB, Anderson EE: Familial camptomelic dwarfism. J Pediatr 83:841, 1973.
13. Winter R, Rosenkranz W, Hofmann H, et al.: Prenatal diagnosis of campomelic dysplasia by ultrasonography. Prenat Diagn 5:1, 1985.

Chondroectodermal Dysplasia

Synonyms
Ellis–van Creveld syndrome, mesodermal dysplasia, and six-fingered dwarfism.

Incidence
More than 120 cases have been reported.[2] In the United States, the disorder is prevalent in the inbred Amish communities in Pennsylvania.[4]

Etiology
It is inherited in an autosomal recessive pattern.[4–6]

Pathology
The typical findings are shortening of the forearm and lower leg (acromesomelic dwarfism), postaxial polydactyly (generally of fingers but occasionally of the toes), and dysplasia of ectodermal derivates (hypoplastic or absent nails, neonatal teeth, partial anodontia, scant or fine hair). The thorax is long and narrow. In 50 percent of patients, a congenital heart defect (typically atrial septal defect) is found. The spine is normal. Rarer anomalies are hypoplasia of the tibia, talipes equinovarus, and cryptorchidism.

Diagnosis
Prenatal diagnosis of this condition has been reported in three instances.[1,3,8] The first prenatal diagnosis of chondroectodermal dysplasia was made with fetoscopy by demonstrating the presence of polydactyly in a fetus at risk.[3] Fetoscopy was used before the development of high-resolution ultrasound. More recently, an infant with short limb skeletal dysplasia, narrow thorax, ectodermal dysplasia, polydactyly, and cardiac defects was identified antenatally with ultrasound.[8] Sonography demonstrated the short limb dysplasia and the narrow thorax. Although the authors did not label the condition as chondroectodermal dysplasia, their description fits the disorder. An important diagnostic consideration is that polydactyly is a constant finding.[4,7] The supernumerary finger usually has well-formed metacarpal and phalangeal bones.

Prognosis
One third of the infants die in the first month of life due to cardiopulmonary problems. Survivors may reach adulthood, usually with normal intellectual development but quite short stature (40 to 63 inches).[6]

Obstetrical Management
If the diagnosis is made before viability, the option of pregnancy termination should be offered. After viability, standard obstetrical management is not altered by the diagnosis. Echocardiography is indicated.

REFERENCES

1. Bui TH, Marsk .L, Ekloef O: Prenatal diagnosis of chondroectodermal dysplasia with fetoscopy. Prenat Diagn 4:155, 1984.
2. Cremin BJ, Beighton P: Bone Dysplasias of Infancy. A radiological Atlas. Berlin, Springer-Verlag, 1978, pp 33–36.
3. Mahoney MJ, Hobbins JC: Prenatal diagnosis of chondroectodermal dysplasia (Ellis–van Creveld syndrome) with fetoscopy and ultrasound. N Engl J Med 297:258, 1977.
4. McKusick VA, Egeland JA, Eldridge R, Krusen DE: Dwarfism in the Amish. The Ellis-van Creveld syndrome. Bull Johns Hopkins Hosp 115:306, 1964.
5. Metrakos JD, Fraser FC: Evidence for a heredity factor in chondroectodermal dysplasia (Ellis–van Creveld syndrome). Am J Hum Genet 6:260, 1954.
6. Smith DW: Recognizable Patterns of Human Malformation. Genetic, Embryologic and Clinical Aspects. Philadelphia, Saunders, 1982, pp 266–267.
7. Temtamy S, McKusick V: The genetics of hand malformations. Birth Defects 14:393, 1978.
8. Zimmer EZ, Weinraub Z, Raijman A, et al.: Antenatal diagnosis of a fetus with an extremely narrow thorax and short limb dwarfism. J Clin Ultrasound 12:112, 1984.

Chondrodysplasia Punctata

Synonyms
Stippled epiphyses, chondrodystrophia calcificans congenita, and dysplasia epiphysealis punctata.

Definition
Chondrodysplasia punctata includes two different disorders: a rhizomelic, potentially lethal variety, and

a nonrhizomelic variety (Conradi-Hünermann syndrome), which is more common and generally benign. These two conditions have different clinical, genetic, and radiologic characteristics.

Incidence
Chondrodysplasia punctate occurs in 0.09 per 10,000 births (see Table 10–1).

Etiology
The rhizomelic type of chondrodysplasia punctata is inherited with an autosomal recessive pattern.[4,10–12,18,19] The nonrhizomelic type is heterogeneous. An autosomal dominant,[1,16,21] X-linked dominant[6,14] and recessive transmission pattern has been postulated for this type.[7]

Pathology
The rhizomelic type is characterized by marked limb shortening that is maximal in the arms. Contractions may occur, and the fingers are fixed in flexion. The face is flat, with a depressed nasal bridge, and hypertelorism may occur. Some patients have ichthyosiform skin dysplasia and cataract. Radiographically there is calcific stippling of the epiphysis.[3,5] This finding is not pathognomonic for chondrodysplasia punctata, since it may occur with other conditions (multiple epiphyseal dysplasia, spondyloepiphyseal dysplasia, hypothyroidism, trisomy 18, trisomy 21, warfarin embryopathy, and the Zellweger cerebrohepatorenal syndrome).[7,13,15] Metaphyseal splaying is seen, particularly at the level of the knee. The spine has coronal clefts in the lumbar and lower thoracic region.

The nonrhizomelic, or Conradi-Hünermann, type is a milder form of the disease.[2] The limb shortening is mild or absent. Metaphyses are not splayed. Stippling is very fine and may be limited to the tarsal or carpal bones. Joint contractures can be present. Ascites and polyhydramnios have been reported.[20]

Diagnosis
An antenatal sonographic diagnosis of chondrodysplasia punctata has not been reported. Prenatal diagnosis of the rhizomelic variety with radiography has been made. The findings included stippling of pubic, ischium, and femoral epiphyses and abnormal epiphyseal centers of the joints of the knees and ankles.[8] The radiographic changes, however, are not sufficiently specific to permit recognition and separation of the two types in all cases.[7] Figures 10–24 and 10–25 permit the diagnosis of rhizomelia by comparing the length of the humerus or femur to that of the ulna or tibia, respectively. Stippling has not been reported with ultrasound.

Prognosis
The rhizomelic type is frequently fatal. Infants generally die before 1 or 2 years of age because of respiratory failure.[9,17] Severe mental deficiency and psychomotor retardation with spastic tetraplegia are present in most of the late survivors.[7] The nonrhizomelic type is compatible with life. Complications include failure to thrive, orthopedic problems, such as scoliosis, cataracts, retinal detachment, and recurrent infections.[17]

Obstetrical Management
The option of pregnancy termination should be offered if diagnosis is made prior to viability. After viability, standard obstetrical management is not altered.

REFERENCES

1. Bergstrom K, Gustavson KH, Jorulf H: Chondrodystrophia calcificans congenita (Conradi's disease) in a mother and her child. Clin Genet 3:158, 1972.
2. Conradi E: Vorzeitiges auftreten von knochen-und eigenartigen verkalkungskernen bei chondrodystrophie foetalis hypoplastica: Histologische und Rontgenuntersuchungen. JB Kinderh 80:86, 1914.
3. Fairbank HAT: Some general diseases of the skeleton. Br J Surg 15:120, 1927.
4. Fraser FC, Scriver JB: A hereditary factor in chondrodystrophia calcificans congenita. N Engl J Med 250:272, 1954.
5. Gilberg EF, Opitz JM, Spranger JW, et al.: Chondrodysplasia punctata — rhizomelic form. Pathologic and radiologic studies of three infants. Eur Pediatr 123:89, 1976.
6. Happle R, Matthiass HH, Macher E: Six-linked chondrodysplasia punctata? Clin Genet 11:73, 1977.
7. Heselson NG, Cremin BJ, Beighton P: Lethal chondrodysplasia punctata. Clin Radiol 29:679, 1978.
8. Hyndman WB, Alexander DS, Mackie KW: Chondrodystrophia calcificans congenita (Conradi-Hunermann syndrome). Report of a case recognized antenatally. Clin Pediatr 15:317, 1976.
9. Kaufmann HJ, Mahboubi S, Spackman TJ, et al.: Tracheal stenosis as a complication of chondrodysplasia punctata. Ann Radiol 19:203, 1976.
10. Mason RC, Kozlowski K: Chondrodysplasia punctata. A report of 10 cases. Radiology 109:145, 1973.
11. Melnick JC: Chondrodystrophia calcificans congenita. Am J Dis Child 110:218, 1965.
12. Mosekilde E: Stippled epiphyses in the newborn and in infants. Acta Radiol 37:291, 1952.
13. Pauli RM, Madden JD, Kranzler KJ, et al.: Warfarin therapy initiated during pregnancy and phenotypic chondrodysplasia punctata. J Pediatr 88:506, 1976.
14. Sheffield LJ, Danks DM, Mayne V, et al.: Chondrodysplasia punctata — 23 cases of a mild and relatively common variety. J Pediatr 89:916, 1976.

15. Silverman FN: Dysplasie epiphysaires: Entities protei-forme. Ann Radiol 4:833, 1961.
16. Silverman FN: Discussion on the relation between stippled epiphyses and the multiplex form of epiphyseal dysplasia. Birth Defects 5:68, 1969.
17. Smith DW: Recognizable Patterns of Human Malformation. Genetic, Embryologic and Clinical Aspects. Philadelphia, Saunders, 1982, pp 277–279.
18. Spranger JW, Bidder U, Voelz C: Chondrodysplasia punctata (chondrodystrophia calcificans). II. Der rhizo-mele Type. Fortschr Geb Roentgenstr Nuklearmed 114:327, 1971.
19. Spranger J, Opitz JM, Bidder U: Heterogeneity of chondrodysplasia punctata. Humangenetik 11:190, 1971.
20. Straub W, Zarabi M, Mazer J: Fetal ascites associated with Conradi's disease (chondrodysplasia punctata): Report of a case. J Clin Ultrasound 11:234, 1983.
21. Vinke TH, Duffy FP: Chondrodystrophia calcificans congenita: Report of two cases. J Bone Joint Surg 29:509, 1947.

Diastrophic Dysplasia

Synonyms
Diastrophic nanism syndrome and diastrophic dwarfism.

Definition
Diastrophic dysplasia is characterized by micromelia, clubfoot, hand deformities, multiple joint flexion contractures, and scoliosis. The term "diastrophic" means *twisted* and refers to the twisted habitus present in this condition.

Etiology
The disorder is inherited as an autosomal recessive trait.[3,5,9,11]

Pathology
The disease may be recognized at birth, but milder cases are diagnosed later.[1,2,12] The clinical features at birth include short stature, micromelia (predominantly of the rhizomelic type), multiple joint flexion contractures (notably of the major joints), hand deformities, with short and widely spaced fingers and abducted position of the thumbs (hitchhiker thumb) (Fig. 10–59) and severe talipes equinovarus. The head and skull are normal. Micrognathia and cleft palate are frequently observed.[11]

With time, the affected infants develop progressive kyphoscoliosis with a potential for respiratory compromise. The gait is characterized by a twisting motion because of hip dislocation and genu varum deformities of the knee. Inflammation of the pinna of the ear results in a typical deformation known as "cauliflower ear."[1,11]

Diastrophic dysplasia is a generalized disorder of cartilage. There is a destructive process of chondrocytes and cartilage matrix. This is followed by the formation of fibrous scar tissue and ossification. The latter process is responsible for the contractures. Growth plates are also affected.[10] No known biochemical defects have been demonstrated.[12]

Diagnosis
Antenatal diagnoses of diastrophic dysplasia have been reported in fetuses at risk for the disorder.[4,6,8,15]

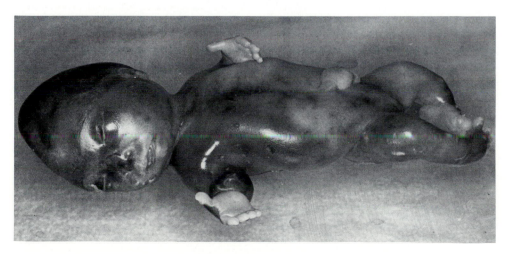

Figure 10–59. Abortus with hitchhiker thumbs.

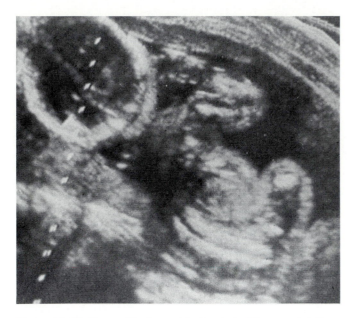

Figure 10–60. Fetus with diastrophic dysplasia. The prenatal diagnosis was based on the detection of shortened limbs. *(Reproduced with permission from Mantagos et al.: Am J Obstet Gynecol 139:111, 1981.)*

We have made this diagnosis by ultrasound, demonstrating rhizomelic dwarfism at 20 weeks' gestation[6] (Figs. 10–60, 10–61). O'Brien et al. made the diagnosis at 16 weeks with a combination of ultrasound and fetoscopy.[8] Sonography demonstrated shortening of the long bones, and fetoscopy showed a cleft palate and micrognathia. Wladimiroff et al. diagnosed the condition at 17 weeks by visualizing with ultrasound the severe shortening and bowing of all long bones.[15] Kaitila et al. reported a diagnosis at 18 weeks by demonstrating shortening of the limbs and lateral projection of the thumb with ultrasound in a patient at risk.[4] They also reported the exclusion of the

diagnosis in three fetuses at risk who were examined between 15 and 16 weeks of gestation.

The spectrum of the disease is wide,[2] and some cases of diastrophic dysplasia may not be diagnosable in utero. Besides short limb dysplasia, the most characteristic feature of diastrophic dysplasia is the presence of multiple contractures in the upper and lower extremities. However, this finding can occur in other disorders, such as arthrogryposis multiplex congenita (p. 380), and the Nievergelt type of mesomelic dysplasia (p. 361). A skeletal dysplasia that should be considered as part of the differential diagnosis is Weissenbacher-Zweymuller syndrome, which consists of the association of short limb dysplasia and micrognathia (other facial features of the syndrome may include cleft palate, hypertelorism, and a depressed nasal bridge). In this condition, contracture deformities are not expected.[7,14]

Prognosis
Increased neonatal mortality has been reported in these patients. Respiratory distress and aspiration pneumonia are the leading causes.[1,13] The disorder is nonlethal, and intellect is not affected. The progressive kyphoscoliosis and arthropathy lead to severe physical handicap and, in extreme cases, to restrictive respiratory distress.[13]

Obstetrical Management
The option of pregnancy termination can be offered when diagnosis is made before viability. After viability, diagnosis of diastrophic dysplasia does not alter standard obstetrical management.

REFERENCES

1. Hollister DW, Lachman RS: Diastrophic dwarfism. Clin Orthop 114:61, 1976.
2. Horton WA, Rimoin DL, Lachman RS, et al.: The

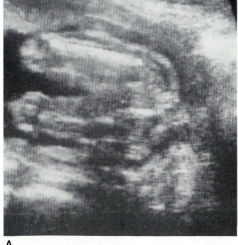
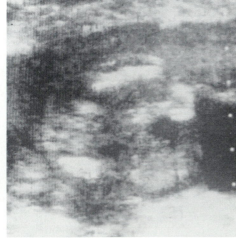

Figure 10–61. A comparison between the normal femur (*left*) and those of a fetus with diastrophic dysplasia (*right*) for the same gestational age.

A   B

phenotypic variability of diastrophic dysplasia. J. Pediatr 93:609, 1978.

3. Jackson WPU: An irregular familial chondro-osseous defect. J Bone Joint Surg 33B:420, 1951.

4. Kaitila I, Ammala P, Karjalainen O, et al.: Early prenatal detection of diastrophic dysplasia. Prenat Diagn 3:237, 1983.

5. Lamy M, Maroteaux P: Le nanisme diastrophique. Presse Med 68:1977, 1960.

6. Mantagos S, Weiss RR, Mahoney M, Hobbins JC: Prenatal diagnosis of diastrophic dwarfism. Am J Obstet Gynecol 139:111, 1981.

7. Maroteaux P, Roux C, Fruchter Z: Le nanisme micrognathe. Presse Med 78:2371, 1970.

8. O'Brien G, Rodeck C, Queenan JT: Early prenatal diagnosis of diastrophic dwarfism by ultrasound. Br Med J 280:1300, 1980.

9. Paul SS, Rao PL, Mullick P, et al.: Diastrophic dwarfism. A little known disease entity. Clin Pediatr 4:95, 1965.

10. Rimoin DL: The chondrodystrophies. Adv Genet 5:1, 1975.

11. Taybi H: Diastrophic dwarfism. Radiology 80:1, 1963.

12. Vasquez AM, Lee FA: Diastrophic dwarfism. J Pediatr 72:234, 1968.

13. Walker BA, Scott CI, Hall JG, et al.: Diastrophic dwarfism. Medicine 51:41, 1972.

14. Weissenbacher VG, Zweymuller E: Coincidental occurrence of Pierre Robin and fetal chondrodysplasia. Monatschr Kinderh 112:315, 1964.

15. Wladimiroff JW, Niermeijer MF, Laar J, et al.: Prenatal diagnosis of skeletal dysplasia by real-time ultrasound. Obstet Gynecol 63:360, 1984.

Metatropic Dysplasia

Synonyms

Hyperplastic achondroplasia and metatropic dwarfism.

Definition

Metatropic dysplasia is a short limb skeletal dysplasia characterized by dumbbell-like configuration of the long bones, a narrow but normal length thorax, and, occasionally, a coccygeal appendage similar to a tail.

Etiology

Some familial cases have been reported, suggesting an autosomal recessive pattern of inheritance.[1] However, most cases occur sporadically.

Pathology

The term "metatropic" means *changeable* and was suggested by Maroteaux et al.[4] to indicate the change in proportions of the trunk to the limbs that occurs over time.

The newborns have a normal trunk length with a restricted thorax and short limb dwarfism. The long bones have a characteristic broadening of their metaphyses (trumpet-shaped long bones). With time, the pelvis develops a typical battle-axe configuration. The intervertebral disk spaces are widened, and a typical tail-like appendage can be seen at the level of the coccyx. Although inconstant, this finding is very characteristic of the disorder.[2,3,5]

In childhood there is growth retardation of the spine and kyphoscoliosis develops, resulting in a trunk shorter than the limbs.

Cleft palate has been reported in association with metatrophic dysplasia.

Diagnosis

Not all cases are identifiable at birth. The diagnosis should be suspected when shortening of the limbs is associated with a trumpet-shaped widening of the metaphyses. A prenatal diagnosis of this condition has not been reported.

Another disorder associated with a dumbbell configuration of long bones is the Weisenbacher-Zweymuller syndrome characterized by severe micromelia, micrognathia, and coronal cleft in the vertebrae. Other disorders with metaphyseal flaring include fibrochondrogenesis (p. 339), Kniest syndrome (p. 364), and dyssegmental dysplasia (p. 365).

Prognosis

This disorder is compatible with life. However, with age, there is increased disability because of progressive kyphoscoliosis. In some patients, death occurs during infancy.

Obstetrical Management

If the diagnosis is made before viability, the option of pregnancy termination should be offered to the parents. Diagnosis after viability does not change standard obstetrical management.

REFERENCES

1. Crowle P, Astley R, Insley J: A form of metatropic dwarfism in two brothers. Pediatr Radiol 4:172, 1976.

2. Gefferth K: Metatropic dwarfism. In: Kaufman HJ (ed). Progress in Pediatric Radiology. Basel, Karger, 1973, vol 4, p 137.

3. Jenkins P, Smith MB, McKinnel JS: Metatropic dwarfism. Br J Radiol 43:561, 1970.
4. Maroteaux P, Spranger J, Wiedemann HR: Metatropische Zwergwuchs. Arch Kinderheil 173:211, 1966.
5. Rimoin DL, Siggers DC, Lachman RS, Silberberg R: Metatropic dwarfism, the Kniest syndrome and the pseudoachondroplastic dysplasias. Clin Orthop 114:70, 1976.

Skeletal Dysplasias Characterized by Bone Demineralization

OSTEOGENESIS IMPERFECTA

Synonyms
Van der Hoeve syndrome, trias fragilitas osseum, Eddowe's syndrome, osteopsathyrosis idiopathica of Lobstein, and Ekman-Lobstein disease.

Definition
Osteogenesis imperfecta (OI) is a heterogeneous group of collagen disorders characterized by bone fragility, blue sclerae, and dentinogenesis imperfecta.

Incidence
The overall incidence of OI is 1 in 28,500 live births.[19] The most frequent variety ascertained in newborns is OI type II, with an incidence of 1 in 54,000 births.[4]

Etiology
OI is a heterogeneous disorder of production, secretion, or function of collagen. A detailed discussion of the nature of the biochemical alterations is beyond the scope of this text. The interested reader is referred to other reviews on the subject.[3]

Pathology
Several classifications of OI have been proposed, but the most widely accepted is one based on phenotype suggested by Sillence et al.[19] and subsequently modified.[3]

OI Type I. This type is inherited in an autosomal dominant pattern. Patients have blue sclerae and bone fragility and are deaf or have a family history of presenile deafness. Infants are of normal weight and length at birth and do not have multiple fractures. Vertebral malalignment and deformation of tubular bones are uncommon complications. OI type I is subdivided into type A and type B according to the presence or absence of abnormal dentinogenesis, respectively.

OI Type II. This form is the lethal variety of OI. It is claimed to be inherited as an autosomal recessive trait, but the lack of affected siblings in different series suggests, in some cases, a new mutation of a dominant gene or a nongenetic etiology.[22] Therefore, the empiric recurrence risk should be somewhat below the expected 25 percent. Infants are either stillborn or die during the neonatal period. Multiple fractures occur in utero, and the long bones are shortened, broad, and crumpled. The thorax is short but not narrowed. The skull is poorly ossified, and blue sclerae are present. Infants are frequently small for gestational age. Sillence et al.[20] proposed a subdivision of type II OI into three varieties based on radiologic criterion. The first variety is characterized by short, broad, "crumpled" long bones, angulation of tibiae and beaded ribs, the second type by broad, "crumpled" femora but minimal or no rib fractures, and the third by narrow fractured femora and thin, beaded ribs.

OI Type III. Type III can be transmitted as an autosomal recessive or an autosomal dominant disorder. Patients have bluish sclerae during infancy and normal or pale blue sclerae later in life. Long bones are shortened and bowed, and multiple fractures are present at birth in most patients. The skull has decreased ossification. The disease is characterized by progressive deformity of the long bones and spine.

OI Type IV. This type is the mildest form of the disease and is inherited as an autosomal dominant disorder. Patients' sclerae are blue at birth, but with time they become white. Tubular bones are normal in length, but mild femoral bowing may occur. According to the presence or absence of dentinogenesis imperfecta, the disease is subclassified into subtype A or B, respectively. Although this classification encompasses most cases of the disease, some do not fit the proposed subdivision.[22]

Diagnosis
The diagnosis of OI type II has been reported several times with ultrasound.[11–14,24,25] This condition has been diagnosed before 20 weeks' gestation,[6,7,9,15,18,23] and no false negative diagnoses have been reported. The sonographic findings may be present in all skeletal districts. Long bones may show fractures (Fig.

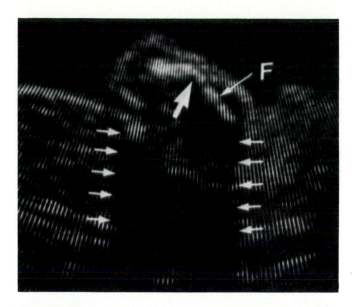

Figure 10–62. Fracture (*large white arrow*) of a femur (F) in a fetus with osteogenesis imperfecta.

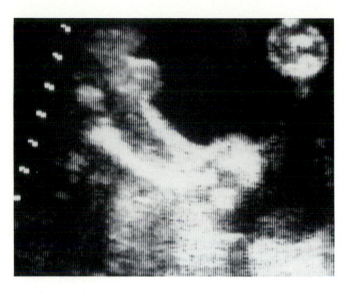

Figure 10–64. Bowing of the femur at 24 weeks of gestation in a fetus with osteogenesis imperfecta. *(Reproduced with permission from Chervenak et al.: Am J Obstet Gynecol 143:228, 1982.)*

10–62), angulations, shortening (Fig. 10–63), localized thickening secondary to callous formation, and bowing and demineralization (Fig. 10–64). These findings are usually more evident in the femurs but have been described in the upper limbs as well. In rare instances, the limbs are so shortened that they become impossible to measure.[13] The skull may be thinner than usual, and the weight of the ultrasound probe may deform the head quite easily. In severe cases, the cranial vault has a wavy outline and is easily compressible. Multiple fractures of the ribs result in a bell-shaped or narrow chest. Seldom does the spine

show decreased echogenicity. Fetal movements are decreased.[7,9]

Type I OI diagnosis has been attempted as well.[5,10,17] An early diagnosis was possible in some fetuses,[10,17] but in others, even serial sonographic scans failed to diagnose the condition with certainty.[5]

Type III OI was diagnosed once in a fetus at risk because of a previous affected sibling.[1] At 15½ weeks of gestation, the long bones were normal in length, but a fracture was suspected. At 19 weeks, long bones of the lower extremities were shortened, whereas bones of the upper extremities were within normal limits.*

There are limitations to the evaluation of bone mineralization with sonography (Figs. 10–65 and 10–66).

Although a biochemical approach to the diagnosis by measuring pyrophosphate concentration in amniotic fluid has been proposed,[21] this method has been reported to be unreliable.[8] As molecular defects are identified, prenatal diagnosis is likely to shift to molecular biology techniques.

Prognosis

There is limited information available on the prognosis of OI diagnosed in utero, since most of these pregnancies have been electively terminated. Of the 16 fetuses diagnosed in utero, 12 were type II (the lethal form), 3 were type I, and 1 was type III.

OI is a disease with a wide range of clinical presentations. Multiple fractures and intracranial bleeding may lead to intracranial hemorrhage and

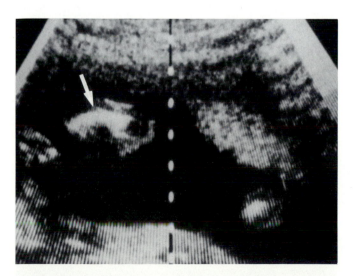

Figure 10–63. Left femur at 18 weeks of gestation is 1.9 cm in length. Note the marked bowing and shortening of the shaft and breakage (*arrow*). *(Reproduced with permission from Ghosh et al.: Prenat Diagn 4:235, 1984.)*

*A similar case has been reported.[16]

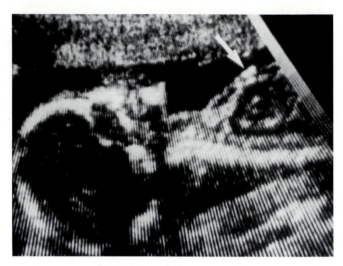

Figure 10–65. This image illustrates the limitations of sonography in the evaluation of bone mineralization. It is a longitudinal scan of an 18-week fetus showing normal shape of the head, spine, and chest. Note the normal echogenicity of the skull bones. *(Reproduced with permission from Ghosh et al.: Prenat Diagn 4:235, 1984.)*

death in utero or during the neonatal period. The quality of life of survivors is extremely variable. Multiple fractures may require repeated surgery and lead to serious handicaps. Spinal deformities, otosclerosis, and deafness can occur in long-term survivors.[2]

The classification proposed by Sillence does not have a reliable prognostic significance. Spranger et al. have proposed a radiographic scoring system based on the severity of underossification and bone deformities and fractures.[22] The scoring system should be used during the neonatal period to predict prospective mortality. Infants with a score of more than 2.6 have an 88 percent mortality rate, whereas those with a score of 2.6 or less have a 90 percent chance of survival.

Type II OI is lethal. Type I and type III are compatible with life, but affected individuals may suffer significant handicaps because of multiple and recurring fractures and deformities. Type IV has the best prognosis, since fractures and deformities are uncommon.

Obstetrical Management

The option of pregnancy termination can be offered any time a type II OI is diagnosed. For other varieties, the option of pregnancy termination should be offered before viability. After viability, consideration should be given to the mode of delivery. Theoretically, skull fractures could occur during the passage of the infant through the birth canal. Therefore, delivery by cesarean section has been proposed.[25] This view seems reasonable, although there are no empirical data to prove the benefit of this approach.

REFERENCES

1. Aylsworth AS, Seeds JW, Bonner-Guilford W, et al.: Prenatal diagnosis of a severe deforming type of osteogenesis imperfecta. Am J Med Genet 19:707, 1984.
2. Benson DR, Donaldson DH, Millar EA: The spine in osteogenesis imperfecta. J Bone Joint Surg 60:925, 1978.
3. Byers PH, Bonadio JF, Steinmann B: Osteogenesis imperfecta: Update and perspective. Am J Med Genet 17:429, 1984.
4. Camera G, Mastroiacovo P: Birth prevalence of skeletal dysplasias in the Italian multicentric monitoring system for birth defects. Prog Clin Biol Res 104:441, 1982.
5. Chervenak FA, Romero R, Berkowitz RL, et al.: Antenatal sonographic findings of osteogenesis imperfecta. Am J Obstet Gynecol 143:228, 1982.
6. Dinno ND, Yacoub UA, Kadlec JF, et al.: Midtrimester

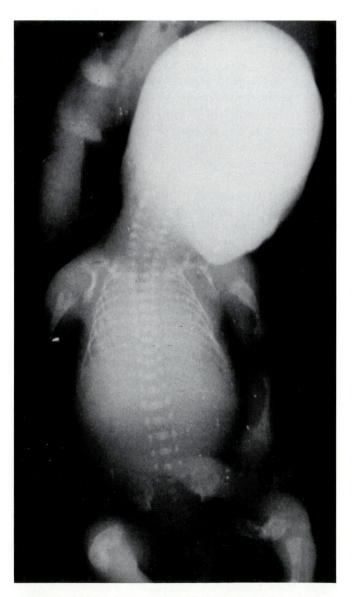

Figure 10–66. Radiogram of the fetus shown in Figure 10–65. Note the poorly calcified skull. *(Reproduced with permission from Ghosh et al.: Prenat Diagn 4:235, 1984.)*

diagnosis of osteogenesis imperfecta, type II. Birth Defects 18(3A):125, 1982.

7. Elejalde BR, de Elejalde MM: Prenatal diagnosis of perinatally lethal osteogenesis imperfecta. Am J Med Genet 14:353, 1983.

8. Garver KL, Blitzer MG, Ibezim G, et al.: Evaluation of inorganic pyrophosphate in amniotic fluid as a mode of prenatal diagnosis of osteogenesis imperfecta. Prenat Diagn 4:109, 1984.

9. Ghosh A, Woo JSK, Wan CW, et al.: Simple ultrasonic diagnosis of osteogenesis imperfecta type II in early second trimester. Prenat Diagn 4:235, 1984.

10. Hobbins JC, Bracken MB, Mahoney MJ: Diagnosis of fetal skeletal dysplasias with ultrasound. Am J Obstet Gynecol 142:306, 1982.

11. Kurtz AB, Wapner RJ: Ultrasonographic diagnosis of second trimester skeletal dysplasias: A prospective analysis in a high-risk population. J Ultrasound Med 2:99, 1983.

12. Mertz E, Goldhofer W: Sonographic diagnosis of lethal osteogenesis imperfecta in the second trimester: Case report and review. J Clin Ultrasound 14:380, 1986.

13. Milsom I, Mattsson LA, Dahlen-Nilsson I: Antenatal diagnosis of osteogenesis imperfecta by real-time ultrasound: Two case reports. Br J Radiol 55:310, 1982.

14. Miskin M, Rothberg R: Prenatal detection of congenital anomalies by ultrasound. Semin Ultrasound 1:281, 1980.

15. Patel ZM, Shah HL, Madon PF, et al.: Prenatal diagnosis of lethal osteogenesis imperfecta (OI) by ultrasonography. Prenat Diagn 3:261, 1983.

16. Robinson LP, Worthen NJ, Lachman RS, et al.: Prenatal diagnosis of osteogenesis imperfecta type III. Prenat Diagn 7:7, 1987.

17. Rumack CM, Johnson ML, Zunkel D: Antenatal diagnosis. Clin Diagn Ultrasound 8:210, 1981.

18. Shapiro JE, Phillips JA, Byers PH, et al.: Prenatal diagnosis of lethal perinatal osteogenesis imperfecta (OI type II). J Pediatr 100:127, 1982.

19. Sillence DO, Senn A, Danks DM: Genetic heterogeneity in osteogenesis imperfecta. J Med Genet 16:101, 1979.

20. Sillence DO, Barlow KK, Garber AP, et al.: Osteogenesis imperfecta type II: Delineation of the phenotype with reference to genetic heterogeneity. Am J Med Genet 17:407, 1984.

21. Solomons CC, Gottesfeld K: Prenatal biochemistry of osteogenesis imperfecta. Birth Defects 15(5):69, 1976.

22. Spranger J, Cremin B, Beighton P: Osteogenesis imperfecta congenita. Features and prognosis of a heterogeneous condition. Pediatr Radiol 12:21, 1982.

23. Stephens JD, Filly RA, Callen PW, et al.: Prenatal diagnosis of osteogenesis imperfecta type II by real-time ultrasound. Hum Genet 64:191, 1983.

24. Woo JSK, Ghosh A, Liang ST, et al.: Ultrasonic evaluation of osteogenesis imperfecta congenita in utero. J Clin Ultrasound 11:42, 1983.

25. Zervoudakis IA, Strongin MJ, Schrotenboer KA, et al.: Diagnosis and management of fetal osteogenesis imperfecta congenita in labor. Am J Obstet Gynecol 121:116, 1978.

HYPOPHOSPHATASIA

Definition
Hypophosphatasia is a congenital disease usually inherited in an autosomal recessive pattern and characterized by demineralization of bones and low activity of serum and other tissue alkaline phosphatase.

Incidence
The incidence of hypophosphatasia is 1 in 100,000.[2]

Etiology
Autosomal recessive. Some familial cases of the mild form have been attributed to an autosomal dominant trait.[10]

Pathology
There are four clinical forms of the disease depending on the age of onset: neonatal, juvenile, adult, and latent. The neonatal (also known as "congenital" or "lethal") variety is associated with a high incidence of intrauterine fetal demise or early neonatal death. In the juvenile or severe variety, the onset of symptoms takes place within weeks or months. The adult or mild form is recognized later in childhood, adolescence, or even during adulthood. It seems to be inherited with an autosomal dominant pattern with variable expressivity and penetrance.[10] The latent form (heterozygote state) is characterized by normal or borderline levels of alkaline phosphatase and no other pathologic features. It is unclear whether these clinical varieties represent different forms of the same genetic defect or rather different diseases. It has been suggested that recurrences within a family are type specific.[2]

The mechanism for the development of bone fragility in hypophosphatasia is not clearly understood. Alkaline phosphatase normally acts on pyrophosphates and other phosphate esters and leads to the accumulation of inorganic phosphates, which are critical for the formation of bone crystals. A deficiency in alkaline phosphatase leads to deficient generation of bone crystals.

Diagnosis
The variety relevant to antenatal diagnosis is the congenital form. It is characterized by marked demineralization of the calvarium.[1,4,7,9,11] The skull appears soft and is called "caput membranaceum" (Fig. 10-67). An increased echogenicity of the falx cerebri has been attributed to enhanced sound transmission through a poorly mineralized skull.[5] Tubular bones are short, bowed, and demineralized, and multiple fractures can be present. Amniotic fluid volume is characteristically increased.[3,6,8]

The amniotic fluid alpha-fetoprotein concentra-

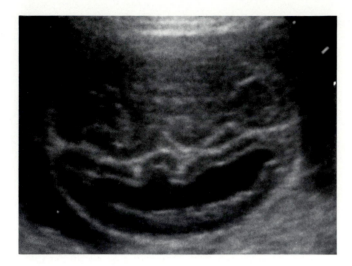

Figure 10–67. Congenital hypophosphatasia. Note the demineralized skull.

tion has been used for the differential diagnosis between hypophosphatasia and anencephaly. With modern ultrasound equipment, this should not be a diagnostic problem.[3,9]

A precise differential diagnosis with other skeletal dysplasias may be difficult purely on clinical or radiologic findings. It has been suggested that a specific diagnosis could be made by demonstrating a low level of alkaline phosphatase.[1,8] However, alkaline phosphatase measurement in amniotic fluid is not a reliable means of making a diagnosis because most of the alkaline phosphatase activity in amniotic fluid is of intestinal origin.[7,9] The involved enzymes in hypophosphatasia are bone and liver alkaline phosphatase. These isoenzymes contribute only 16 percent of the total amniotic fluid enzymatic activity.[7] Another alternative involves culturing amniotic fluid cells obtained by amniocentesis and examining their alkaline phosphatase activity.[7] Another means is to measure alkaline phosphatase in fetal blood, since Mulivor et al. have reported differences in activities between heterozygote carriers and controls by examining cord blood enzymatic activity.[7] Recently, a prenatal diagnosis in the first trimester has been made by assaying alkaline phosphatase activity in tissues obtained by chorionic villous sampling.[9a]

Prognosis
The congenital variety of hypophosphatasia is uniformly fatal.

Obstetrical Management
When a confident diagnosis of the lethal variety is made, the option of pregnancy termination can be offered any time during gestation.

REFERENCES

1. Benzie R, Doran TA, Escoffery W, et al.: Prenatal diagnosis of hypophosphatasia. Birth Defects 12(6):271, 1976.
2. Fraser D: Hypophosphatasia. Am J Med 22:730, 1957.
3. Kousseff BG, Mulivor RA: Prenatal diagnosis of hypophosphatasia. Obstet Gynecol 57:9S, 1981.
4. Kurtz AB, Wapner RJ: Ultrasonographic diagnosis of second-trimester skeletal dysplasias: A prospective analysis in a high-risk population. J Ultrasound Med 2:99, 1983.
5. Laughlin CL, Lee TG: The prominent falx cerebri: New ultrasonic observation in hypophosphatasia. J Clin Ultrasound 10:37, 1982.
6. Leroy JG, Vanneuville FJ, De Schepper AM, et al.: Prenatal diagnosis of congenital hypophosphatasia: Challenge met most adequately by fetal radiography. Prog Clin Biol Res 104:525, 1982.
7. Mulivor RA, Mennuti M, Zackai EH, et al.: Prenatal diagnosis of hypophosphatasia: Genetic, biochemical, and clinical studies. Am J Hum Genet 30:271, 1978.
8. Rattenbury JM, Blau K, Sandler M, et al.: Prenatal diagnosis of hypophosphatasia. Lancet 1:306, 1976.
9. Rudd NL, Miskin M, Hoar DI, et al.: Prenatal diagnosis of hypophosphatasia. N Engl J Med 1:146, 1976.
9a. Warren RC, McKenzie CF, Rodeck CH, et al.: First trimester diagnosis of hypophosphatasia with a monoclonal antibody to the liver/bone/kidney isoenzyme of alkaline phosphatase. Lancet 2:856, 1985.
10. Whyte MP, Teitelbaum SL, Murphy WA, et al.: Adult hypophosphatasia. Medicine 58:329, 1979.
11. Wladimiroff JW, Niermeijer MF, Van-der-Harten JJ, et al.: Early prenatal diagnosis of congenital hypophosphatasia: Case report. Prenat Diagn 5:47, 1985.

Heterozygous Achondroplasia

Definition
The term "achondroplasia" was used in the past for defining all short limb dysplasias. With recognition of the heterogeneity of these disorders, this term is used currently to describe a specific disease characterized by predominantly rhizomelic dwarfism, limb bowing, lordotic spine, bulky head, and depressed nasal bridge. The disorder is compatible with normal life.

Incidence
A birth prevalence of 1 in 66,000 in the United States has been reported.[12] These figures probably represent an overestimate of the real incidence of the condition because other skeletal dysplasias were probably confused with achondroplasia and included in the calculations.

Etiology
Achondroplasia is transmitted with an autosomal dominant pattern with invariable penetrance. However, in 80 percent of cases, the parents are not affected, suggesting the occurrence of a new mutation.[13] Achondroplasia is one of the few diseases in which advanced paternal age probably plays a role.[8] The disease is lethal in the homozygous state.

Parents can be informed that after the birth of one achondroplastic infant, the chance of recurrence is extremely small. However, familial cases with normal parents have been reported.[1,10] If one parent is affected, the likelihood of an infant being affected is 50 percent. If both parents are affected, there is a 25 percent chance of an unaffected infant, a 50 percent chance of heterozygous achondroplasia, and a 25 percent risk of homozygous achondroplasia.

Pathology
The disease was regarded as the result of anomalous growth of cartilage (hence the term "achondroplasia"), followed by abnormal endochondral ossification,[12] but it has been demonstrated that the disorder is not qualitative but quantitative.[6] Defective endochondral bone formation is responsible for the shortness of long bones, whereas normal periosteal bone formation gives the impression of abnormally thickened long bones. Moreover, long bones are enlarged at the end and frequently bowed. The bones of the hands and feet are short (brachydactyly). The fingers are divergent, and the infants are unable to approximate the third and fourth fingers (trident hand) (Fig. 10–68). Progressive narrowing of the interpedicular space in the anteroposterior x-ray projection is a typical finding in the spine. Marked lordosis in the lumbar area results in a prominent buttocks (Fig. 10–69). The head is large with a shortened cranial base and frequently a small foramen magnum. Facial features include a flattened nasal bridge, frontal bossing, and a broad mandible (Fig. 10–70). The chest shows decreased dimensions, and the pelvic bones appear square-shaped with a tombstone configuration.

Associated Anomalies
Hydrocephalus has been reported in some patients and may be related to a narrowed foramen magnum.

Diagnosis
Prenatal diagnosis of achondroplasia has been reported by several authors.[2,3,5,7] The diagnosis has relied on identification of shortened long bones, particularly the femur. An extremely important observation is that alterations in long bone growth may not be observed until the third trimester, and, therefore, a diagnosis before viability may only be possible in the most severe cases. Kurtz et al. recently reviewed their experience with seven cases of prenatal diagnosis of heterozygous achondroplasia.[5] None had an abnormally short femur in early second trimester. Using the relationship between femur and biparietal diameter, all fetuses with serial examinations (six) fell below the 1st percentile between 20.9 and 27 weeks of gestation. The shape of long bones

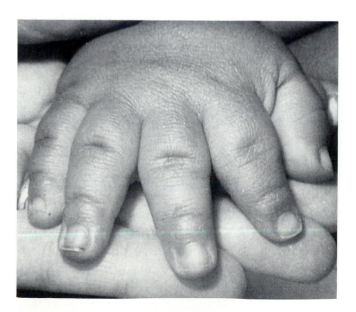

Figure 10–68. Hand of an achondroplastic child, showing the typical trident appearance and stubby fingers.

was normal. Spine and head abnormalities were not identified in utero.

Prognosis

Achondroplasia may be compatible with a normal life span. However, affected individuals experience significant morbidity. Recurrent ear infections during early childhood are attributed to poor development of the facial bones, with constriction and inadequate drainage of the eustachian tube. Unrecognized or incompletely treated infections are probably responsible for hearing loss. Orthodontic care may be required to alleviate crowded dentition and problems of malocclusion. The mean adult height for men is 52 inches and for women 49 inches. Obesity is frequent. Hydrocephalus as well as syringomyelia may result from a small foramen magnum.[4] However, hydrocephaly is rarely a serious problem and is generally managed conservatively. Sudden infant death and respiratory compromise have been attributed to compression of the upper cervical spine.[11,14] Indeed, a recent study using somatosensory evoked potentials showed that up to 44 percent of asymptomatic achondroplasts had abnormal findings secondary to spinal compression.[9] The most significant handicaps suffered by achondroplastic patients are neurologic complications secondary to spinal cord compression, which may range from paresthesias to complete paraplegia. Genu varum and tibia vara are more frequent with advancing age.

Obstetrical Management

At present, it is doubtful whether a confident diagnosis can be made before viability. In the third trimester, fetal head growth should be monitored because of the possible development of macrocrania. The method of choice for delivery of achondroplastic mothers is elective cesarean section.

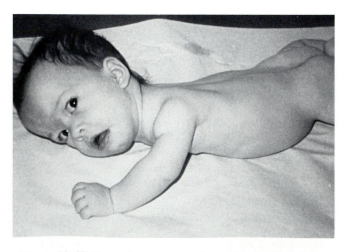

Figure 10–69. General appearance of an achondroplastic baby.

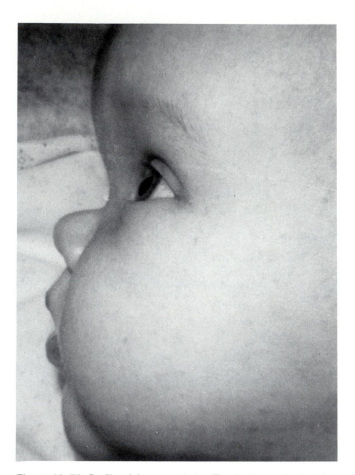

Figure 10–70. Profile of the same baby. The features of achondroplasia are evident.

REFERENCES

1. Bowen P: Achondroplasia in two sisters with normal parents. Birth Defects 10:31, 1974.
2. Elejalde BR, de Elejalde MM, Hamilton PR, et al.: Prenatal diagnosis in two pregnancies of an achondroplastic woman. Am J Med Genet 15:437, 1983.
3. Filly RA, Golbus MS, Carey JC, et al.: Short-limbed dwarfism: Ultrasonographic diagnosis by mensuration of fetal femoral length. Radiology 138:653, 1981.
4. Hecht JT, Butler IJ, Scott CI: Long-term neurological sequelae in achondroplasia. Eur J Pediatr 143:58, 1984.
5. Kurtz AB, Filly RA, Wapner RJ, et al.: In utero analysis of heterozygous achondroplasia: Variable time of onset as detected by femur length measurements. J. Ultrasound Med 5:137, 1986.
6. Langer LO Jr, Baumann PA, Gorlin RJ: Achondroplasia. AJR 100:12, 1967.
7. Leonard CO, Sanders RC, Lau HL: Prenatal diagnosis of the Turner syndrome, a familial chromosomal rearrangement and achondroplasia by amniocentesis and ultrasonography. Johns Hopkins Med J 145:25, 1979.
8. Murdoch JL, Walker BA, Hall JG, et al.: Achondroplasia — A genetic and statistical survey. Ann Hum Genet 33:227, 1970.
9. Nelson FW, Goildie WD, Hecht JT, et al.: Short-latency

somatosensory evoked potentials in the management of patients with achondroplasia. Neurology 34:1053, 1984.

10. Opitz, JM: Delayed mutation in achondroplasia? Birth Defects 5/4:20, 1969.

11. Pauli RM, Scott CI, Wassman ER Jr, et al.: Apnea and sudden unexpected death in infants with achondroplasia. J. Pediatr 104:342, 1984.

12. Potter EL, Coverstone VA: Chondrodystrophy fetalis. Am J Obstet Gynecol 56:790, 1948.

13. Scott, CI: Achondroplastic and hypochondroplastic dwarfism. Clin Orthop 114:18, 1976.

14. Stokes DC, Phillips JA, Leonard CO, et al.: Respiratory complications of achondroplasia. J Pediatr 102:534, 1983.

Mesomelic Dysplasia

Definition

The term "mesomelic dysplasia" refers to a group of disorders in which limb shortening is most pronounced in the middle segment (forearm and leg) of the extremities. It includes dyschondrosteosis, Nievergelt mesomelic dysplasia, Langer mesomelic dysplasia, Robinow (fetal face syndrome) mesomelic dysplasia, Reinhardt mesomelic dysplasia, and Werner mesomelic dysplasia.

Incidence

Rare.

Etiology

Mesomelic dysplasias are inherited with an autosomal dominant pattern, with the exception of the Langer variety which is inherited as an autosomal recessive trait.[1,5]

Pathology

The most prominent findings of the different varieties are described as follows.[3,13]

Langer Mesomelic Dysplasia. Hypoplastic ulna, fibula, and mandible; the mesomelia is more marked in the lower extremities. The ulna is shorter than the radius. The degree of mandibular hypoplasia is variable and can be mild. There is marked ulnar deviation of the hand. Some authors have considered the Langer type as the homozygous state of dyschondrosteosis, a mesomelic dysplasia that is not recognized until late childhood and is characterized by mesomelic dwarfism and Madelung deformity or dinner fork deformity of the forearm (short radius with lateral and dorsal bowing).[4,6,8]

Robinow Mesomelic Dysplasia. Acromelic brachymelia (short hands and feet with stubby fingers and toes), mesomelic shortening predominantly of the upper extremities, abnormal facies resembling that of an 8-week fetus (with macrocephaly, prominent forehead, hypertelorism, hypoplastic mandible), and mental retardation. Additional features include hemivertebra formation and fusion anomalies of the spine and ribs. Small genitalia are present.[7,12,15,16]

Nievergelt Mesomelic Dysplasia. Besides mesomelia, it is characterized by clubfeet, flexion deformities of the fingers and elbows, and genu valgum. The tibia

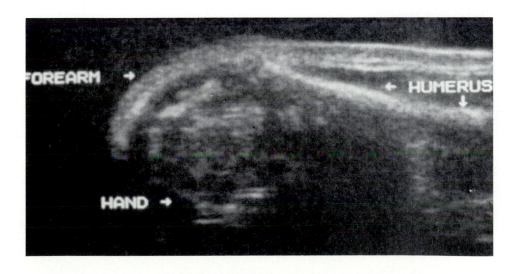

Figure 10–71. Mesomelic shortening of the upper extremity. Note the normal humerus, extremely short forearm bones, and deformed hand.

TABLE 10–10. MESOMELIC DYSPLASIAS

Syndrome	Clinical Features	Radiographic Features	References
Nievergelt	Flexion deformities	Rhomboidal tibia	Young and Wood[17]
Langer	Mandibular hypoplasia	Madelung deformity	Langer[8]
Robinow (fetal face syndrome)	Abnormal facies and genitals	Hemivertebrae and rib fusions	Robinow et al.[12]
			Giedon et al.[7]
Reinhardt	Limb bowing	Synostosis in the carpus and tarsus	Reinhardt and Pfeiffer[11]
Werner	Polydactyly and absence of thumbs	Gross tibial hypoplasia	Pashayan et al.[10]

Reproduced with permission from Cremin, Beighton: Bone Dysplasias of Infancy. A Radiological Atlas. Berlin, Springer-Verlag, 1978.

may be flattened and rhomboid.[17] Although the disease was originally described in a man and his three affected sons (from different mothers),[9] the disorder has also been reported in a nonfamilial case.[14]

Reinhardt Mesomelic Dysplasia. This disorder is characterized by mesomelic shortening of the upper extremities, bowing of the forearm bones, and ulnar deviation of the arm. The fibula is hypoplastic, and there is synostosis of the carpus and tarsus.[11]

Werner Mesomelic Dysplasia. This is characterized by extreme bilateral hypoplasia of the tibia, polydactyly, absence of the thumbs, and frequently webbing of the fingers.[10]

Diagnosis

Of the mesomelic dysplasias, dyschondrosteosis is generally recognized late in childhood and may not be detected prenatally. The other varieties are recognized at birth and are, therefore, amenable to prenatal diagnosis. However, a prenatal diagnosis of any of the mesomelic dysplasias has not been reported. Diagnosis is feasible by comparing the dimensions of the long bones of the leg with the femur and the long bones of the forearm with the humerus (see Figs.

10–24, 10–25; Fig. 10–71). Table 10–10 shows the major characteristics of the mesomelic dysplasias. Some of these findings are identifiable with ultrasound (e.g., hemivertebrae, tibial hypoplasia). Figure 10–72 illustrates a prenatal diagnosis of hemivertebrae.[2]

Prognosis

With the exception of the Robinow type, these disorders are usually associated with normal intelligence. Some orthopedic problems could result from the associated skeletal deformities and stress in the affected bones.

Obstetrical Management

It is unknown whether the diagnosis of mesomelic dysplasia can be made before viability. A diagnosis after viability does not alter standard obstetrical management.

REFERENCES

1. Beighton P: Autosomal recessive inheritance in the mesomelic dwarfism of Campailla and Martinelli. Clin Genet 5:363, 1974.
2. Benacerraf BR, Greene MF, Barss VA: Prenatal sonographic diagnosis of congenital hemivertebra. J Ultrasound Med 5:257, 1986.
3. Cremin BJ, Beighton P: Bone Dysplasias of Infancy. A Radiological Atlas. Berlin, Springer-Verlag, 1978, pp 73–77.
4. Dannenberg M, Anton JL, Spiegel MD: Madelung's deformity. Consideration of its roentgenological diagnostic criteria. AJR 42:671, 1939.
5. Espiritu C, Chen H, and Wooley PV: Mesomelic dwarfism as the homozygous expression of dyschondrosteosis. Am J Dis Child 129:375, 1975.
6. Felman AH, Kirkpatrick JA: Madelung's deformity: Observations in 17 patients. Radiology 93:1037, 1969.
7. Giedon A, Battaglia GF, Bellini F, et al.: The radiological diagnosis of the fetal-face (Robinow) syndrome (mesomelic dwarfism and small genitalia). Report of 3 cases. Helv Paediatr Acta 30:409, 1975.
8. Langer LO: Mesomelic dwarfism of of the hypoplastic ulna, fibula, mandibula type. Radiology 89:654, 1967.
9. Nievergelt K: Positiver Vaterschaftsnachweis auf

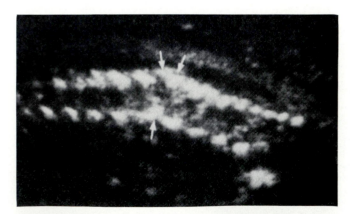

Figure 10–72. Hemivertebra. Longitudinal view of the lower thoracic spine showing the two abnormal ossification centers of the posterior elements, opposite a single ossification center. *(Reproduced with permission from Benacerraf et al.: J Ultrasound Med 5:257, 1986.)*

Grund erblicher Missbildungen der Extremitaten. Arch Julius Klaus-Stiftung 19:157, 1944.

10. Pashayan H, Fraser FC, McIntyre JM, et al.: Bilateral aplasia of the tibia, polydactyly and absent thumbs in father and daughter. J Bone Joint Surg 53B:495, 1971.

11. Reinhardt K, Pfeiffer RA: Ulno-fibulare Dysplasie. Eine autosomal-dominant vererbte Mikromesomelie ahnlich dem Nievergeltsyndrom. Fortschr Roentgenstr 107:379, 1967.

12. Robinow M, Silverman FN, Smith HD: A newly recognized dwarfing syndrome. Am J Dis Child 117:645, 1969.

13. Silverman FN: Mesomelic dwarfism. Prog Pediatr Radiol 4:546–562, 1975.

14. Solonen KA, Sulamaa M: Nievergelt syndrome and its treatment. Ann Chir Gynaecol Fenn 47:142, 1958.

15. Vera-Roman JM: Robinow dwarfing syndrome accompanied by Penile agenesis and hemivertebrae. Am J Dis Child 126:206, 1973.

16. Wadlington WB, Tucker VL, Schimke RN: Mesomelic dwarfism with hemivertebrae and small genitalia (the Robinow syndrome). Am J Dis Child 126:202, 1973.

17. Young LW, Wood BP: Nievergelt syndrome (mesomelic dwarfism type Nievergelt). Birth Defects 10:81, 1975.

Spondyloepiphyseal Dysplasia

Definition

"Spondyloepiphyseal dysplasia" refers to a heterogeneous group of disorders involving the spine and the epiphyses. Two varieties have been described: congenita and tarda. Only the congenital variety is apparent at birth.

Etiology

The congenital form is inherited with an autosomal dominant pattern with considerable variability of expression.[3,4]

Pathology

The disease is characterized by ovoid vertebral bodies and severe platyspondyly (flattened vertebral bodies). There is also hypoplasia of the odontoid process, which may cause cervical myelopathy with significant neurologic compromise. The limbs may or may not be shortened, but severe dwarfism is not seen. The thorax is bell-shaped in the anteroposterior projection.[2]

Morphologic and histochemical studies suggest an unknown disorder of metabolism of mucopolysaccharide in the chondrocytes.[4,5]

Diagnosis

Antenatal diagnosis of spondyloepiphyseal dysplasia congenita has not been reported. Even at birth, a diagnosis may be difficult because the radiographic changes can be subtle. Therefore, the condition seems very difficult to diagnose antenatally with ultrasound but should probably be suspected when mild shortening of the limbs, flattened vertebral bodies, and bell-shaped thorax are seen in a patient at risk.

Prognosis

The disease is often compatible with life. Adults are usually less than 140 cm tall. Secondary arthritis develops in weightbearing joints. Ophthalmologic problems occur in 50 percent of patients,[4] and retinal detachment and myopia can seriously impair vision.[2] The progressive spinal deformities lead to kyphoscoliosis and eventually to cardiorespiratory compromise.

Obstetrical Management

It is unclear if the diagnosis can be made in the second trimester. If the diagnosis is made after viability, standard obstetrical management should not be altered.

REFERENCES

1. Maroteaux P: Spondyloepiphyseal dysplasias and metatropic dwarfism. Birth Defects 5(4):35, 1969.

2. Spranger J, Langer LO: Spondyloepiphyseal dysplasia congenita. Radiology 94:313, 1970.

3. Spranger J, Wiedemann HR: Dysplasia spondyloepiphysaria congenita. Helv Pediatr Acta 21:598, 1966.

4. Van Regemorter N, Rooze M, Milaire J, et al.: Spondyloepiphyseal dysplasia congenita: Case report. In Papadatos CJ, Bartsocas CS (eds): Skeletal Dysplasias. New York, Alan R. Liss, 1982, pp 81–88.

5. Yang SS, Chen H, Williams P, et al.: Spondyloepiphyseal dysplasias congenita: A comparative study of chondrocytic inclusions. Arch Pathol Lab Med 104:208, 1980.

Kniest Syndrome

Synonyms
Metatropic dwarfism type II,[10] and pseudometatropic dwarfism.[11]

Definition
Kniest syndrome is a skeletal dysplasia characterized by involvement of the spine (platyspondyly and coronal cleft) and the tubular bones (shortened and metaphyseal flaring), with a broad and short thorax. The entity has been confused with metatropic dysplasia because both entities share dumbbell-shaped, short, tubular bones and platyspondyly.

Etiology
The original cases reported by Kniest were sporadic,[7] but an autosomal dominant inheritance has been suggested by other authors.[5,8]

Pathology
The disorder affects tubular bones and the spine. Long bones are short and demonstrate metaphyseal enlargement. The thorax is broad and short. Platyspondyly and vertical clefting of the vertebral bodies are present. With time, the spinal involvement may lead to scoliosis. A deep posterior fossa of the skull can also be present. Facial features include a flat midface, flat nasal bridge, wide-set and prominent eyes, and cleft palate.[1,4,7,13]

Associated Anomalies
Inguinal hernia, deafness, myopia, and retinal detachment.

Diagnosis
Prenatal diagnosis of Kniest syndrome has not been reported. The disease should be considered as part of the differential diagnosis of skeletal dysplasias associated with metaphyseal flaring (metatropic dysplasia, fibrochondrogenesis, Weissenbacher-Zweymuller syndrome). In metatropic dysplasia, the thorax is long and narrow and is not associated with the facial features of Kniest syndrome. Weissenbacher-Zweymuller syndrome consists of micromelia with dumbbell configuration of long bones, micrognathia, and coronal clefting of the vertebrae rather than platyspondyly. Another condition that is virtually identical to Kniest dysplasia is dyssegmental dysplasia. This disorder is inherited with an autosomal recessive pattern and has similar radiologic and histologic findings as Kniest dysplasia.[3,6,9,12] Some authors have suggested that Kniest syndrome and dyssegmental dysplasia represent different manifestations of the same disorder.[2]

Prognosis
This disorder is compatible with life. However, progressive disability develops mainly because of kyphoscoliosis. Deafness and ophthalmologic complications are major incapacitating complications.

Obstetrical Management
It is not clear if this diagnosis can be made before viability. After viability, a diagnosis would not alter standard obstetrical management.

REFERENCES

1. Brill, JA: Forms of dwarfism recognizable at birth. Clin Orthop 76:150, 1971.
2. Chen H, Yang SS, Gonzalez E: Kniest dysplasia: Neonatal death with necropsy. Am J Med Genet 6:171, 1980.
3. Dinno ND, Shearer L, Weisskopf B: Chondrodysplastic dwarfism, cleft palate and micrognathia in a neonate. A new syndrome? Eur J Pediatr 123:39, 1976.
4. Eteson DJ, Stewart RE: Craniofacial defects in the human skeletal dysplasias. Birth Defects 20(3):19, 1984.
5. Gnamey D, Farriaux JP, Fontaine G: La maladie de Kniest. Une observation familiale. Arch Franc Pediatr 33:143, 1976.
6. Gruhn JG, Gorlin RJ, Langer LO Jr: Dyssegmental dwarfism. A lethal anisospondylic camptomicromelic dwarfism. Am J Dis Child 132:382, 1978.
7. Kniest W: Zur Abgrenzung der Dysostosis enchondralis von der Chondrodystrophie. Zeitschr Kinderheil 70:633, 1952.
8. Lachman RS, Rimoin DL: Kniest Dysplasia. In: Bergsma D (ed): Birth Defects Compendium, 2d ed. New York, Alan R. Liss, 1979, pp 614–615.
9. Langer LO Jr, Gonzalez-Ramos M, Chen H, et al.: A severe infantile micromelic chondrodysplasia which resembles Kniest disease. Eur J Pediatr 123:29, 1976.
10. McKusick VA: Mendelian Inheritance in Man: Catalogs of autosomal dominant, autosomal recessive and X-linked phenotypes, 4th ed. Baltimore, Johns Hopkins University Press, 1975, p. 496.
11. Rimoin DL, Hughes GNF, Kaufman RL, et al.: Metatropic dwarfism: Morphological and biochemical evidence of heterogeneity. Clin Res 17:317, 1969.
12. Rolland JC, Laugier J, Grenier B, et al.: Nanisme chondrodystrophique et division palatine chez un nouveau-né. Ann Pediatr (Paris) 19:139, 1972.
13. Siggers D, Rimoin D, Dorst J, et al.: The Kniest syndrome. Birth Defects 10(9):193, 1974.

Dyssegmental Dysplasia

Synonyms
Rolland-Langer-Dinno syndrome,[1,6,8] Rolland-Desquois syndrome,[8] and dyssegmental dwarfism.

Definition
Dyssegmental dysplasia is a lethal short limb dysplasia characterized by micromelia, marked disorganization of the vertebral bodies and, frequently, an occipital cephalocele.

Incidence
The disorder was first recognized as a distinct entity in 1977, when four cases (one new and three from the literature) were discussed.[4] Since then, occasional cases have been reported.[2,5]

Etiology
Autosomal recessive.

Pathology
Dyssegmental dysplasia is characterized by severe micromelia with bowing and metaphyseal flaring of long bones, narrow thorax, vertebral segmentation defects, and variable limited mobility at the elbow, wrist, knee, and ankle joints. The hallmark of the condition is the disorganization of the vertebral bodies, with varying vertebral body size and vertical clefts. The frequent encephalocele is probably the result of defective segmentation at the level of the occiput.

Associated Anomalies
Inguinal hernia, hydronephrosis, hydrocephalus, patent ductus arteriosus, and cleft palate.[4]

Diagnosis
Prenatal identification of dyssegmental dysplasia has been reported once in a patient at risk.[5] The disorder should be suspected when micromelia with metaphyseal flaring is associated with a cephalocele and there is an abnormal spine. The differential diagnosis includes other causes of micromelia and metaphyseal flaring, such as Weissenbacher-Zweymuller syndrome and fibrochondrogenesis.[3] Some authors have suggested that dyssegmental dysplasia is a variety of the Kniest syndrome.[7] Other conditions associated with vertebral disorganization are Jarcho-Levin syndrome (p. 382) and mesomelic dysplasia (p. 361).

Prognosis
This is a uniformly lethal disorder.

Obstetrical Management
A certain diagnosis of dyssegmental dysplasia can be made if there has been a previously affected child. The option of pregnancy termination should be offered to the parents before viability. As dyssegmental dysplasia is considered a lethal disorder, the option of pregnancy termination after viability could be offered. Only a few cases of this disorder have been reported in the literature, however.

REFERENCES

1. Dinno ND, Shearer L, Weisskopf B: Chondrodysplastic dwarfism, cleft palate and micrognathia in a neonate. A new syndrome? Eur J Pediatr 123:39, 1976.
2. Gruhn JG, Gorlin RJ, Langer LO Jr: Dyssegmental dwarfism. A lethal anisospondylic camptomicromelic dwarfism. Am J Dis Child 132:382, 1978.
3. Haller JO, Berdon WG, Robinow M, et al.: The Weissenbacher-Zweymuller syndrome of micrognathia and rhizomelic chondrodysplasia at birth with subsequent normal growth. AJR 125:936, 1975.
4. Handmaker SD, Campbell IA, Robinson LD, et al.: Dyssegmental dwarfism: A new syndrome of lethal dwarfism. Birth Defects 13(3D):79, 1977.
5. Kim HJ, Costales F, Bouzouki M, et al.: Prenatal diagnosis of dyssegmental dwarfism. Prenat Diagn 6:143, 1986.
6. Langer LO Jr, Gonzalez-Ramos M, Chen H, et al.: A severe infantile micromelic chondrodysplasia which resembles Kniest disease. Eur J Pediatr 123:29, 1976.
7. Opitz JM: Editorial comment to reference 4. Birth Defects 13(3D):89, 1977.
8. Rolland JC, Laugier J, Grenier B, et al.: Nanisme chondrodystrophique et division palatine chez un nouveau-né. Ann Pediatr (Paris) 19:139, 1972.

Larsen Syndrome

Definition
Larsen syndrome is a skeletal dysplasia characterized by a flat face, multiple joint laxities, and a supernumerary ossification center of the calcaneous.

Etiology
Although the original report included six sporadic cases,[4] subsequent communications suggest both autosomal recessive and dominant patterns of inheritance.[2,5,7] The severe type (associated with cardiac and vertebral abnormalities) seems to be inherited with an autosomal recessive pattern, whereas the mild form is probably an autosomal dominant disease.[1]

Pathology
Infants have a flat face, with a depressed nasal bridge, and joint laxity with multiple dislocations. Hypertelorism and clubfoot are frequently present. Cleft palate has been reported. A supernumerary ossification center in the calcaneous is pathognomonic of the disease, but it does not appear until the end of the first year of life. Scoliosis may develop with time.[6] Tubular bones are not shortened.[3,7]

Diagnosis
A prenatal diagnosis has not been reported. The diagnosis could be suspected by the combination of hypertelorism and joint dislocation in patients with a positive family history. Since the syndrome is characterized by joint laxity and these deformations are present at birth,[7] Larsen syndrome is potentially identifiable in patients at risk.

Prognosis
The autosomal dominant type is relatively benign. The recessive type is potentially lethal. Prognosis is generally related to the presence of cardiac lesions and spinal cord compression. An insufficient number of cases have been reported to permit adequate counseling of parents about the long-term prognosis of the disease.

Obstetrical Management
It is unclear if a prenatal diagnosis could be made before viability. In this case, the option of pregnancy termination should be offered to the parents. After viability, a diagnosis does not demand a change in standard obstetrical management.

REFERENCES

1. Cremin BJ, Beighton P: Bone Dysplasias of Infancy. Berlin, Springer-Verlag, 1978, pp 79–81.
2. Habermann ET, Sterling A, Dennis RI: Larsen syndrome: A heritable disorder. J Bone Joint Surg 58:558, 1976.
3. Kozlowski K, Robertson F, Middleton R: Radiographic findings in Larsen's syndrome. Aust Radiol 18:336, 1974.
4. Larsen LJ, Schottstaedt ER, Bost FD: Multiple congenital dislocations associated with a characteristic facial abnormality. J Paediatr 37:574, 1950.
5. Maroteaux P: Heterogeneity of Larsen's syndrome. Arch Fr Pediatr 32:597, 1975.
6. Micheli LJ, Hall JE, Watts HG: Spinal instability in Larsen's syndrome: Report of three cases. J Bone Joint Surg 58:562, 1976.
7. Oki T, Terashima Y, Murachi S, et al.: Clinical features and treatment of joint dislocations in Larsen's syndrome. Report of three cases in one family. Clin Orthop 119:206, 1976.

Otopalatodigital Syndrome Type II

Definition
This is a syndrome characterized by the combination of cleft palate, hearing loss, and skeletal abnormalities, including polydactyly, syndactyly, and bowed long bones.

Incidence
At least eight cases have been reported in the literature.[2,3]

Etiology
This disease seems to be transmitted as an X-linked recessive trait,[1,4] but an autosomal dominant pattern with variable expressivity has not been ruled out.[4]

Pathology
This syndrome has been recognized at birth in three infants.[1] The most prominent features include cleft palate, microstomia, micrognathia, flattened bridge of the nose, hypertelorism, flexed overlapping fingers, finger syndactyly and polydactyly, toe syndactyly, and short thumbs and short big toes.[4] The bones of forearms and legs are curved, and the fibula is frequently either absent or hypoplastic. The ribs are short and wavy. Some of the findings may change with growth (e.g., the curved long bones may disappear).

Diagnosis

A prenatal diagnosis of this condition has not been reported. The disorder should be suspected in the presence of micrognathia, polydactyly, syndactyly, clinodactyly, and curved long bones. The differential diagnosis should include campomelic syndrome, which may affect both males and females and has hypoplastic or absent scapulae, nonmineralized thoracic pedicles, and vertically narrow iliac bones.[2]

Prognosis

Six of the eight affected infants died shortly after birth. Of the survivors, one is mentally retarded,[5] and the other developed aseptic meningitis, multiple respiratory tract infections, and profound hearing loss but is reported to have normal psychomotor development and intelligence for his age.[3]

Obstetrical Management

The option of pregnancy termination should be offered if diagnosis is made before viability in a family at risk. After viability, no change in standard obstetrical management seems warranted.

REFERENCES

1. André M, Vigneron J, Didier F: Abnormal facies, cleft palate, and generalized dysostosis: A lethal X-linked syndrome. J Pediatr 98:747, 1981.
2. Brewster TG, Lachman RS, Kushner DC, et al.: Oto-palato-digital syndrome, Type II — An X-linked skeletal dysplasia. Am J Med Genet 20:249, 1985.
3. Fitch N, Jequier S, Gorlin R: The oto-palato-digital syndrome, proposed type II. Am J Med Genet 15:655, 1983.
4. Fitch N, Jequier S, Papageorgiou A: A familial syndrome of cranial, facial, oral and limb anomalies. Clin Genet 10:226, 1976.
5. Kozlowski K, Turner G, Scougall J, et al.: Oto-palato-digital syndrome with severe x-ray changes in two half brothers. Pediatr Radiol 6:97, 1977.

Cleidocranial Dysplasia

Synonyms

Cleidocranial dysostosis, mutational dysostosis.

Definition

This disorder is characterized mainly by absence or hypoplasia of the clavicles and by skull abnormalities.

Etiology

The disease is inherited as an autosomal dominant trait,[2,3] although some authors have suggested an autosomal recessive transmission.[1,5]

Pathology

Cleidocranial dysplasia is characterized by varying degrees of clavicular hypoplasia and skull abnormalities.[7] Absence of the clavicle occurs in only 10 percent of affected infants.[9] The thorax may be narrow, which could lead to respiratory distress. Other thoracic findings include supernumerary ribs and incompletely ossified sternum. The pubic bones are characteristically not ossified. Iliac bones are generally hypoplastic,[3] and long bones are of normal length.

TABLE 10–11. NOMOGRAM FOR EVALUATION OF CLAVICULAR SIZE

Gestational Age (weeks)	Clavicle Length (mm) Percentile		
	5th	50th	95th
15	11	16	21
16	12	17	22
17	13	18	23
18	14	19	24
19	15	20	25
20	16	21	26
21	17	22	27
22	18	23	28
23	19	24	29
24	20	25	30
25	21	26	31
26	22	27	32
27	23	28	33
28	24	29	34
29	25	30	35
30	26	31	36
31	27	32	37
32	28	33	38
33	29	34	39
34	30	35	40
35	31	36	41
36	32	37	42
37	33	38	43
38	34	39	44
39	35	40	45
40	36	41	46

Reproduced with permission from Yarkoni et al.: J Ultrasound Med 4:467, 1985.

TABLE 10–12. CONDITIONS ASSOCIATED WITH CLAVICULAR HYPOPLASIA OR AGENESIS

Finding	Condition
Minimal, inconsistent, rare hypoplasia	Sprengel deformity, Klippel-Feil, many others

Significant hypoplasia or agenesis	Skeletal dysostosis
	  Chromosome disorder (11q partial trisomy, 11q/22q partial trisomy, 20p trisomy)
	  Multiple congenital anomalies
	  Dysplasia cleidofacialis [8]
	  Digit–mandible–clavicle hypoplasia[11]
	  Microcephaly–micrognathia–contracture dwarfism[1]
	  Imperforate anus–psoriasis–clavicle deficiency[4]

Associated with significant upper limb deficiency	Roberts syndrome, Holt-Oram syndrome, thrombocytopenia–radial aplasia, many others
Associated with lethal neonatal dwarfism	Achondrogenesis, hyperplastic osteogenesis imperfecta, others

Modified from Hall. In: Papadatos, Bartsocas (eds): Skeletal Dysplasias. New York, Liss, 1982.

The skull shows wide sutures and multiple wormian bones (small and irregular bones in the course of the cranial sutures). The foramen magnum is enlarged, and paranasal sinuses are absent. The anterior fontanel remains open. Scoliosis is a rare but serious complication.[3]

Diagnosis

Although a prenatal diagnosis of cleidocranial dysplasia has not been reported, its identification seems feasible, since the clavicles are easily imaged with ultrasound (see Fig. 10–1). The diagnosis does not depend on absence of the clavicles. In fact, in most instances, clavicles are hypoplastic. Figure 10–17 displays the growth of the clavicle during gestation. Table 10–11 is a nomogram for the assessment of clavicular size. Hypoplastic or absent clavicles are not pathognomonic

of cleidocranial dysplasia, and other entities with such findings are listed in Table 10–12.

Prognosis

This condition does not seriously affect the individual and frequently goes unrecognized. Problems associated with the disease include occasional luxation of the shoulder and hip and scoliosis.

Obstetrical Management

Standard obstetrical management is not altered by diagnosis of this condition.

REFERENCES

1. Bixler D, Antley RM: Microcephalic dwarfism in sisters. Birth Defects 10(7):161, 1974.
2. Faure C, Maroteaux P: Progress in Pediatric Radiology. Intrinsic Diseases of Bones,. Cleidocranial Dysplasia. Basel, Karger, 1973, Vol 4, p 211.
3. Forland, M: Cleidocranial dysostosis. Am Med 33:792, 1962.
4. Fukuda K, Miyanomae T, Nakata E, et al.: Two siblings with cleidocranial dysplasia associated with atresia ani and psoriasis-like lesions: A new syndrome? Eur J Pediatr 136:109, 1981.
5. Goodman RM, Tadmor R, Zaritsky A, et al.: Evidence for an autosomal recessive form of cleidocranial dysostosis. Clin Genet 8:20, 1975.
6. Hall BD: Syndromes and situations associated with congenital clavicular hypoplasia or agenesis. In: Papadatos CJ, Bartsocas CS (eds): Skeletal Dysplasias. New York, Alan R. Liss, 1982, pp 279–288.
7. Jarvis LJ, Keats TE: Cleidocranial dysostosis, a review of 40 new cases. AJR 121:5, 1974.
8. Kozlowski K, Hanicka M, Zygulska-Machowa H: Dysplasia cleido-facialis. Z Kinderheilk 108:331, 1970.
9. Soule AB: Mutational dysostosis (cleidocranial dysostosis) J Bone Joint Surg 28:81, 1946.
10. Yarkoni S, Schmidt W, Jeanty P, et al.: Clavicular measurement: A new biometric parameter for fetal evaluation. J Ultrasound Med 4:467, 1985.
11. Yunis E, Varon H: Cleidocranial dysostosis, severe micrognathism, bilateral absence of thumbs and first metatarsal bone and distal aphalangia. A new genetic syndrome. Am J Dis Child 134:649, 1980.

Dysostoses

Dysostoses refer to malformations or absence of individual bones singly or in combination. Any bone can be affected. Table 10–2 shows the classification of

dysostosis of the International Nomenclature Group of Skeletal Dysplasias. There are three main groups, depending on the most affected part of the skeleton:

dysostosis with craniofacial involvement, dysostosis with predominant axial involvement, and dysostosis with predominant involvement of the extremities.

Diagnosis

Some of the listed conditions have been diagnosed in utero by fetoscopy or ultrasound or are amenable to prenatal detection. A definitive diagnosis is possible in cases at risk.[1-3] The most frequent conditions are discussed in subsequent sections.

REFERENCES

1. Filkins K, Russo J, Bilinki I, et al.: Prenatal diagnosis of thrombocytopenia absent radius syndrome using ultrasound and fetoscopy. Prenat Diagn 4:139, 1984.
2. Nicolaides KH, Johansson D, Donnai D, et al.: Prenatal diagnosis of mandibulofacial dysostosis. Prenat Diagn 4:201, 1984.
3. Savoldelli G, Schinzel A: Prenatal ultrasound detection of humero-radial synostosis in a case of Antley-Bixler syndrome. Prenat Diagn 2:219, 1982.

TABLE 10–13. CLASSIFICATION OF CRANIOSYNOSTOSES

I. Idiopathic craniosynostosis
  A. Scaphocephaly
    1. Leptocephaly
    2. Clinocephaly
    3. Sphenocephaly
    4. Bathmocephaly
  B. Brachycephaly–acrobrachycephaly–turricephaly
  C. Plagiocephaly
  D. Trigonocephaly
  E. Pachycephaly
  F. Oxycephaly
II. Craniosynostosis as part of other known syndromes
  A. Chromosomal syndromes
    1. 1q− syndrome
    2. 3q+ syndrome
    3. 5p+ syndrome
    4. 6q+ syndrome
    5. 7p− syndrome
    6. 9p− syndrome
    7. 11q− syndrome
    8. 12p− syndrome
    9. 13q− syndrome
    10. Triploidy
  B. Monogenic syndromes
    11. Apert syndrome
    12. Armendares syndrome
    13. Baller-Gerold syndrome
    14. Berant syndrome
    15. Carpenter syndrome
    16. Christian syndrome type I
    17. Christian syndrome type II
    18. Cloverleaf skull anomaly
    19. Cranioectodermal dysplasia
    20. Craniofacial dyssynostosis
    21. Craniofrontonasal dysplasia
    22. Crouzon syndrome
    23. Elejalde syndrome
    24. Escobar-Bixler syndrome
    25. Gorlin-Chaudhry-Moss syndrome
    26. Hootnick-Holmes syndrome
    27. Jones syndrome
    28. Lowry syndrome
    29. Opitz-Kaveggia FG syndrome
    30. Pfeiffer syndrome
    31. Seathre-Chotzen syndrome
    32. San Francisco syndrome
    33. Summit syndrome
    34. Ventruto syndrome
    35. Washington syndrome type I
    36. Washington syndrome type II
    37. Weiss syndrome
  C. Teratogenically induced syndromes
    38. Amniopterin syndrome
    39. Fetal hydantoin syndrome
  D. Unknown genesis syndromes
    40. Antley-Bixler syndrome
    41. Campomelic syndrome
    42. Craniotelencephalic dysplasia
    43. Fairbanks syndrome
    44. Hall syndrome
    45. Hausam syndrome
    46. Herrmann-Opitz syndrome
    47. Herrmann-Pallister-Opitz syndrome
    48. Idaho syndrome type I
    49. Idaho syndrome type II
    50. Lacheretz-Allain syndrome
    51. Lowry-Maclean syndrome
    52. McGillivray syndrome
    53. Montefiore syndrome
    54. Pederson syndrome
    55. Sakati-Nyhan-Tisdale syndrome
    56. Say-Meyer syndrome
    57. Waardenburg craniosynostosis syndrome
    58. Wardinsky syndrome
    59. Wisconsin syndrome
III. Craniosynostosis in association with other conditions
  A. Hematologic disorders
    1. Thalassemia
    2. Sickle cell anemia
    3. Polycythemia vera
    4. Congenital hemolytic icterus
  B. Metabolic disorders
    1. Calcium metabolism alterations
      a. Idiopathic hypercalcemia
      b. Vitamin D deficiency rickets
      c. Vitamin D resistant rickets
      d. Hypophosphatasia
    2. Hyperthyroidism
    3. Mucopolysaccharidosis
      a. Hurler syndrome
      b. Morquio syndrome
      c. β-Glucurondiase deficiency
    4. Mucolipidosis III
  C. Iatrogenic disorders
    1. CSF diversion procedures
  D. Various disorders
    1. Epidermal nevus syndrome
    2. Job's syndrome
    3. Microcephaly
IV. Craniosynostosis induced by mechanical compression
  A. Fetal constraint
  B. Postnatal deformities
    1. Postural deformities
    2. Intentional deformations

Reproduced with permission From David et al.: The Craniosynostoses. Causes, Natural History, and Management. Berlin, Springer-Verlag, 1982.

Craniosynostoses

Synonym
Craniostenoses.

Definition
Craniosynostosis is an abnormal shape or dimension of the skull caused by premature closure of one or more skull sutures. It includes scaphocephaly, brachycephaly, oxycephaly, plagiocephaly, trigonocephaly, turricephaly, and cloverleaf skull.

Incidence
Since craniosynostoses are not lethal or always diagnosed at birth, a birth prevalence cannot be provided. Neurosurgical files provide an incidence of 1 in 4000 births.[1]

Etiology
Craniosynostoses can be due to an idiopathic developmental error (primary craniosynostoses) or part of other syndromes that involve other abnormalities, such as chromosomal, metabolic, inherited mendelian disorders, teratogenic (e.g., aminopterin), or infectious. Table 10–13 provides a list of conditions associated with craniosynostoses. For further details, references 1 and 2 are excellent texts on the subject.

Pathogenesis and Pathology
The names and locations of skull sutures are shown in Figure 10–73. All sutures close anatomically after the fourth decade of life, with the exception of the frontal or metopic suture that closes during infancy in 90 percent of people (in the remaining 10 percent, it never closes). Premature closure of skull sutures results in alteration of the shape of the skull, but, more importantly, craniosynostosis prohibits normal growth of the brain and leads to intracranial hypertension, brain dysfunction, and visual impairment. The brain increases in weight by 85 percent during the first 6 months after birth and by 135 percent during the first year. Visual symptoms are attributed to traction and distortion of the optic nerve.

During intrauterine life, the skull bones are separated by fibrous tissue that remains from the original membranous constitution of the calvarium. The mechanisms responsible for the physiologic closure of the skull sutures are not known. Several hypotheses have been proposed to explain the occurrence of craniosynostosis: (1) hypoplasia of the fibrous tissue normally interposed between the bones, (2) primary decrease in intracranial pressure, (3) anomalous ossification process, and (4) primary anomaly in the base of the skull interfering with venous outflow or the architectural growth of the vault.

When craniosynostosis occurs, growth of adjacent bones is inhibited in a direction perpendicular to the closed suture. This results in a compensatory growth of the vault in the direction of the open sutures and fontanelles. The nomenclature of craniosynostoses refers to the shape of the head. Craniosynostoses are commonly classified according to the involved suture (Fig. 10–74).

Diagnosis
Physiologic molding of the fetal head occurs frequently due to changes in intrauterine pressure, position, intrauterine tumors, and oligohydramnios. The two most frequent types are dolicocephaly and brachycephaly. Diagnosis of these conditions is made by the cephalic index, which describes the relationship between the biparietal and the occipitofrontal diameters. The normal range is 75 to 85 percent when an outer-to-inner biparietal diameter and a midecho-to-midecho occipitofrontal diameter are used. The cranial sutures can be imaged with ultrasound (Fig. 10–75). Dolicocephaly is diagnosed when the cephalic index is below 75 percent, and brachycephaly is diagnosed when the index is above 85 percent. In either case, biparietal diameter should not be used for

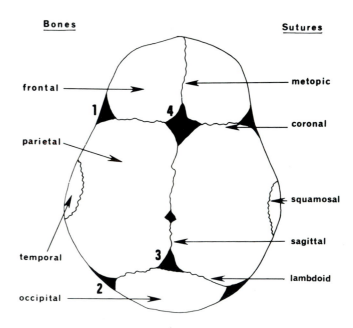

Figure 10–73. Schematic arrangement of the bones, sutures, and fontanelles. The fontanelles are: 1, sphenoidal, 2, mastoid, 3, occipital, 4, frontal. *(Reproduced with permission from David et al.: The Craniosynostoses. Causes, Natural History, and Management. Berlin, Springer-Verlag, 1982.)*

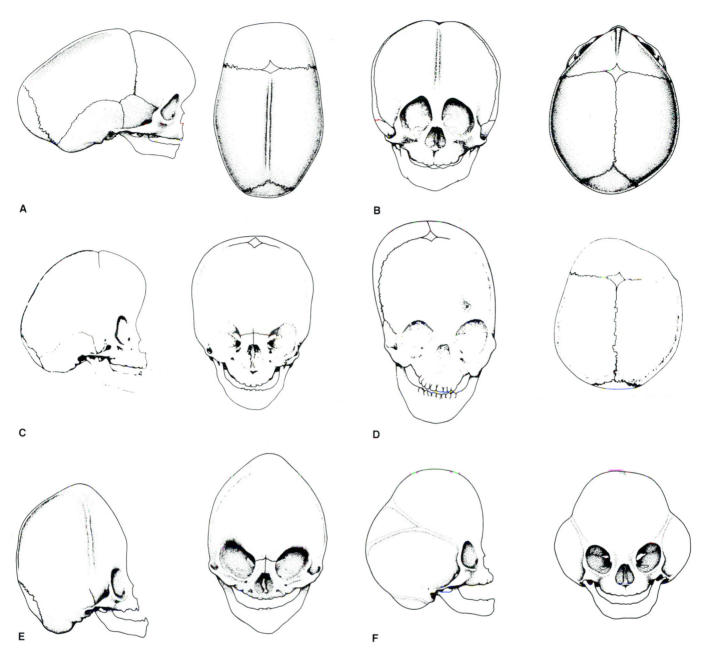

Figure 10–74. Schematic representation of the most common craniosynostoses. **A**. Scaphocephaly. **B**. Trigonocephaly. **C**. Turricephaly. **D**. Frontal plagiocephaly. **E**. Oxycephaly with bregmatic prominence. **F**. Cloverleaf skull. *(Reproduced with permission from David et al: The Craniosynostoses. Causes, Natural History, and Management. Berlin, Springer-Verlag, 1982.)*

gestational age prediction. Since the head perimeter does not change with molding, this parameter can be used to assess gestational age when an abnormal cephalic index is present.

A specific diagnosis of craniosynostosis in utero is extremely difficult (except for cloverleaf skull and trigonocephaly). There is no information about the natural history of craniostenoses in utero. Antenatal diagnosis of these conditions has barely been discussed in the literature. Some practical diagnostic guidelines follow.

Premature closure of the sagittal suture (scapho-

cephaly) is characterized by a disproportionately large occipitofrontal and short biparietal diameter.

Premature closure of the coronal suture (brachycephaly) is characterized by a cephalic index above 85 percent. Still, the differential diagnosis with molding appears difficult. A sagittal scan of the fetal face can be helpful by demonstrating a very prominent forehead. Hypertelorism is sometimes associated with this type of craniosynostosis.

Premature closure of the metopic or frontal suture (trigonocephaly) is characterized by a triangular or egg-shaped head (oocephaly) (Figs. 10–76, 10–77).

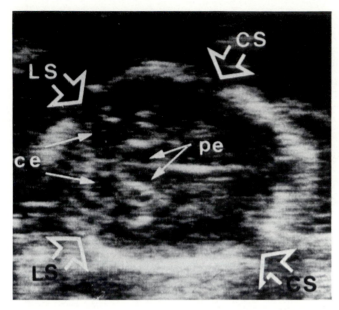

Figure 10–75. Skull sutures in an axial scan of the fetal head. CS, coronal sutures; LS, lambdoid suture; ce, cerebellar hemispheres; pe, cerebral peduncles. *(Reproduced with permission from Jeanty, Romero: Obstetrical Ultrasound. New York, McGraw-Hill, 1983.)*

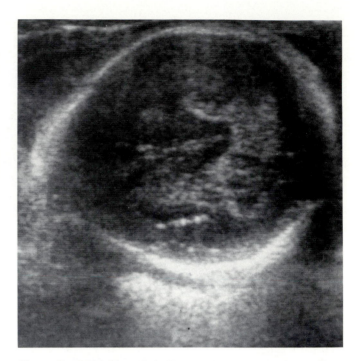

Figure 10–76. Trigonocephaly diagnosed in utero at 28 weeks. Note the egg-shaped appearance of the skull.

Since the upper portion of the orbits are formed by the frontal bone, premature closure of the metopic suture frequently leads to hypotelorism.

Oxycephaly is a craniosynostosis that results from fusion of multiple sutures and leads to a high, conical, pointed head (Fig. 10–78). Different head shapes can result depending on the involved sutures. If the main involved suture is the sagittal, a form of scaphocephaly will result. A variety of turricephaly occurs if the coronal suture is primarily affected. Cloverleaf skull is a variety of oxycephaly.

Cloverleaf skull syndrome, or Kleeblattschadel, is characterized by the association of premature closure of the coronal, lambdoid, and sagittal sutures and hydrocephalus (usually a communicating type or aqueductal stenosis). As a consequence of this craniosynostosis, grotesque bulging of the temporal, occipital, and frontal bones occurs (Figs. 10–42, 10–43, 10–46, 10–47). This diagnosis can be made easily with ultrasound.

Turricephaly is an abnormally broad head with a high forehead and is due to premature closure of the coronal suture. Plagiocephaly is due to asymmetrical synostosis of a suture—the coronal suture (frontal plagiocephaly), the lambdoid suture (occipital plagiocephaly)—or more than one suture (hemicranial plagiocephaly).

Associated Anomalies

Craniosynostoses are frequently associated with other anomalies (Table 10–13). Therefore, the sonographer must perform a throrough fetal examination.

Prognosis

The prognosis is dependent primarily on the presence of associated anomalies. Secondarily, there are some differences in neurologic and intellectual performance according to the type of craniosynostosis.

Scaphocephaly is not usually associated with

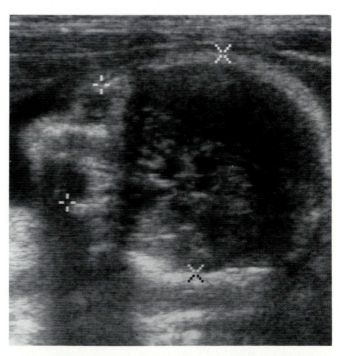

Figure 10–77. Axial scan at the level of the orbits of the fetus shown in Figure 10–76. Hypotelorism is apparent.

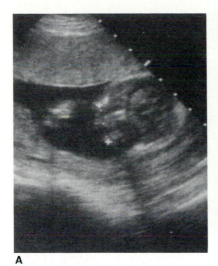
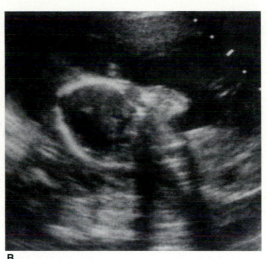

A   B

Figure 10–78. Oxycephaly. **A.** The picture on the left is a transverse scan demonstrating hypothelorism. **B.** On the right, a sagittal scan of the head of the same fetus. Note a reduction in the occipitofrontal diameter and the cone-shaped appearance of the head.

symptoms of intracranial pressure, and its relationship with mental retardation is unclear. Most infants seem to do well, but ocular problems have been reported. Prognosis is, however, different for those patients with associated Apert, Cruzon, and Carpenter syndromes.

Brachycephaly is frequently associated with symptoms of elevated intracranial pressure and ophthalmologic problems, including exophthalmos, strabismus, and optic nerve atrophy.

Trigonocephaly is associated with a higher incidence of mental retardation than the other types. In addition, other congenital anomalies are frequently associated with this syndrome (holoprosencephaly, cleft palate, microphthalmos).

Surgical procedures to accomplish decompression of the intracranial content and cosmetic changes are available. Their value in altering the course of neurologic impairment in these syndromes seems promising.

Obstetrical Management

Detection of an abnormally shaped head is an indication for a careful search for associated anomalies. Amniocentesis to look for chromosomal anomalies is indicated. The diagnosis of craniosynostosis per se does not change obstetrical management. However, the etiology of the disorder may alter obstetrical management (e.g., a chromosomal disorder).

REFERENCES

1. David DJ, Poswillo D, Simpson D: The Craniosynostoses. Causes, Natural History, and Management. Berlin, Springer-Verlag, 1982.
2. Galli G: Craniosynostosis. Boca Raton, FL, CRC Press, 1984.

LIMB REDUCTION ABNORMALITIES

The term "limb reduction abnormalities" refers to the absence of a limb or a segment of a limb. These defects are usually nongenetic in origin except for a few rare syndromes.

Terms frequently used to refer to limb reduction abnormalities include:

- Amelia: absence of a limb or limbs
- Hemimelia: absence of a longitudinal segment of a limb (e.g., radial aplasia, radial hypoplasia)
- Phocomelia: hypoplasia of the limbs, with hands and feet attached to the shoulder and hips
- Acheira: absence of a hand or hands
- Apodia: absence of a foot or feet

- Acheiropodia: absence of hands and feet

The prenatal diagnosis of isolated limb reduction abnormalities is technically simple. It is our opinion that identification of all segments of both extremities should be an integral part of a routine sonographic examination. This approach must be taken because limb reduction abnormalities are by and large a nongenetic group of disorders.

We will discuss only three entities with important genetic and diagnostic value that we have encountered in our prenatal diagnostic practice: Roberts syndrome, Holt-Oram syndrome, and thrombocytopenia with absent radius.

Roberts Syndrome

Synonyms
Tetraphocomelia with cleft lip and palate, Appelt–Gerken syndrome, hypomelia–hypotrichosis–facial hemangioma syndrome.

Definition
This disorder is characterized by the association of tetraphocomelia with midfacial clefting or hypoplastic nasal alae.[2,3]

Etiology
Autosomal recessive.

Pathology
The most important finding is the reduction deformity of the four limbs. Reduction is more prominent in the upper than lower extremities and may consist of absence or severe micromelia. Toes and fingers may be absent or reduced in number. Other limb abnormalities include bowing of long bones, flexion contractures of knees and elbows, and clubfoot deformities.[1,4] Severe growth retardation is a prevalent feature.

Facial abnormalities are also prominent and include hypertelorism and cleft lip or palate, which may be bilateral or in the midline. Polyhydramnios has been described. Other findings are hypoplasia of the alae nasi, ocular proptosis, and microcephaly. The phallus or clitoris can be prominent.[3]

Associated Anomalies
Hydrocephaly, encephalocele, spina bifida, and polycystic and horseshoe kidneys.

Diagnosis
The diagnosis can be made in patients at risk by demonstrating the severe limb reduction abnormalities and the described facial features. Specific diagnosis of a sporadic case would be extremely difficult.

Prognosis
The condition is associated with a high perinatal mortality. The syndrome has been reviewed by Freeman et al., who found that 15 of 19 patients were either stillborn or died within the first month of life.[1] Survivors have a short life span, and mental retardation is common.

Obstetrical Management
The option of pregnancy termination should be offered before viability.

REFERENCES

1. Freeman MVR, Williams DW, Schimke N, et al: The Roberts syndrome. Clin Genet 5:1, 1974.
2. Roberts JB: A child with double cleft of lip and palate, protrusion of the intermaxillary portion of the upper jaw and imperfect development of the bones of the four extremities. Ann Surg 70:252, 1919.
3. Smith DW: Recognizable Patterns of Human Malformation. Genetic, Embryologic and Clinical Aspects. Philadelphia, Saunders, 1982, p 221.
4. Waldenmaier C, Aldenhoff P, Klemm T: The Roberts syndrome. Hum Genet 40:345, 1978.

Holt-Oram Syndrome

Synonyms
Atriodigital dysplasia, cardiac limb syndrome, upper limb cardiovascular syndrome, cardiomelic syndrome, and heart upper limb syndrome.

Definition
The Holt-Oram syndrome is characterized by the association of aplasia or hypoplasia of the radial structures and congenital heart disease, mainly atrial septal defect secundum type.[1,3]

Etiology
The disorder is inherited with an autosomal dominant pattern with variable degree of penetrance.[2]

Pathology
The skeletal abnormalities encompass a wide spectrum of defects. Basically, they affect the radial structures, which include the thumb, the first metacarpal, the carpal bones, and the radius. The defects range

from absence, hypoplasia, or triphalangism of the thumb to upper limb hemimelia.

The most common cardiac abnormality is an atrial septal defect secundum type. Other reported cardiac anomalies include ventricular septal defect, tetralogy of Fallot, and coarctation of the aorta. In some family members, only the cardiac or skeletal abnormalities are present.[3]

Diagnosis

The diagnosis can be made in a patient at risk by demonstrating the skeletal anomaly. It is doubtful that a small ostium secundum defect can be recognized by ultrasound. A specific diagnosis of Holt-Oram syndrome in fresh mutations seems extremely difficult.

Prognosis

The prognosis depends on the severity of the cardiac congenital abnormality. Functional impairment depends on the extent of the skeletal defect.

Obstetrical Management

The option of pregnancy termination should be offered before viability. After viability standard obstetrical management is not altered.

REFERENCES

1. Holt M, Oram S: Familial heart disease with skeletal malformations. Br Heart J 22:236, 1960.
2. Kaufman RL, Rimoin DL, McAlister WH, et al.: Variable expression of the Holt-Oram syndrome. Am J Dis Child 127:21, 1974.
3. Smith DW: Recognizable Patterns of Human Malformation. Genetic, Embryologic and Clinical Aspects. Philadelphia, Saunders, 1982, p 232.

Thrombocytopenia with Absent Radius

Synonyms

TAR syndrome, amegakaryocytic thrombocytopenia and bilateral absence of the radii, and phocomelia with congenital thrombocytopenia.

Definition

This syndrome is characterized by thrombocytopenia (platelet count of less than 100,000/mm³) and bilateral absence of the radius.

Etiology

The disease is inherited with an autosomal recessive pattern.

Pathology

The radius is absent bilaterally in all cases. The ulna and humerus may be unilaterally or bilaterally absent or hypoplastic. Clubfoot and hand deformations have been described.[4]

Thrombocytopenia is present in all patients. It is due to a decreased production of platelets by bone marrow. The platelet count fluctuates and can be sometimes within normal range. Stress associated with surgery or infections can induce thrombocytopenia.

Associated Anomalies

Cardiac anomalies are found in 33 percent of patients.[2] The most common defects are tetralogy of Fallot and atrial septal defects. Other anomalies include renal malformations, spina bifida, brachycephaly, micrognathia, and syndactyly.[1,5]

Diagnosis

The diagnosis can be made in a patient at risk in whom radial aplasia is detected with ultrasound.[1,3] Thrombocytopenia may be absent at presentation.

Prognosis

The disease is associated with a high fatality rate within the first months of life. Ten of 40 patients reviewed by Hall et al. died in that period of time.[2] After 1 year, prognosis improves considerably. Mental retardation is present in 8 percent of the patients, and it is usually mild.[2] Intracranial bleeding associated with thrombocytopenia is the proposed mechanism. Long-term disability is related to the skeletal deformity. Some patients develop nerve compression and arthritis because of the hand deformations.

Obstetrical Management

Diagnosis before viability would make elective termination of pregnancy possible. After viability, the most important consideration is to avoid the intracranial hemorrhage that could be associated with a traumatic delivery. Therefore, an elective cesarean section can be performed or, alternatively, a percutaneous umbilical cord puncture may be used to assess the fetal platelet count. In the presence of a normal value, labor may be allowed.

REFERENCES

1. Filkins K, Russo J, Bilinki I, et al.: Prenatal diagnosis of thrombocytopenia absent radius syndrome using ultrasound and fetoscopy. Prenat Diagn 4:139, 1984.
2. Hall JG, Levin J, Kuhn JP, et al.: Thrombocytopenia with absent radius (TAR). Medicine 48:411, 1969.
3. Luthy DA, Hall JG, Graham CB, et al.: Prenatal diagnosis of thrombocytopenia with absent radii. Clin Genet 15:495, 1979.
4. Ray R, Zon E, Kelly T, et al.: Brief clinical report: Lower limb anomalies in the thrombocytopenia absent-radius (TAR) syndrome. Am J Med Genet 7:523, 1980.
5. Smith DW: Recognizable Patterns of Human Malformation. Genetic, Embryologic and Clinical Aspects. Philadelphia, Saunders, 1982, p 236.

Polydactyly

Definition
Presence of extra digits.

Epidemiology
The incidence varies in different ethnic groups.

Etiology
Polydactyly is a feature of many genetic syndromes. Table 10–14 shows the most common associations. Isolated postaxial polydactyly, polydactyly of the index finger, and polydactyly of the triphalangeal thumb are inherited as autosomal dominant traits with variable penetrance.[1]

Pathology
Polydactyly can be classified as preaxial and postaxial, depending on the presence of the extra digit on the ulnar side (postaxial) or on the radial side (preaxial) of the hand. The same concept applies to the foot. The former is more common than the latter. In some cases, the extra digit is a simple cutaneous appendage, whereas in others, it contains a full bony complement.[2]

Diagnosis
Diagnosis of polydactyly can be made with ultrasound provided the extra digit contains bony structures (Fig. 10–79). The ideal means for imaging the hands is in a coronal view where all the fingers can be counted. The same approach can be used with the feet.

Prognosis
The prognosis is dependent on the presence or absence of associated congenital anomalies. A careful search for other defects is necessary both prenatally and postnatally.

Obstetrical Management
Management is dependent on the associated disorder.

REFERENCES

1. Beighton P: Inherited disorders of the skeleton. Edinburgh, Churchill Livingstone, 1978, pp 192–194.
2. Smith DW, Jones KL: Recognizable Patterns of Human Malformation. Genetic, Embryologic and Clinical Aspects, 3d ed. Philadelphia, Saunders, 1982, p 633.

TABLE 10–14. SYNDROMES FEATURING POLYDACTYLY

Frequent Finding	Occasional Finding
Carpenter syndrome	Bloom syndrome
Ellis–van Creveld syndrome	Conradi-Hunermann syndrome
Meckel-Gruber syndrome	Goltz syndrome
Polysyndactyly syndrome	Klippel-Trenaunay-Weber syndrome
Towne syndrome	
Trisomy 13 syndrome	Oral–Facial–digital syndrome
Short rib–polydactyly syndrome	Partial trisomy 10q syndrome
	Rubinstein-Taybi syndrome
	Smith-Opitz syndrome
	Trisomy 4p syndrome

Reproduced with permission from Smith, Jones: Recognizable Patterns of Human Malformation, 3d ed. Philadelphia, Saunders, 1982.

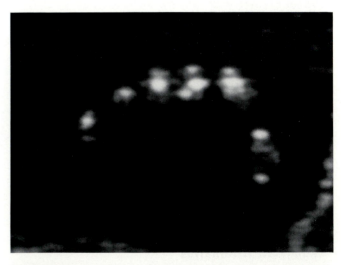

Figure 10–79. Scan of the hand of a fetus with short rib–polydactyly syndrome. Six digits are clearly identified.

Congenital Contractures: Clubfoot

Synonyms
Equinovarus and talipes.

Definition
This defect is characterized by medial deviation and inversion of the sole of the foot.

TABLE 10–15. SYNDROMES ASSOCIATED WITH CLUBFEET

Frequent
  Amyoplasia congenita disruptive sequence
  Diastrophic dysplasia syndrome
  Distal arthrogryposis syndrome
  Escobar syndrome
  Femoral hypoplasia—unusual facies syndrome
  Fetal aminopterin effects (varus)
  Freeman-Sheldon syndrome (varus with contracted toes)
  Hecht syndrome
  Larsen syndrome
  Meckel-Gruber syndrome
  Moebius sequence
  Partial trisomy 10q syndrome
  Pena-Shokeir I syndrome
  Triploidy syndrome
  Trisomy 9 mosaic syndrome
  Trisomy 9p syndrome
  Trisomy 20p syndrome
  Zellweger syndrome
  4p– syndrome
  9p– syndrome
  13q– syndrome
  18q– syndrome
Occasional
  Aarskog syndrome
  Bloom syndrome
  Conradi-Hunermann syndrome
  Dubowitz syndrome
  Ehlers-Danlos syndrome
  Ellis–van Creveld syndrome (valgus)
  Generalized gangliosidosis syndrome
  Homocystinuria syndrome (pes cabus, everted feet)
  Hunter syndrome
  Mietens syndrome
  Nail–patella syndrome
  Noonan syndrome
  Popliteal web syndrome
  Radial aplasia–thrombocytopenia syndrome
  Riley-Day syndrome
  Schwartz syndrome
  Seckel syndrome
  Steinert myotonic dystrophy syndrome
  Trisomy 4p syndrome
  Trisomy 13 syndrome
  Trisomy 18 syndrome
  Weaver syndrome
  XXXXX syndrome
  XXXXY syndrome
  Zellweger syndrome
  18 p– syndrome

Reproduced with permission from Smith: *Recognizable Patterns of Human Deformations.* Philadelphia, Saunders, 1982.

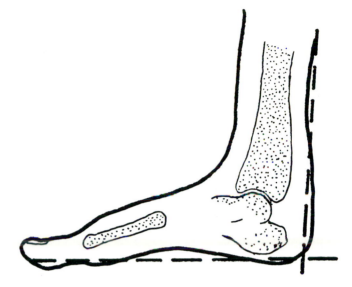

Figure 10–80. Diagram of a normal foot. A lateral longitudinal scan of the leg would show two bones and the heel.

Epidemiology
The overall incidence is reported to be 1.2 in 1000.[6] The male to female ratio is 2:1. When the mild forms of postural clubfoot are considered, the ratio is reversed.[6]

Etiology
Clubfoot can be caused by genetic or environmental causes. There may be a genetic predisposition to laxity of the joint ligaments.[2] Indeed, a tendency toward dislocation of hips and shoulders has been documented in first degree relatives.[1] Other congenital diseases, such as skeletal dysplasias (e.g., dias-

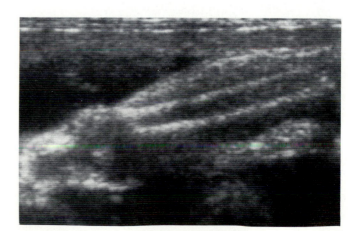

Figure 10–81. Sonogram taken in the lateral longitudinal plane. Note the two bones in the leg and the heel.

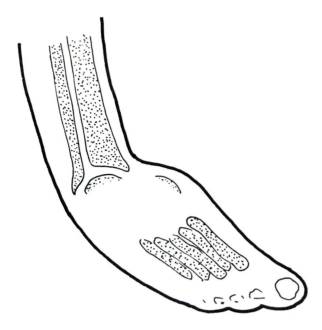

Figure 10–82. Diagram of a clubfoot. *(Reproduced with permission from Jeanty, et al.: J Ultrasound Med 4:595, 1985.)*

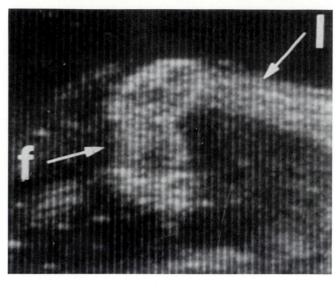

Figure 10–84. Clubfoot. l, leg; f, foot. *(Reproduced with permission from Jeanty, Romero: Obstetrical Ultrasound. New York, McGraw-Hill, 1984.)*

trophic dysplasia), limb deficiencies, or neurologic disorders (e.g., spina bifida), are associated with this condition.

Environmental causes are those associated with intrauterine constraint (oligohydramnios, amniotic band syndrome, and uterine tumors).

Clubfoot is a feature of many genetic syndromes, which are listed in Table 10–15.

Pathology

The basic pathology is inversion of the foot and flexion of the sole. The navicular bone comes closer to the medial portion of the calcaneous.

Diagnosis

Diagnosis is based on knowledge of the relative orientation of the leg bones and the heel of the foot. When a normal lower extremity is scanned in the lateral axis, the two bones of the leg and the heel are imaged (Figs. 10–80, 10–81). In clubfoot, a similar view will demonstrate the leg bones and both the heel and forefoot (Figs. 10–82 through 10–85).[3,4]

Another approach to the diagnosis is to use the anteroposterior view of the leg, which allows visualization of both the leg and the entire foot. In a fetus with clubfoot deformity, only the heel will be seen. The diagnosis of clubfoot in the presence of oligohy

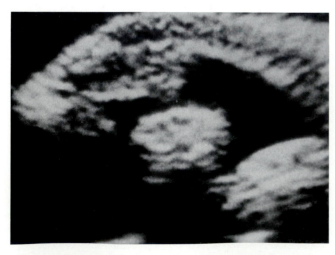

Figure 10–83. Clubfoot. *(Reproduced with permission from Jeanty, Romero: Obstetrical Ultrasound. New York, McGraw-Hill, 1984.)*

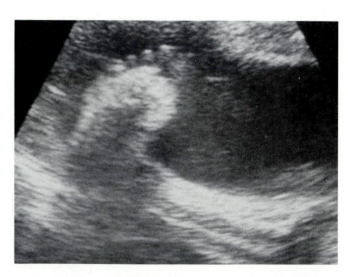

Figure 10–85. Clubfoot.

dramnios is difficult. Recognition of a clubfoot deformity should prompt a careful search for associated
anomalies, particularly a neural tube defect.

Prognosis

The prognosis is dependent on the etiology of the
equinovarus. Cases secondary to intrauterine constraint have a better prognosis than those associated
with true malformations.[5]

Obstetrical Management

This defect does not alter obstetrical management at
any time in gestation.

REFERENCES

1. Carter C, Sweetnam R: Recurrent dislocation of the
patella and of the shoulder. J Bone Joint Surg 42B:721,
1960.
2. Carter C, Wilkinson JA: Persistent joint laxity and congenital dislocation of the hip. J Bone Joint Surg 46B:40,
1964.
3. Jeanty P, Romero R: Obstetrical Ultrasound. New York,
McGraw-Hill, 1984, pp 195–198.
4. Jeanty P, Romero R, d'Alton M, et al.: In utero
sonographic detection of hand and foot deformities. J
Ultrasound Med 4:595, 1985
5. Smith DW: Recognizable Patterns of Human Deformations. Philadelphia, Saunders, 1982, pp 12–15.
6. Wynne-Davis R: Family studies and aetiology of club
foot. J Med Genet 2:227, 1965.

Rocker-Bottom Foot

Definition
This defect is characterized by a prominent heel with
a convex sole.

Etiology
This anomaly is associated with trisomy 18, 18q–
syndrome, and cerebrooculofacioskeletal syndrome.[1]

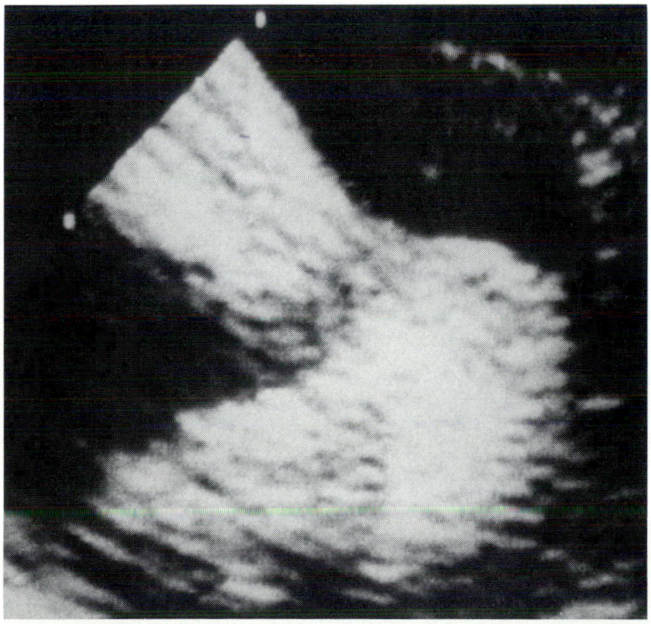

Epidemiology
Unknown.

Pathology
The defect is due to a prominent calcaneus. The sole
adopts a rounded or convex shape.

Diagnosis
Sonographic imaging of the foot and leg in the
anteroposterior axis may allow the diagnosis. Figure
10–86 shows an image of a rocker-bottom foot.[2]

Identification of this deformity should prompt a
careful search for associated congenital anomalies.
An amniocentesis to exclude chromosomal abnormalities should be considered.

Prognosis
Prognosis depends on the presence and severity of
associated anomalies.

Figure 10–86. Typical image of a rocker-bottom foot. *(Reproduced with permission from Jeanty, Romero: Obstetrical Ultrasound. New York, McGraw-Hill, 1984.)*

REFERENCES

1. Bergsma D. Birth Defects Compendium, 2d ed. New
York, Alan R. Liss, 1979, pp 180, 200, 201, 1062.
2. Jeanty P, Romero R: Obstetrical Ultrasound. New York,
McGraw-Hill, 1984.

Arthrogryposis Multiplex Congenita

Synonyms

Classic arthrogryposis, myodystrophia fetalis deformans, multiple congenital rigidities, congenital arthromyodysplasia, myophagism congenita, and amyoplasia congenita.

Definition

The term "arthrogryposis multiplex congenita" (AMC) refers to multiple joint contractures present at birth.[6] AMC is not a specific disorder but is the consequence of neurologic, muscular, connective tissue, and skeletal abnormalities or intrauterine crowding, which may lead to limitation of fetal joint mobility and the development of contractures (Fig. 10–87).[6]

Incidence

The incidence of AMC varies widely because different definitions and heterogeneous conditions have been grouped under the term AMC, and the accuracy of these figures is open to question.

Etiology

Normal intrauterine movement is essential for the development of fetal joints, which occurs during the 3d month of gestation.[11] Any process that impairs fetal motion around this critical time leads to congenital contractures.[3] Administration of curare to chick embryos[2] or fixation of the ankle joint[4] has resulted in the development of contractures. In the human, prolonged administration of curare to a mother with tetanus has been reported to lead to AMC.[7] The role of timing and duration of immobilization in the pathogenesis of AMC has not been clearly established. Table 10–16 illustrates the different conditions that have been reported to cause limitation of movement in the fetus and AMC.[6]

Cases of AMC are sporadic. However, some cases suggesting an autosomal dominant[12] and recessive pattern of inheritance have been reported.[1,9] The multiple etiology of AMC is responsible for this heterogeneity.

Pathology

In most cases of AMC, all four limbs are involved. However, patients with bimelic or asymmetrical involvement have been reported.[6] Knees and elbows are the joints most frequently involved. The typical deformities are flexure contractures of hips, knees, and elbows, adduction of the scapulohumeral joint, pronated clubhands and equinovarus. Among the causes of AMC, neurologic disorders are the most common (e.g., loss of anterior horn cells and amyoplasia congenita). Pathologic examination may

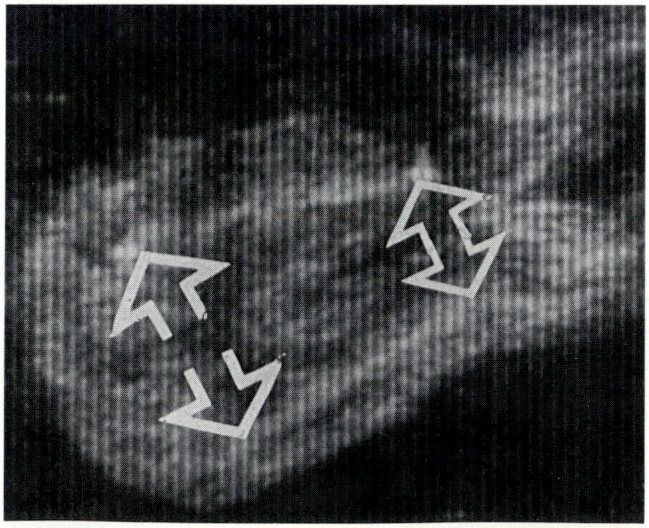

Figure 10–87. In arthrogryposis, the internal rotation of the femur contributes to a much smaller intercondyle distance (*small double arrow*) than the distance between the two femoral heads (*separated double arrows*). (*Reproduced with permission from Jeanty, Romero: Obstetrical Ultrasound. New York, McGraw-Hill, 1984.*)

TABLE 10–16. DISORDERS OF THE DEVELOPING MOTOR SYSTEM ON ALL LEVELS, LEADING TO IMMOBILIZATION

Disorders of the developing neuromuscular system
    Loss of anterior horn cells
    Radicular disease with collagen proliferation
    Peripheral neuropathy with neurofibromatosis
    Congenital myasthenia
    Neonatal myasthenia (maternal myasthenia gravis)
    Amyoplasia congenita
    Congenital muscular dystrophy
    Central core disease
    Congenital myotonic dystrophy
    Glycogen accumulation myopathy
Disorders of developing connective tissue or connective tissue
    disease
    Muscular and articular connective tissue dystrophy
    Articular defects by mesenchymal dysplasia
    Increased collagen synthesis
Disorders of developing medulla or medullar disease
    Congenital spinal epidural hemorrhage
    Congenital duplication of the spinal canal
Disorders of brain development (e.g., porencephaly) or brain
    disease (e.g., congenital encephalopathy)

TABLE 10–17. CONGENITAL ANOMALIES ASSOCIATED WITH AMC

Cleft palate	Polydactyly
Klippel-Feil syndrome	Hypertelorism
Meningomyelocele	Microphthalmia
Hyperostosis frontalis	Congenital heart defect
Intestinal abnormalities	Kidney defects
Glaucoma and cataract	Carpal fusion
Esophageal atresia	Spondylohypoplasia

allow differentiation between neurogenic and myophathic forms of AMC.

Associated Anomalies

Table 10–17 shows some of the anomalies associated with AMC. Ten percent of patients with AMC have associated anomalies of the CNS, including hydrocephaly, porencephaly, lissencephaly, cortical atrophy, micropolygyria, cerebellar vermal agenesis, and agenesis of the corpus callosum.[6]

Diagnosis

The prenatal diagnosis of AMC with ultrasound has been reported twice. The first fetus was examined with fetoscopy at 16 weeks of gestation because a previous infant was affected with the condition.[10] During endoscopic visualization, fetal motion was seen, and the extremities looked normal. Subsequently, real-time examinations at 18 weeks also showed normal motion of the extremities. However, serial scans at 23, 28, and 35 weeks failed to show any fetal movement. The infant died shortly after birth, and autopsy showed dropout of anterior horn cells. The muscles demonstrated findings consistent with neurogenic atrophy. This case suggests that the diagnosis of AMC due to a neurologic lesion may not be possible before 20 weeks. The other prenatal diagnosis was reported in a fetus examined because of preterm labor.[5] At 30 weeks, the fetus showed significant limb shortening and flexion and crossing of lower extremities. The elbow joints and one hand were also flexed. No movement was seen during a 1-hour examination. Polyhydramnios has been reported in association with AMC.[5,10]

Although real-time examination permits the detection of joint contracture (see the section on clubfoot) and the assessment of fetal motion, its sensitivity for early diagnosis of AMC remains to be established (Fig. 10–87).

The Pena-Shokeir syndrome can present with manifestations of AMC. This condition is inherited with an autosomal recessive pattern and is characterized by intrauterine growth retardation, polyhydramnios, absent breathing movement, pulmonary hypoplasia, hypertelorism, low-set ears, depressed nasal bridge, micrognathia, camptodactyly, and clubfoot or rocker-bottom foot. We have diagnosed this condition in a fetus at risk who failed to show any breathing or body movement and had typical contracture deformities of the upper and lower extremities. The syndrome is usually lethal within a few days of birth. The cause of death is pulmonary hypoplasia, which is probably caused by lack of chest wall movement during intrauterine life.

Prognosis

The prognosis for AMC is related to the specific etiology. In some severe cases, the disease is lethal, and death occurs shortly after birth. In other cases, musculoskeletal impairment is minimal, and intelligence is normal. Between these extremes, affected infants may have handicaps of different severity. Treatment should begin shortly after birth, and surgery may be required to correct incapacitating deformities.

Obstetrical Management

If a diagnosis is made before viability, the option of pregnancy termination should be offered to the parents. The optimal mode of delivery has not been established. Infants with AMC are at risk for severe birth trauma because of fixed joints. Cesarean section seems to be the best method of delivery.

REFERENCES

1. Bhatnagar DP, Sidhu LS, Aggarwal ND: Family studies for the mode of inheritance in arthrogryposis multiplex congenita. Z Morph Antrop 68:233, 1977.
2. Drachman DB, Coulombre AJ: Experimental clubfoot and arthrogryposis multiplex comgenita. Lancet 2:523, 1962.
3. Drachman DB, Sokoloff L: The role of movement in embryonic joint development. Dev Biol 14:401, 1966.
4. Fuller DJ: Immobilization of foetal joints as a cause of progressive prenatal deforming. J Bone Joint Surg 57B:115, 1975.
5. Goldberg JD, Chervenak FA, Lipman RA, et al.: Antenatal sonographic diagnosis of arthrogryposis multiplex congenita. Prenat Diagn 6:45, 1986.
6. Hageman G, Willemse J: Arthrogryposis multiplex congenita. Review with comment. Neuroped 14:6, 1983.
7. Jago RH: Arthrogryposis following treatment of maternal tetanus with muscle relaxants. Arch Dis Child 45:277, 1970.
8. Jeanty P, Romero R: Obstetrical Ultrasound. New York, McGraw-Hill, 1984.
9. Lebenthal E, Shochet SB, Adam A, et al.: Arthrogryposis multiplex congenita: 23 cases in an Arab kindred. Pediatrics 46:891, 1970.

10. Miskin M, Rothberg R, Rudd NL, et al.: Arthrogryposis multiplex congenita—Prenatal assessment with diagnostic ultrasound and fetoscopy. J Pediatr 95:463, 1979.
11. Murray PDF, Drachman DB: The role of movement in the development of joints and related structures: The head and neck in the chick embryo. J Embryol Exp Morphol 22:349, 1969.
12. Radu H, Stenzel K, Bene M, et al.: Das arthrogrypotische Syndrom. Deutsh Z Nervenheilk 193:118, 1968.

Jarcho-Levin Syndrome

Synonyms
Occipitofacial-cervicothoracic-abdominodigital dysplasia,[7] spondylocostal dysplasia,[4] costovertebral dysplasia,[2] spondylothoracic dysostosis,[6] spondylocostal dysostosis,[11] and spondylothoracic dysplasia.[3]

Definition
Jarcho-Levin syndrome is a congenital disorder of the skeleton inherited in an autosomal recessive pattern and characterized by disorganization of the spine (hemivertebrae, fused vertebrae) and a crablike appearance of the rib cage.

Etiology
Autosomal recessive.

Incidence
In a recent review of the literature, 35 cases were reported.[1] Probands of Puerto Rican descent constitute a significant number of these cases.

Pathology
Spondylocostal dysplasia has been subdivided into two types. Type I is inherited with an autosomal recessive pattern, often occurs in families of Puerto Rican descent, is characterized by severe involvement of the spine, and generally causes respiratory failure and death in affected children before they reach 15 months of age.[7,9] Type II is inherited as an autosomal dominant trait, is found most often in Caucasians, is characterized by milder involvement, and is associated with nearly normal longevity.[2,3,10] Because it is not known if type II can be diagnosed in utero, this section is confined to the description of type I.

A recent classification of spondylocostal dysplasia was proposed by Ayme and Preus.[1] Using cluster analysis of all informative cases in the literature, they suggested that spondylocostal dysplasia be subdivided into a severe form inherited with an autosomal recessive pattern and a mild form inherited with an autosomal recessive or dominant pat-

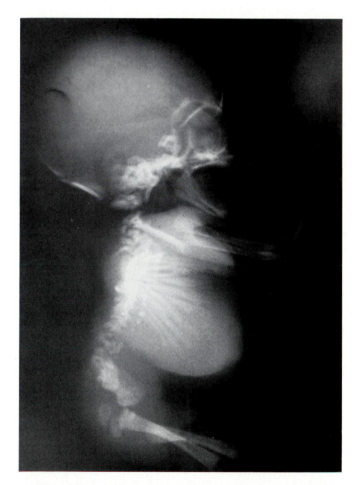

Figure 10–88. Lateral x-ray of a fetus with Jarcho-Levin syndrome. Note the characteristic chest deformity with posterior fusion and anterior flaring of the ribs. Disorganization of the vertebral bodies is apparent.

tern. They admit, however, that more data are required for further delineation between the mild autosomal recessive and dominant forms.

Spinal involvement is characterized by multiple fused vertebrae and hemivertebrae in the cervical, thoracic, and lumbar regions (Fig. 10–88). This leads to a short neck and to characteristic changes in the rib cage described as a "crab-chest" deformity (Fig. 10–89). This deformity is the result of posterior fusion and anterior flaring of the ribs. The rest of the skeleton is spared.

Associated Anomalies

The following anomalies have been reported: prominent occiput (37 percent), microcephaly (15 percent), triangular opening of the mouth (15 percent), cleft palate (10.5 percent), spina bifida occulta (31.5 percent), lordosis (26.3 percent), abdominal wall defect (26.3 percent), anal defects (10.5 percent), long arms (37 percent), syndactyly (15 percent), and camptodactyly (31.5 percent).[1,9]

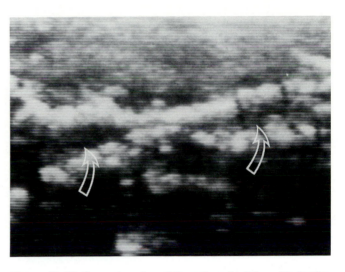

Figure 10–90. Coronal section of the spine of a fetus with Jarcho-Levin syndrome at 23 weeks. Note the shortening of the spine and flaring of the vertebral canal (*arrows*).

Diagnosis

The condition should be suspected when spinal disorganization is associated with an abnormal chest configuration. Spinal disorganization consists of fused vertebrae or hemivertebrae (Figs. 10–90, 10–91). A more precise diagnosis can be made in a family with previous affected probands.

The prenatal diagnosis of spondylocostal dysplasia type I has been made in families at risk by radiograph.[8,9] We have recently made this diagnosis using ultrasonography in a 23-week-old fetus with no positive family history.

The differential diagnosis of spinal disorganization in a fetus includes spondylocostal dysplasia, dyssegmental dysplasia, spondyloepiphyseal dysplasia congenita, the VACTERL association, and the costovertebral segmentation defect with mesomelia (COVESDEM) association. Dyssegmental dysplasia is characterized by severe micromelia (extreme shortening of all segments of the extremities) and occipital cephalocele, and it lacks the crablike appearance of the chest. The VACTERL association is characterized by vertebral anomalies, anal atresia, tracheoesophageal fistula, cardiac anomalies (generally a ventricular septal defect), and radial limb dysplasia (including preaxial polydactyly, syndactyly, radial hypoplasia, and thumb hypoplasia). A single umbilical artery can also be observed. A diagnosis of this condition requires the presence of at least 3 of the 7 cardinal anomalies of the association. Spondyloepiphyseal dysplasia congenita is characterized by ovoid vertebral bodies and severe platyspondyly (flattening of vertebral bodies). Hemivertebrae are absent. The limbs may or may not be shortened, but severe dwarfism is not seen. The thorax is bell-shaped in the anteroposterior projection, but lacks the crablike mor-

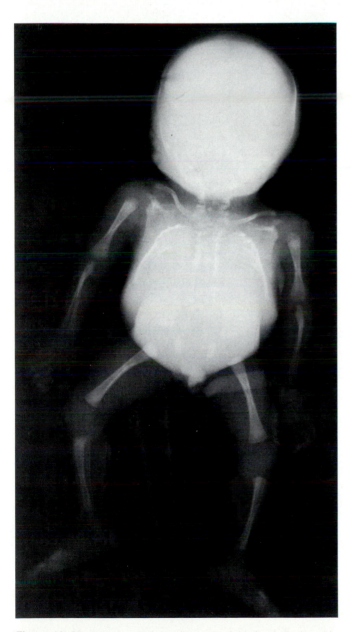

Figure 10–89. Anteroposterior radiograph of the fetus displayed in the previous figure. It is a 24-week-old fetus with Jarcho-Levin syndrome. Note the dramatic spinal shortening, chest deformity, and unaffected long bones.

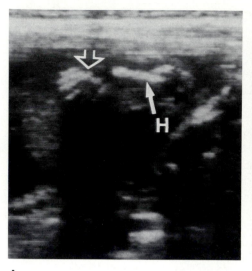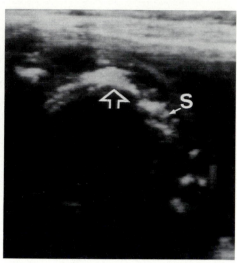

Figure 10–91. Ultrasound images in a fetus with Jarcho-Levin syndrome. **A.** The left panel of the figure represents an oblique section through the fetal chest. Note the posterior fusion of the ribs (*empty arrow*). H, humerus. **B.** The right panel shows a transverse section through the fetal chest. Posterior fusion of the ribs is visible (*empty arrow*). S, spine.

A   **B**

phology seen in Jarcho-Levin syndrome. Another condition to be considered is the COVESDEM association.[12] This condition includes mesomelic dysplasia (particularly of the upper extremities), costovertebral segmentation defects (hemivertebrae, vertebral fusion, and butterfly vertebrae), and facial abnormalities (hypertelorism, depressed nasal bridge, large bony upper lip, constantly open mouth, and peg teeth). Mesomelia is absent in Jarcho-Levin syndrome.

Prognosis
The severe form of spondylocostal dysplasia is considered a uniformly lethal condition. Death occurs from respiratory failure generally caused by recurrent pneumonia by 15 months of age.

Obstetrical Management
If a prenatal diagnosis of type I spondylocostal dysplasia is made before viability, the option of pregnancy termination should be offered to the parents. Cases identified after viability constitute a difficult ethical dilemma and we recommend that the issue be discussed with the parents. A nonaggressive management for cases with fetal distress may be considered, as the condition seems to be uniformly lethal.

REFERENCES

1. Ayme S, Preus M: Spondylocostal/spondylothoracic dysostosis: The clinical basis for prognosticating and genetic counseling. Am J Med Gen 24:599, 1986.
2. Casamassima AC, Casson Morton C, Nance WE, et al: Spondylocostal dysostosis associated with anal and urogenital anomalies in a mennonite sibship. Am J Med Gen 8:117, 1981.
3. Heilbronner DM, Renshaw TS: Spondylothoracic dysplasia. A case report. J Bone Joint Surg 66:302, 1984.
4. Kozlowski K: Spondylocostal dysplasia. A further report—review of 14 cases. ROFO 140:204, 1984.
5. Li DFH, Woo JSK: Fractional spine length: A new parameter for assessing fetal growth. J Ultrasound Med 5:379, 1986.
6. Moseley JE, Bonforte RJ: Spondylothoracic dysplasia — a syndrome of congenital anomalies. AJR 106:166, 1969.
7. Perez-Comas A, Garcia-Castro JM: Occipito-facial-cervico-thoracic-abdomino-digital dysplasia: Jarco-Levin syndrome of vertebral anomalies. J Pediatrics 85:388, 1974.
8. Perez-Comas A, Garcia-Castro JM: Prenatal diagnosis of OFCTAD dysplasia or Jarcho-Levin syndrome. Birth Defects 15(5):39, 1979.
9. Poor MA, Alberti O Jr, Griscom NT, et al.: Nonskeletal malformations in one of three siblings with Jarcho-Levin syndrome of vertebral anomalies. J Pediatrics 103:270, 1983.
10. Rimoin DL, Fletcher BD, McKusick VA: Spondylocostal dysplasia. A dominantly inherited form of short-trunked dwarfism. Am J Med 45:948, 1968.
11. Young ID, Moore JR: Spondylocostal dysostosis. J Med Gen 21:68, 1984.
12. Wadia RS, Shirole DB, Dikshit MS: Recessively inherited costovertebral segmentation defect with mesomelia and peculiar facies (COVESDEM syndrome). A new genetic entity? J Med Genet 15:123, 1978.

The Umbilical Cord

Normal Anatomy of the Umbilical Cord

The umbilical cord normally contains three vessels, two arteries and one vein, surrounded by a connective tissue known as "Wharton's jelly" (Figs. 11–1, 11–2, 11–3). At term, the mean length of the umbilical cord is 55 cm. A short cord is less than 35 cm in length (lower 6th percentile), and a long cord measures more than 80 cm (upper 6th percentile).[3] The mean umbilical cord circumference at 40 weeks is 3.6 cm (range 2.6 to 6.0 cm).[2] The 90th percentile for the area of the umbilical cord at term is 1.3 cm square.[4]

Sonographic Biometry of the Umbilical Cord
There is a paucity of data concerning the biometry of the umbilical cord during gestation. The only nomogram available concerning the umbilical cord refers to the size of the umbilical vein in a free-floating cord (Fig. 11–4).[1]

REFERENCES

1. DeVore GR, Mayden K, Tortora M, et al.: Dilation of the fetal umbilical vein in rhesus hemolytic anemia: A predictor of severe disease. Am J Obstet Gynecol 141:464, 1981.
2. Dooley SL, Lamb R, Helseth DL Jr: Umbilical cord circumference as a measure of Wharton's jelly: Clinical correlates. Abstract 32, Sixth Annual Meeting of the Society of Perinatal Obstetricians. January 30–February 1, 1986, San Antonio, Texas.
3. Rayburn WF, Beynen A, Brinkman DL: Umbilical cord length and intrapartum complications. Obstet Gynecol 57:450, 1981.
4. Scott JM, Jordan JM: Placental insufficiency and the small-for-dates baby. Am J Obstet Gynecol 113:823, 1972.

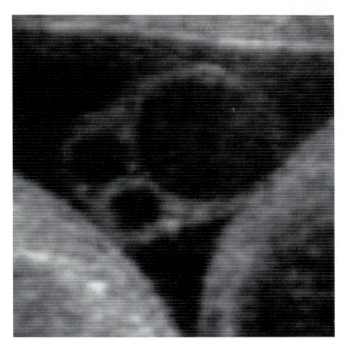

Figure 11–1. Transverse section of the umbilical cord showing two arteries and one vein.

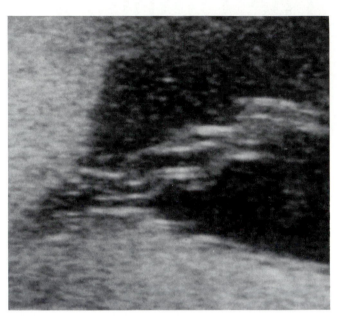

Figure 11–3. Insertion of the umbilical cord in the placental mass. Demonstration of the insertion site is important for percutaneous umbilical cord sampling. This section excludes velamentous insertion.

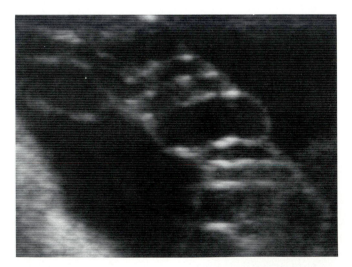

Figure 11–2. Longitudinal section of the umbilical cord showing the typical braided appearance.

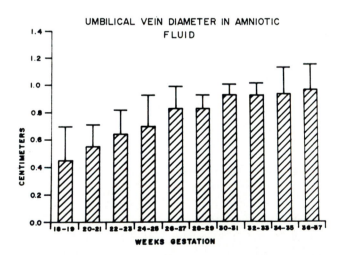

Figure 11–4. Nomogram for the umbilical vein diameter. (*Reproduced with permission from DeVore et al.: Am J Obstet Gynecol 141:464, 1981.*)

Single Umbilical Artery

Synonyms
Absence of an umbilical artery, umbilical artery agenesis, umbilical artery atrophy, and missing umbilical artery.

Definition
Single umbilical artery (SUA) is the absence of one umbilical artery.

Epidemiology
Prospective studies indicate that SUA is present in 1 percent of all deliveries. The method of examination of the umbilical cord and the patient's race are important factors in determining the prevalence of this anomaly. For example, gross examination of the umbilical cord underestimates the prevalence.[14,18,21] The location of the section is also important, since the two arteries may fuse close to the placental insertion of the cord,[2,8,32] and examination at this point would overestimate the prevalence of this anomaly.[2,22] SUA is less common in Japanese and blacks and more common in eastern Europeans.[11,12,14,15,26,31] SUA is more common in autopsy series and in stillbirths.[10,29] The prevalence is higher in the third trimester than in very early embryos (less than 8 weeks old).[10,33] This suggests that a developmental atrophy of a normally formed umbilical artery may occur in some fetuses.[28,34] The male to female ratio is

0.85:1.[5,13,15,16,18,21,27,39] There is a greater tendency of males to be malformed in prospective series. The prevalence of SUA is three to four times higher in multiple gestations.[4,13,15,16,21,27] There is no evidence of an epidemiologic association between maternal age, parity,[15,21,38] month of the last menstrual period,[7,14-16] and the prevalence of SUA.

Etiology
There is no evidence of a familial tendency of this disorder. A genetic etiology is unlikely. The increased incidence in twin gestations is not observed in monozygotic twins.[14]

The three theories about the pathogenesis of SUA are (1) primary agenesis of one of the umbilical arteries, (2) secondary atrophy of a previously normal artery, and (3) persistence of the original single allantoid artery of the body stalk. There is no statistical difference between atrophy and aplasia in SUA and associated malformations.[1]

Prenatal Diagnosis
The normal umbilical cord contains two arteries and one vein readily visible in transverse or longitudinal sections.[17,35] In longitudinal sections, the helicoidal shape provides a typical braided appearance to the umbilical cord. A single umbilical artery can be seen readily in transverse sections by identifying a cord

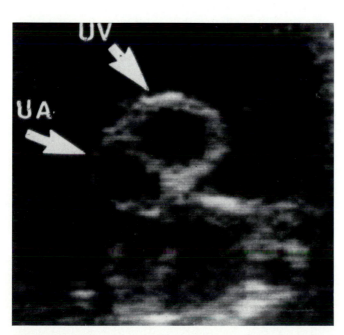

Figure 11–5. Transverse section of the umbilical cord demonstrating only two vessels. UA, umbilical artery; UV, umbilical vein.

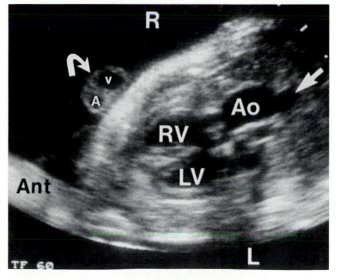

Figure 11–6. Transverse section of the fetal chest in a fetus with double outlet right ventricle. The umbilical cord is seen anterior to the chest (*curved arrow*). RV, right ventricle; LV, left ventricle; Ao, aorta; Ant, anterior; L, left; R, right; V, umbilical vein; A, single umbilical artery.

with only two vessels (Figs. 11–5, 11–6). The vein is typically larger than the artery. In longitudinal sections, a loss of the braided pattern of the umbilical cord can be visualized (Figs. 11–2, 11–3).

Identification of an SUA is an indication for a careful search for associated anomalies including echocardiography (see section on associated anomalies). These infants are also at risk for intrauterine growth retardation, and serial examinations are recommended.

Associated Anomalies

Infants with SUA have a higher prevalence of congenital anomalies, intrauterine growth retardation,[1,4,5,13,15,26] prematurity,[1,4,5,13,20] and a higher perinatal mortality[1,5,13,15,25,31] than infants born with two umbilical arteries. Twenty-one percent of infants with SUA have associated anomalies in prospective series,[1,4,5,7,11,13,15,18,22,24,26,31,36,37] and the incidence is three times higher in autopsy series.[20,29] Heifetz has estimated that the risk of anomalies is seven times greater in infants with SUA than in control infants with two umbilical arteries.[14] Table 11–1 illustrates the associated anomalies in 158 autopsy cases examined at the Armed Forces Institute of Pathology and reported by Heifetz.[14] It is clear that many of these anomalies are subtle (e.g., absence of the uvula) and, therefore, nondetectable with ultrasound. In other cases, the severity of the anomaly is such (e.g., bilateral renal agenesis) that identification of SUA is practically irrelevant. The mean number of malformations per infant varies between 2 and 5.

Abnormalities that are detectable with ultrasound and are most commonly associated with SUA include cardiovascular abnormalities (particularly ventricular septal defects and conotruncal anomalies), cleft lip, ventral wall defects, esophageal atresia, spina bifida, central nervous system defects (hydrocephaly, holoprosencephaly), diaphragmatic hernia, cystic hygromas, genitourinary abnormalities (hydronephrosis, dysplastic kidneys), and digital abnormalities (polydactyly, syndactyly). All fetuses with SUA should have echocardiography performed, since cardiovascular abnormalities are among the most frequent defects.

SUA is associated with a higher incidence of marginal and velamentous insertion of the umbilical cord while these anomalies have been found in 5.9 percent and 1.2 percent of all placentas, respectively,[30] in SUA, their incidence is 18 percent and 9.3 percent, respectively.[4,13,15,22,24–26] In two different series, the association of SUA with velamentous insertion of the umbilical cord slightly increased the risk for other anomalies.[9,14] The prevalence of chromosomal abnormalities in term infants with SUA is unknown. Isolated reports have documented that

SUA can occur in association with autosomal trisomies.[1–3,19,20,23,26,27] A recent pathologic study examining fetuses with SUA delivered before the 28th week of gestation reported an incidence of chromosomal anomalies of 67 percent (6 out of 9).[6] This is higher than the 31 percent (24 out of 74) observed in infants born with malformations other than SUA.[6] In this small series ($n = 9$), all infants with SUA and chromosomal anomalies had severe malformations. From these data, performance of amniocentesis seems justified when SUA is associated with severe anomalies.

Prognosis

The mean perinatal mortality for infants with SUA has been reported to be 20 percent.[14] Two thirds of the perinatal deaths are stillbirths,[12,15,21,37,39] and among these, three quarters have occurred antepartum and one quarter intrapartum.[9,13] The main cause of death is the presence of associated anomalies. However, the perinatal mortality remains elevated in infants with SUA but without associated malformations.[5,12,13] This is mainly due to prematurity and intrauterine growth retardation.

Infants with SUA are at risk for internal malformation even if external anomalies cannot be detected.[11,25] However, if these infants remain asymptomatic during the neonatal period, their risk for lethal or serious anomalies is not higher than that of non-SUA infants.[5,11,26,37] The long-term prognosis for growth-retarded infants with SUA is good, since these infants attain growth rates comparable to nonaffected infants.[11]

Obstetrical Management

The detection of a single umbilical artery should prompt a search for associated anomalies. Echocardiography is indicated. Karyotype determination should be performed if associated anomalies are detected. The risk of chromosomal abnormalities in SUA without gross anomalies detected by ultrasound has not been established. Serial sonography for identification of IUGR is recommended. Intrapartum fetal heart monitoring is indicated, since some series suggest that these infants are at risk for intrapartum fetal distress and death. Pediatricians should be alerted to the diagnosis of SUA, and noninvasive techniques like neonatal ultrasound should be used freely to detect subclinical anomalies. Invasive procedures for diagnostic purposes in an otherwise asymptomatic infant do not seem justified. Data from the Collaborative Perinatal project show that infants born with SUA had a higher incidence of inguinal hernias (5.5 percent versus 1.1 percent) than a control group in a follow-up period of 4 years. The IQ of nonmalformed infants with SUA is not different from that of infants with two umbilical arteries.[5,11,26,36]

TABLE 11-1. MALFORMATIONS IDENTIFIED IN 158 AFIP AUTOPSY CASES OF SUA

1. Urogenital Tract		**4. Gastrointestinal Tract**	
Renal agenesis or hypoplasia	18	Agenesis of uvula	1
Renal dysplasia or dysgenesis	30	Tracheoesophageal fistula	12
Horseshoe kidney	16	Esophageal atresia or stenosis	6
Pelvic kidney	2	Gastric atresia	1
Hydroureter and hydronephrosis	17	Duodenal atresia	1
Other ureteral anomalies	6	Midgut aplasia or stenosis	2
Urethral anomalies	12	Meckel's diverticulum	4
Persistent cloaca	7	Malrotation	10
Urachal anomalies	2	Intestinal duplication	1
Malformed or absent ext. genitalia	15	Imperforate anus	25
Testicular agenesis	3	Colorectal atresia or stenosis	3
Hypospadias	4	Liver anom./gallbladder agenesis	5
Agenesis of vas and prostate	1	Miscellaneous	1
Hydrocele	1		72
Agenesis of ovary and tube	4		
Cervical agenesis	3	**5. Central Nervous System**	
Uterine fundal anomalies	9	Anencephaly	17
Vaginal anomalies	3	Meningocele, spina bifida	12
	153	Hydrocephalus	4
		Holoprosencephaly, cebocephaly	7
2. Cardiovascular System		Microcephaly	2
Patent ductus arteriosus	21	Cerebellar anomalies	6
Patent foramen ovale	10	Microphthalmia	4
Atrial septal defect	14	Cranial nerve abnormalities	3
Ventricular septal defect	33	Miscellaneous	7
Hypoplastic left ventricle	5		62
Tetralogy of Fallot	2		
Truncus anomalies	11	**6. Respiratory System**	
Transposition	3	Choanal atresia	2
Anomalous pulmonary venous return	2	Atresia nasal septum	1
Coarctation	7	Laryngeal sten./trach. agenesis	3
Dextrocardia	3	Pulmonary hypoplasia	26
Dextroposition of aorta	3	Abnormal lobation	14
Valve anomalies	11	Pulmonary aplasia	1
Subaortic stenosis	1	Diaphragmatic hernia	12
Coronary artery anomalies	4		59
Other thoracic vessel anomalies	12		
	142	**7. Integument**	
		External ear abnormalities	47
3. Musculoskeletal System		Skin tags	4
High arched palate	2	Epicanthal folds	5
Cleft lip and palate	27	Hemangiomas	2
Rib and sternal anomalies	12	Lymphang./cystic hygroma/web	14
Vertebral anomalies	15	Hydrops	2
Sacral agenesis	2	Hypoplastic fingernails	1
Amelia and phocomelia	4		75
Other long bone anomalies	8		
Wrist and ankle deformities	4	**8. Miscellaneous**	
Talipes	19	Endocrine gland anomalies	7
Rocker bottom feet	5	Accessory spleen	4
Hip dislocation	5	Situs inversus	1
Polydactyly	12	Sacrococcygeal teratoma	4
Syndactyly or clinodactyly	6	Pharyngeal teratoma	1
Other finger or toe anomalies	15		17
Mandibular hypoplasia	4		
Abnormal sphenoid	1		
Achondroplasia	1	**Total**	753
Prune belly	4		
Abdominal wall hernia	1		
Femoral hernia	1		
Omphalocele	21		
Gastroschisis	4		
	173		

Reproduced with permission from Heifetz: Perspect Pediatr Pathol 8:345, 1984.

REFERENCES

1. Altshuler G, Tsang RC, Ermocilla R: Single umbilical artery. Correlation of clinical status and umbilical cord histology. Am J Dis Child 129:697, 1975.
2. Benirschke K, Driscoll SG: The Pathology of the Human Placenta. Berlin, Springer-Verlag, 1974.
3. Bjoro K Jr: Vascular anomalies of the umbilical cord. II. Perinatal and pediatric implications. Early Hum Dev 8:279, 1983.
4. Broussard P, Raudrant D, Picaud JJ, et al: Artere ombilicale unique. Etude de 45 cas. J Gynecol Obstet Biol Reprod 1:551, 1972.
5. Bryan EM, Kohler HG: The missing umbilical artery. I. Prospective study based on a maternity unit. Arch Dis Child 49:844, 1974.
6. Byrne J, Blanc WA: Malformations and chromosome anomalies in spontaneously aborted fetuses with single umbilical artery. Am J Obstet Gynecol 151:340, 1985.
7. Cederqvist L: Die Bedeutung des Fehlens einer Arterie in der Nabelschnur: Eine prospektive endemiologische Studie. Acta Obstet Gynecol Scand 49:113, 1970.
8. Chantler C, Baum JD, Wigglesworth JS, et al: Giant umbilical cord associated with a patent urachus and fused umbilical arteries. J Obstet Gynaecol Br Commonw 76:273, 1969.
9. Dellenbach P, Leissner P, Philippe E, et al.: Artere ombilicale unique, insertion velamenteuse du cordon ombilical et malformations foetales. Rev Fr Gynecol Obstet 63:603, 1968.
10. Ezaki K, Tanimura T, Fujikura T: Genesis of single umbilical artery. Teratology 6:105, 1972.
11. Froehlich LA, Fujikura T: Follow-up of infants with single umbilical artery. Pediatrics 52:6, 1973.
12. Froehlich LA, Fujikura T: Significance of a single umbilical artery. Report from the collaborative study of cerebral palsy. Am J Obstet Gynecol 94:274, 1966.
13. Giraud JR, Allal A, Payard J, et al.: Artere ombilicale unique et pathologie perinatale. Gynecol Obstet 70:433, 1971.
14. Heifetz SA: Single umbilical artery. A statistical analysis of 237 autopsy cases and review of the literature. Perspect Pediatr Pathol 8:345, 1984.
15. Itoh H, Nishimura K, Iwatsubo T: Single umbilical artery—A review of 37 cases. Acta Obstet Gynecol Jpn 23:96, 1976.
16. Jean C, Dupre A, Carrier C: L'artere ombilicale unique: Etude de 112 observations. Can Med Assoc J 100:1088, 1969.
17. Jeanty P, Romero R: Obstetrical Ultrasound. New York, McGraw-Hill, 1984.
18. Johnsonbaugh RE: Unilateral short lower extremity and single umbilical artery. Absence of a relationship. Am J Dis Child 126:186, 1973.
19. Khudr G, Benirschke K: Pure gonadal dysgenesis associated with a single umbilical artery. Obstet Gynecol 38:697, 1971.
20. Konstantinova B: Malformations of the umbilical cord. Acta Genet Med Gemellol 26:259, 1977.
21. Kristoffersen K: The significance of absence of one umbilical artery. Acta Obstet Gynecol Scand 48:195, 1969.
22. LeMarec B, Kerisit J, DeVillartay A, et al.: L'artere ombilicale unique. Etude de 31 cas. J Gynecol Obstet Biol Reprod 1:825, 1972.
23. Matayoshi K, Yoshida K, Soma H, et al: Placental pathology associated with chromosomal anomalies of the human neonate. A survey of seven cases. Congen Anom 17:507, 1977.
24. Matheus M, Sala MA: The importance of placental examination in newborns with single umbilical artery. Z Geburtshilfe Perinatol 184:231, 1980.
25. Mikulandra F: Occurrence of aplasia of the umbilical artery in fetuses with intrauterine retardation. Jugosl Ginekol Opstet 16:295, 1976.
26. Nishimura K, Iwatsubo T: Clinical observations of children with a single umbilical artery (Abstr). Teratology 16:86, 1977.
27. Pageaut G, Oppermann A, Carbillet JP: L'absence d'une artere ombilicale (a propos de 57 observations). Rev CHU 13:26, 1970.
28. Philippe E, Ritter J, Dehalleux JM, et al.: De la pathologie des avortements spontanes. Gynecol Obstet 67:97, 1968.
29. Satow Y: The relation between single umbilical artery and associated anomalies (Abstr). Teratology 16:86, 1977.
30. Shanklin DR: The influence of placental lesions on the newborn infant. Pediatr Clin North Am 17:25, 1970.
31. Soma H: Single umbilical artery with congenital malformations. Curr Top Pathol 66:159, 1979.
32. Szpakowski M: Morphology of arterial anastomoses in the human placenta. Folia Morphol 33:53, 1974.
33. Tanimura T: Abnormalities of embryos and their membranes (Abstr). Teratology 16:86, 1977.
34. Tanimura T, Ezaki KI: Single umbilical artery found in Japanese embryos. Proc Cong Anom Res Assoc Jpn 8:27, 1968.
35. Tortora M, Chervenak FA, Mayden K, et al.: Antenatal sonographic diagnosis of single umbilical artery. Obstet Gynecol 63:693, 1984.
36. Trutt B: L'artere ombilicale unique. Thesis, Strasbourg, 1967. Cited by Le Marec et al., Ref. 22.
37. Vlietinck RF, Thiery M, Orye E, et al: Significance of the single umbilical artery. A clinical, radiological, chromosomal and dermatoglyphic study. Arch Dis Child 47:639, 1972.
38. Wentworth P: Some anomalies of the fetal vessels of the human placenta. J Anat 99:273, 1965.
39. Zeman V: Aplazie umbilikalni arterie. Cesk Pediatr 27:78, 1972.

CYSTIC LESIONS OF THE UMBILICAL CORD

Omphalomesenteric Cyst

Synonym
Omphalomesenteric duct cyst.

Definition
A cystic lesion of the umbilical cord due to persistence and dilatation of a segment of the omphalomesenteric duct lined by epithelium of gastrointestinal origin.

Embryology
The omphalomesenteric duct joins the embryonic gut and the yolk sac. It is formed during the 3d week of gestation and is closed by the 16th week of gestation. Small vestigial remnants of this duct are found frequently in normal umbilical cords.[2]

Incidence
A total of nine cases have been described in the literature.[2] The male to female ratio is 3:5, which is consistent with the predominance of omphalomesenteric anomalies seen in males (e.g., Meckel's

diverticula, intraabdominal mesenteric cysts, fistulas, polyps or cysts of the umbilicus, polyps or cysts of the umbilical cord).

Pathology
The cysts are generally located in close proximity to the fetus. Cysts vary in size, with the largest being 6 cm in diameter. The lining is epithelium of the gastrointestinal type (stomach, small intestine, and colon). On occasion, the surface of the cysts may have an angiomatoid appearance.[2]

Diagnosis
Identification of an umbilical cord cyst, which at pathology proved to be an omphalomesenteric cyst, has been reported.[3] The cyst was identified at 20 weeks and did not change in dimensions during pregnancy (Fig. 11–7). The infant was normal. Differential diagnosis includes other hypoechogenic lesions of the umbilical cord, like allantoid cysts, and hematomas of the umbilical cord.

Prognosis
The prognosis is excellent. One exception is a case reported by Blanc and Allan, in which acid produced by a cyst lined by gastric mucosa eroded the umbilical vein and caused fetal exsanguination.[1]

Infants with other types of remnants of the omphalomesenteric duct have been found to have a 62 percent incidence of internal lesions, of which the most common is Meckel's diverticulum.[4] Therefore, identification of this lesion should be called to the attention of parents and pediatricians. If abdominal symptoms develop later in life, Meckel's diverticulum should be considered as part of the differential diagnosis.

Obstetrical Management
The diagnosis of a cystic lesion of the umbilical cord should be an indication for serial examinations to verify normal growth of the fetus and changes in the size of the lesion. A theoretical risk is the development of vascular compression by an expanding cyst. Doppler examination may be helpful in these instances. Delivery could be recommended as soon as lung maturity is documented in patients with sizable lesions.

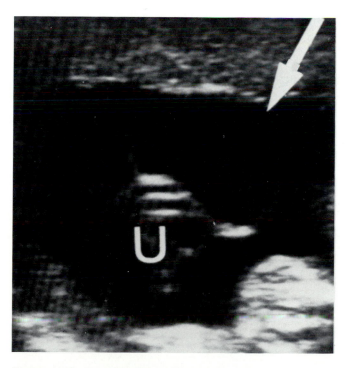

Figure 11–7. An omphalomesenteric cyst can be seen as a hypoechogenic mass *(arrow)* protruding from the umbilical cord (U). *(Reproduced with permission from Rosenberg, et al.: J Ultrasound Med 5:719, 1986.)*

REFERENCES

1. Blanc WA, Allan GW: Intrafunicular ulceration of persistent omphalomesenteric duct with intra-amniotic hemorrhage and fetal death. Am J Obstet Gynecol 82:1392, 1961.
2. Heifetz SA, Rueda-Pedraza ME: Omphalomesenteric duct cysts of the umbilical cord. Pediatr Pathol 1:325, 1983.
3. Rosenberg JC, Chervenak FA, Walker BA, et al.: Antenatal sonographic appearance of omphalomesenteric duct cyst. J Ultrasound Med 5:719, 1986.
4. Steck WD, Helwig EB: Cutaneous remnants of the omphalomesenteric duct. Arch Dermatol 90:463, 1964.

Allantoid Cyst

Definition
A cystic dilatation of an allantoid remnant.

Embryology
The allantoid is one of the four fetal adnexa (amnion, chorion, yolk sac, and allantoid). It becomes a fibrous band after the 3d month of gestation.[2]

Pathology
These cysts are generally located close to the fetus. They are lined by a flattened epithelium or in some areas by transitional epithelium.[1] In one case, analysis of the cystic fluid revealed a specific gravity of 1.016, BUN of 22 mg/100 ml, and no protein content.

Diagnosis
This entity appears as a cystic structure of the umbilical cord close to the fetus[2] (Fig. 11–8). The differential diagnosis with other cystic lesions, such as omphalomesenteric cysts and old hematomas of the umbilical cord, is not possible. Visualization of a patent urachus in the abdomen should raise the index of suspicion.

Associated Anomalies
It may be associated with a patent urachus and lower genitourinary obstruction.

Prognosis
We are aware of only one case reported in the literature.[2] The infant was born without complications.

Obstetrical Management
The diagnosis of a cystic lesion of the umbilical cord should be an indication for serial examinations to verify normal growth of the fetus and changes in the size of the lesion. A theoretical risk is the development of vascular compression by an expanding cyst. Doppler examination may be helpful in these instances. Delivery could be recommended as soon as lung maturity is documented in patients with sizable lesions.

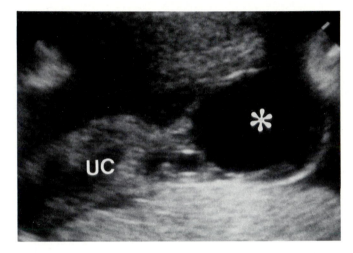

Figure 11–8. Cystic lesion of the umbilical cord (∗) corresponds to an allantoid cyst. UC, umbilical cord.

REFERENCES

1. Fox H: Pathology of the Placenta. London, Saunders, 1978.
2. Sachs L, Fourcroy JL, Wenzel DJ, et al.: Prenatal detection of umbilical cord allantoic cyst. Radiology 145:445, 1982.

VASCULAR LESIONS OF THE UMBILICAL CORD

Thrombosis of the Umbilical Vessels

Definition
Occlusion of one[6] or more[3] vessels of the umbilical cord. This entity refers primarily to thrombosis of the umbilical vein, since this vessel is the only source of oxygenated blood coming from the placenta.

Incidence
Approximately 20 cases have been reported in the literature.[6,10,16] Only 3 cases were found in an autopsy series of 4000 neonatal deaths and stillbirths weighing more than 400 g.[12] The incidence of umbilical cord thrombosis is higher in infants born to diabetic mothers (1:82) than in infants born to nondiabetic mothers (2:3918).[12] Also, the incidence of systemic thrombosis is higher in infants with diabetic mothers.

Etiology and Pathology
Thrombosis of the umbilical vessels may be a primary event[16] or may be secondary to localized increased resistance in the umbilical circulation (torsion, knotting, looping, compressions, hematoma).[2,6,7,11,13,15] Usually, the anatomic abnormality is close to the thrombus. However, in one fetus the thrombosis occurred at the opposite end of the torsion.[3] Aneurysmic dilatation has also been reported in association with this disorder.[5,8]

Other etiologic factors could be phlebitis and arteritis.[10] In one documented case, the mother had rheumatoid arthritis.[1] The incidence of systemic thrombotic accidents has been reported to be higher in infants born to mothers with overt diabetes than to nondiabetic mothers (15.8 percent versus 0.8 percent).[12]

Thrombosis of the umbilical vein has been observed in association with nonimmune hydrops.[1,4,14] Tense ascites could impair blood flow in the abdominal portion of the umbilical vein and create conditions favoring the development of thrombosis.

Diagnosis
The sonographic visualization of a thrombosed umbilical vein has been demonstrated in a report in which three fetal demises were carefully examined for thrombosis. Increased echogenecity of umbilical vessels was the diagnostic finding. In one case, this occurred in the intraabdominal portion of the umbilical vein. This condition has been prenatally diagnosed in live fetuses.

Associated Anomalies
In most reports, no associated anomalies have been reported. In one patient, dysmorphic features, such as low set ears, hypertelorism, and long limbs, were reported.[16] A report at variance with the literature is that of Konstantinova, who cited eight patients with varices and thrombosis of the umbilical cord having severe associated anomalies (hydrocephaly, anencephaly, trisomy 21, renal agenesis, spina bifida, cor triloculare, and phocomelia).[9]

Prognosis
There are only four infants who have survived thrombosis of the umbilical vein.[8,10,13,16] The prognosis in all other patients is understandably poor.

REFERENCES
1. Abrams SL, Callen PW, Filly RA: Umbilical vein thrombosis: Sonographic detection in utero. J Ultrasound Med 4:283, 1985.
2. Benirschke K, Driscoll SG: The Pathology of the Human Placenta. New York, Springer-Verlag, 1968, pp 63–73, 334–339.
3. Colgan TJ, Luk SC: Umbilical cord torsion, thrombosis and intrauterine death of a twin fetus. Arch Pathol Lab Med 106:101, 1982.
4. Driscoll SG: Hydrops fetalis. N Engl J Med 275:1432, 1966.
5. Fischer A: Fetale Atrophie bei fehlerhafter Anlage der Nabelarterien und Kleinheit der Placenta: Ein Beitrag zur Frage nichterblicher Missbildungen. Frankfurt Z Pathol 68:497, 1957.
6. Fritz MA, Christopher CR: Umbilical vein thrombosis and maternal diabetes mellitus. J Reprod Med 26:320, 1981.
7. Gardner RF, Trussell RR: Ruptured hematoma of the umbilical cord. Obstet Gynecol 24:791, 1964.
8. Ghosh A, Woo JSK, MacHenry C, et al.: Fetal loss from umbilical cord abnormalities—A difficult case for prevention. Eur J Obstet Gynecol 18.183, 1984.
9. Konstantinova B: Malformations of the umbilical cord. Acta Genet Med Gemellol 26:259, 1977.
10. Lednar A, Arfwedson H, Havu N: Die Trombose der Umbilikalgefasse. Zentralbl Gynaekol 92:435, 1970.
11. Nayak SK: Thrombosis of the umbilical cord vessels. Aust NZ J Obstet Gynaecol 7:148, 1967.
12. Oppenheimer EH, Esterly JR: Thrombosis in the new-

born: Comparison between infants of diabetic and nondiabetic mothers. J Pediatr 67:549, 1965.

13. Perrin EVD, Kahn-Vander Bel J: Degeneration and calcification of the umbilical cord. Obstet Gynecol 26: 371, 1965.

14. Turkel SB: Conditions associated with nonimmune hydrops fetalis. Clin Perinatol 9:613, 1982.

15. Weber J: Constriction of the umbilical cord as a cause of fetal death. Acta Obstet Gynecol Scand 42:259, 1963.

16. Wolfman WL, Purohit DM, Self SE: Umbilical vein thrombosis at 32 weeks' gestation with delivery of a living infant. Am J Obstet Gynecol 146:468, 1983.

Hemangiomas of the Umbilical Cord

Synonyms
Angiomyxomas of the umbilical cord, cavernous hemangioma, hemangiofibromyxoma, myxoangioma, and telangioectasic myxosarcoma.

Definition
Hemangioma of the umbilical cord is a tumor arising from the endothelial cells of the vessels of the umbilical cord.

Incidence
After excluding those cases in which the tumor does not arise along the umbilical cord (placental hemangiomas) or lacks an endothelial component (representing, therefore, hematomas), only 18 cases are reported in the literature.[3–11,13]

Etiology and Pathology
The lesions can measure up to 15 cm. They consist of an angiomatous nodule surrounded by edema and myxomatous degeneration of the Wharton's jelly. The tumor is more frequently located toward the placental end of the umbilical cord. The sites of origin are the main vessels of the umbilical cord, in order of frequency: arteries, veins, and vitelline capillaries. The lesions may involve more than one vessel. The typical microscopic appearance is that of multiple channels lined by benign endothelium accompanied by edema and myxoid degeneration of the stroma of the cord. The differential diagnosis between hemangiomas and hematomas of the umbilical cord is provided by the presence in the former of capillaries lined by endothelium and showing a positive immunoperoxidase staining for factor VIII–related antigen.

Associated Anomalies
This entity has been associated with nonimmune hydrops.[2,11,12] In one case, there was an association between a hemangioma of the umbilical cord and severe diffuse skin hemangiomas.[11] In placental hemangiomas, the incidence of associated vascular neoplasms is 10 percent. Although the same risk has not been reported with umbilical cord hemangiomas, it is possible that these infants are at a greater risk.[8]

Diagnosis
We have made a prenatal diagnosis of this tumor in a 34-week-old fetus. The lesion appeared as a hyperechogenic mass, extending from the fetal umbilicus for a distance of about 5 cm. The cord appeared edematous for most of its length, and a localized collection of edematous fluid (pseudocyst) could be seen close to the nodule (Fig. 11–9). Three umbilical vessels were present with normal wave form at Doppler examination.

A hemangioma of the umbilical cord appears as a hyperechogenic mass. Differential diagnosis for this type of lesion includes teratomas and an umbilical cord hematoma (see respective sections in this chapter). Associated localized edema of the umbilical cord has been noted in the two cases identified prenatally with ultrasound. In one case, the solid component of the lesion was not recognized because of its small size.[11] The mechanism responsible for the pseudocyst formation is unknown. It has been suggested that it results from transudation of fluid. A precise diagnosis of hemangioma of the umbilical cord may not be possible.

An umbilical cord hemangioma has been associated with elevated alphafetoprotein.[1] However, in our case, maternal serum alphafetoprotein determination in midtrimester was normal.

Prognosis
Data are limited because of the rarity of the disease. The development of hydrops would logically suggest compromise. Increased morbidity (12 of 18) and mortality (7 of 18) have been observed.[3,4] It is unclear whether this represents a truly poor prognosis or detection biases. The excessive mortality is due to other seemingly unrelated complications, such as

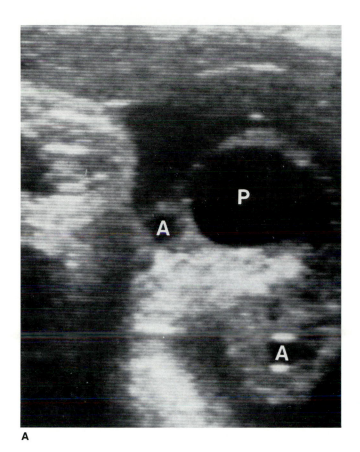
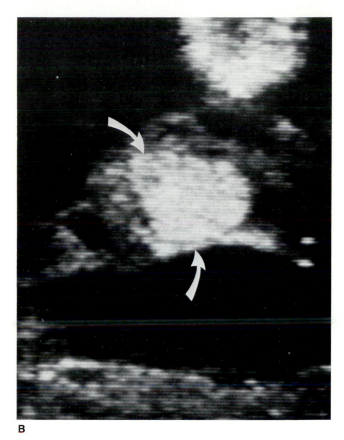

A B

Figure 11–9. A. Umbilical cord close to the level of insertion into the fetal abdomen. A hyperechogenic nodule is clearly visible within the cord. A, umbilical arteries, P, pseudocyst due to localized accumulation of fluid within the Wharton's jelly. **B.** Loop of cord free floating. The dense nodule is visible, surrounded by edema of the Wharton's jelly.

prematurity, postmaturity, birth trauma, preeclampsia, or short umbilical cord. The mechanism by which this tumor causes fetal compromise is probably mechanical impairment of the fetal circulation.

Obstetrical Management

The diagnosis of a lesion of the umbilical cord should probably be an indication for serial examinations to verify normal growth of the fetus, changes in the size of the lesion and signs of non-immune hydrops. A theoretical risk is the development of vascular compression by an expanding lesion. Doppler examination may be helpful in these instances. Delivery could be recommended as soon as lung maturity is documented in patients with sizable lesions.

REFERENCES

1. Barson AJ, Donnai P, Ferguson A, et al: Haemangioma of the cord: Further cause of raised maternal serum and liquor alpha-fetoprotein. Br Med J 281:1252, 1980.
2. Becker MJ: Proceedings: Hydrops fetalis. Arch Dis Child 50:665, 1975.
3. Benirschke K, Dodds JP: Angiomyxoma of the umbilical cord with atrophy of an umbilical artery. Obstet Gynecol 30:99, 1967.
4. Buettner HH, Goecke H: Kavernoeses Haemangiom der Nabelschnur. Zentralbl Gynakol 97:439, 1975.
5. Carvounis EE, Dimmick JE, Wright VJ: Angiomyxoma of umbilical cord. Arch Pathol Lab Med 102:178, 1978.
6. Dohmen W, Bubenzer J: Haematom als Komplikation eines kavernoesen Haemangioms der Nabelschnur. Fallbericht mit Literaturuebersicht. Z Geburtshilfe Perinatol 182:312, 1978.
7. Fortune DW, Ostor AG: Angiomyxomas of the umbilical cord. Obstet Gynecol 55:375, 1980.
8. Heifetz SA, Rueda-Pedraza ME: Hemangiomas of the umbilical cord. Pediatr Pathol 1:385, 1983.
9. Jakobovits A, Herezeg J: Haemangioma of the umbilical cord. Ann Chir Gynaecol Fenn 59:159, 1970.
10. Schlaeder G, Irrmann M, Philippe E: Un cas d'hemangiome du cordon avec hematome. Bull Fed Gynecol Obstet Fr 16:208, 1964.
11. Seifer DB, Ferguson JE, Behrens CM, et al: Nonimmune hydrops fetalis in association with hemangioma of the umbilical cord. Obstet Gynecol 66:283, 1985.
12. Turkel SB: Conditions associated with nonimmune hydrops fetalis. Clin Perinatol 9:613, 1982.
13. Zeman V, Rauchenberg M: Cavernous and capillary hemangiomas of umbilical cord. Cesk Pediatr 25:603, 1970.

Hematoma of the Umbilical Cord

Definition
Extravasation of blood into the Wharton's jelly.

Incidence
Between 1 in 5505[5] and 1 in 12,699.[4]

Etiology and Pathology
There is no adequate explanation for this phenomenon. A traumatic insult (torsion, loops, knots, traction, and prolapse) in an area of local weakness of the vessel wall has been advocated by some.[3,5,14] With the use of invasive techniques of prenatal diagnosis, such as fetoscopy and percutaneous umbilical cord puncture, it is possible that this entity occurs iatrogenically.[12] The dimensions of the reported hematomas have ranged from 1 to 4 cm, and the length has been up to 42 cm. The most frequently involved vessel is the umbilical vein, with a vein: artery ratio of 9:1.[5] The vitelline vessels could also be involved. In 11 of 61 cases, the hematoma was multiple.[2,5] The most common site was near the fetal insertion of the cord,[3,6,14] but hematomas have been reported also in its central portion.[7,9] A serious complication is the rupture of the hematoma into the amniotic cavity, since this may lead to exsanguination.[2] Another complication, reported by Fletcher,[7] is neonatal myocardial infarction attributed to embolization of fragments released from the hematoma.

Diagnosis
Prenatal identification of this condition has been reported twice (Fig. 11–10).[13,15] The first case presented as a 6- by 8-cm hypoechogenic septated mass.[13] The hypoechogenic nature of the mass suggests that the clot was old, because a fresh clot is expected to be hyperechogenic. The second case showed a hyperechogenic lesion, which was recognized after an initially bloody amniocentesis.[15] The differential diagnosis between this entity and other masses of the umbilical cord is difficult. Hematomas may be more irregular than other cystic lesions.

Prognosis
The fetal mortality reported by Dippel is 47 percent.[5] The overall perinatal mortality in all reported cases is 52 percent (26 of 50).[1,3,5,7,8–11,13,14] Death is caused mainly by exsanguination and compression of the vessels.

Obstetrical Management
If a hematoma is suspected in a fetus, an amniocentesis should be performed to establish lung maturity. In the presence of a mature fetus, there would be little advantage to prolonging the pregnancy. The optimal mode of delivery has not been established. However, 10 of 17 fetal deaths have occurred during labor. It is not known whether the accident occurs predominantly during labor or whether labor per se is dangerous for the infant with an umbilical cord hematoma. Doppler examination may provide a non-invasive means of examining umbilical vascular resistance.

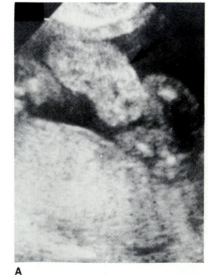 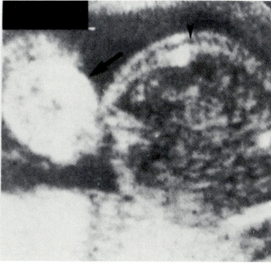

Figure 11–10. A. Sausage-shaped umbilical cord hematoma (*arrow*) is hyperechoic and markedly thickened. **B.** Cross-section of umbilical cord hematoma (*arrow*) adjacent to but not contiguous with the fetal abdomen at the level of the intrahepatic umbilical vein. *(Reproduced with permission from Sutro et al.: AJR 142:802, 1984.)*

A   B

REFERENCES

1. Breen JL, Riva HL, Hatch RP: Hematoma of the umbilical cord. A case report. Am J Obstet Gynecol 76:1288, 1958.
2. Bret AJ, Bardiaux M: Hematoma of the umbilical cord. Rev Franc Gynecol Obstet 55:81, 1960.
3. Clare NM, Hayashi R, Khodr G: Intrauterine death from umbilical cord hematoma. Arch Pathol Lab Med 103:46, 1979.
4. Corkill TF: The infant's vulnerable life-line. Aust NZ J Obstet Gynaecol 1:154, 1961.
5. Dippel AL: Hematomas of the umbilical cord. Surg Gynecol Obstet 70:51, 1940.
6. Elhassani SB: The umbilical cord: Care, anomalies, and diseases. South Med J 77:730, 1984.
7. Fletcher MA, Meyer M, Kirkpatrick SE, et al.: Myocardial infarction associated with umbilical cord hematoma. J Pediatr 89:806, 1976.
8. Gardner RF, Trussell RR: Ruptured hematoma of the umbilical cord. Obstet Gynecol 24:791, 1964.
9. Lupovitch A, McInerney TS: Hematoma of the umbilical cord: A dissecting aneurysm of the umbilical vein. Am J Obstet Gynecol 102:902, 1968.
10. Ratten GJ: Spontaneous haematoma of the umbilical cord. Aust NZ J Obstet Gynaecol 9:125, 1969.
11. Roberts-Thomson ME: The hazards of umbilical cord haematoma. Med J Aust 1:648, 1973.
12. Romero R, Chervenak FA, Coustan D, et al.: Antenatal sonographic diagnosis of umbilical cord laceration. Am J Obstet Gynecol 143:719, 1982.
13. Ruvinsky ED, Wiley TL, Morrison JC, et al.: In utero diagnosis of umbilical cord hematoma by ultrasonography. Am J Obstet Gynecol 140:833, 1981.
14. Schreier R, Brown S: Hematoma of the umbilical cord: Report of a case. Obstet Gynecol 20:798, 1962.
15. Sutro WH, Tuck SM, Loesevitz A, et al.: Prenatal observation of umbilical cord hematoma. AJR 142:801, 1984.

OTHER PATHOLOGIC CONDITIONS OF THE UMBILICAL CORD

Strictures or Coarctation of the Umbilical Cord

Synonyms

Constriction of the umbilical cord,[11] umbilical cord occlusion,[7] and fibrosis circumscripta of the umbilical cord.[6]

Definition

Coarctation is characterized by a localized narrowing of the cord with disappearance of the Wharton's jelly, thickening of the vascular walls, and narrowing of their lumens.[10] Generally, torsion of the umbilical cord is present.[9]

Incidence

Approximately 30 cases have been described in the literature. However, this may not represent the real incidence of this entity. Tavares-Fortuna and Lourdes-Pratas conducted a prospective study and reported an incidence of 1 in 250 deliveries.[10]

Etiology and Pathology

The mechanisms responsible for coarctation of the umbilical cord are not understood. Edmonds[1] suggested that coarctation and subsequent torsion are a postmortem event caused by necrobiosis of the Wharton's jelly. Weber[11] pointed out the following objections to this hypothesis: (1) liveborn fetuses have been reported to have constrictions and (2) coarctations are extremely rare in stillbirths. Perhaps this complication should be viewed as a local failure of Wharton's jelly development that creates a weak point in the umbilical cord. Fetal motion could lead to torsion around this point.

The site of the torsion is generally close to the fetus.[3] A localized edematous area is frequently reported distal to the torsion point.[8] Multiple strictures along the length of the umbilical cord can be found.[4,10]

Diagnosis

To date, this condition has not been diagnosed with ultrasound, although recognition should be possible.

Associated Anomalies

The following anomalies have been reported with coarctation of the umbilical cord: type C tracheoesophageal fistula, cleft lip,[5] anencephaly, anophthalmia and exophthalmos,[6] polyhydramnios, ventricular septal defect and trisomy 18,[2] and generalized subcutaneous edema.[7]

Prognosis
Most reported cases of coarctation result in stillbirths. However, this may represent reporting biases. Recurrences in subsequent pregnancies have not been noted in the literature.[3,11]

Obstetrical Management
Should this diagnosis be made, serial monitoring of preterm infants would be indicated. Delivery as soon as there is a reasonable chance for survival would seem logical.

REFERENCES

1. Edmonds HW: The spiral twist of the normal umbilical cord in twins and in singletons. Am J Obstet Gynecol 67:102, 1954.
2. Ghosh A, Woo JSK, MacHenry C, et al.: Fetal loss fromumbilical cord abnormalities—A difficult case for prevention. Eur J Obstet Gynecol 18:183, 1984.
3. Gilbert EF, Zugibe FT: Torsion and constriction of the umbilical cord. Arch Pathol 97:58, 1974.
4. Javert CT, Barton B: Congenital and acquired lesions of the umbilical cord and spontaneous abortion. Am J Obstet Gynecol 63:1065, 1952.
5. Kiley KC, Perkins CS, Penney LL: Umbilical cord stricture associated with intrauterine fetal demise. J Reprod Med 31:154, 1986.
6. Konstantinova B: Malformations of the umbilical cord. Acta Genet Med Gemellol 26:259, 1977.
7. Shenker L, Anderson W, Anderson C: Short communications. Ultrasound demonstration of masses in a 15-week fetus: Hydrops in a fetus with umbilical cord occlusion. Prenat Diagn 1:217, 1981.
8. Speck G, Palmer RE: Torsion of the umbilical cord: A cause of fetal death. South Med J 54:48, 1961.
9. Virgilio LA, Spangler DB: Fetal death secondary to constriction and torsion of the umbilical cord. Arch Pathol Lab Med 102:32, 1978.
10. Tavares-Fortuna JF, Lourdes-Pratas M: Coarctation of the umbilical cord: A cause of intrauterine fetal death. Int J Gynaecol Obstet 15:469, 1978.
11. Weber J: Constriction of the umbilical cord as a cause of fetal death. Acta Obstet Gynecol Scand 42:259, 1963.

Teratomas

Definition
A germ cell tumor containing elements from the three germinal layers.

Incidence
Four cases have been reported in the literature.[2–5]

Embryology
Germ cells arise in the dorsal wall of the yolk sac; from there they migrate to the genital ridge. During the course of this process, germ cells are found in the wall of the primitive gut. Since in early pregnancy, the primitive gut sends an evagination into the umbilical cord, germ cells may reach the cord at this stage.[1]

It is possible that some teratomas are indeed acardiac twins, and vice versa.[4]

Pathology
This tumor has been reported to measure up to 9 cm in diameter. Histologically, it shows elements originating from the three germinal layers, and it may undergo calcification. Teratomas are found at any point along the length of the umbilical cord. The differential diagnosis with an acardiac twin is based on the following: (1) the acardiac twin has a separate, although rudimentary, umbilical cord, (2) the twin cannot be entirely intrafunicular, and (3) the twin shows some evidence of body organization (e.g., cranium, spine) whereas teratomas are completely disorganized.

Diagnosis
An umbilical cord teratoma has not been diagnosed prenatally. The entity must be considered as part of the differential diagnosis, of a complex lesion of the umbilical cord.

Prognosis
In one of the three available cases for review, the fetus died.[4]

Obstetrical Management
Diagnosis of a lesion of the umbilical cord should probably be an indication for serial examinations to verify normal growth of the fetus, changes in the size of the lesion, and development of nonimmune hydrops. A theoretical risk is the development of vascular compression by an expanding lesion. Doppler examination may be helpful in these instances. Delivery could be recommended as soon as lung

maturity is documented in patients with sizable lesions.

REFERENCES

1. Fox H: Pathology of the Placenta. London, Saunders, 1978.
2. Haendly P: Teratom der Nabelschnur. Arch Gynakol 116:578, 1922.
3. Heckmann U, Cornelius HV, Freudenberg V: Das Teratom der Nabelschnur: ein kasuistischer Beitrag zu den echten Tumoren der Nabelschnur. Geburtshilfe Fraunheilk 32:605, 1972.
4. Kreyberg L: A teratoma-like swelling in the umbilical cord possibly of acardius nature. J Pathol Bacteriol 75:109, 1958.
5. Perrin EVDK: Anatomy of the umbilical cord. In: Perrin E, Roth LM (eds.): Contemporary Issues in Surgical Pathology. Pathology of the Placenta. New York, Churchill Livingstone, 1984, pp 122–139.

True Knots of the Umbilical Cord

Definition
Knots of the umbilical cord are classified as false or true. The former consist of simple dilatations of the umbilical vessels that look like knots but are considered devoid of any clinical significance. True knots are formed when the fetus passes through a loop of umbilical cord.

Incidence
In recent prospective series, it varied from 0.04 to 1 percent.[2-7]

Etiology and Pathology
Factors predisposing to true knots are commonly believed to include monoamniotic twins, long cords, and polyhydramnios. It seems logical that knots are formed in early pregnancy, when it is possible for the fetus to go through a loop of umbilical cord. Tightening of the knot can occur during labor. Knots can be single or multiple.

Diagnosis
This diagnosis is feasible with ultrasound. We have seen one fetus with isolated ascites who later proved to have a true knot of the umbilical cord.

Associated Anomalies
A recent study has suggested that infants with true knots of the umbilical cord have an increased incidence of congenital anomalies.[1]

Prognosis
Perinatal mortality varies from 8 to 11 percent.[4,7]

Obstetrical Management
A cesarean section would seem the most logical approach if a diagnosis is made.

REFERENCES

1. Bronsteen RA, Bottoms SF: Perinatal implications of umbilical cord abnormalities. Presented at the Sixth Annual Meeting of the Society of Perinatal Obstetricians, January 30–February 1, 1986, San Antonio, Texas.
2. Chasnoff IJ, Fletcher MA: True knot of the umbilical cord. Am J Obstet Gynecol 117:425, 1977.
3. Corkill TF: The infant's vulnerable life-line. Aust NZ J Obstet Gynaecol 1:154, 1961.
4. di Terlizzi G, Rossi GF: Studio clinico-statistico sulle anomalie del funicolo. Ann Ostet Ginecol 77:459, 1955.
5. Earn AA: The effect of congenital abnormalities of the umbilical cord and placenta on the newborn and mother: A survey of 5676 consecutive deliveries. J Obstet Gynaecol Br Emp 58:456, 1951.
6. Ragucci N, Morandi C: Le distocie del funicolo ombelicale (contributo clinico-statistico). Min Ginecol 21:653, 1969.
7. Scheffel T, Langanke D: Die Nabelschnurkomplikationen an der Universitats-Frauenklinik Leipzig von 1955 bis 1967. Zentralbl Gynaekol 92:429, 1970.

Cord Presentation

Synonym
Occult prolapse.

Definition
Prolapse refers to protrusion of the umbilical cord through the cervix into the vagina. Occult prolapse occurs when the cord lies alongside the presenting part. Cord presentation is defined as a cord lying between the presenting part and the lower pole of the intact membranes.

Incidence
The mean incidence of cord prolapse is 1 in 200 births. The frequency of cord presentation (diagnosed with ultrasound) is 0.61 percent.[1]

Etiology
Predisposing factors include abnormal presentation, prematurity, polyhydramnios, unengaged present-

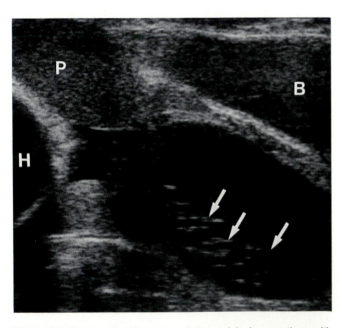

Figure 11–11. Longitudinal scan of the pelvis in a patient with preterm labor at 27 weeks. Note the multiple loops of umbilical cord (*arrows*), which are in front of the fetal head. B, bladder; H, head; P, placenta.

ing part, and long umbilical cord.[2] Prolapse occurs after either artificial or spontaneous rupture of the membranes.

Diagnosis
The diagnosis is easily made by demonstrating loops of umbilical cord in the lower segment below the presenting part (Fig. 11–11).

Prognosis
Lange et al.[1] have conducted a prospective study demonstrating that 9 of 1471 (0.61 percent) patients had cord presentation. This diagnosis was based on the demonstration of loops of umbilical cord in the lower uterine segment below the presenting part. Of the nine patients diagnosed to have cord presentation, seven were delivered by cesarean section and two vaginally. In four of the seven cases delivered by cesarean section, a cord presentation was found. In the other three it was suspected. Of the two vaginal deliveries, one was a stillbirth associated with a cord prolapse and the other underwent a spontaneous version with resolution of cord presentation.

Obstetrical Management
In patients at risk for cord presentation (malpresentation, polyhydramnios), a specific evaluation of the position of the cord should be performed. If a cord presentation is found in a term infant, admission to the hospital for delivery is recommended. Delivery can be accomplished by cesarean section. If the diagnosis is made in a viable but preterm gestation, expectant management is the most prudent approach. Serial examinations are recommended.

REFERENCES

1. Lange IR, Manning FA, Morrison I, et al.: Cord prolapse: Is antenatal diagnosis possible? Am J Obstet Gynecol 151:1083, 1985.
2. Rayburn WF, Beynen A, Brinkman DL: Umbilical cord length and intrapartum complications. Obstet Gynecol 57:450, 1981.

Velamentous Insertion

Definition
The term "velamentous insertion" refers to attachment of the cord to the membranes rather than to the placental mass. Marginal insertions refer to implantation of the cord into the edge of the placenta.

Incidence
The incidence is 0.09 to 1.8 percent.[5,6,8] This condition is more common in multiple pregnancies.

Etiology
Benirschke and Driscoll[1] favor the concept of trophotropism. This view proposes that velamentous insertion occurs when most of the placental tissue grows laterally, leaving the initially centrally located umbilical cord in an area that will become atrophic. An alternative hypothesis suggests that there is a primary defect in the implantation of cord that occurs in a site of trophoblast in front of the decidua capsularis instead of the area of trophoblast that forms the placental mass.[9]

Pathology
Implantation of the umbilical vessels occurs in the chorion laeve, and therefore, the umbilical vessels lie on the membrane surface.

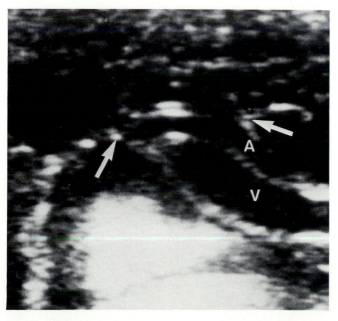

Figure 11–12. Velamentous insertion *(arrows)* of the umbilical cord on the amnion. A, umbilical artery, V, umbilical vein.

Associated Anomalies
The incidence of associated anomalies is increased and varies from 5.9 percent[3] to 8.5 percent.[7] The reported anomalies have included esophageal atresia, obstructive uropathies, congenital hip dislocation, asymmetrical head shape, spina bifida, ventricular septal defects, cleft palate, and trisomy 21 (one case). Bilobated placenta has also been found in association with the velamentous insertion of the umbilical cord. The birth weight of infants with velamentous insertion is lower than that of a control group even when malformed infants are excluded (3098 g, SD = 765, versus 3416 g, SD = 712).[2,4] The incidence of intrauterine growth retardation (defined as 2 SD below the mean for gestational age) is 7.5 percent,[2,8] and the incidence of premature births is 17.2 percent.[2] In twin gestations, the twin with velamentous insertion has a lower birth weight than the unaffected twin.[2]

Diagnosis
This diagnosis has been made several times in our institution. The critical point is establishing the relationship between the insertion of the umbilical cord and the placental mass (Fig. 11–12).

Prognosis
Infants with velamentous insertion are at increased risk for IUGR, preterm birth, and congenital anomalies.[6] Data collected in Norway between 1969 and 1981 showed that infants with low birth weight and velamentous insertion had some difficulty in attaining normal weight and length.[3] There were also some anomalies detected in childhood that were missed at birth, including esophagobranchial fistula, tetralogy of Fallot, obstructive uropathy, osteogenesis imperfecta, and muscle dystrophia.[3]

Obstetrical Management
If this diagnosis is made, a careful examination for associated anomalies is required. It is important to demonstrate a stomach, since esophageal atresia has been the most common anomaly detected in a large series (4 of 305). Echocardiography should be included. Serial sonographic examinations are indicated to exclude IUGR. Labor is a critical period of time because the umbilical vessels could be ruptured (vasa previa). For velamentous insertions located in the uterine fundus, no change in standard obstetrical management seems to be required. If the velamentous insertion is located in the lower uterine segment,

an elective section to avoid rupture of a vasa previa may be considered.

REFERENCES

1. Benirschke K, Driscoll SG: The Pathology of the Human Placenta. New York, Springer-Verlag, 1974.
2. Bjoro K Jr: Vascular anomalies of the umbilical cord: I. Obstetric implications. Early Hum Dev 8:119, 1983.
3. Bjoro K Jr: Vascular anomalies of the umbilical cord. II. Perinatal and pediatric implications. Early Hum Dev 8:279, 1983.
4. Bjoro K, Jr: Gross pathology of the placenta in intra-uterine growth retardation. Ann Chir Gynaecol 6:316, 1981.
5. di Terlizzi G, Rossi GF: Studio clinico-statistico sulle anomalie del funicolo. Ann Ostet Ginecol 77:459, 1955.
6. Fox H: Pathology of the Placenta. London, Saunders, 1978.
7. Robinson LK, Jones KL, Benirschke K: The nature of structural defects associated with velamentous and marginal insertion of the umbilical cord. Am J Obstet Gynecol 146:191, 1983.
8. Scott JM, Jordan JM: Placental insufficiency and the small-for-dates baby. Am J Obstet Gynecol 113:823, 1972.
9. von Franque O: Zur Pathologie der Nachgeburtsheile. Geburtshilfe Gynaekol 43:463, 1950.

12

Other Anomalies

Twin Pregnancies

Definition

Monozygotic (MZ) or "identical" twins derive from a single fertilized ovum. They are of the same sex and have identical genotypes. Dizygotic (DZ) or "fraternal" twins arise from two different ova fertilized by two different sperms. Their genetic similarity is the same as with siblings.

Incidence

There is considerable geographic variation in the incidence of twin births ranging from 1:25 in the Yoruba tribe in Nigeria to 1:150 in Japan. The incidence in the United States is 1:88.[2] This difference is attributable to changes in the rate of DZ twinning, as the MZ twinning rate remains stable (0.35 to 0.45 per 100 births) throughout different populations. Factors that alter the rate of DZ twinning include race, maternal age, use of ovulation-inducing agents, and a positive family history. Twins are more common in blacks than in whites. The incidence of twinning increases with maternal age up to the age of 35, and then decreases.[1] The use of clomiphene citrate is associated with a multiple pregnancy rate of 5 percent, almost all of which are twins.[9] Pergonal therapy is associated with a twinning rate of 30 percent, of which triplets or higher conceptional rates account for 5 percent.[9] The tendency for multiple ovulation seems to be an inherited trait expressed only in females. Therefore, the recurrence risk for twinning in a sibship is constant for MZ twins (0.35 to 0.4 per 1000 births), while it rises to three times that of the normal population for DZ twins.[10] Among white North Americans, 35 percent of all twins are unlike-sexed DZ, 35 percent are like-sexed DZ, and 30 percent are MZ.

Embryology-Pathology

DZ twinning is determined at ovulation, as it requires the availability of two ova. MZ twinning occurs after fertilization and is confined to the earliest stages of embryogenesis, because the embryo is incapable of fission once it is formed. Figure 12–1 illustrates the timing of monozygotic twinning events. If the separation occurs at the two-cell stage (approximately 60 hours after fertilization), the twins will be dichorionic diamniotic. If it occurs between the 3d and 8th days after fertilization, the twins will be monochorionic diamniotic. Separation between the 8th and 10th days results in monochorionic monoamniotic twins. Conjoined twins constitute the last type of event in the spectrum of monozygotic twinning.[2]

Determination of Twin Zygocity

Determination of zygocity is important. Zygocity information will be helpful later in life if one twin develops a disease such as diabetes or requires a transplant. Zygocity assessment, therefore, should be attempted at birth. A simple approach consists of first looking at the sex of the twins, because discordant sex (35 percent of twins) indicates dizygocity. If the sex is the same, information should be obtained from microscopic placental examination. The critical area for study is a section of the dividing membranes at the placental insertion, also known as the T-zone. Twenty percent of all twins will have a monochorionic placenta, which is always a sign of monozygocity. (Sixty-five percent of MZ twins have monochorionic placentation.) For the remaining 45 percent, i.e., those of the same sex and without a monochorionic placenta, genetic studies including

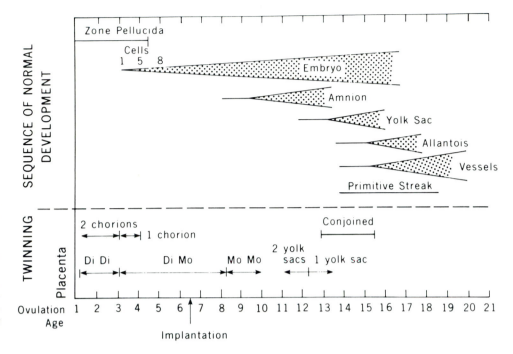

Figure 12–1. The timing of the monozygotic twinning process. On the horizontal axis are days after fertilization. The types of placenta expected from embryonic events are: Di Di, diamniotic dichorionic; Di Mo, diamniotic monochorionic; Mo Mo, monoamniotic monochorionic. (*Reproduced with permission from Benirschke, Kim: N Engl J Med 288:1276, 1973.*)

blood typing and chromosomal marking will be required to determine zygocity. Molecular biology studies may help in this assessment.

Associated Anomalies

The prevalence of congenital anomalies in twin pregnancies is higher than in singleton pregnancies. All twins are at risk for constraint deformities as a consequence of intrauterine crowding. The excess in structural congenital anomalies observed in multiple pregnancies is attributable to MZ twins.[3,6,8] Congenital defects in multiple pregnancies can be classified into three groups: (1) anomalies unique to multiple conception, such as conjoined twins and twin reversed arterial perfusion (TRAP) sequence; (2) anomalies not unique to multiple conception, but that occur more often in twins, such as hydrocephalus, congenital heart disease, single umbilical artery, and neural tube defects; and (3) anomalies not unique to twins, but observed with increased frequency because of mechanical or vascular factors associated with twinning, such as talipes, skull asymmetry, and congenital dislocation of the hip. The rate of concordance for congenital anomalies in twins varies from 3.6 percent to 18.8 percent.[5] These figures are influenced by zygocity and the specific anomaly. For example, the incidence of concordance for facial clefting is 40 percent in MZ twins and 8 percent in DZ twins.

Discrepancy for chromosomal anomalies is the rule for DZ twins and surprisingly, also occasionally for MZ twins.[5] Heterokaryotypes refer to the discrepant chromosomal constitution observed in some MZ twins. Some genotypes may also be expressed differently in MZ twins. While phenotypic concordance is the rule for MZ twins with trisomy 21 or Klinefelter's syndrome, MZ twins with gonadal dysgenesis are often discordant.[4,7]

REFERENCES

1. Benirschke K: Multiple gestation: Incidence, etiology, and inheritance. In: Creasy RK, Resnik R (eds): Maternal-Fetal Medicine: Principles and Practice. Philadelphia, Saunders, 1984, pp 511–526.
2. Benirschke K: The pathophysiology of the twinning process. In: Iffy L, Kaminetzy HA (eds): Principles and Practice of Obstetrics and Gynecology. New York, Wiley, 1981, pp 1165–1170.
3. Hay S, Wehrung DA: Congenital malformations in twins. Am J Hum Genet 22:662, 1970.
4. Karp L, Bryant JI, Tagatz G, et al.: The occurrence of gonadal dysgenesis in association with monozygotic twinning. J Med Genet 12:70, 1975.
5. Little J, Bryan E: Congenital anomalies in twins. Semin Perinatol 10:50, 1986.
6. Myrianthopoulos NC: Congenital malformations in twins: Epidemiologic survey. Birth Defects 11(8):1, 1975.
7. Pedersen IK, Philip J, Sele V, et al.: Monozygotic twins with dissimilar phenotypes and chromosome complements. Acta Obstet Gynecol Scand 59:459, 1980.
8. Schinzel AA, Smith DW, Miller JR: Monozygotic twinning and structural defects. J Pediatr 95:921, 1979.
9. Speroff L, Glass RH, Kase NG (eds): Clinical Gynecologic Endocrinology and Infertility. Baltimore, Williams & Wilkins, 1983, pp 531–538.
10. Thompson JS, Thompson MW: Genetics in Medicine. Philadelphia, Saunders, 1986, pp 273–282.

Conjoined Twins

Incidence

The incidence is from 1 in 30,000 to 1 in 100,000 live births.[3,4,8] Seventy-five percent of conjoined twins are females.

Etiology

Unknown. Monozygotic twins arise from a single blastocyst that undergoes duplication between the 1st and 10th day after ovulation. Conjoined twins are commonly regarded as an abnormality of the process of monozygotic twinning, because of an incomplete division of the embryonic cell mass at one pole or at a point between the poles. Conjoined twins are a sporadic event that tends not to recur.

Pathology

A classification of conjoined twins is provided in Table 12–1. The most frequent types of conjoined twins are thoracoomphalopagus (28 percent), thoracopagus (18 percent), omphalopagus (10 percent), incomplete duplication (10 percent), and craniopagus (6 percent).[3]

Anatomic abnormalities are the rule in conjoined twins. In most cases, it is possible to assume that they derive directly as a consequence of the presumed abnormal division of the embryonic mass. In other cases, the origin of the malformation cannot be explained on a purely mechanical basis (e.g., facial clefting), and it suggests a more diffuse disturbance of morphogenesis. Figure 12–2 illustrates the different varieties of conjoined twins.

Craniopagus. Craniopagus may be classified, according to the area of junction, into frontal, parietal, temporal, or occipital varieties. Parietal craniopagus is twice as common as all other types combined. For surgical and prognostical purposes, craniopagus may also be subdivided into partial and complete types. In the former, brains are separated by bone or dura, and each brain has separate leptomeninges. In total craniopagus, brains are connected. Cerebral connection is most frequent in temporoparietal varieties. Successful separation depends upon the degree of connection between the brains and the presence of a superior sagittal sinus for each brain, as this is critical for adequate venous drainage.

Thoracopagus. Congenital heart disease is found in about 75 percent of patients. In 90 percent of cases, there is some degree of fusion of the pericardial sac.

The most frequent abnormality is a conjoined heart, with two ventricles and a varying number of atria (1 to 4), although a number of permutations have been reported. Ventricular septal defects are found in virtually all patients in addition to other deformities.[13,14]

Omphalopagus–Xiphopagus. A review of the literature indicates that the liver is conjoined in 81 percent of patients, the sternal cartilage in 26 percent, the diaphragm in 17 percent, and the genitourinary tract in 3 percent.[6] The anomalies not obviously linked to the abnormal division process of the embryonic mass include malformations of the abdominal wall (usually omphalocele) in at least one of the twins in 33 percent of cases, and congenital heart disease (most frequently ventricular septal defects and tetralogy of Fallot) in at least one of the twins in 25 percent of cases. Only one of nine sets of twins had concordance of the cardiac defect in both twins.[6]

Pygopagus. Pygopagus accounts for 20 percent of all conjoined twins. They are joined at the buttocks and lower spine, and face away from each other. They may share part of the sacral spinal canal, may have a common rectum and anus, and the external genitalia are often fused.

TABLE 12–1. CLASSIFICATION OF CONJOINED TWINS

Duplicata incompleta: Duplication occurring in only one part or region of the body. Examples:
  Diprosopus: one body, one head, two faces
  Dicephalus: one body, two heads
  Dipygus: one head, thorax and abdomen with two pelvis, and/or external genitalia, and/or four legs

Duplicata completa: Two complete conjoined twins
  Terata catadidyma: Conjunction in the lower part of the body
    Ischiopagus: Joined by inferior portion of coccyx and sacrum
    Pygopagus: Joined by lateral and posterior portion of coccyx and sacrum
  Terata anadidyma: Conjunction in the upper part of the body
    Syncephalus: Joined by the face
    Craniopagus: Joined at homologous portion of the cranial vault
  Terata anacatadidyma: Conjunction in the midpart of the body
    Thoracopagus: Joined at thoracic wall
    Xiphopagus: Joined at xyphoid process
    Omphalopagus: Joined in the area between the umbilicus and the xiphoid cartilage
    Rachipagus: Joined at any level of the spines above the sacrum

Adapted with permission from Guttmacher, Nichols: Birth Defects 3(1):3, 1967.

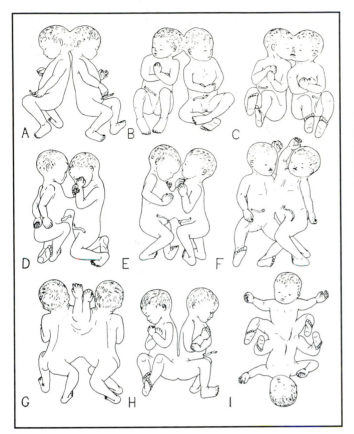
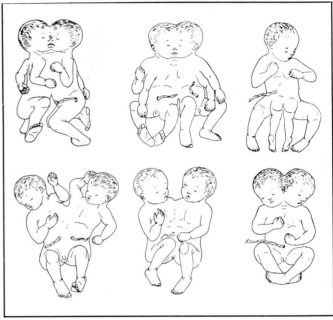

Figure 12–2. Drawing of the different types of conjoined twins. **Left.** This diagram illustrates cases of duplicata completa (conjoined twins where heads and limbs maintain their identity). **A-C.** Craniopagus. **D-G.** Thoracopagus. **H, I.** Pygopagus. **Right.** This diagram shows cases of duplicata incompleta (conjoined twins in which more extensive fusion takes place). *(Reproduced with permission from Patten: Human Embryology, 3d ed. New York, McGraw-Hill, 1968.)*

Ischiopagus. Ischiopagus represents 5 percent of all conjoined twins. They are joined at the inferior part of the sacrum and coccyx, and often have a common large pelvic ring formed by the union of the two pelvic girdles. Ischiopagus may have four legs (ischiopagus tetrapus) or three legs (ischiopagus tripus). These twins frequently share the lower gastrointestinal tract, so that the intestines join at the terminal ileum and empty into a single colon. They may have a single bladder and urethra, and the anus can be displaced. Vaginal anomalies and rectovaginal communications are quite common.[19]

Diagnosis

A detailed ultrasound examination to exclude the possibility of conjoined twins is mandatory in all multiple pregnancies. The index of suspicion should be raised when an interamniotic membrane cannot be identified, because all conjoined twins are monoamniotic. Other signs include difficulties in completely separating the twins (Figs. 12–3, 12–4), fetal spines in unusual extension or proximity, more than three vessels in the umbilical cord, and single cardiac motion. Discordant presentation does not exclude conjoined twins. The prenatal diagnosis has been reported several times[1,4,6,10,11,16,17] and can be made as early as the first trimester of pregnancy.[11] Polyhydramnios is present in 75 percent of thoracopagus twins.[8] A complete examination of the twins is indicated because of the high frequency of associated anomalies. Neural tube defects, orofacial clefts, imperforate anus, and diaphragmatic hernia are the most common defects not associated with fusion. Echocardiography is indicated in all cases as congenital heart disease is a major prognostic factor for survival. Evaluation of the visceral situs is important, because abnormalities of the disposition of the abdominal organs are highly suggestive of cardiac defects.[13] If the diagnosis is not certain, other imaging techniques can be considered including plain radiography or amniography. Radiography may show a bony connection, but is otherwise less detailed than sonography. Amniography, especially when performed with oil soluble dyes, may allow a

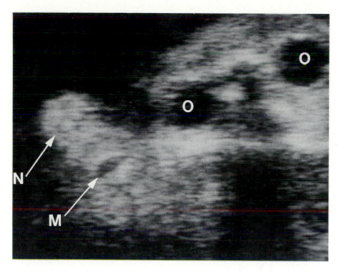

Figure 12–3. Conjoined twins were suspected in view of the proximity between the two faces. Note the ocular fossae of one twin (O) and the mouth (M) and nose (N) of the other. The twins were thoracopagus.

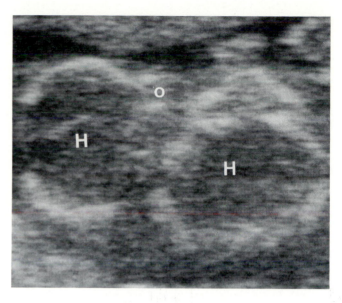

Figure 12–4. Craniopagus diagnosed in the midtrimester. The two heads are joined at the level of the face. H, head; O, orbit.

Zbetter delineation of the bridge between the twins, because these dyes adhere to the fetal skin surface.

Prognosis

Thirty-nine percent of conjoined twins are stillborn, and 34 percent die within the first day of life. Survival depends upon the type of conjunction and the presence of associated anomalies.

Omphalopagus twins have a reasonable chance for survival and surgical separation, unless severe associated anomalies are found. Data published in 1967 document survival of 19 of 22 twins (11 pairs). The prognosis is worse if an omphalocele is present.[20]

In thoracopagus (Fig. 12–5), the degree of fusion of the heart determines the prognosis. When a common heart is present, the chances for a successful surgical separation are negligible. Xiphopagus twins have a better prognosis than thoracopagus, because the former has a lower incidence of cardiac lesions.

Outcome for craniopagus is unpredictable and depends mainly on the degree of fusion of intracranial structures and on the extent of venous connections at the junction site.[2,18] A cerebral connection is present in 43 percent of cases, but cannot be reliably diagnosed preoperatively even with modern imaging techniques, such as CT scan and MNR. In a recent review of 21 cases of craniopagus, the site of junction was an important prognostic factor for mortality and morbidity; temporoparietal and occipital junctions had a worse outcome than frontal and parietal junctions.[2] The perioperative mortality rate in craniopagus operated on in the past decade is 36 percent. Quality of life for the same group was good

(only 1 out of 9 had a severe neurological deficit), suggesting that separation of craniopagus should always be considered.[2] The prognosis improves when surgery is performed in the neonatal period and when craniopagus twins are separated in stages rather than in one procedure.[2] Improved results have been reported with the use of a shunt to prevent postoperative increase in intracranial pressure and cerebrospinal fluid leakage. Tissue expanders may help to achieve primary closure.[2,18]

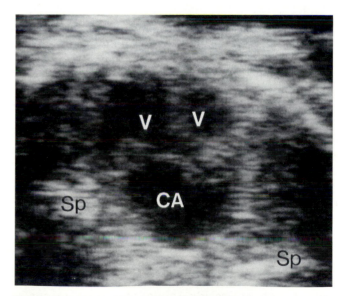

Figure 12–5. Transverse section at 23 weeks of gestation at the level of the chest in a set of thoracopagus twins. Sp represents two spines. Note the single heart. V, ventricles; CA, common atrium.

Among twins conjoined in the lower part of the body, pygopagus have a fairly good outcome, because sharing of organs critical for life (e.g., heart, brain) does not occur. Although data for ischiopagus are scanty, separation is frequently difficult, because these twins often share abdominal viscera. Rehabilitation is required in most cases because of residual orthopedic, gynecologic, and intestinal disabilities. Tripus ischiopagus will need orthopedic prostheses. If male genitalia are shared, one infant will need to be raised as a female. Colostomies and suprapubic drainage may also be required to deal with the problems of a shared genitourinary and intestinal tract.[5]

Obstetrical Management

When the diagnosis of conjoined twins is made before viability, the option of pregnancy termination should be offered to the parents.

After viability, serial examinations are indicated to monitor fetal growth and the development of hydrops, and to detect fetal demise. Scheduled delivery in a tertiary care center is ideal so that procedures required to evaluate the twins can be carried out shortly after birth. There is a paucity of data to assess the reliability of lung maturity studies in monoamniotic twins. The method of delivery depends upon the prenatal assessment of the likelihood of survival. Although vaginal delivery is possible,[15] dystocia occurs frequently[12]; in omphalopagus twins, it has been reported in 36 percent of cases.[8] Vaginal delivery should be reserved for stillbirths and for varieties that are incompatible with life. A destructive procedure (embryotomy) can be considered for stillbirths. Cesarean section is the method of choice to maximize survival of the twins, because it decreases the risk of birth trauma and hypoxia. A vertical uterine incision is recommended. In cephalic/cephalic presentation, the heads should be delivered before the rest of the bodies. The same principle is applicable to breech/breech and cephalic/breech conjoined twins.

After birth, evaluation of both twins should be conducted to assess the extent of organ system sharing. The following studies have been employed: plain and contrasted radiography, echocardiography, angiography, sonography, and CT scans.[9] Twins born alive fall into two categories: infants who thrive despite being conjoined, and infants whose lives are jeopardized because of the union or coexisting congenital anomalies. The former group includes twins like xiphopagus, pygopagus, and ischiopagus, whose union does not result in physiologic compromise, because they do not share critical organs. The impulsive desire to achieve separation as soon as possible

in these cases should be resisted. Over time the infants will be larger, other congenital anomalies may be identified, the risks of anesthesia should decrease, and the procedure can be carefully planned. The surgical challenges include the separation of important shared organs (e.g., liver) and the closure of the soft tissue and bony defect. The second group is constituted by those conjoined twins requiring emergency separation. Indications for this include: (1) one twin is stillborn or its critical condition threatens the other, (2) a congenital anomaly incompatible with life is present and can be corrected, and (3) there is significant damage to the connecting bridge.

REFERENCES

1. Austin E, Schifrin BS, Pomerance JJ, et al.: The antepartum diagnosis of conjoined twins. J Pediatr Surg 15:332, 1980.
2. Bucholz RD, Yoon KW, Shively RE: Temporoparietal craniopagus: Case report and review of the literature. J Neurosurg 66:72, 1987.
3. Edmonds LD, Layde PM: Conjoined twins in the United States, 1970–1977. Teratology 25:301, 1982.
4. Fagan CJ: Antepartum diagnosis of conjoined twins by ultrasonography. AJR 129:921, 1977.
5. Filler RM: Conjoined twins and their separation. Semin Perinatol 10:82, 1986.
6. Gore RM, Filly RA, Parer JT: Sonographic antepartum diagnosis of conjoined twins. Its impact on obstetrical management. JAMA 247:3351, 1982.
7. Guttmacher AF, Nichols BL: Teratology of conjoined twins. Birth Defects 3(1):3, 1967.
8. Harper RG, Kenigsberg K, Sia CG, et al.: Xiphopagus conjoined twins: A 300-year review of the obstetric, morphopathologic, neonatal, and surgical parameters. Am J Obstet Gynecol 137:617, 1980.
9. Herbert NP, Cephalo RC, Koontz WL: Perinatal management of conjoined twins. Am J Perinatol 1:58, 1983.
10. Koontz WL, Herbert WN, Seeds JW, et al.: Ultrasonography in the antepartum diagnosis of conjoined twins: A report of two cases. J Reprod Med 28:627, 1983.
11. Maggio M, Callan NA, Hamod KA, et al.: The first trimester ultrasonographic diagnosis of conjoined twins. Am J Obstet Gynecol 152:883, 1985.
12. Nichols BL, Blattner RJ, Rudolph AJ: General clinical management of thoracopagus twins. Birth Defects 3(1):38, 1967.
13. Noonan JA: Twins, conjoined twins, and cardiac defects. Am J Dis Child 132:17, 1978.
14. Patel R, Fox K, Dawson J, et al.: Cardiovascular anomalies in thoracopagus twins and the importance of preoperative cardiac evaluation. Br Heart J 39:1254, 1977.
15. Rudolph AJ, Michaels JP, Nichols BL: Obstetric management of conjoined twins. Birth Defects 3(1):28, 1967.

16. Sanders, SP, Chin AJ, Parness IA, et al.: Prenatal diagnosis of congenital heart defects in thoracoabdominally conjoined twins. N Engl J Med 313:370, 1985.
17. Schmidt W, Heberling D, Kubli F: Antepartum ultrasonographic diagnosis of conjoined twins in early pregnancy. Am J Obstet Gynecol 139:961, 1981.
18. Shively RE, Bermant MA, Bucholz RD: Separation of craniopagus twins utilizing tissue expanders. Plast Reconstr Surg 76:765, 1985.
19. Somasundaram K, Wong KS: Ischiopagus tetrapus conjoined twins. Br J Surg 73:738, 1986.
20. Votteler TP: Conjoined twins. In: Welch KJ, Randolph JG, Ravitch MM, et al. (eds): Pediatric Surgery. Chicago, Year Book, 1986, pp 771–779.

Twin Reversed Arterial Perfusion Sequence

Synonyms

Acardius, acardiac monster, acephalus, pseudocardiac anomaly, acephalus acardia, and holoacardius.

Definition

Twin reversed arterial perfusion (TRAP) sequence is a specific anomaly of multiple gestations characterized by vascular communications between fetuses, a total or partial absence of the heart, and a spectrum of malformations and reduction anomalies that may affect all tissues.[10]

Incidence

The incidence is 1 in 35,000 births.[5] This figure may represent an underestimate of the real frequency of the problem, since TRAP sequence can be lethal for both twins in early pregnancy.[10] TRAP sequence is found only in twin pregnancies with fused placentas. Seventy-five percent of cases occur in monozygotic triplets and the rest in monozygotic twins.[6] Since fusion of the placenta may be found in dizygotic twins, there is a theoretical possibility that TRAP sequence occurs in these twins, and a few cases have been reported.[2,10] This condition is sporadic and family recurrences have not been reported.[11]

Etiopathogenesis

The pathogenesis of TRAP sequence is controversial. Umbilical anastomoses have been found in all cases where placentas were available for examination.[10] This finding suggests two main etiopathogenetic hypotheses: (1) anastomosis of the umbilical arteries of the two twins in early embryogenesis would lead to reversed circulation in the perfused twin, with secondary disruption of organ morphogenesis caused by deficient oxygen and nutrient contents in the perfused blood, and (2) a primary disorder in the development of one twin early in embryogenesis, because of chromosomal abnormality, polar body twinning,

or other reasons, usually leads to reabsorption of the embryo or, if demise occurs later, to a fetus papyraceous. However, if a vascular anastomosis is present between the two circulations, the failing twin would be saved and become the malformed perfused fetus.

Pathology

The members of a TRAP sequence are known as the perfused twin and the pump twin. The perfused twin exhibits a wide range of abnormalities, while the pump fetus is morphologically normal. Figure 12–6A illustrates representative examples of perfused twins. A wide range of anomalies involving virtually all organ systems has been reported in the perfused twin. They include total or partial absence of the cranial vault, holoprosencephaly, anencephaly, absent facial features, anophthalmia, microphthalmia, cleft lip/cleft palate, absent or rudimentary limbs, absent thorax, diaphragmatic defects, absent lungs and heart, esophageal atresia, short intestine, omphalocele, gastroschisis, ascites, absent liver, gallbladder, and pancreas, exstrophy of the cloaca, edema of the skin, and single umbilical artery.[10] Typically the most severe abnormalities are found in the upper part of the body. This has been attributed to the retrograde pattern of fetal perfusion through the umbilical and iliac arteries, which would relatively spare the lower part of the body. An absent or rudimentary heart is frequently found in these fetuses, explaining the term "acardius," which is classically used in referring to such fetuses. In a series of 14 cases, no heart tissue could be found in 5, an unfolded heart tube was seen in 7, and a folded heart with a common chamber was seen in 2.[10]

Chromosomal abnormalities have been found in 50 percent of cases.[1,2,3,10] However, the pattern of abnormalities did not conform to the expected phenotype of the chromosomal aberrations. It has been suggested that the abnormal karyotype per se is not responsible for the malformation complex but rather that it increases the likelihood of a discordant development between the twins, thus creating a favorable

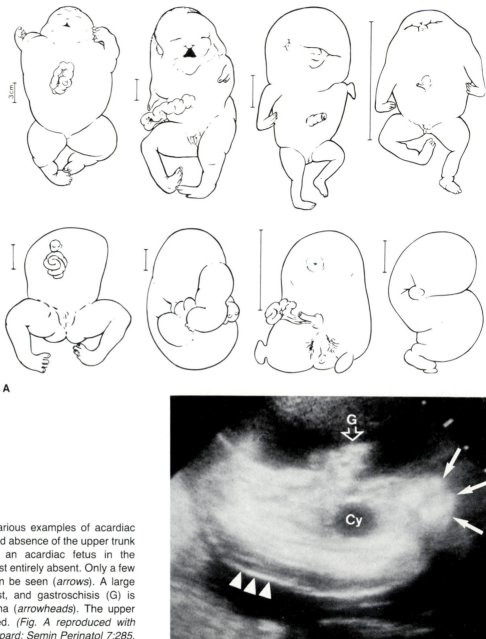

Figure 12–6. A. Drawings showing various examples of acardiac monster. Note the presence of limbs and absence of the upper trunk and head. **B.** Longitudinal scan of an acardiac fetus in the midtrimester. The cephalic pole is almost entirely absent. Only a few remnants of the splanchnocranium can be seen (*arrows*). A large cyst (Cy) occupies most of the chest, and gastroschisis (G) is present. Note diffuse soft tissue edema (*arrowheads*). The upper extremities could not be demonstrated. *(Fig. A reproduced with permission from Van Allen, Smith, Shepard: Semin Perinatol 7:285, 1983.)*

ground for the TRAP sequence to occur.[10] In a pregnancy complicated by TRAP sequence, analysis of the histocompatibility antigen haplotypes indicated that the perfused acardiac twin was probably derived from the fertilization of a polar body.[2]

The pump twin was morphologically and chromosomically normal in all the reported cases. However, signs of intrauterine cardiac overload, including overt hydrops, intrauterine growth retardation, hypertrophy of the right ventricle, and hepatosplenomegaly, were always present. Ascites may result in

overdistention of the abdominal wall and prune-belly phenotype.

Diagnosis

The prenatal diagnosis of TRAP sequence has been made in a handful of cases,[4,8,9] but it is not always an easy task. The condition should be suspected when one of the members of a multiple gestation has a grotesque malformation (unidentifiable head, trunk, or extremities) (Fig. 12–6B). TRAP sequence should also be considered in singleton gestations associated with an intraamniotic tumor. The identification of a pulsating heart in the malformed twin does not exclude the diagnosis. We have seen one case in which the perfused twin presented with a sonographic image similar to cystic hygromas and oligohydramnios. Death occurs in utero and progressive skin edema develops. Polyhydramnios is a frequent finding. Signs of congestive heart failure may be present in the pump twin.[4,9]

Prognosis
The mortality rate of the perfused twin is 100 percent. The mortality rate of the pump twin is 50 percent.[10] Causes of death include intrauterine heart failure and prematurity. Parents may be reassured that embolic phenomena from the perfused twin do not occur in the pump twin.

Obstetrical Management
Serial ultrasound scans are mandatory to assess the growth rate and the cardiovascular status of the pump twin. A detailed investigation for signs of heart failure (polyhydramnios, enlargement of the cardiac chambers, hepatosplenomegaly, ascites, hydrothorax, pericardial effusion) and IUGR should be performed at each examination. Tocolytic agents to treat preterm labor are indicated, preferably magnesium sulfate, since beta-adrenergic agents could exert adverse effects on the cardiovascular system of the pump fetus. Therapeutic amniocentesis may be considered in cases of preterm labor associated with hydramnios. The development of signs of congestive heart failure in the pump twin is serious. Maternal digoxin administration has been effective in controlling the heart failure of the pump twin in a case diagnosed at 28 weeks of gestation. Pregnancy was continued for 6 weeks, allowing the survival of the pump infant.[9] A surgical approach could be considered for those cases in which medical therapy has failed. Ligature of the umbilical circulation could be

undertaken by hysterotomy or under endoscopic control. Some experimental evidence in animal models suggests that laser electrocoagulation may be of use for intrauterine surgery. The delivery of a perfused twin may be associated with significant soft tissue dystocia. In one case, delivery occurred 8 hours after the birth of the pump twin and required oxytocin administration, drainage of multiple cystic structures under ultrasonic guidance, and intrauterine manipulation.[10] Delivery of a perfused twin is one of the few indications in obstetrics for a destructive procedure (embryotomy) to avoid a cesarean section.

REFERENCES

1. Benirschke K, Harper VDR: The acardiac anomaly. Teratology 15:311, 1977
2. Bieber FR, Nance WE, Morton CC, et al.: Genetic studies of an acardiac monster: Evidence of polar body twinning in man. Science 213:775, 1981.
3. Deacon JS, Machin GA, Martin JM, et al.: Investigation of acephalus. Am J Med Genet 5:85, 1980.
4. Gewolb IH, Freedman RM, Kleinman CS, et al.: Prenatal diagnosis of human pseudoacardiac anomaly. Obstet Gynecol 61:657, 1983.
5. Gillim DL, Hendricks CH: Holoacardius. Review of the literature and case report. Obstet Gynecol 2:647, 1953.
6. James WH: A note on the epidemiology of acardiac monsters. Teratology 16:211, 1977.
7. Jirasek J: Personal communication (quoted in reference 10).
8. Napolitani FD, Schreiber I: The acardiac monster: A review of the world literature and presentation of 2 cases. Am J Obstet Gynecol 80:582, 1960.
9. Simpson PC, Trundinger BJ, Walker A, et al.: The intrauterine treatment of fetal cardiac failure in a twin pregnancy with an acardiac acephalic monster. Am J Obstet Gynecol 147:842, 1983.
10. Van Allen MI, Smith DW, Shepard TH: Twin reversed arterial perfusion (TRAP) sequence: A study of 14 twin pregnancies with acardius. Semin Perinatol 7:285, 1983.
11. Wilson EA: Holoacardius. Obstet Gynecol 40:740, 1972.

Amniotic Band Syndrome

Synonyms
Aberrant tissue bands, Adam complex, amniochorionic mesoblastic fibrous strings, amniogenic bands, amniotic band disruption complex, congenital annular bands, congenital annular constrictions, congenital constriction band syndrome, congenital ring constrictions, and congenital transverse defects.

Incidence
The incidence is 1 in 1,200 to 1 in 15,000 live births.[9]

TABLE 12–2. ABNORMALITIES ASSOCIATED WITH AMNIOTIC BAND SYNDROME

Limb defects, multiple, asymmetrical
 Constriction rings of limbs or digits
 Amputation of limbs or digits
 Pseudosyndactyly
 Abnormal dermal ridge patterns
 Simian creases
 Clubfeet
Craniofacial defects
 Encephalocele, multiple, asymmetrical
 Anencephaly
 Facial clefting—lip, palate
  Embryologically appropriate
  Embryologically inappropriate
 Severe nasal deformity
 Asymmetrical microphthalmia
 Incomplete or absent cranial calcification
Visceral defects
 Gastroschisis
 Omphalocele

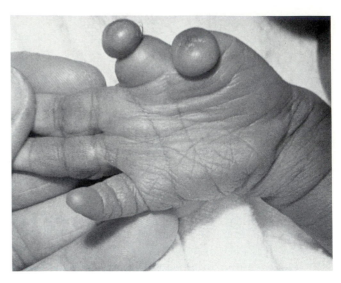

Figure 12–8. Amputation of fingers in a fetus with amniotic band syndrome.

Etiology
Amniotic band syndrome is a sporadic condition.

Etiopathogenesis
Although several theories have been proposed to explain the genesis of amniotic band syndrome, the most widely accepted view is that early rupture of the amnion results in mesodermic bands that emanate from the chorionic side of the amnion and insert on the fetal body, leading to amputations, constrictions, and postural deformities secondary to immobilization.[10] It has been suggested that the earlier the insult occurs, the more severe the lesion. Amniotic rupture in the first weeks of pregnancy results in craniofacial and visceral defects, whereas during the second trimester, it may lead to limb and digital constriction

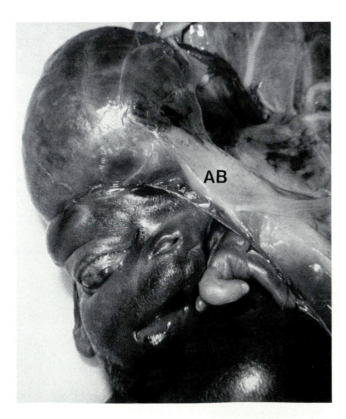

Figure 12–7. Amniotic band syndrome. An amniotic band is seen inserting on the fetal head. There is great distortion of the fetal face. The hand is forced against the fetal face and deformed. AB, amniotic band.

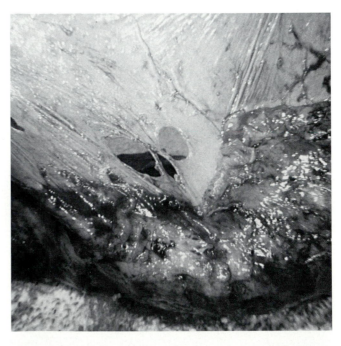

Figure 12–9. Fibrous strings originating from the surface of the placenta.

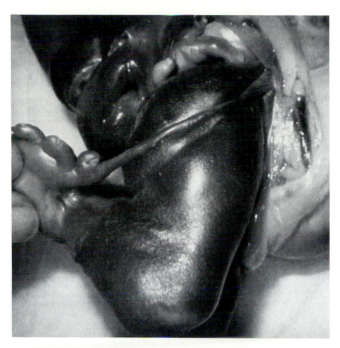

Figure 12–10. Fibrous string inserting into the fetal body.

and amputations.[4] An alternative view is that amniotic band syndrome is the consequence of an insult that results in typical malformations as well as ectodermal and mesenchymal disruption. Vascular compromise may have a pathogenetic role in the genesis of external deficits. Amniotic band syndrome has been reported after amniocentesis.[1,7,8]

Pathology

The pathologic findings of amniotic band syndrome have been extensively described.[4,9] Table 12–2 illustrates the abnormalities most commonly associated with this condition. Multiple anomalies are present in 77 percent of cases.[2] When encephaloceles are present, they are often asymmetrical and may be multiple (Fig. 12–7). Such a configuration is almost pathognomonic of amniotic band syndrome, since these lesions are usually single and located in the midline (see section on cephaloceles). Grotesque facial anomalies, including anophthalmia, microphthalmia, and irregular and multiple clefts, may be found (Fig. 12–7). Ring deformities encompass two groups of lesions: those that can be related to the disruptive effect of the amniotic bands, such as amputations and ring constrictions (Fig. 12–8) and those related to immobilization of the fetus, such as clubfoot, which is seen in two-thirds of the cases.[9] Internal organs are generally normal. However, if amniotic disruption occurs around the time of physiologic evisceration of abdominal contents, entanglement with mesodermic bands can result in ventral wall defects, such as gastroschisis and, less frequently, omphaloceles. Kyphoscoliosis can be seen.[9]

Fibrous strings originating from the surface of the placenta (Fig. 12–9) are frequently seen inserting into the fetal body at the level of the defects (Fig. 12–10). In some fetuses, amniotic rupture allows communication between the amniotic cavity and the extraembryonic coelom. The fetus may escape from the amniotic cavity (extraamniotic pregnancy), and the amnion does not grow and can be found after delivery as a small sac connected to the umbilical cord.[10]

Diagnosis

Prenatal diagnosis of this condition has been made.[3,6] Amniotic band syndrome encompasses a broad constellation of anomalies that are different in each case. Suspicion should arise when two or more of the anomalies indicated in Table 12–2 are encountered.

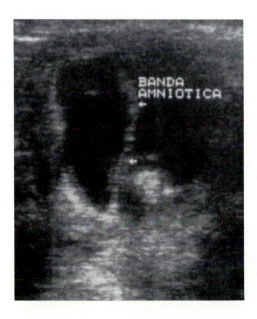

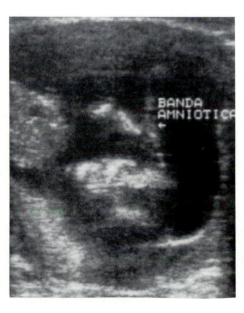

Figure 12–11. Sonogram of a fetus with amniotic band syndrome. Note a thick band inserting into the uterine wall (*left*) and fetal body (*right*). The fetus was born with multiple congenital amputations. (*Courtesy of Dr. Heriberto Alarcon and Dr. Carlos Alarcon, Puebla, Mexico.*)

Asymmetrical or multiple encephaloceles in combination with amputations, ventral wall defects, and postural deformities should strongly raise the index of suspicion.

At times, amniotic bands can be seen as linear echoes floating in the amniotic fluid and connected to the fetal body (Fig. 12–11).[6] However, oligohydramnios may interfere with visualization of the bands. Confusion may arise with two conditions that may cause linear echoes crossing the amniotic cavity: chorioamniotic separation and intrauterine synechiae. In these cases, meticulous scanning will demonstrate that these structures do not insert into the fetal body and that there are no structural anomalies.

Prognosis

The prognosis depends on the severity of the anomalies. The spectrum varies from individuals with normal intelligence whose only defect is a minor digital constriction to multiple severe anomalies incompatible with life.

Obstetrical Management

Fetal karyotype is indicated because the multiple congenital anomalies may be due to a chromosomal abnormality. The option of pregnancy termination should be offered before viability. In those cases diagnosed after viability, obstetrical management is not altered unless associated anomalies incompatible with life are visualized (e.g., anencephaly). In such instances the option of pregnancy termination can be offered to the parents any time in gestation.

REFERENCES

1. Ashkenazy M, Borenstein R, Katz Z, et al.: Constriction of the umbilical cord by an amniotic band after midtrimester amniocentesis. Acta Obstet Gynecol Scand 61:89, 1982.
2. Baker CJ, Rudolph AJ: Congenital ring constrictions and intrauterine amputations. Am J Dis Child 121:393, 1971
3. Fiske CE, Filly RA, Golbus MS: Prenatal ultrasound diagnosis of amniotic band syndrome. J Ultrasound Med 1:45, 1982.
4. Higginbottom MC, Jones KL, Hall BD, et al.: The amniotic band disruption complex: Timing of amniotic rupture and variable spectra of consequent defects. J Pediatr 95:544, 1979.
5. Hughes RM, Benzie RJ, Thompson CL: Amniotic band syndrome causing fetal head deformity. Prenat Diagn 4:447, 1984.
6. Mahony BS, Filly RA, Callen PW, et al.: The amniotic band syndrome: Antenatal sonographic diagnosis and potential pitfalls. Am J Obstet Gynecol 152:63, 1985.
7. Moessinger AC, Blanc WA, Byrne J, et al.: Amniotic band syndrome associated with amniocentesis. Am J Obstet Gynecol 141:588, 1981.
8. Rehder H, Weitzel H: Intrauterine amputations after amniocentesis. Lancet 1:382, 1978.
9. Seeds JW, Cefalo RC, Herbert WN: Amniotic band syndrome. Am J Obstet Gynecol 144:243, 1982.
10. Torpin R: Amniochorionic mesoblastic fibrous strings and amniotic bands: Associated constricting fetal malformation or fetal death. Am J Obstet Gynecol 91:65, 1965.
11. Worthen NJ, Lawrence D, Bustillo M: Amniotic band syndrome: Antepartum ultrasonic diagnosis of discordant anencephaly. J Clin Ultrasound 8:453, 1980.

Nonimmune Hydrops Fetalis

Incidence

Nonimmune hydrops (NIH) fetalis has been reported with an incidence of 1 in 1500 to 1 in 4000 deliveries.[59,60,70,74,80,109]

Definition

NIH implies an excess of total body water, which is usually evident as extracellular accumulation of fluid in tissues and serous cavities, without any identifiable circulating antibody against red blood cell (RBC) antigen. With the decreasing frequency of Rh isoimmunization, NIH has become a relatively more frequent cause of hydrops.[90]

Diagnosis

The sonographic diagnosis of hydrops is easy. The excessive body fluid accumulation can be seen as subcutaneous edema (skin thickness 5 mm), pleural and pericardial effusions, ascites, polyhydramnios, or placental thickening (>6 cm). Fluid accumulation must involve more than one site for the term "hydrops" to be used (Figs. 12–12 through 12–17). When the fluid accumulation is limited to only one cavity, the situation should be described in terms of the involved site (e.g., ascites), since this may be helpful in narrowing the differential diagnosis. The first site to show excessive fluid accumulation may

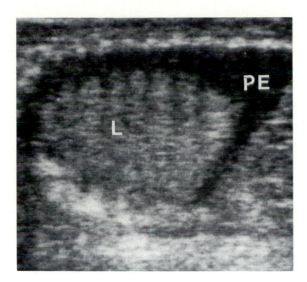

Figure 12–12. Longitudinal scan of a fetus with nonimmune hydrops showing pleural effusion (PE) surrounding lung tissue (L).

vary with the cause of the hydrops. For example, cystic adenomatoid tumor of the lung will first cause a pleural effusion. When the intrathoracic pressure is sufficiently elevated to impair venous return, generalized hydrops will develop. Therefore, depending on when the fetus is examined, it may be possible to detect excessive fluid accumulation in a single site before it becomes generalized. In systemic conditions (anemia, congestive heart failure), fluid accumulation tends to be more evenly distributed and can be detected simultaneously in multiple sites. Many factors, such as lymphatic drainage, venous return, surface area and potential volume of serosal cavities, tissue pressure in the skin, and, finally, accessibility to ultrasound evaluation, affect the detection of fluid accumulation with ultrasound. A pericardial effusion may be the first sign of fluid overload. This is probably due to the volume limitations of the pericardial

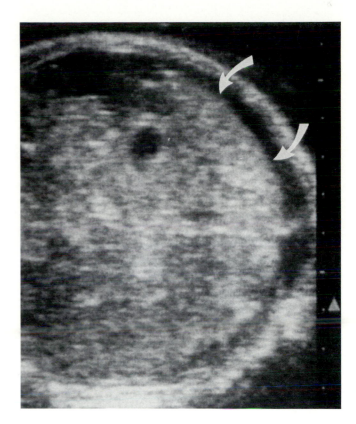

Figure 12–14. Ascites (*arrows*) in abdomen of fetus with NIH.

cavity as opposed to the ease of fluid distribution within the pleural and abdominal cavities.[90]

Fetal ascites may be so large as to cause prune belly.[69,94] Several cases of isolated ascites have been reported. Meconium peritonitis and viral infections (CMV) can present in this form. Isolated ascites can also be the first stage of NIH in progress. The workup for isolated ascites is similar to that of NIH (see Table

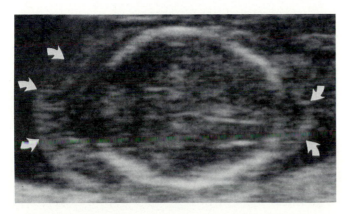

Figure 12–13. Skull of fetus with NIH. Edema is indicated by arrows.

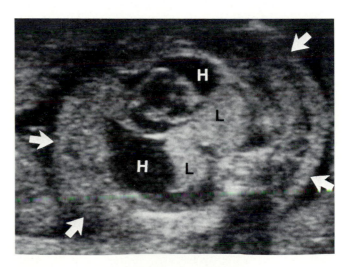

Figure 12–15. Cross section of a fetal thorax with hydrothorax (H) and subcutaneous edema (*arrows*). L, lungs.

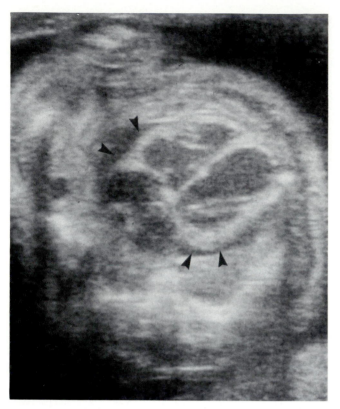

Figure 12–16. Transverse section across the chest of a fetus with NIH. Note the pericardial effusion (*arrowheads*) surrounding the fetal heart.

12–5). In some instances this condition has resolved spontaneously.

Polyhydramnios is associated with hydrops fetalis in about 75 percent of cases studied.[70] When polyhydramnios is detected, incipient hydrops fetalis should be excluded by careful examination of the fetal serosal cavities. In some cases, the amount of fluid may be so massive as to preclude appropriate visualization of the fetus with real-time ultrasound because the infant is beyond the depth field of the transducer. This problem can be solved either by using a static scanner or by examining the patient in the knee-chest position with real-time ultrasound.

Etiology

In about 44 percent of fetuses, NIH is an idiopathic condition, and no cause can be elicited.[59] Table 12–3 is an outline of conditions associated with the presence of NIH. For some of these, a direct pathophysiologic mechanism has been postulated, whereas in others, a mere association has been reported without implying a causal relationship.

Hematologic Causes. The common pathway of NIH of hematologic origin is fetal anemia. This can be the

result of hemoglobinopathies, hemolysis, fetal blood loss, or in one report, red blood cell (RBC) aplasia.[85]

Among hemoglobinopathies, alpha-thalassemia is the leading cause of NIH fetalis. The globin portion of hemoglobin is normally built from two pairs of polypeptide chains. In the adult, the predominant form is hemoglobin A, consisting of two alpha-chains and two beta-chains, whereas the predominant form in the fetus is hemoglobin F, formed from two alpha-chains and two gamma-chains. If the synthesis of one of the chains is decreased or completely absent, abnormal hemoglobins are produced, giving rise to the clinical syndromes called "thalassemias." The two major groups of thalassemias are called "alpha" and "beta," corresponding to the involved chain. Thalassemias have a wide clinical spectrum ranging from the asymptomatic carrier (e.g., beta-thalassemia minor) to the invariably fatal disease.

Alpha-thalassemia is due to the absence of one or more of the genes controlling the synthesis of alpha-chains. In the homozygotic condition, all four genes are deleted, and, therefore, no alpha-chains are produced. Consequently, no hemoglobin F or A can be produced, and the result is that tetramers of gamma-chains are formed (beta-chains are not produced in significant quantities during fetal life). These tetramers are called "hemoglobin Bart," which has a higher affinity for oxygen than hemoglobin F—so high that it does not release its oxygen to fetal tissues sufficiently. Fetal tissue hypoxia leads to a high output cardiac failure state and hydrops fetalis.[17,24,53,59,71,73,81]

Beta-thalassemias do not become clinically evident until approximately the third month after birth. This is because the switch from hemoglobin F to reliance on hemoglobin A (requiring beta-chains) does not occur until the postnatal period.

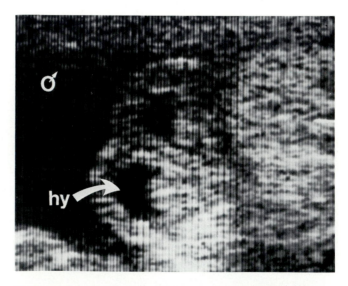

Figure 12–17. Hydrocele (hy), fluid accumulation in the scrotum.

TABLE 12–3. CONDITIONS ASSOCIATED WITH NONIMMUNE HYDROPS FETALIS

Hematologic
  Anemia due to maternal acquired pure red cell aplasia[85]
  Anemia due to blood loss
    Fetomaternal bleeding[33,73,80,88,117]
    Twin-to-twin transfusion[37,56,59,60,69–71,80,120,122]
  Hemolysis: Glucose-6-phosphate dehydrogenase deficiency[76,87]
  Hemoglobinopathy: Homozygous alpha-thalassemia[24,53,59,71,73,81]
Pulmonary
  Congenital cystic adenomatoid malformation
    (CCAM)[12,32,37,48,51,59,67,77]
  Pulmonary lymphangiectasia[59,73]
  Pulmonary leiomyosarcoma[48]
  Alveolar cell adenoma of the lung[29]
  Diaphragmatic hernia[50,59,70,88]
  Extralobar pulmonary sequestration[97]
  Enlargement of one lung[89]
  Chylothorax[4,34,62,114]
Neurologic
  Fetal intracranial hemorrhage[18]
  Encephalocele[59]
  Porencephaly with absent corpus callosum[59]
Gastrointestinal
  Midgut volvulus[103]
  Diaphragmatic hernia[12,42,45,59,70,88]
  Atresia
    Esophageal with imperforate anus[57]
    Duodenal[38,59]
    Bowel[73]
    Ileal with meconium peritonitis[12,37]
  Meconium peritonitis with gut herniated into peritoneal sac[12]
  Meconium peritonitis of unknown etiology[59,68]
  Duodenal diverticulum[59]
  Imperforate anus[59]
Hepatic
  Cirrhosis with portal hypertension[59]
  Giant cell hepatitis[12]
  Hepatic necrosis[59]
  Hemangioendothelioma of the liver[23,50]
Genitourinary
  Congenital nephrotic syndrome (Finnish type)[54,80]
  Pelvic kidney[70]
  Hypoplastic kidney (with microcephaly)[70]
  Urethral obstruction with renal dysplasia[32]
  Hypoplastic uterus, imperforate hymen, bilateral accessory renal
    arteries[70]
  Polycystic kidneys, vaginal atresia, and hydrocolpos[12,59]
  Urogenital sinus, hydronephrosis, bifid uterus, hydrocolpos[59]
  Adult polycystic kidney disease[124]
Infectious
  Coxsackievirus pancarditis[9]
  Secondary syphilis[22,70]
  Toxoplasmosis[7]
  Cytomegalovirus hepatitis, myocarditis, encephalitis[37,40,59,80,91]
  Parvovirus[21]
  Herpes simplex type I[60]
  Respiratory syncytial virus[50]
Neoplastic
  Neuroblastoma[3,64,79,83,88,111,115]
  Teratoma
    Sacral[59,80,88]
    Mediastinal[12,42,48]
    Malignant[59]
  Congenital leukemia with Down syndrome[32]
  Hemangioendothelioma of the liver[23]
  Pulmonary leiomyosarcoma[48]
  Tuberous sclerosis[59,86,116,121]

Cardiovascular
  Cardiac structure
    Atrioventricular canal defect
      With abdominal situs inversus and complete heart block[67]
      With transposition of great arteries[50]
      With transposition of the great vessels and asplenia[67]
      With transposition of the great vessels and polysplenia[74]
      With double outlet right ventricle and pulmonic stenosis[108]
      With overriding aorta, tracheoesophageal fistula[12]
      With complex bradyarrhythmia, AV valve insufficiency,
        interrupted IVC[108]
      Complete communication with common AV valve[88]
    Tetralogy of Fallot[67,73]
    Absent pulmonary valve or pulmonary atresia[67,108]
    Aortic atresia, diminutive left ventricle and mitral valve[73,108]
    Aortic valve stenosis with mitral insufficiency[110]
    Aortic arch interruption[75]
    Tricuspid dysplasia[32] and Ebstein's anomaly[108]
    Tricuspid and pulmonary atresia[50]
    Myocardial infarction with coronary artery embolus[6]
    Intrapericardial teratoma[8,73,80]
    Cardiac rhabdomyoma[50,67]
    Myocardial tumors involving ventricular septum, aortic outflow
      and left atrium, not requiring surgery[118]
    Intrauterine closure of foramen ovale[14]
    Intrauterine closure of ductus arteriosus[5]
    Endocardial fibroelastosis[12,38,50]
      With mitral valve insufficiency[78]
      With subaortic stenosis[70]
    Ventricular septal defect (VSD)[12,73]
      With atrial septal defect (ASD)[70]
      With ASD and right atrial conduction system hamartoma[116]
      With patent ductus arteriosus[37]
      With absent right hemidiaphragm[12]
  Cardiac Rhythm
    Atrial
      Bradycardia and bradyarrhythmia[60,107]
      Tachycardia[19,23,52,73,82,105,116]
        Paroxysmal (PAT)[28,42,59,60,67,92,107,118]
        Wolff-Parkinson-White (WPW)[81]
      Flutter with block[58,67,107]
    Complete heart block[2,26,55,73]
Vascular
  Vena cava thrombosis[99]
  Hemangioendothelioma[30]
  Arterial calcification[12,31,50,59]
  Arterovenous malformation[49,113]
  Cerebral angioma[50]
Metabolic
  Gaucher's disease[46,60,80]
  Sialidosis[11,113]
  Gangliosidosis GM1[37]
  Mucopolysaccharidosis[73]
Skeletal dysplasias
  Achondroplasia[113]
  Achondrogenesis
    Parenti-Fraccaro (or type I)[13,15,47,80]
    Langer-Saldino (or type II)[15]
  Osteogenesis imperfecta[59,80]
  Thanatophoric dwarfism[113]
  Short rib–polydactyly syndrome
    Saldino-Noonan type[74]
    Majewski type[15]
  Asphyxiating thoracic dysplasia[59]
Chromosomal
  Triploidy[59]

(Continued)

TABLE 12–3. (*Continued*)

Trisomies	45XO (Turner syndrome)[60,80,84]
13[73]	dup(11p)[44]
21 (Down syndrome)[32,59,60,73,80,84,88,108]	Hereditary
E[12]	Pena-Shokeir type I[25,72]
18 (Edward's syndrome)[12]	Lethal multiple pterygium syndrome[41,61,73]
Translocation E[12,70]	Idiopathic[101]
47XY+der,[22] t(11:21)(q23:q11)mat[84]	Noonan syndrome with congenital heart defect[123]
Abnormal chromosome 11[67]	Placental
Mosaic 46XX/XY[32]	Chorioangioma[10,12,50,55,60,70,74,112]
Mosaic 46XY/92XXYY[84]	

Thalassemia syndromes are transmitted as autosomal recessive traits. For a fetus to be affected with alpha-thalassemia, both the parents must be carriers. A simple screen for the carrier of thalassemia is to check the complete blood count with RBC indices. If the mean corpuscular volume (MCV) is above 80 femtoliters, the diagnosis is effectively excluded. If the MCV is less than 80, microcytosis is present, and the differential diagnosis includes iron deficiency anemia, anemia of chronic disease, thalassemia, and sideroblastic anemia. Performing serum iron studies (iron concentration, total iron-binding capacity and saturation) will permit differentiation of these syndromes. The most common cause of microcytic anemia is iron deficiency, but if the serum iron concentration is greater than 50 μg/dl and the saturation greater than 15 percent, this diagnosis is excluded. At this point, a hemoglobin A_2 level determination should be ordered. If the concentration is above 3.5 percent, the diagnosis is beta-thalassemia, which is not a cause of hydrops. If the concentration is below 3.5 percent, the diagnosis is alpha-thalassemia-1 (two of the four genes are missing). Since this mother is at risk of having an infant with homozygous alpha-thalassemia, the father must be similarly evaluated. Unless the father is also affected with alpha-thalassemia-1, the fetus cannot have alpha-thalassemia major as the cause of hydrops. Fetal diagnosis can be accomplished via percutaneous umbilical blood sampling or by amniocentesis, and culturing of amniotic fluid cells and DNA analysis for the alpha-chain gene.[95]

Glucose-6-phosphate dehydrogenase (G-6PD) deficiency has been reported as causing NIH in two fetuses.[76,87] The mechanism of hydrops appears to be intrauterine hemolysis related to the impaired production of reduced glutathione by the affected RBC. This compound is essential to protect the RBC membrane from oxidative agents. Hemolysis can occur spontaneously or in response to maternal ingestion of oxidative agents that cross the placenta. A list of frequently encountered compounds that can trigger a hemolytic crisis is given in Table 12–4.

G-6PD is inherited as an X-linked recessive disorder. The frequency of the gene in the population is highly variable. In Southern China it is 5.5 percent, in American blacks 10 to 15 percent, in Greece 30 percent, and in some areas of Sardinia 35 percent.[119] The two reported cases of NIH apparently related to G-6PD, involved carrier mothers ingesting oxidative agents; one ingested fava beans,[76] the other sulfisoxazole.[87]

Diagnosis of G-6PD deficiency in the fetus would require examination of fetal blood, which is rarely justified. If the fetus is female and the father is not affected, the diagnosis is excluded. The most sensitive test for detection of the carrier state is the hemoglobin reduction test, which unfortunately is positive in only 75 percent of carriers.[20]

Another cause of severe anemia fetalis has been reported in a woman with acquired pure RBC aplasia.[85] In this disease, there are serum inhibitors of erythropoiesis, probably IgG antibodies, directed against bone marrow erythroblasts, erythroid stem cell differentiation, or erythropoietin. These antibodies may be transferred to the fetus, leading to severe anemia. The Coombs test remains negative both in the mother and in the fetus. Should the baby survive, the RBC aplasia lasts for about 3 months.

Fetal anemia due to blood loss has been described in association with hydrops fetalis in two circumstances: fetomaternal bleeding and twin-to-twin transfusion syndrome.

Fetal erythrocytes have been found in the maternal blood at least once during pregnancy in 39 percent of normal subjects.[100] However, the volume of such bleeding is small in virtually all cases (98 percent <0.1 ml). Perlin et al.[88] reported well-documented cases of NIH associated with severe fetomaternal hemorrhage. The magnitude of the hemorrhage must not be enough to produce death due to acute hypovolemia and is generally chronic.

TABLE 12–4. COMPOUNDS ASSOCIATED WITH HEMOLYSIS IN G-6PD

Acetylsalicylic acid (aspirin)

Phenacetin

Sulfas

Antimalarials
 Primaquine
 Quinidine

Nitrofurantoin

Chloramphenicol

Paraaminosalicylic acid

Naphthalene (mothballs)

Methylene blue

Nalidixic acid

Ascorbic acid (vitamin C, massive doses required)

Quinine

Quinidine

Dapsone

Several tests are available to screen for fetal bleeding into the maternal circulation. The Kleihauer-Betke test is an acid elution test based on the relative sensitivity of adult and fetal hemoglobin to the presence of a strong acid. When maternal erythrocytes are exposed to an acid solution, adult hemoglobin is washed through the cell membrane, whereas fetal hemoglobin is not. After fixation and staining, the maternal RBCs appear as unstained ghost cells and are easily distinguished from the stained fetal cells. The volume of the transplacental hemorrhage (TPH) can be calculated using the following formula:

$$\text{TPH (ml)} = \text{Estimated maternal blood volume)} \times (\text{\# Stained cells}) \div (\text{\# Maternal cells})$$

Other available tests to quantify fetomaternal bleeding include the Fetaldex (Ortho Diagnostics) and BMC Reagent Set (Boehringer Mannheim Corporation), both of which are variations on the original Kleihauer-Betke methodology and are of sufficient accuracy for clinical use.[100] Measurement of the serum alphafetoprotein has been used to quantify transplacental hemorrhage.[39] If a significant fetomaternal bleed has occurred, it is important to carefully examine the placenta at the time of delivery, since such macrotransfusions have been reported in association with placental chorioangiomas and choriocarcinomas.[39]

Another cause of hydrops related to blood loss occurs in monozygotic twins with twin-to-twin transfusion. Although the traditional concept has been that the recipient, or plethoric, infant is the one to become hydropic, NIH has also been described in the donor twin.[37,69,70,122] The mechanism for the development of hydrops has not been clearly established. Anemia has been suggested as the etiology of NIH in the donor, although the extent of the hydrops is greater than that observed in isoimmunized infants with comparable hemoglobin levels.[70] Volume overload may be the explanation of hydrops in the recipient.[113] NIH has also been described in the donor twin when the recipient is an acardius with parabiotic parasitism.[56] A twin-to-twin transfusion can be suspected antenatally in the presence of a weight difference greater than 20 percent of the weight of the larger twin and with a single placenta. NIH can be identified in one member of a multiple gestation, but it is important to bear in mind that this does not necessarily represent a twin-to-twin transfusion syndrome. The diagnosis can be confirmed postnatally by a blood hemoglobin difference of more than 5 g/100 ml, a higher reticulocyte count in the donor twin, and contrast studies showing anastomotic links between the two circulations in the placenta.

Cardiac Causes. Cardiac problems are relatively common causes of NIH,[113] accounting for 40 percent of cases in the series of Allan et al.[1] Some of them are amenable to intrauterine medical therapy.[19,58,66,67,107,118] They can be divided into those related to cardiac dysrhythmias and those due to structural abnormalities. The common mechanism in the development of hydrops regardless of the specific cause is intrauterine congestive heart failure. Chapter 4 provides a detailed discussion of the diagnostic approach to fetal congenital abnormalities and arrhythmias by echocardiography.

When a cardiac dysrhythmia is suspected, its nature can best be elucidated with M-mode echocardiography.[36,66] It should be stressed that both tachyarrhythmias and bradyarrhythmias can be the cause of NIH and can be treated with transplacental pharmacologic manipulation. These fetuses have the best prognosis. An intrauterine dysrhythmia should be suspected when postmortem examination fails to show a cause for NIH. Identification of a fetal third degree heart block is an indication for screening the mother for manifestations and laboratory evidence of connective tissue disorders, such as systemic lupus erythematosus[55] and Sjogren's syndrome,[108] since these associations have been well established. Digoxin, propranolol, and procainamide all cross the placenta and have been used to treat tachyarrhythmias.

The association of a structural cardiac abnormality and NIH usually has a poor prognosis. Of the reported cases, the only long-term survivor was an infant born with an intrapericardial teratoma that was successfully resected in the neonatal period.[8] Intrinsic cardiac defects are generally associated with poor perinatal outcome. This observation may be a reflection of the severity of the defects (serious enough to cause intrauterine congestive heart failure), as well as the condition of these frequently premature babies at delivery. Neonatal congestive heart failure with pulmonary edema may aggravate the severity of respiratory distress syndrome and delay permanent surgical correction of the underlying structural defect. It should be added that intrauterine myocardial infarction has been reported in association with NIH.[6] This may be diagnosed postnatally by electrocardiographic changes, creatine-phosphokinase elevation in the case of a recent event, or at autopsy.

Calcifications in the pericardial sac can occur with intrauterine Coxsackie B3 viral infection.[9] If such calcifications are seen, a viral infection should be suspected, and acute phase viral titers drawn on the mother.

The underlying mechanism in the development of most NIH of vascular etiology is high output cardiac failure. Vascular tumors increase cardiac work, as do arteriovenous malformations, and occur in a variety of sites, including the pulmonary artery system,[113] the great vein of Galen,[49] and the celiac trunk.[30] The antenatal detection of a tumor mass should prompt Doppler ultrasound examination to investigate the possibility of a vascular tumor. Other causes, such as thrombosis of the inferior vena cava,[99] have been reported, although the mechanism for the development of NIH remains obscure.

Infectious Causes. NIH has been associated with a number of viral, bacterial, and spirochetal organisms without any clear pathophysiologic mechanisms. Isolated case reports of toxoplasmosis,[7] parvovirus,[21] cytomegalovirus,[37,40,59,80,91] Coxsackievirus,[9] and syphilis[22,70] are available with good documentation. Less certain are passing references in some reviews to associations with trypanosomiasis, herpes simplex type 1, respiratory syncytial virus, and leptospirosis.[32,36,50,60] Intrauterine infections with human parvovirus leading to NIH seem to be associated with aplastic crisis in the fetus and may be suspected by raised maternal serum alphafetoprotein.

Toxoplasmosis was reported in a series of three cases in association with NIH, each of which appeared to have excessive extramedullary hematopoiesis.[7] Since most cases of maternal toxoplasmosis are asymptomatic, the diagnosis rests on serologic changes or pathologic demonstration of the organisms.[102] A twofold increase in titer is significant and suggests acute infection. The inability to demonstrate acute seroconversion in the mother does not exclude toxoplasmosis as a cause of NIH, since the infection could have occurred some weeks earlier. If, however, the mother was known to have a positive toxoplasmosis titer before conception, the diagnosis of congenital infection can be ruled out. Any patient with a positive titer should have the placenta carefully examined histologically for the presence of toxoplasma cysts. For this examination, the placenta should be immediately fixed in formalin and not refrigerated or frozen, since this may cause lysis of the organisms and lead to false negative results. A positive identification of the characteristic cysts is predictive of neonatal toxoplasmosis. Cord blood for IgM toxoplasma serology should be obtained, but 50 percent of infants with definitive congenital toxoplasmosis have negative serology by fluorescent antibody testing for IgM.[102]

Cytomegalovirus infections of the fetus can occur with primary infection and reinfections of the mother. Maternal serologic results are of little help unless they are negative.[102] Viral isolation from neonatal urine, cerebrospinal fluid, nasopharynx, or conjunctiva remains the best method of establishing the diagnosis.

Screening for syphilis can be performed with VDRL or RPR tests, with confirmation by specific treponemal antibody testing (e.g., FTA-ABS).

Renal Disorders. Congenital nephrotic syndrome (Finnish type) with resultant hypoproteinemia is a cause of NIH, reported primarily from the Scandinavian countries.[54,80] It is inherited with an autosomal recessive pattern, and over 100 kindreds have been reported. The infants have normal or slightly elevated BUN values, but massive proteinuria is uniformly present, and microscopic hematuria is often seen as well.

Although other abnormalities of the urinary tract, such as obstructive uropathy,[32,43] polycystic kidney disease with hydrometrocolpos,[12,59] hypoplastic kidney,[70] and pelvic kidney[70] have been reported in association with NIH, these are likely to reflect reporting bias because an underlying mechanism is unclear. In our experience with relatively large numbers of fetuses with obstructive uropathy and infantile polycystic kidney disease, NIH is uncommon.[98]

Gastrointestinal Disorders. A number of gastrointestinal disorders have been associated with NIH, including diaphragmatic hernia,[12,42,45,59,70,88] midgut volvulus,[103] gastrointestinal obstructions,[12,37,38,57,59,73] meconium peritonitis secondary to herniation of the gut into a peritoneal sac,[12] and meconium peritonitis of unknown etiology.[59,68] Whether these represent mere associations or an underlying common etiology has not been determined.

Hepatic disorders, such as cirrhosis and hepatic necrosis, were reported by Hutchinson et al.[59] along with NIH. A single case of giant cell hepatitis has also appeared in the literature.[12] These are all pathologic diagnoses and were not made antenatally. The common mechanism in the development of hydrops may be hypoproteinemia,[113] although analbuminemia alone is not a sufficient cause.[27] Two reports of hemangioma of the liver associated with NIH may be explained by arteriovenous shunting within the hepatic mass, leading to heart failure.[23,50]

Chromosomal Abnormalities. Turner syndrome (45XO) is one of the most common causes of NIH among the chromosomal abnormalities associated with hydrops.[60,80,84] In this syndrome there are often multiple, septated cysts in the paracervical region ("cystic hygroma"), related to a lack of communication between the lymphatic system and venous drainage in the neck. For unclear reasons, infants with Turner syndrome may also have lymphedema of the hands and feet as well as chylothorax, giving a picture resembling NIH.

NIH has been reported in association with other genetic abnormalities, including trisomy 13,[73] trisomy 18,[12] trisomy 21,[32,59,60,73,80,84,88,108], dup(11p),[44] mosaicisms, unbalanced translocations, and triploidy.[12,32,59,70,84]

The diagnosis of NIH is an indication for genetic amniocentesis. The identification of trisomy 18 (Edward's syndrome) could change the management, since 50 percent of these infants die within 2 months of birth, and only 10 percent survive the first year as severely mentally handicapped infants.[15] Of course, early identification offers the parents the option of elective termination of pregnancy.

Hereditary Syndromes. Pena-Shokeir syndrome type 1 is an autosomal recessive condition characterized by neurogenic arthrogryposis, pulmonary hypoplasia, and hypertelorism, which has been described in association with hydrops fetalis.[25,72] Another autosomal recessive disorder associated with NIH is the lethal type of multiple pterygium syndrome.[41,61,73] A recurrent NIH within a sibship of idiopathic origin has been described as well.[101] In one case, Noonan's syndrome has been associated with NIH, but the cause of the fetal effusions was probably the associated heart anomalies.[123]

Neoplasms. Neoplastic diseases can occur in utero, and two in particular have been associated with NIH: neuroblastomas[3,64,79,83,88,111,115] and teratomas.[12,42,48,59,80,88] Single cases of NIH associated with congenital leukemia,[32] pulmonary leiomyosarcoma,[48] and hemangioendothelioma of the liver[23] have also been reported. This latter tumor causes a hemodynamic state similar to that of an arteriovenous mal-

formation or an obstruction to venous return. The reported cases of teratomas were localized in the mediastinum, in the pericardial sac, and in the sacrococcygeal area. These tumors are potentially identifiable if they are of sufficient size or if they cause a shift in the location of other organs (e.g., the heart). Hutchinson et al.[59] noted one case of malignant teratoma without reporting any details of the case.

Tuberous sclerosis is an autosomal dominant disease characterized by fibroangiomatous tumors in multiple organs of the body. The most frequently affected organs are the cortex of the brain, the skin, and the kidneys. Occasionally, the heart may be involved with rhabdomyomas. Fibrosis of the liver may occur as well. The mechanism for the development of hydrops is probably heart failure in those with intracardiac rhabdomyomas or hepatic failure in those with cirrhosis. Antenatal diagnosis is not possible, and although the disease is inherited as an autosomal recessive disorder, 86 percent of the cases represent new mutations. Therefore, the parents are not involved in the disease process. Several cases of NIH in association with tuberous sclerosis have been reported.[59,86,116] In a series of 21 cases of tuberous sclerosis diagnosed within 1 week of birth, there was only 1 with NIH.[86]

Metabolic Disorders. The metabolic derangements associated with NIH are drawn from a number of pathways that involve either synthesis or storage disorders. The mechanisms for the development of hydrops in cases of storage diseases may involve visceromegaly and obstruction of venous return.[11] The storage diseases that have been reported include Gaucher disease (cerebrosidosis), gangliosidosis GM1 type I, Hurler syndrome (mucopolysaccharidosis type I), and mucolipidosis type I (sialidosis).

Gaucher disease results from an accumulation of glucocerebrosides in the histiocytes due to a tissue deficiency of beta-glucosidase. It is an autosomal recessive disease that can be diagnosed in cell culture of fibroblasts from amniotic fluid.[95] Heterozygote (carrier) identification can be accomplished by beta-glucosidase analysis of white blood cells or culture of skin fibroblasts. NIH is rare in infants with Gaucher disease. This diagnosis should be considered primarily in patients of Ashkenazi-Jewish ancestry, since two thirds of cases occur in this group.[15]

Gangliosidosis GM1 is an autosomal recessive disorder that is due to the absence of beta-galactosidase, and gangliosides collect diffusely in storage cells in many organs.[15]

Hurler syndrome is an autosomal recessive condition characterized by an accumulation of acid mucopolysaccharides due to deficiency in alpha-L-iduronidase.[15]

Sialidosis (mucolipidosis type I) is an autosomal recessive disease due to a deficiency in alpha-N-acetylneuraminidase, leading to accumulation of sialic acid.[15]

It is unclear if these metabolic disorders are associated with NIH or simply with soft tissue excess that leads to gross appearance resembling NIH.

These conditions are amenable to prenatal diagnosis and to detection of the carrier state.[95] In patients with NIH of unknown origin, a screening of urine by thin-layer chromatography and enzymatic assays on cultured fibroblasts is essential for accurate genetic counseling and prenatal diagnosis in subsequent pregnancies.

Skeletal Dysplasias. Skeletal dysplasias associated with NIH are achondroplasia,[113] achondrogenesis,[13,47,80] osteogenesis imperfecta,[59,80] thanatophoric dwarfism,[113] short rib–polydactyly syndrome,[74] and asphyxiating thoracic dysplasia.[59] In all of these, the mechanism for the production of NIH is unknown.

When performing real-time ultrasound evaluation of the hydropic fetus, careful attention to proximal and distal long bone lengths and mineralization will permit screening for some of these disorders.[63] Further discussion is available in Chapter 10.

Neurologic Conditions. There have been isolated reports of NIH along with an encephalocele[59] and with porencephaly and absence of the corpus callosum.[59] All of these probably represent chance associations. An additional case documents the occurrence of NIH in an infant with intracranial hemorrhage and severe anemia.[18]

Pulmonary Causes. The most frequent cause of NIH among pulmonary lesions is congenital cystic adenomatoid malformation (CCAM).[12,32,37,48,51,59,67,77] Antenatal diagnosis of this condition has been reported (see Chapter 5). Other conditions that have been associated with NIH include pulmonary lymphangiectasia,[59,73] pulmonary leiomyosarcoma,[48] alveolar cell adenoma of the lung,[29] extralobar pulmonary sequestration,[97] and diaphragmatic hernia.[50,59,70,88] An unusual cause of NIH is enlargement of one lung with shift of the mediastinal structures.[89] The mechanism for hydrops in all these conditions is probably obstruction of venous return. Congenital chylothorax may lead to hydrops as well.[4,34,62,114]

The Placenta. Chorioangiomas of the placenta act as high volume arteriovenous shunts to produce hydrops.[10,12,50,55,60,70,74,112] Small chorioangiomas may

TABLE 12–5. LABORATORY TESTS FOR HYDROPIC FETUS

Blood tests
  CBC with differential and RBC indices
  Kleinhauer-Betke stain
  ABO type and rhesus antigen status
  Indirect Coombs (antibody screen) test
  Acute phase titers
    Toxoplasmosis
    Cytomegalovirus
  Serologic test for syphilis (VDRL or RPR)
  G-6PD deficiency screen
Amniotic fluid tests
  Karyotype
  L:S ratio after viability

not be visualized, and the true incidence of these placental tumors may be higher than has been determined in the past.[106] In the larger lesions, there may be vascular stasis, with resultant loss of plasma proteins into the amniotic fluid and hydrops.[112]

Prognosis

Although some cases of spontaneous intrauterine remission of NIH fetalis are reported in the literature,[68,93,96,104] the prognosis for the majority of these infants is gloomy. The perinatal mortality rate in these infants is very high, ranging from 70 to 90 percent.[37,50,59,60,73]

Obstetrical Management

Identification of the hydropic infant is not a diagnostic challenge. The real problem is to establish the underlying cause and to determine appropriate therapy and optimal timing of delivery. Once a hydropic infant is identified, the first step is to investigate the possibility of isoimmunization and whether it is due to rhesus or other irregular antibodies. This can be done easily by performing an indirect Coombs test on maternal serum. A negative Coombs test rules out isoimmunization.

A comprehensive ultrasound examination is the next step in the management of the pregnancy, along with appropriate investigative blood and amniotic fluid tests, as outlined in Table 12–5. Interpretation of these blood tests was discussed in the preceding sections. Ultrasound examination should include fetal echocardiography and a careful survey for congenital anomalies of the fetus and placenta. Most commonly, the workup (both ultrasound and laboratory) fails to reveal the etiology. Management decisions at this juncture are dependent on gestational age.

Before viability, the option of pregnancy termination should be offered to the parents. They should be counseled that the prognosis in cases of previable NIH is poor. If a decision to continue the pregnancy is made, the clinician is faced with the dilemma of either delivering the baby to prevent intrauterine death or continuing expectant management to allow fetal maturation. Immediate delivery of an immature fetus is likely to result in a newborn with increased total lung water, thus compounding the problems in treating respiratory distress syndrome by adding pulmonary edema.

Expectant management, on the other hand, raises the questions of ensuring fetal well-being and defining the end-point for delivery. Obstetricians usually elect to defer delivery until fetal lung maturity appears as measured by the lecithin:sphingomyelin (L:S) ratio. However, the natural evolution of surfactant production in hydropic infants is unknown. In other conditions associated with pulmonary hypoplasia, such as diaphragmatic hernia, immature L:S ratios have been obtained close to term.[16] Furthermore, NIH is often associated with polyhydramnios, and uterine overdistention may precipitate premature labor.

A reasonable approach to management of the very premature infant is to follow the fetus with frequent ultrasound evaluations, including biophysical profiles, and to defer delivery until the clinical picture appears to deteriorate. If such a course is chosen and premature labor due to polyhydramnios occurs, the option of therapeutic amniocentesis is available. In 40 to 50 percent of the cases, preeclampsia occurs with NIH for unclear reasons.[70] We consider the appearance of this complication to be an indication for delivery, since the mother's health may be seriously threatened and the chance of the infant's survival is extremely small.

If the pregnancy is close to term, elective delivery would decrease the risk of intrauterine fetal demise. Because fetal ascites may cause soft tissue dystocia, cesarean section should be considered as a way of minimizing birth trauma and maximizing the likelihood of survival. On the other hand, patients should be informed that the chances of survival for these infants are minimal. Thoracentesis and abdominal paracentesis may be considered prior to delivery.

The prognosis for the hydropic fetus is improved in selected groups. Cardiac dysrhythmias amenable to transplacental medical therapy usually carry a good prognosis, provided they are not associated with a serious congenital anomaly. Another potentially treatable cause in the antepartum period is a significant fetomaternal hemorrhage, which may be treated with current techniques of in utero transfusion. This is possible when the risks of prematurity outweigh the risks of transfusion. Alternatively, elective delivery and neonatal transfusion may be chosen. In the rare case of G-6PD as a cause of hemolysis, it should be sufficient to remove the offending agent

and depending on the gestational age, either deliver or transfuse the fetus.

It is necessary to develop a systematic approach to establish the etiology. Autopsy should be performed in every case to help reach this goal.

REFERENCES

1. Allan LD, Crawford DC, Sheridan R, et al.: Aetiology of non-immune hydrops: The value of echocardiography. Br J Obstet Gynaecol 93:223, 1986
2. Altenburger KM, Jedziniak M, Roper WL, et al.: Congenital complete heart block associated with hydrops fetalis. J Pediatr 91:618, 1977.
3. Anders D, Kindermann G, Pfeifer U: Metastasizing fetal neuroblastoma with involvement of the placenta simulating fetal erythroblastosis. J Pediatr 82:50, 1973.
4. Anderson EA, Hertel J, Pedersen SA, et al.: Congenital chylothorax: Management by ligature of the thoracic duct. Scand J Thorac Cardiovasc Surg 18:193, 1984.
5. Arcilla RA, Thilenius OG, Ranniger K: Congestive heart failure from suspected ductal closure in utero. J Pediatr 75:74, 1969.
6. Arthur A, Cottom D, Evans R, et al.: Myocardial infarction in a newborn infant. J Pediatr 73:110, 1968.
7. Bain AD, Bowie JH, Flint WF, et al.: Congenital toxoplasmosis simulating haemolytic disease of the newborn. J Obstet Gynaecol Br Commonw 63:826, 1956.
8. Banfield F, Dick M, Behrendt DM, et al.: Intrapericardial teratoma: A new and treatable cause of hydrops fetalis. Am J Dis Child 134:1174, 1980.
9. Bates HR: Coxsackie virus B3 calcific pancarditis and hydrops fetalis. Am J Obstet Gynecol 106:629, 1970.
10. Battaglia FC, Woolever CA: Fetal and neonatal complications associated with recurrent chorioangiomas. Pediatrics 41:62, 1968.
11. Beck M, Bender SW, Reiter HL, et al.: Neuraminidase deficiency presenting as non-immune hydrops fetalis. Eur J Pediatr 143:135, 1984.
12. Beischer NA, Fortune DW, Macafee J: Nonimmunologic hydrops fetalis and congenital abnormalities. Obstet Gynecol 38:86, 1971.
13. Benacerraf B, Osathanondh R, Bieber FR: Achondrogenesis type I: Ultrasound diagnosis in utero. J Clin Ultrasound 12:357, 1984.
14. Benner MC: Premature closure of foramen ovale: Report of 2 cases. Am Heart J 17:437, 1939.
15. Bergsma D: Birth Defects Compendium, 2nd ed. New York, Alan R. Liss, 1979, pp 32, 33, 201, 484, 724, 727, 953.
16. Berk C: ''High-risk'' lecithin/sphingomyelin ratios associated with neonatal diaphragmatic hernia. Case reports. Br J Obstet Gynaecol 89:250, 1982.
17. Boer HR, Anido G: Hydrops fetalis caused by Bart's hemoglobin. South Med J 72:1623, 1979.
18. Bose C: Hydrops fetalis and in utero intracranial hemorrhage. J Pediatr 93:1023, 1978.

19. Boutte P, Bourlon F, Tordjman C, et al.: Tachycardie supraventriculaire et anasarque foetales: A propos de deux observations. Arch Fr Pediatr 42:777, 1985.

20. Brewer GJ, Tarlov AR, Alving AS: The methemoglobin reduction test for primaquine-type sensitivity of erythrocytes. A simplified procedure for detecting a specific hypersusceptibility to drug hemolysis. JAMA 180:386, 1962.

21. Brown T, Anand A, Ritchie LD, et al.: Intrauterine parvovirus infection associated with hydrops fetalis. Lancet 2:1033, 1984.

22. Bulova SI, Schwartz E, Harrer WV: Hydrops fetalis and congenital syphilis. Pediatrics 49:285, 1972.

23. Caldwell CC, Hurley RM, Anderson CL, et al.: Nonimmune hydrops fetalis managed with peritoneal dialysis. Am J Perinatol 2:211, 1985.

24. Chan V, Chan TK, Liang ST, et al.: Hydrops fetalis due to an unusual form of Hb H disease. Blood 66:224, 1985.

25. Chen H, Blumberg B, Immken L, et al.: The Pena-Shokeir syndrome: Report of five cases and further delineation of the syndrome. Am J Med Genet 16:213, 1983.

26. Cooke RW, Mettau JW, Van Capelle AW, et al.: Familial congenital heart block and hydrops fetalis. Arch Dis Child 55:479, 1980.

27. Cormode EJ, Lyster DM, Israels S: Analbuminemia in a neonate. J Pediatr 86:862, 1975.

28. Cowan RH, Waldo AL, Harris HB, et al.: Neonatal paroxysmal supraventricular tachycardia with hydrops. Pediatrics 55:428, 1975.

29. Dadak C, Gerstner L, Schaller A: Hydrops universalis und Respiratory distress infolge angeborener Lungengeschwulst. Zentralbl Gynaekol 106:55, 1984.

30. Daniel SJ, Cassady G: Non-immunologic hydrops fetalis associated with a large hemangioendothelioma. Pediatrics 42:828, 1968.

31. Darnell-Jones DE, Pritchard KI, Giovannini CA, et al.: Hydrops fetalis associated with idiopathic arterial calcification. Obstet Gynecol 39:435, 1972.

32. Davis CL: Diagnosis and management of nonimmune hydrops fetalis. J Reprod Med 27:594, 1982.

33. Debelle GD, Gillam GL, Tauro GP: A case of hydrops foetalis due to foeto–maternal haemorrhage. Aust Pediat J 13:131, 1977.

34. Defoort P, Thiery M: Antenatal diagnosis of congenital chylothorax by gray scale sonography. J Clin Ultrasound 6:47, 1978.

35. DeVore GR, Siassi B, Platt LD: Fetal echocardiography. III. The diagnosis of cardiac arrhythmias using real-time-directed M-mode ultrasound. Am J Obstet Gynecol 146:792, 1983.

36. Driscoll S: Hydrops fetalis. N Engl J Med 275:1432, 1966.

37. Etches PC, Lemons JA: Nonimmune hydrops fetalis: Report of 22 cases including three siblings. Pediatrics 64:326, 1979.

38. Evron S, Yagel S, Samueloff A, et al.: Nonimmunologic hydrops fetalis: A review of 11 cases. J Perinat Med 13:147, 1985.

39. Fay RA: Feto-maternal haemorrhage as a cause of fetal morbidity and mortality. Br J Obstet Gynaecol 90:443, 1983.

40. Filloux F, Kelsey DK, Bose CL, et al.: Hydrops fetalis with supraventricular tachycardia and cytomegalovirus infection. Clin Pediatr 24:534, 1985.

41. Fitch N, Rochon L, Srolovitz H, et al.: Vascular abnormalities in a fetus with multiple pterygia. Am J Med Genet 21:755, 1985.

42. Fleischer AC, Killam AP, Boehm FH, et al.: Hydrops fetalis: Sonographic evaluation and clinical implications. Radiology 141:163, 1981.

43. France NE, Back EH: Neonatal ascites associated with urethral obstruction. Arch Dis Child 29:565, 1954.

44. Fryns JP, Kleczkowska A, Vandenberghe K, et al.: Cystic hygroma and hydrops fetalis in dup (11p) syndrome. Am J Med Genet 22:287, 1985.

45. Gilsanz V, Emons D, Hansmann M, et al.: Hydrothorax, ascites, and right diaphragmatic hernia. Radiology 158:243, 1986.

46. Ginsberg SJ, Groll M: Hydrops fetalis due to infantile Gaucher's disease. J Pediatr 82:1046, 1973.

47. Glenn LW, Teng SS: In utero sonographic diagnosis of achondrogenesis. J Clin Ultrasound 13:195, 1985.

48. Golladay ES, Mollitt DL: Surgically correctable fetal hydrops. J Pediatr Surg 19:59, 1984.

49. Gomez MR, Whitten CF, Nolke A, et al.: Aneurysmal malformation of the great vein of Galen causing heart failure. Report of five cases. Pediatrics 31:400, 1963.

50. Gough JD, Keeling JW, Castle B, et al.: The obstetric management of non-immunological hydrops. Br J Obstet Gynaecol 93:226, 1986.

51. Graham D, Winn K, Dex W, et al.: Prenatal diagnosis of cystic adenomatoid malformation of the lung. J Ultrasound Med 1:9, 1982.

52. Guntheroth WG, Cyr DR, Mack LA, et al.: Hydrops from reciprocating atrioventricular tachycardia in a 27-week fetus requiring quinidine for conversion. Obstet Gynecol 66:29S, 1985.

53. Guy G, Coady DJ, Jansen V, et al.: Alpha-Thalassemia hydrops fetalis: Clinical and ultrasonographic considerations. Am J Obstet Gynecol 153:500, 1985.

54. Hallman N, Norio R, Rapola J: Congenital nephrotic syndrome. Nephron 11:101, 1973.

55. Hardy JD, Solomon S, Banwell GS, et al.: Congenital complete heart block in the newborn associated with maternal systemic lupus erythematosus and other connective tissue disorders. Arch Dis Child 54:7, 1979.

56. Harkavy KL, Scanlon JW: Hydrops fetalis in a parabiotic, acardiac twin. Am J Dis Child 132:638, 1978.

57. Hatjis CG: Nonimmunologic fetal hydrops associated with hyperreactioluteinalis. Obstet Gynecol 65:11S, 1985.

58. Hirata K, Kato H, Yoshioka F, et al.: Successful treatment of fetal atrial flutter and congestive heart failure. Arch Dis Child 60:158, 1985.

59. Hutchison AA, Drew JH, Yu VYH, et al.: Nonimmunologic hydrops fetalis: A review of 61 cases. Obstet Gynecol 59:347, 1982.

60. Im SS, Rizos N, Joutsi P, et al.: Nonimmunologic hydrops fetalis. Am J Obstet Gynecol 148:566, 1984.

61. Isaacson G, Gargus JJ, Mahoney MJ: Brief clinical report: Lethal multiple pterygium syndrome in an 18-week fetus with hydrops. Am J Med Genet 17:835, 1984.

62. Jaffa AJ, Barak S, Kaysar N, et al.: Case report. Antenatal diagnosis of bilateral congenital chylothorax with pericardial effusion. Acta Obstet Gynecol Scand 64:455, 1985.

63. Jeanty P. Romero R: Fetal limbs, normal anatomy and congenital malformations. Semin Ultrasound 5:3, 1984.

64. Johnson AT, Halbert D: Congenital neuroblastoma presenting as hydrops fetalis. NC Med J 35:289, 1974.

65. Jones CEM, Rivers RPA, Taghizadeh A: Disseminated intravascular coagulation and fetal hydrops in a newborn infant in association with a chorioangioma of placenta. Pediatrics 50:901, 1972.

66. Kleinman CS, Donnerstein RL: Ultrasonic assessment of cardiac function in the intact human fetus. J Am Coll Cardiol 5:84S, 1985.

67. Kleinman CS, Donnerstein RL, DeVore GR, et al.: Fetal echocardiography for evaluation of in utero congestive heart failure. N Engl J Med 306:568, 1982.

68. Leppert PC, Pahlka BS, Stark RI, et al.: Spontaneous regression of fetal ascites in utero in an adolescent. J Adolescent Health Care 5:286, 1984.

69. Lubinsky M, Rapport P: Transient fetal hydrops and "prune belly" in one identical female twin. N Engl J Med 308:256, 1983.

70. Macafee CAJ, Fortune DW, Beischer NA: Non-immunological hydrops fetalis. J Obstet Gynaecol Br Commonw 77:226, 1970.

71. Machin GA: Differential diagnosis of hydrops fetalis. Am J Med Genet 9:341, 1981.

72. MacMillan RH, Harbert GM, Davis WD, et al.: Prenatal diagnosis of Pena-Shokeir syndrome type I. Am J Med Genet 21:279, 1985.

73. Mahony BS, Filly RA, Callen PW, et al.: Severe nonimmune hydrops fetalis: Sonographic evaluation. Radiology 151:757, 1984.

74. Maidman JE, Yeager C, Anderson V, et al.: Prenatal diagnosis and management of nonimmunologic hydrops fetalis. Obstet Gynecol 56:571, 1980.

75. Marasini M, Pongiglione G, Lituania M, et al.: Aortic arch interruption: Two-dimensional echocardiographic recognition in utero. Pediatr Cardiol 6:147, 1985.

76. Mentzer WC, Collier E: Hydrops fetalis associated with erythrocyte G-6-PD deficiency and maternal ingestion of fava beans and ascorbic acid. J Pediatr 86:565, 1975.

77. Merenstein GB: Congenital cystic adenomatoid malformation of the lung. Report of a case and review of the literature. Am J Dis Child 118:772, 1969.

78. Moller JH, Lynch RP, Edwards JE: Fetal cardiac failure resulting from congenital anomalies of the heart. J Pediatr 68:699, 1966.

79. Moss TJ, Kaplan L: Association of hydrops fetalis with congenital neuroblastoma. Am J Obstet Gynecol 132:905, 1978.

80. Mostoufi-Zadeh M, Weiss LM, Driscoll SG: Nonimmune hydrops fetalis: A challenge in perinatal pathology. Hum Pathol 16:785, 1985.

81. Nakayama R, Yamada D, Steinmiller V, et al.: Hydrops fetalis secondary to Bart hemoglobinopathy. Obstet Gynecol 67:177, 1986.

82. Newburger JW, Keane JF: Intrauterine supraventricular tachycardia. J Pediatr 95:780, 1979.

83. Newton ER, Louis F, Dalton ME, et al.: Fetal neuroblastoma and catecholamine-induced maternal hypertension. Obstet Gynecol 65:49s, 1985.

84. Nicolaides KH, Rodeck CH, Gosden CM: Rapid karyotyping in non-lethal fetal malformations. Lancet 1:283, 1986.

85. Oie BK, Hertel J, Seip M, et al.: Hydrops foetalis in 3 infants of a mother with acquired chronic pure red cell aplasia: Transitory red cell aplasia in 1 of the infants. Scand J Haematol 33:466, 1984.

86. Ostor AG, Fortune DW: Tuberous sclerosis initially seen as hydrops fetalis. Arch Pathol Lab Med 102:34, 1978.

87. Perkins RP: Hydrops fetalis and stillbirth in a male glucose-6-phosphate dehydrogenase-deficient fetus possibly due to maternal ingestion of sulfisoxazole: A case report. Am J Obstet Gynecol 111:379, 1971.

88. Perlin BM, Pomerance JJ, Schifrin BS: Nonimmunologic hydrops fetalis. Obstet Gynecol 57:584, 1981.

89. Phillips RR, Batcup G, Vinall PS: Non-immunologic hydrops fetalis. Arch Dis Child 60:84, 1985.

90. Platt LD, DeVore GR: In utero diagnosis of hydrops fetalis: ultrasound methods. Clin Perinatol 9:3:627, 1982.

91. Price JM, Fisch AE, Jacobson J: Ultrasonic findings in fetal cytomegalovirus infection. J Clinical Ultrasound 6:268, 1978.

92. Radford DJ, Izukawa T, Rowe RD: Congenital paroxysmal atrial tachycardia. Arch Dis Child 51:613, 1976.

93. Ramzin MS, Napflin S: Transient intrauterine supraventricular tachycardia associated with transient hydrops fetalis. Case report. Br J Obstet Gynaecol 89:965, 1982.

94. Rementeria JL, Gulrajani MR, Stankewick WR: Fetal hydrops and "prune belly" in one identical twin. N Engl J Med 309:52, 1983.

95. Roberts NS, Dunn LK, Weiner S, et al.: Midtrimester amniocentesis: indications, technique, risks and potential for prenatal diagnosis. J Reprod Med 28:167, 1983.

96. Robertson L, Ott A, Mack L, et al.: Sonographically documented disappearance of nonimmune hydrops fetalis associated with maternal hypertension. West J Med 143:382, 1985.

97. Romero R, Chervenak FA, Kotzen J, et al.: Antenatal sonographic findings of extralobar pulmonary sequestration. J Ultrasound Med 1:131, 1982.

98. Romero R, Cullen M, Grannum PAT, et al.: Antenatal diagnosis of renal anomalies with ultrasound. III. Bilateral renal agenesis. Am J Obstet Gynecol 151:38, 1985.

99. Rudolph N, Levin EJ: Hydrops fetalis with vena caval thrombosis in utero. NY State J Med 77:421, 1977.

100. Scott JR, Warenski JC: Tests to detect and quantitate fetomaternal bleeding. Clin Obstet Gynecol 25:2:277, 1982.

101. Seeds JW, Herbert WNP, Bowes WA et al.: Recurrent idiopathic fetal hydrops: Results of prenatal therapy. Obstet Gynecol 64:30S, 1984.

102. Sever JL, Larsen JW, Grossman JH: Handbook of Perinatal Infections. Boston, Little, Brown, 1979, pp 157–163.

103. Seward JF, Zusman J: Hydrops fetalis associated with small-bowel volvulus. Lancet 2:52, 1978.

104. Shapiro I, Sharf M: Spontaneous intrauterine remission of hydrops fetalis in one identical twin: Sonographic diagnosis. J Clin Ultrasound 13:427, 1985.

105. Silber DL, Durnin RE: Intrauterine atrial tachycardia, associated with massive edema in a newborn. Am J Dis Child 117:722, 1969.

106. Sieracki JC, Panke TW, Horvat BL, et al.: Chorioangiomas. Obstet Gynecol 46:155, 1975.

107. Silverman NH, Enderlein MA, Stanger P, et al.: Recognition of fetal arrhythmias by echocardiography. J Clin Ultrasound 13:255, 1985.

108. Silverman NH, Kleinman CS, Rudolph AM, et al.: Fetal atrioventricular valve insufficiency associated with nonimmune hydrops: A two-dimensional echocardiographic and pulsed Doppler ultrasound study. Circulation 72:825, 1985.

109. Spahr RC, Botti JJ, MacDonald HM, et al.: Nonimmunologic hydrops fetalis: A review of 19 cases. Int J Gynaecol Obstet 18:303, 1980.

110. Strasburger JF, Kugler JD, Cheatham JP, et al.: Nonimmunologic hydrops fetalis associated with congenital aortic valvular stenosis. Am Heart J 108:1380, 1984.

111. Strauss L, Driscoll SG: Congenital neuroblastoma involving the placenta. Reports of two cases. Pediatrics 34:23, 1964.

112. Sweet L, Reid WD, Robertson NRC: Hydrops fetalis in association with chorioangioma of the placenta. Pediatrics 82:91, 1973.

113. Turkel SB: Conditions associated with nonimmune hydrops fetalis. Clin Perinatol 9:613, 1982.

114. Van Aerde J, Campbell AN, Smyth JA, et al.: Spontaneous chylothorax in newborns. Am J Dis Child 138:961, 1984.

115. Van der Slikke JW, Balk AG: Hydramnios with hydrops fetalis and disseminated fetal neuroblastoma. Obstet Gynecol 55:250, 1980.

116. Wedemeyer AL, Breitfeld V: Cardiac neoplasm, tachyarrhythmia, and anasarca in an infant, Am J Dis Child 129:738, 1975.

117. Weisert O, Marstrander J: Severe anemia in a newborn caused by protracted feto-maternal "transfusion." Acta Pediatr 49:426, 1960.

118. Wiggins JW, Bowes W, Clewell W, et al.: Echocardiographic diagnosis and intravenous digoxin management of fetal tachyarrhythmias and congestive heart failure. Am J Dis Child 140:202, 1986.

119. Wintrobe MM, Lee GR, Boggs DR, et al.: Clinical Hematology, 8th ed. Philadelphia, Lea & Febiger, 1981, pp 786–800, 869–900.

120. Wittmann BK, Baldwin VJ, Nichol B: Antenatal diagnosis of twin transfusion syndrome by ultrasound. Obstet Gynecol 58:123, 1981.

121. Wright VJ, Dimmick JE: Hydrops fetalis due to tuberose sclerosis. Proc Interim Meet Pediatr Pathol Club, October 1977.

122. Young LW, Wexler HA: Radiological case of the month. Am J Dis Child 132:201, 1978.

123. Zarabi M, Mieckowski GC, Mazer J: Cystic hygroma associated with Noonan's syndrome. J Clin Ultrasound 11:398, 1983.

124. Zerres K, Hansmann M, Knopfle G, et al.: Clinical case reports. Prenatal diagnosis of genetically determined early manifestation of autosomal dominant polycystic kidney disease. Hum Genet 71:368, 1985.

Sacrococcygeal Teratoma

Definition
Sacrococcygeal teratoma (SCT) is a congenital germ cell tumor arising from the presacral area.

Incidence
SCT is the most common tumor encountered in the newborn. The estimated incidence is 1 in 40,000 births. Eighty percent of affected infants are females.[5]

Etiopathogenesis
SCTs arise from the primitive knot or Hensen's node. Hensen's node is an aggregation of totipotential cells that are the primary organizers of embryonic development (Fig. 12–18). Originally located in the posterior portion of the embryo, it migrates caudally during the first weeks of life inside the tail of the embryo, finally resting anterior to the coccyx.[11] Segregation of totipotential cell from Hensen's node probably gives rise to SCTs. This theory provides an explanation for the more frequent occurrence of teratomas in the sacral area rather than in other parts of the body.[11]

Although the majority of SCTs occurs sporadically, the association of SCT, anorectal stenosis, and sacrococcygeal defects has been reported and appears to be inherited in an autosomal dominant pattern.[2,16]

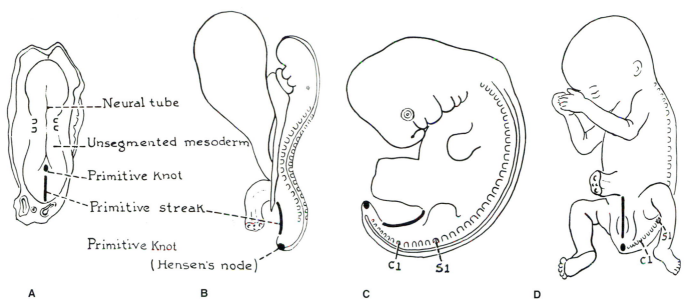

A   B   C   D

Figure 12–18. Sacrococcygeal teratomas presumably arise from totipotential cells that are initially derived from the primitive knot (Hensen's node). These primordial cells are most apt to be found close to the pathway traversed by the primitive node or to its final resting place in the sacrococcygeal area. **A.** The human embryo at the beginning of somite formation. The primitive node is located at the caudal end of the neural tube. **B.** A 17-somite human embryo demonstrates the apparent caudal migration of the primitive knot while somites are formed and pushed cephalad. The primitive streak is now ventral. The primitive node remains at the tip of the neural tube. **C.** Human embryo at the middle of the 6th week, at which time the tail is of maximal length. Forty-two somites are present, and the primitive node is now pushed to the tip of the tail. **D.** The fetal form reached in the 10th week after the resorption of the tail. Thirty-four somites, including the coccyx, remain. The tail does not drop off, but a retraction of it takes place as fragmentation and resorption of the ependymal canal somites and tail duct take place. The primitive knot comes to lie at the tip of the coccyx, and any teratoma arising from it would be similarly located. *(Reproduced with permission from Gonzalez-Crussi et al.: Arch Pathol Lab Med 102:420, 1978.)*

However, it is unclear if the SCT in these cases is congenital or arises in the postnatal period.

Pathology

The American Academy of Pediatrics[1] classifies SCTs into four types: type I, a predominant external lesion protruding from the perineal region and covered by skin with a minimal presacral component; type II, a predominant external tumor with a significant presacral component; type III, a tumor with a predominant sacral component and external extension; type IV, a presacral tumor with no external component. Types I and II account for more than 80 percent of cases.[10,21] In 15 percent of patients, the lesion is entirely cystic. In the remaining patients, it is either solid or mixed.[7] A histopathologic classification similar to that used for ovarian teratomas has been suggested.[10,27] Three types of SCT can thus be distinguished. (1) Mature (or benign) teratomas consist of tissues markedly similar to normal, well-developed structures. A variety of tissues, usually derived from all three germ layers, can be found in these cases. Glia, bowel, pancreas, bronchial mucosa, skin appendages, and striated and smooth muscle have been described.[5,10,27] Fully formed organs may be present. Bowel loops,[12] limb components, such as metacarpal

bones and digits,[20] and well-formed teeth[5] have been documented. Choroid plexus structures are frequently found, and their production of cerebrospinal fluid is responsible for the cysts within the tumor. (2) Immature teratomas are usually graded from 0 to 3

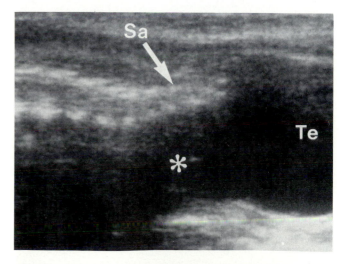

Figure 12–19. Longitudinal scan demonstrating a cystic lesion (Te) arising from the sacrum (Sa). The integrity of the sacrum and the intraabdominal extension of the lesion (∗) allow a diagnosis of sacrococcygeal teratoma.

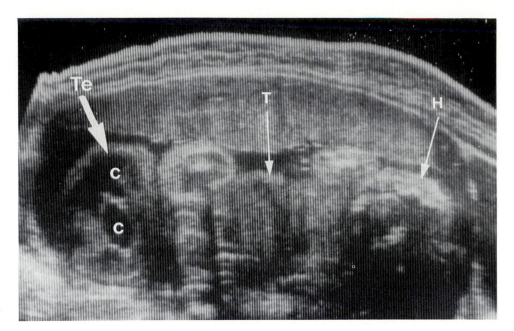

Figure 12–20. Longitudinal scan passing through the head (H) and trunk (T) of a fetus affected by a large, partly cystic (c), partly solid teratoma (Te).

depending upon the proportion of immature or embryonal tissues. The immature component is almost exclusively of neuroepithelial origin or, less frequently, of renal origin.[10,27] (3) Malignant teratomas are of the yolk sac or endodermal sinus tumor type and are characterized by production of alphafetoprotein.

Mature, immature, and malignant forms account for 55 to 75 percent, 11 to 28 percent, and 7 to 13 percent of all SCTs, respectively.[27] Mature and immature forms are frequently cystic (72 percent and 62 percent, respectively). Malignant forms are predominantly solid.[27] Hypervascularity is a frequent finding[26] and may result in severe spontaneous and intraoperative hemorrhage.

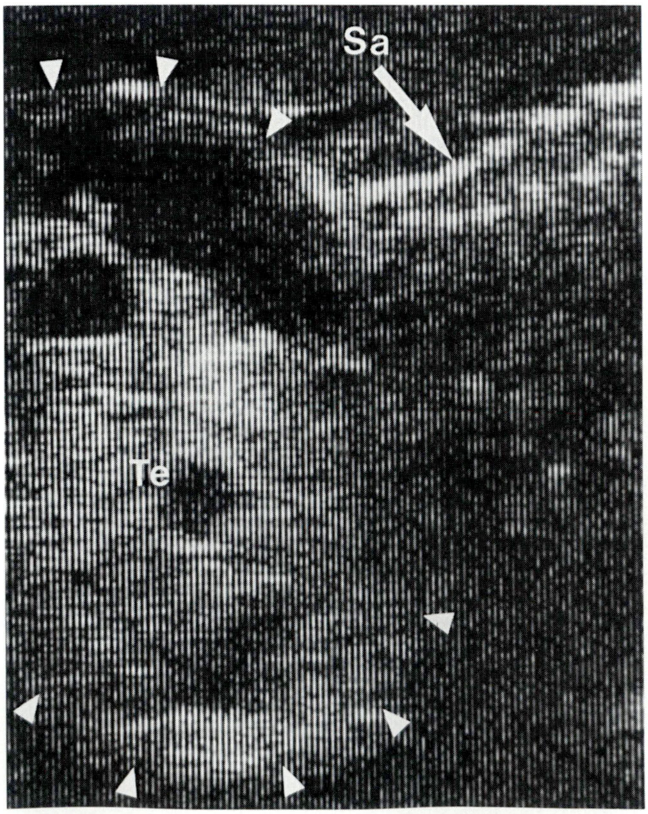

Associated Anomalies
The frequency of associated anomalies ranges from 5 to 25 percent in different series.[1,3,7,10,11] No specific pattern has been identified. Anomalies have included

Figure 12–21. Longitudinal scan passing through the sacrum (Sa) of a fetus with very large, mixed sacrococcygeal teratoma (Te, *arrowheads*).

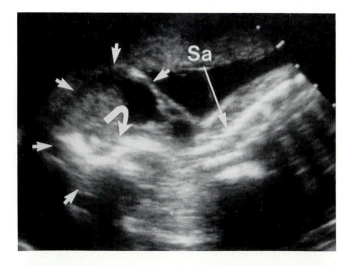

Figure 12–22. Longitudinal scan passing through the sacrum (Sa) in a midtrimester fetus with a large, predominantly solid sacrococcygeal teratoma. Calcifications are seen within the tumor (*arrowheads*). At necropsy, a well-formed foot was found inside the mass.

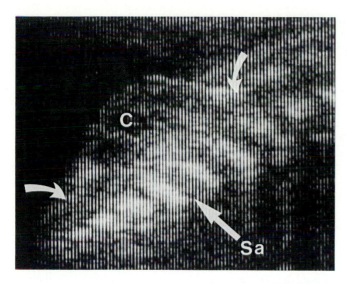

Figure 12–23. Myelomeningocele. A cystic lesion (c) with internal septa is seen arising from the posterior aspect of the sacrum (Sa). Note the defect of the vertebrae below the cystic structure (*curved arrows*).

spina bifida, obstructive uropathy, cleft palate, and calcaneous valgus deformity. Severe hemorrhage inside the tumor leading to anemia and NIH has been reported in a fetus.[9]

Prenatal Diagnosis

The experience in prenatal diagnosis of SCT has been reviewed recently.[14] A total of 20 cases[4,6,8,9,13–15,17,19,22–25,28,29] has been reported, to which we can add 7 cases from our own experience.

The diagnosis of types I, II, and III is easy and depends on demonstration of a mass arising from the sacral area and protruding through the perineum. The mass may be either cystic (Fig. 12–19), solid, or mixed (Figs. 12–20, 12–21). Calcifications are present in 36 percent of cases[7] (Fig. 12–22). Identification of type IV SCT appears difficult, since this type occurs as intraabdominal masses, and establishing their origin may be impossible. A careful investigation of the intraabdominal cavity in search of tumor extension is critical for the assessment of the type of SCT. Evaluation of fetal bladder function has been suggested, in an effort to identify involvement of the pelvic nerves.[14] The accuracy of ultrasound in recognizing such dysfunction remains to be established.

In some patients, an elevation of the amniotic fluid alphafetoprotein level and the presence of acetylcholinesterase have been reported.[13,14] Polyhydramnios has been found in association with SCT.

In the fetus, a large myelomeningocele may closely mimic SCT. However, a distinction can be made by demonstrating in the latter that the spine is intact, the tumor has intraabdominal or perineal extensions, and derives from the anterior portion of the sacrum (Fig. 12–23). Alphafetoprotein and acetylcholinesterase may have limited value in the differential diagnosis between a neural tube defect and SCT. A differentiation between SCT and more rare conditions, such as neuroenteric cysts and tumors of various origins (e.g., chordoma, sarcoma, ependymoma), may be impossible in prenatal ultrasound studies.

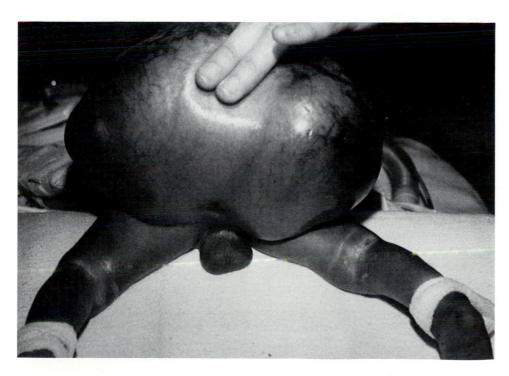

Figure 12–24. Newborn with a large sacrococcygeal teratoma.

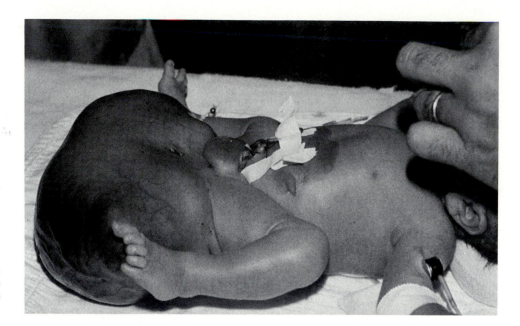

Figure 12–25. The same infant as in Figure 12–24. This mass was resected with no difficulties in the immediate neonatal period.

Prognosis

The prognosis is related to the histology and size of the tumor. The histologic type predicts the likelihood of malignancies, and the size of the tumor relates to the occurrence of complications during surgical extirpation (Figs. 12–24, 12–25). According to Altman et al.,[1] no patient with type I tumor had metastasis, whereas types II, III, and IV were associated with spread in 6 percent, 20 percent, and 76 percent, respectively. Malignant tumors are uniformly and rapidly fatal. The average time of survival after diagnosis is 8.9 months,[27] with only one reported case of long-term survival.[18] Malignancies should be differentiated from local recurrences of benign SCT after extirpation.[3] The mortality rate of patients with immature SCT varies between 55 percent[10] and 37 percent.[27] Benign SCT carries a good prognosis and its mortality rate varies between 3 percent[5] and 12 percent.[7] The main cause of death in these patients is uncontrolled hemorrhage at the time of surgery. Even though entire cystic lesions and those with calcifications are likely to be benign, such correlation is not always correct.[7] The size of the tumor does not seem to predict malignancy. However, very large SCT may be associated with significant intraoperative morbidity. There is limited experience with the intrauterine growth of these lesions. We have seen one rapidly growing tumor that was benign in nature. A review of the prenatally diagnosed cases indicates a much higher mortality rate than that expected from the pediatric series. Of a total of 27 patients, an elective termination was performed in 7. The perinatal mortality rate in the remaining patients was 45 percent (9/20). It is remarkable that in the 7 fatalities for which histopathologic examination was available, the SCT was benign in 6 and immature in 1.

Obstetrical Management

Before viability, the option of pregnancy termination should be offered to the parents. A careful search for associated anomalies is indicated. In continuing pregnancies, serial scans are indicated to evaluate the growth of the tumor and to detect the appearance of hydrops. SCT can vary greatly in size. Dystocia has complicated 6 to 13 percent of labors. With a large tumor, a cesarean section would seem prudent. Aspiration of a massive cystic lesion to permit cesarean delivery has been reported.[19]

REFERENCES

1. Altman RP, Randolph JG, Lilly JR: Sacrococcygeal teratoma. American Academy of Pediatrics Surgical Section Survey, 1973. J Pediatr Surg 9:389, 1974.
2. Ashcraft KW, Holder TM: Hereditary presacral teratoma. J Pediatr Surg 9:691, 1974.
3. Carney JA, Thompson DP, Johnson CL, et al.: Teratomas in children: Clinical and pathologic aspects. J Pediatr Surg 7:271, 1972.
4. Cousins L, Benirschke K, Porreco R, et al.: Placentomegaly due to fetal congestive failure in a pregnancy with a sacrococcygeal teratoma. J Reprod Med 25:142, 1980.
5. Donnellan WA, Swenson O: Benign and malignant sacrococcygeal teratomas. Surgery 64:834, 1968.

6. Dube S, Legros G, Rosenfeld R, et al.: Sacrococcygeal tumor in infancy. Can J Surg 23:363, 1980.

7. Ein SH, Adeyemi SD, Mancer K: Benign sacrococcygeal teratomas in infants and children. A 25-year review. Ann Surg 191:382, 1980.

8. Feige A, Gille J, von Maillot K, et al.: Praenatale diagnostik eine steissbeinteratoms mit hypertrophie der plazenta. Geburtshilfe Frauenheilkd 42:20, 1982.

9. Gergely RZ, Eden R, Schifrin BS, et al.: Antenatal diagnosis of congenital sacral teratoma. J Reprod Med 24:229, 1980.

10. Gonzalez-Crussi F, Winkler RF, Mirkin DL: Sacrococcygeal teratomas in infants and children: Relationship of histology and prognosis in 40 cases. Arch Pathol Lab Med 102:420, 1978.

11. Gross RE, Clatworthy HW Jr, Meeker IA: Sacrococcygeal teratomas in infants and children. A report of 40 cases. Surg Gynecol Obstet 92:341, 1951.

12. Hatteland K, Knutrud O: Sacrococcygeal teratomata in children. Acta Chir Scand 119:444, 1960.

13. Hecht F, Hecht B, O'Keefe D: Sacrococcygeal teratoma: Prenatal diagnosis with elevated alpha-fetoprotein and acetylcholinesterase in amniotic fluid. Prenat Diagn 2:229, 1982.

14. Holzgreve W, Mahony BS, Glick PL, et al.: Sonographic demonstration of fetal sacrococcygeal teratoma. Prenat Diagn 5:245, 1985.

15. Horger EO, McCarter LM: Prenatal diagnosis of sacrococcygeal teratoma. Am J Obstet Gynecol 134:228, 1979.

16. Hunt PT, Davidson KC, Ashcraft KW, et al.: Radiography of hereditary presacral teratoma. Radiology 122:187, 1977.

17. Lees RF, Williamson BR, Brenbridge NA, et al.: Sonog-

raphy of benign sacral teratoma in utero. Radiology 134:717, 1980.

18. Mahour GH, Woolley MM, Trivedi SN, et al.: Teratomas in infancy and childhood: Experience with 81 cases. Surgery 76:309, 1974.

19. Mintz MC, Mennuti M, Fishman M: Prenatal aspiration of sacrococcygeal teratoma. AJR 141:367, 1983.

20. Nicholson GW: Studies on tumour formation: Sacrococcygeal teratoma with three metacarpal bones and digits. Guy's Hosp Rep 87:46, 1937.

21. Pantoja E, Lopez E: Sacrococcygeal teratomas in infancy and childhood. NY State J Med 78:813, 1978.

22. Rayburn WF, Barr M: Teratomas: Concordance in mother and fetus. Am J Obstet Gynecol 144:110, 1982.

23. Sand H, Bock JE: Prenatal diagnosis of soft-tissue malformations by ultrasound and x-ray. Acta Obstet Gynecol Scand 55:191, 1976.

24. Santos Ramos R, Duenhoelter JH: Diagnosis of congenital fetal abnormalities by sonography. Obstet Gynecol 45:279, 1975.

25. Seeds JW, Mittelstaedt A, Cefalo RC, et al.: Prenatal diagnosis of sacrococcygeal teratoma: An anechoic caudal mass. J Clin Ultrasound 10:193, 1982.

26. Smith WL, Stokka C, Franken EA Jr: Arteriography of sacrococcygeal teratomas. Radiology 137:653, 1980.

27. Valdiserri RO, Yunis EJ: Sacrococcygeal teratomas: A review of 68 cases. Cancer 48:217, 1981.

28. Verma U, Weiss RR, Almonte R, et al.: Early prenatal diagnosis of soft-tissue malformations. Obstet Gynecol 53:660, 1979.

29. Zaleski AM, Cooperberg PL, Kliman MR: Ultrasonic diagnosis of extrafetal masses. J Can Assoc Radiol 30:55, 1979.

Appendix

A–1. COMMON DRUGS AND CHEMICALS DESCRIBED IN ASSOCIATION WITH FETAL MALFORMATIONS

A frequent indication for sonographic examination is exposure to drugs or chemicals during pregnancy. A detailed discussion of the literature for each one of these drugs is out of the scope of this text. As a guide to the sonographer we have reproduced and modified this table published by Koren et al., describing the anomalies that can be detected with ultrasound.

Drug	Central Nervous System	Cardiovascular	Skeleton
Acetaminophen (overdose)			
Acetazolamide			Sacrococcygeal teratoma
Acetylsalicylic acid		Intracranial hemorrhage	
Albuteral		Fetal tachycardia	
Alcohol	Microcephaly		Short nose, hypoplastic maxilla, micrognathia, occasional features of skeleton
Amantadine		Single ventricle with pulmonary atresia	
Aminopterin*	Meningoencephalocele, hydrocephalus, incomplete skull ossification, brachycephaly, anencephaly		Hypoplasia of thumb and fibula, clubfoot, syndactyly, hypognathia
Amitryptyline			Micrognathia
Amobarbital	Anencephaly	Congenital heart malformations	
Antithyroid drugs*			
Azathioprine*		Pulmonary valvular stenosis	
Betamethasone	Reduced head circumference		
Bromides			
Busulfan			
Caffeine			Musculoskeletal defects
Captopril			
Carbon monoxide*	Cerebral atrophy, hydrocephalus		
Carbamazepine	Meningomyelocele	Atrial septal defect, patent ductus arteriosus	Nose hypoplasia, hypertelorism
Chlordiazepoxide	Microcephaly	Congenital defects of heart	
Chloroquine			
Chlorpheniramine	Hydrocephalus		
Chlorpropamide	Microcephaly		
Clomiphene	Meningomyelocele, hydrocephalus, microcephaly, anencephaly		
Codeine	Hydrocephalus	Congenital cardiac defects	Musculoskeletal malformations
Cortisone	Hydrocephalus	Ventricular septal defect, coarctation of aorta	
Coumadin*	Encephalocele, anencephaly, spina bifida	Congenital heart disease	Nasal hypoplasia, scoliosis, skeletal deformities
Cyclophosphamide*	Tetralogy of Fallot		Flattened nasal bridge

Extremities	Gastrointestinal	Genitourinary	Miscellaneous	Source
			Polyhydramnios	CR
				CR
			Growth retardation	CR
				RS
				PS
				PS
			Growth retardation	CR
				RS
				PS
				CR
				CR
Limb reduction, swelling of hands and feet		Urinary retention		CR
Severe limb deformities, congenital hip dislocation, polydactyly, clubfoot	Oral cleft	Intersex	Soft tissue deformity of neck	CR
				PS
				RS
			Goiter	CR
				RS
Polydactyly				CR
				AS
Polydactyly, clubfoot, congenital dislocation of hip				CR
				PS
	Pyloric stenosis, cleft palate		Microphthalmia, growth retardation	CR
		Hydronephrosis		PS
Leg reduction				CR
			Stillbirth	CR
Congenital hip dislocation	Cleft lip			CR
				PS
				RS
	Duodenal atresia			RS
			Hemihypertrophy	CR
Polydactyly, congenital dislocation of hip				PS
Dysmorphic hands and fingers				CR
Syndactyly, clubfoot, polydactyly	Esophageal atresia			CR
				RS
Dislocated hip	Pyloric stenosis, oral cleft		Respiratory malformations	PS
Clubfoot	Cleft lip			RS
				CR
Stippled epiphysis, chondroplasia punctata, short phalanges, toe defects	Incomplete rotation of gut		Growth retardation, bleeding	CR
				RS
Four toes on each foot, hypoplastic midphalanx, syndactyly				CR

(Continued)

A–1.(*Continued*)

Drug	Central Nervous System	Cardiovascular	Skeleton
Cytarabine*	Anencephaly	Tetralogy of Fallot	
Daunorubicin*	Anencephaly	Tetralogy of Fallot	
Dextroamphetamine	Exencephaly	More cardiac defects than controls, atrial septal defect	
Diazepam	Spina bifida	More cardiac defects than controls	
Diphenhydramine			
Disulfiram			Vertebral fusion
Diuretics			
Estrogens		Congenital cardiac malformation	
Ethanol*	Microcephaly	Ventral septal defect, atrial septal defect, double outlet of right ventricle, pulmonary atresia, dextrocardia, patent ductus arteriosus, tetralogy of Fallot	Short nose, hypoplastic philtrum, micrognathia, pectus excavatum, radioulnar synostosis, bifid xyphoid, scoliosis
Ethosuximide	Hydrocephalus		Short neck
Fluorouracil			
Fluphenazine			Poor ossification of frontal bone
Haloperidol			
Heparin*			
Hormones, progestogenic	Anencephaly, hydrocephalus	Tetralogy of Fallot, truncus arteriosus, ventral septal defect	Spina bifida
Imipramine	Exencephaly		
Indomethacin			
Isoniazid	Meningomyelocele		
Lithium	Hydrocephalus, meningomyelocele	Ventral septal defect, Ebstein's anomaly, mitral atresia, patent ductus arteriosus, dextrocardia	Spina bifida
Lysergic acid diethylamide	Hydrocephalus, encephalocele, meningomyelocele		
Meclizine		Hypoplastic left heart	
Meprobamate		Congenital heart malformations	
Methotrexate*	Oxycephaly, absence of frontal bone, large fontanelles	Dextrocardia	Hypoplastic mandible
Methyl mercury*	Microcephaly, asymmetric head		
Metronidazole			Midline facial defects
Nortriptyline			
Oral contraceptives	Meningomyelocele, hydrocephalus, anencephaly	Cardiac anomalies	Vertebral malformations
Paramethadione		Tetralogy of Fallot	
Penicillamine		Ventral septal defect	
Phenobarbital	Hydrocephalus, meningomyelocele		
Phenothiazines	Microcephaly		
Phenylephrine			Eye and ear abnormalities
Phenylpropanolamine			Pectus excavatus

Extremities	Gastrointestinal	Genitourinary	Miscellaneous	Source
Lobster claw of 3 digits, missing feet digits, syndactyly				CR
Syndactyly			Growth retardation	CR
				CR
				RS
Absence of arm, syndactyly, absence of thumbs	Cleft lip-palate			CR
				RS
Clubfoot	Cleft palate			PS
				CR
Clubfoot, radial aplasia, phocomelia	Tracheoesophageal fistula			CR
			Respiratory malformations	PS
Limb reduction				CR
				PS
	Oral cleft		Growth retardation, diaphragmatic hernia	RS
				PS
	Oral cleft			CR
Radial aplasia, absent thumbs	Aplasia of esophagus and duodenum		Hypoplasia of lungs	CR
	Oral cleft			CR
Limb deformities				RS
			Bleeding	CR
				RS
Absence of thumbs				CR
Limb reduction	Cleft palate	Renal cystic degeneration	Diaphragmatic hernia	CR
Phocomelia			Stillbirth, hemorrhage	CR
				CR
				CR
				PS
Limb deficiencies				CR
				RS
			Respiratory defects	RS
Bilateral defects of limbs				RS
				CR
Long webbed fingers			Growth retardation, low-set ears	CR
				RS
				CR
				CR
Limb reduction				CR
Limb reduction	Tracheoesophageal malformations		Growth retardation	CR
				RS
			Growth retardation	CR
	Pyloric stenosis		Growth retardation	CR
Digital anomalies	Cleft palate, ileal atresia		Growth retardation, pulmonary hypoplasia	CR
Syndactyly, clubfoot	Omphalocele, abdominal distention			CR
				PS
Syndactyly, clubfoot, congenital dislocation of hip	Umbilical hernia			PS
Polydactyly, congenital dislocation of hip				PS

(*Continued*)

A–1. (*Continued*)

Drug	Central Nervous System	Cardiovascular	Skeleton
Phenytoin*	Microcephaly, wide fontanelles	Congenital heart malformation	Rib-sternal abnormalities, short nose, broad nasal bridge, wide fontanelle, broad alveolar ridge, short neck, hypertelorism, low-set ears
Polychlorinated biphenyls*			Spotted calcification in skull, fontanelle and sagittal suture
Primidone		Ventral septal defect	Webbed neck, small mandible
Procarbazine*	Cerebral hemorrhage		
Quinine	Hydrocephalus	Congenital heart defects	Facial defects, vertebral anomalies
Retinoic acid*	Hydrocephalus, microcephaly	Various congenital heart defects	Malformations of cranium, ear, face, ribs
Spermicides			
Sulfonamide			
Tetracycline			
Thalidomide*		Congenital heart malformations	Spine malformation
Thioguanine			
Tobacco			
Tolbutamide			
Trifluoperazine		Transposition of great arteries	
Trimethadione*	Microcephaly	Atrial septal defect, ventral septal defect	Low-set ears, broad nasal bridge
Valproic acid*	Lumbosacral meningomyelocele, microcephaly, wide fontanelle	Tetralogy of Fallot	Depressed nasal bridge, hypoplastic nose, low-set ears, small mandibles

Since only malformations that can be visualized by current ultrasonographic techniques are listed, the guide cannot be used as a complete list of drug-induced reratogenicity. CR = case reports: RS = retrospective studies; PS = prospective studies; AS = animal studies.

* Proved to be teratogenic.

Reproduced with permission from Koren G, Edwards MB, Miskin M: Antenatal sonography of fetal malformations associated with drugs and chemicals: A guide. Am J Obstet Gynecol 176(1):79, 1987.

Extremities	Gastrointestinal	Genitourinary	Miscellaneous	Source
Hypoplastic distal phalanges, digital thumb, dislocated hip	Cleft palate-lip		Growth retardation	CR PS
			Stillbirth, growth retardation	PS
				RS
				CR
Oligodactyly				CR
Dysmelias				CR
Limb deformities			Stillbirth	RS PS
Limb reduction				RS
Hypoplasia of limb or part of it, foot defects		Urethral obstructions		PS
Hypoplasia of limb or part of it, clubfoot				CR PS
Limb reduction (amelia, phocomelia), hypoplasia	Duodenal stenosis or atresia, pyloric stenosis		Microtia	RS PS
Missing digits				CR
			Growth retardation	PS
				RS
Finger-toe syndactyly, absent toes, accessory thumb				CR
Phocomelia				CR
Malformed hands, clubfoot	Esophageal atresia		Growth deficiency	CR PS
	Oral cleft		Growth deficiency	CR

A–2. BIPARIETAL DIAMETER (BPD) VERSUS GESTATIONAL AGE

BPD (cm)	Gestational age (weeks)	BPD (cm)	Gestational age (weeks)	BPD (cm)	Gestational age (weeks)	BPD (cm)	Gestational age (weeks)
2.0	12.2	4.0	18.0	6.0	24.6	8.0	32.5
2.1	12.5	4.1	18.3	6.1	25.0	8.1	32.9
2.2	12.8	4.2	18.6	6.2	25.3	8.2	33.3
2.3	13.1	4.3	18.9	6.3	25.7	8.3	33.8
2.4	13.3	4.4	19.2	6.4	26.1	8.4	34.2
2.5	13.6	4.5	19.5	6.5	26.4	8.5	34.7
2.6	13.9	4.6	19.9	6.6	26.8	8.6	35.1
2.7	14.2	4.7	20.2	6.7	27.2	8.7	35.6
2.8	14.5	4.8	20.5	6.8	27.6	8.8	36.1
2.9	14.7	4.9	20.8	6.9	28.0	8.9	36.5
3.0	15.0	5.0	21.2	7.0	28.3	9.0	37.0
3.1	15.3	5.1	21.5	7.1	28.7	9.1	37.5
3.2	15.6	5.2	21.8	7.2	29.1	9.2	38.0
3.3	15.9	5.3	22.2	7.3	29.5	9.3	38.5
3.4	16.2	5.4	22.5	7.4	29.9	9.4	38.9
3.5	16.5	5.5	22.8	7.5	30.4	9.5	39.4
3.6	16.8	5.6	23.2	7.6	30.8	9.6	39.9
3.7	17.1	5.7	23.5	7.7	31.2	9.7	40.5
3.8	17.4	5.8	23.9	7.8	31.6	9.8	41.0
3.9	17.7	5.9	24.2	7.9	32.0	9.9	41.5
						10.0	42.0

A–3. HEAD CIRCUMFERENCE VERSUS GESTATIONAL AGE

Circumference (mm)	Number of Fetuses	Mean Age (weeks)	Standard Deviation	Circumference (mm)	Number of Fetuses	Mean Age (weeks)	Standard Deviation
90	13	15.1	0.3	230	40	26.2	1.3
100	3	15.0	0	240	46	26.9	2.3
110	11	15.4	0.8	250	58	28.3	1.5
120	20	16.2	1.1	260	76	29.6	1.9
130	21	17.2	1.4	270	88	31.0	1.9
140	17	17.9	0.9	280	106	33.0	2.3
150	27	18.8	1.3	290	111	34.1	2.5
160	27	20.1	1.4	300	135	35.9	2.2
170	29	20.5	1.1	310	140	36.7	3.9
180	23	21.3	1.1	320	92	37.5	1.8
190	28	22.2	1.2	330	48	38.1	2.0
200	33	23.3	1.2	340	17	39.3	2.1
210	27	24.1	1.2	350	7	38.7	1.8
220	35	24.7	1.2				

Reproduced with permission from Ott WJ: The use of ultrasonic fetal head circumference for predicting expected date of confinement. J Clin Ultrasound 12:411, 1984.

A–4. GESTATIONAL AGES AS OBTAINED FROM THE LONG BONES (IN WEEKS + DAYS)

Bone Length (mm)	Femur Percentile			Humerus Percentile			Ulna Percentile			Tibia Percentile		
	5th	50th	95th	5th	50th	95th	5th	50th	95th	5th	50th	95th
10	10 + 3	12 + 4	14 + 6	9 + 6	12 + 4	15 + 2	10 + 1	13 + 1	16 + 1	10 + 4	13 + 3	16 + 2
11	10 + 5	12 + 6	15 + 1	10 + 1	12 + 6	15 + 4	10 + 4	13 + 4	16 + 4	10 + 6	13 + 5	16 + 4
12	11 + 1	13 + 2	15 + 4	10 + 3	13 + 1	15 + 6	10 + 6	13 + 6	16 + 6	11 + 1	14 + 1	17
13	11 + 3	13 + 4	15 + 6	10 + 6	13 + 4	16 + 1	11 + 1	14 + 1	17 + 2	11 + 4	14 + 3	17 + 2
14	11 + 5	13 + 6	16 + 1	11 + 1	13 + 6	16 + 4	11 + 4	14 + 4	17 + 5	11 + 6	14 + 6	17 + 5
15	12	14 + 1	16 + 3	11 + 3	14 + 1	16 + 6	11 + 6	15	18	12 + 1	15 + 1	18
16	12 + 3	14 + 4	16 + 6	11 + 6	14 + 4	17 + 2	12 + 2	15 + 3	18 + 3	12 + 4	15 + 4	18 + 3
17	12 + 5	14 + 6	17 + 1	12 + 1	14 + 6	17 + 4	12 + 5	15 + 5	18 + 6	13	15 + 6	18 + 6
18	13	15 + 1	17 + 3	12 + 4	15 + 1	18	13 + 1	16 + 1	19 + 1	13 + 2	16 + 1	19 + 1
19	13 + 3	15 + 4	17 + 6	12 + 6	15 + 4	18 + 2	13 + 4	16 + 4	19 + 4	13 + 5	16 + 4	19 + 4
20	13 + 5	15 + 6	18 + 1	13 + 1	15 + 6	18 + 5	13 + 6	16 + 6	20	14 + 1	17	19 + 6
21	14 + 1	16 + 2	18 + 4	13 + 4	16 + 2	19 + 1	14 + 2	17 + 2	20 + 3	14 + 4	17 + 3	20 + 2
22	14 + 3	16 + 4	18 + 6	13 + 6	16 + 5	19 + 3	14 + 5	17 + 5	20 + 6	14 + 6	17 + 6	20 + 5
23	14 + 5	16 + 6	19 + 1	14 + 2	17 + 1	19 + 6	15 + 1	18 + 1	21 + 1	15 + 1	18 + 1	21 + 1
24	15 + 1	17 + 2	19 + 4	14 + 5	17 + 3	20 + 1	15 + 4	18 + 4	21 + 4	15 + 4	18 + 4	21 + 3
25	15 + 3	17 + 4	19 + 6	15 + 1	17 + 6	20 + 4	16	19	22 + 1	16	18 + 6	21 + 6
26	15 + 6	18	20 + 1	15 + 4	18 + 1	21	16 + 3	19 + 3	22 + 4	16 + 3	19 + 2	22 + 1
27	16 + 1	18 + 2	20 + 4	15 + 6	18 + 4	21 + 3	16 + 6	19 + 6	22 + 6	16 + 6	19 + 5	22 + 4
28	16 + 4	18 + 5	20 + 6	16 + 2	19	21 + 6	17 + 2	20 + 2	23 + 3	17 + 1	20 + 1	23
29	16 + 6	19	21 + 1	16 + 5	19 + 3	22 + 1	17 + 5	20 + 6	23 + 6	17 + 4	20 + 4	23 + 4
30	17 + 1	19 + 3	21 + 4	17 + 1	19 + 6	22 + 4	18 + 1	21 + 1	24 + 2	18 + 1	21	23 + 6
31	17 + 4	19 + 6	22	17 + 4	20 + 2	23	18 + 4	21 + 5	24 + 6	18 + 4	21 + 3	24 + 2
32	17 + 6	20 + 1	22 + 2	18	20 + 5	23 + 4	19 + 1	22 + 1	25 + 1	18 + 6	21 + 6	24 + 5
33	18 + 2	20 + 4	22 + 5	18 + 3	21 + 1	23 + 6	19 + 4	22 + 5	25 + 5	19 + 2	22 + 1	25 + 1
34	18 + 5	20 + 6	23 + 1	18 + 6	21 + 4	24 + 2	20 + 1	23 + 1	26 + 1	19 + 5	22 + 4	25 + 4
35	19	21 + 1	23 + 3	19 + 2	22	24 + 6	20 + 4	34 + 4	26 + 5	20 + 1	23 + 1	26
36	19 + 3	21 + 4	23 + 6	19 + 5	22 + 4	25 + 1	21 + 1	24 + 1	27 + 1	20 + 4	23 + 4	26 + 3
37	19 + 6	22	24 + 1	20 + 1	22 + 6	25 + 5	21 + 4	24 + 4	27 + 5	21	23 + 6	26 + 6
38	20 + 1	22 + 3	24 + 4	20 + 4	23 + 3	26 + 1	22 + 1	25 + 1	28 + 1	21 + 4	24 + 3	27 + 2
39	20 + 4	22 + 5	24 + 6	21 + 1	23 + 6	26 + 4	22 + 4	25 + 4	28 + 5	21 + 6	24 + 6	27 + 5
40	20 + 6	23 + 1	25 + 2	21 + 4	24 + 2	27 + 1	23 + 1	26 + 1	29 + 1	22 + 3	25 + 2	28 + 1
41	21 + 2	23 + 4	25 + 5	22	24 + 6	27 + 4	23 + 4	26 + 5	29 + 5	22 + 6	25 + 5	28 + 4
42	21 + 5	23 + 6	26 + 1	22 + 4	25 + 2	28	24 + 1	27 + 1	30 + 2	23 + 2	26 + 1	29 + 1
43	22 + 1	24 + 2	26 + 4	23	25 + 5	28 + 4	24 + 5	27 + 5	30 + 6	23 + 5	26 + 4	29 + 4
44	22 + 4	24 + 5	26 + 6	23 + 4	26 + 1	29	25 + 1	28 + 2	31 + 2	24 + 1	27 + 1	30
45	22 + 6	25	27 + 1	24	26 + 5	29 + 4	25 + 6	28 + 6	31 + 6	24 + 4	27 + 4	30 + 4
46	23 + 1	25 + 3	27 + 4	24 + 4	27 + 1	30	26 + 2	29 + 3	32 + 3	25 + 1	28	30 + 6
47	23 + 4	25 + 6	28	25	27 + 5	30 + 4	26 + 6	29 + 6	33	25 + 4	28 + 4	31 + 3
48	24	26 + 1	28 + 3	25 + 4	28 + 1	31	27 + 3	30 + 4	33 + 4	26 + 1	29	31 + 6
49	24 + 3	26 + 4	28 + 6	26	28 + 6	31 + 4	28	31 + 1	34 + 1	26 + 4	29 + 3	32 + 2
50	24 + 6	27	29 + 1	26 + 4	29 + 2	32	28 + 4	31 + 4	34 + 5	27	29 + 6	32 + 6
51	25 + 1	27 + 3	29 + 4	27 + 1	29 + 6	32 + 4	29 + 1	32 + 1	35 + 2	27 + 4	30 + 3	33 + 2
52	25 + 4	27 + 6	30	27 + 4	30 + 2	33 + 1	29 + 5	32 + 6	35 + 6	28	30 + 6	33 + 6
53	26	28 + 1	30 + 3	28 + 1	30 + 6	33 + 4	30 + 2	33 + 3	36 + 3	28 + 4	31 + 3	34 + 2
54	26 + 3	28 + 4	30 + 6	28 + 5	31 + 3	34 + 1	30 + 6	34	37	29	31 + 6	34 + 6
55	26 + 6	29 + 1	31 + 2	29 + 1	32	34 + 5	31 + 4	34 + 4	37 + 5	29 + 4	32 + 3	35 + 2
56	27 + 2	29 + 4	31 + 5	29 + 6	32 + 4	35 + 2	32 + 1	35 + 1	38 + 2	30	32 + 6	35 + 6
57	27 + 5	29 + 6	32 + 1	30 + 2	33 + 1	35 + 6	32 + 6	35 + 6	38 + 6	30 + 4	33 + 3	36 + 2
58	28 + 1	30 + 2	32 + 4	30 + 6	33 + 4	36 + 3	33 + 3	36 + 3	39 + 4	31	33 + 6	36 + 6
59	28 + 4	30 + 5	32 + 6	31 + 3	34 + 1	36 + 6	34	37 + 1	40 + 1	31 + 4	34 + 3	37 + 2
60	28 + 6	31 + 1	33 + 2	32	34 + 6	37 + 4	34 + 4	37 + 5	40 + 6	32	34 + 6	37 + 6
61	29 + 3	31 + 4	33 + 6	32 + 4	35 + 2	38 + 1	35 + 2	38 + 2	41 + 3	32 + 4	35 + 3	38 + 2
62	29 + 6	32	34 + 1	33 + 1	35 + 6	38 + 5	35 + 6	39	42	33	35 + 6	38 + 6
63	30 + 1	32 + 3	34 + 4	33 + 6	36 + 4	39 + 2	36 + 4	39 + 4	42 + 5	33 + 4	36 + 4	39 + 3
64	30 + 5	32 + 6	35 + 1	34 + 3	37 + 1	39 + 6	37 + 1	40 + 2	43 + 2	34 + 1	37	39 + 6
65	31 + 1	33 + 2	35 + 4	35	37 + 5	40 + 4				34 + 4	37 + 4	40 + 3
66	31 + 4	33 + 5	35 + 6	35 + 4	38 + 2	41 + 1				35 + 1	38	41
67	32	34 + 1	36 + 3	36 + 1	38 + 6	41 + 5				35 + 5	38 + 4	41 + 4
68	32 + 3	34 + 4	36 + 6	36 + 6	39 + 4	42 + 2				36 + 1	39 + 1	42
69	32 + 6	35	37 + 1	37 + 3	40 + 1	42 + 6				36 + 6	39 + 5	42 + 4
70	33 + 2	35 + 4	37 + 5									
71	33 + 5	35 + 6	38 + 1									
72	34 + 1	36 + 3	38 + 4									
73	34 + 4	36 + 6	39									
74	35 + 1	37 + 2	39 + 4									
75	35 + 4	37 + 5	39 + 6									
76	36	38 + 1	40 + 3									
77	36 + 3	38 + 4	40 + 6									
78	36 + 6	39 + 1	41 + 2									
79	37 + 2	39 + 4	41 + 5									
80	37 + 6	40	42 + 1									

Reproduced with permission from Jeanty P, Rodesch F, Delbeke D, et al.: Estimation of gestational age from measurements of fetal long bones. J Ultrasound Med 3:75, 1984.

A–5. ESTIMATED FETAL WEIGHTS

Biparietal Diameters	Abdominal Circumferences												
	15.5	16.0	16.5	17.0	17.5	18.0	18.5	19.0	19.5	20.0	20.5	21.0	21.5
3.1	224	234	244	255	267	279	291	304	318	332	346	362	378
3.2	231	241	251	263	274	286	299	312	326	340	355	371	388
3.3	237	248	259	270	282	294	307	321	335	349	365	381	397
3.4	244	255	266	278	290	302	316	329	344	359	374	391	408
3.5	251	262	274	285	298	311	324	338	353	368	384	401	418
3.6	259	270	281	294	306	319	333	347	362	378	394	411	429
3.7	266	278	290	302	315	328	342	357	372	388	404	422	440
3.8	274	286	298	310	324	337	352	366	382	398	415	432	451
3.9	282	294	306	319	333	347	361	376	392	409	426	444	462
4.0	290	303	315	328	342	356	371	386	403	419	437	455	474
4.1	299	311	324	338	352	366	381	397	413	430	448	467	486
4.2	308	320	333	347	361	376	392	408	424	442	460	479	498
4.3	317	330	343	357	371	387	402	419	436	453	472	491	511
4.4	326	339	353	367	382	397	413	430	447	465	484	504	524
4.5	335	349	363	377	393	408	425	442	459	478	497	517	538
4.6	345	359	373	388	404	420	436	454	472	490	510	530	551
4.7	355	369	384	399	415	431	448	466	484	503	523	544	565
4.8	366	380	395	410	426	443	460	478	497	517	537	558	580
4.9	376	391	406	422	438	455	473	491	510	530	551	572	594
5.0	387	402	418	434	451	468	486	505	524	544	565	587	610
5.1	399	414	430	446	463	481	499	518	538	559	580	602	625
5.2	410	426	442	459	476	494	513	532	552	573	595	618	641
5.3	422	438	455	472	489	508	527	547	567	589	611	634	657
5.4	435	451	468	485	503	522	541	561	582	604	627	650	674
5.5	447	464	481	499	517	536	556	577	598	620	643	667	691
5.6	461	477	495	513	532	551	571	592	614	636	660	684	709
5.7	474	491	509	527	547	566	587	608	630	653	677	701	727
5.8	488	505	524	542	562	582	603	625	647	670	695	719	745
5.9	502	520	539	558	578	598	619	642	664	688	713	738	764
6.0	517	535	554	573	594	615	636	659	682	706	731	757	784
6.1	532	550	570	590	610	632	654	677	700	725	750	777	804
6.2	547	566	586	606	627	649	672	695	719	744	770	797	824
6.3	563	583	603	624	645	667	690	714	738	764	790	817	845
6.4	580	600	620	641	663	686	709	733	758	784	811	838	867
6.5	597	617	638	659	682	705	728	753	778	805	832	860	889
6.6	614	635	656	678	701	724	748	773	799	826	853	882	911
6.7	632	653	675	697	720	744	769	794	820	848	876	905	935
6.8	651	672	694	717	740	765	790	816	842	870	898	928	958
6.9	670	691	714	737	761	786	811	838	865	893	922	952	983
7.0	689	711	734	758	782	807	833	860	888	916	946	976	1,008
7.1	709	732	755	779	804	830	856	883	912	941	971	1,002	1,033
7.2	730	763	777	801	827	853	880	907	936	965	996	1,027	1,060
7.3	751	775	799	824	850	876	904	932	961	991	1,022	1,054	1,087
7.4	773	797	822	847	874	901	928	957	987	1,017	1,049	1,081	1,114
7.5	796	820	845	871	898	925	954	983	1,013	1,044	1,076	1,109	1,143
7.6	819	844	870	896	923	951	980	1,009	1,040	1,072	1,104	1,137	1,172
7.7	843	868	894	921	949	977	1,007	1,037	1,068	1,100	1,133	1,167	1,202
7.8	868	894	920	947	975	1,004	1,034	1,065	1,096	1,129	1,162	1,197	1,232
7.9	893	919	946	974	1,003	1,032	1,062	1,094	1,126	1,159	1,193	1,228	1,264
8.0	919	946	973	1,002	1,031	1,061	1,091	1,123	1,156	1,189	1,224	1,259	1,296
8.1	946	973	1,001	1,030	1,060	1,090	1,121	1,153	1,187	1,221	1,256	1,292	1,329
8.2	974	1,001	1,030	1,059	1,089	1,120	1,152	1,185	1,218	1,253	1,288	1,325	1,363
8.3	1,002	1,030	1,059	1,089	1,120	1,151	1,183	1,217	1,251	1,286	1,322	1,359	1,397
8.4	1,032	1,060	1,090	1,120	1,151	1,183	1,216	1,249	1,284	1,320	1,356	1,394	1,433
8.5	1,062	1,091	1,121	1,151	1,183	1,216	1,249	1,283	1,318	1,355	1,392	1,430	1,469
8.6	1,093	1,122	1,153	1,184	1,216	1,249	1,283	1,318	1,354	1,390	1,428	1,467	1,507
8.7	1,125	1,155	1,186	1,218	1,250	1,284	1,318	1,353	1,390	1,427	1,465	1,505	1,545
8.8	1,157	1,188	1,220	1,252	1,285	1,319	1,354	1,390	1,427	1,465	1,504	1,543	1,584
8.9	1,191	1,222	1,254	1,287	1,321	1,356	1,391	1,428	1,465	1,503	1,543	1,583	1,625
9.0	1,226	1,258	1,290	1,324	1,358	1,393	1,429	1,456	1,504	1,543	1,583	1,624	1,666
9.1	1,262	1,294	1,327	1,361	1,396	1,432	1,468	1,506	1,544	1,584	1,624	1,666	1,708
9.2	1,299	1,332	1,365	1,400	1,435	1,471	1,508	1,546	1,586	1,626	1,667	1,709	1,752
9.3	1,337	1,370	1,404	1,439	1,475	1,512	1,550	1,588	1,628	1,668	1,710	1,753	1,796
9.4	1,376	1,410	1,444	1,480	1,516	1,554	1,592	1,631	1,671	1,712	1,755	1,798	1,842
9.5	1,416	1,450	1,486	1,522	1,559	1,597	1,635	1,675	1,716	1,758	1,800	1,844	1,889
9.6	1,457	1,492	1,528	1,565	1,602	1,641	1,680	1,720	1,762	1,804	1,847	1,892	1,937
9.7	1,500	1,535	1,572	1,609	1,547	1,686	1,726	1,767	1,809	1,852	1,895	1,940	1,986
9.8	1,544	1,580	1,617	1,654	1,693	1,733	1,773	1,815	1,857	1,900	1,945	1,990	2,037
9.9	1,589	1,625	1,663	1,701	1,740	1,781	1,822	1,864	1,907	1,951	1,996	2,042	2,089
10.0	1,635	1,672	1,710	1,749	1,789	1,830	1,871	1,914	1,958	2,002	2,048	2,094	2,142

Biparietal Diameters	Abdominal Circumferences											
	22.0	22.5	23.0	23.5	24.0	24.5	25.0	25.5	26.0	26.5	27.0	27.5
3.1	395	412	431	450	470	491	513	536	559	584	610	638
3.2	405	423	441	461	481	502	525	548	572	597	624	651
3.3	415	433	452	472	493	514	537	560	585	611	638	666
3.4	425	444	463	483	504	526	549	573	598	624	652	680
3.5	436	455	475	495	517	539	562	587	612	638	666	695
3.6	447	466	486	507	529	552	575	600	626	653	681	710
3.7	458	478	498	519	542	565	589	614	640	667	696	725
3.8	470	490	510	532	554	578	602	628	654	682	711	741
3.9	482	502	523	545	568	592	616	642	669	697	727	757
4.0	494	514	536	558	581	606	631	657	684	713	743	773
4.1	506	527	549	572	595	620	645	672	700	729	759	790
4.2	519	540	562	585	609	634	660	688	716	745	776	807
4.3	532	554	576	600	624	649	676	703	732	762	793	825
4.4	545	567	590	614	639	665	692	719	749	779	810	843
4.5	559	581	605	629	654	680	708	736	765	796	828	861
4.6	573	596	620	644	670	696	724	753	783	814	846	880
4.7	588	611	635	660	686	713	741	770	801	832	865	899
4.8	602	626	650	676	702	730	758	788	819	851	884	919
4.9	617	641	666	692	719	747	776	806	837	870	903	938
5.0	633	657	683	709	736	765	794	824	856	889	923	959
5.1	649	674	699	726	754	783	812	843	876	909	944	980
5.2	665	690	717	744	772	801	831	863	895	929	964	1,001
5.3	682	708	734	762	790	820	851	883	916	950	986	1,023
5.4	699	725	752	780	809	839	870	903	936	971	1,007	1,045
5.5	717	743	771	799	828	859	891	924	958	993	1,030	1,068
5.6	735	762	789	818	848	879	911	945	979	1,015	1,052	1,091
5.7	753	780	809	838	869	900	933	966	1,001	1,038	1,075	1,114
5.8	772	800	829	858	889	921	954	989	1,024	1,061	1,099	1,139
5.9	792	820	849	879	911	943	977	1,011	1,047	1,085	1,123	1,163
6.0	811	840	870	900	932	965	999	1,035	1,071	1,109	1,148	1,189
6.1	832	861	891	922	955	988	1,023	1,058	1,095	1,134	1,173	1,214
6.2	853	882	913	945	977	1,011	1,046	1,083	1,120	1,159	1,199	1,241
6.3	874	904	935	967	1,001	1,035	1,071	1,107	1,145	1,185	1,226	1,268
6.4	896	927	958	991	1,025	1,059	1,096	1,133	1,171	1,211	1,253	1,295
6.5	919	950	982	1,015	1,049	1,084	1,121	1,159	1,198	1,238	1,280	1,323
6.6	942	973	1,006	1,039	1,074	1,110	1,147	1,185	1,225	1,266	1,308	1,352
6.7	965	997	1,030	1,065	1,100	1,136	1,174	1,213	1,253	1,294	1,337	1,381
6.8	990	1,022	1,056	1,090	1,126	1,163	1,201	1,241	1,281	1,323	1,367	1,411
6.9	1,015	1,048	1,082	1,117	1,153	1,190	1,229	1,269	1,310	1,353	1,397	1,442
7.0	1,040	1,074	1,108	1,144	1,181	1,219	1,258	1,298	1,340	1,383	1,427	1,473
7.1	1,066	1,100	1,135	1,171	1,209	1,247	1,287	1,328	1,370	1,414	1,459	1,505
7.2	1,093	1,128	1,163	1,200	1,238	1,277	1,317	1,358	1,401	1,445	1,491	1,538
7.3	1,121	1,156	1,192	1,229	1,267	1,307	1,348	1,390	1,433	1,478	1,524	1,571
7.4	1,149	1,184	1,221	1,259	1,297	1,338	1,379	1,421	1,465	1,511	1,557	1,605
7.5	1,178	1,214	1,251	1,289	1,328	1,369	1,411	1,454	1,499	1,544	1,592	1,640
7.6	1,207	1,244	1,281	1,320	1,360	1,401	1,444	1,487	1,533	1,579	1,627	1,676
7.7	1,238	1,275	1,313	1,352	1,393	1,434	1,477	1,522	1,567	1,614	1,663	1,712
7.8	1,269	1,306	1,345	1,385	1,426	1,468	1,512	1,557	1,603	1,650	1,699	1,749
7.9	1,301	1,339	1,378	1,418	1,460	1,503	1,547	1,592	1,639	1,687	1,737	1,787
8.0	1,333	1,372	1,412	1,453	1,495	1,538	1,583	1,629	1,676	1,725	1,775	1,826
8.1	1,367	1,406	1,446	1,488	1,531	1,575	1,620	1,666	1,714	1,763	1,814	1,866
8.2	1,401	1,441	1,482	1,524	1,567	1,612	1,657	1,704	1,753	1,803	1,854	1,906
8.3	1,436	1,477	1,518	1,561	1,605	1,650	1,696	1,744	1,793	1,843	1,895	1,948
8.4	1,473	1,513	1,555	1,599	1,643	1,689	1,735	1,784	1,833	1,884	1,936	1,990
8.5	1,510	1,551	1,594	1,637	1,682	1,728	1,776	1,825	1,875	1,926	1,979	2,033
8.6	1,548	1,589	1,633	1,677	1,722	1,769	1,817	1,866	1,917	1,969	2,022	2,077
8.7	1,586	1,629	1,673	1,717	1,764	1,811	1,859	1,909	1,960	2,013	2,067	2,122
8.8	1,626	1,669	1,714	1,759	1,806	1,854	1,903	1,953	2,005	2,058	2,113	2,169
8.9	1,667	1,711	1,756	1,802	1,849	1,897	1,947	1,998	2,050	2,104	2,159	2,216
9.0	1,709	1,753	1,799	1,845	1,893	1,942	1,992	2,044	2,097	2,151	2,207	2,264
9.1	1,752	1,797	1,843	1,890	1,938	1,988	2,039	2,091	2,144	2,199	2,255	2,313
9.2	1,796	1,841	1,888	1,936	1,984	2,035	2,086	2,139	2,193	2,248	2,305	2,363
9.3	1,841	1,887	1,934	1,982	2,032	2,083	2,135	2,188	2,242	2,298	2,356	2,414
9.4	1,887	1,934	1,982	2,030	2,080	2,132	2,184	2,238	2,293	2,350	2,407	2,467
9.5	1,935	1,982	2,030	2,080	2,130	2,182	2,235	2,289	2,345	2,402	2,460	2,520
9.6	1,984	2,031	2,080	2,130	2,181	2,233	2,287	2,342	2,398	2,456	2,515	2,575
9.7	2,033	2,082	2,131	2,181	2,233	2,286	2,340	2,396	2,452	2,510	2,570	2,631
9.8	2,085	2,133	2,183	2,234	2,286	2,340	2,395	2,451	2,508	2,567	2,627	2,688
9.9	2,137	2,186	2,237	2,288	2,341	2,395	2,450	2,507	2,565	2,624	2,684	2,746
10.0	2,191	2,241	2,292	2,344	2,397	2,452	2,507	2,564	2,623	2,682	2,743	2,806

(Continued)

A–5. (*Continued*)

Biparietal Diameters	Abdominal Circumferences												
	28.0	28.5	29.0	29.5	30.0	30.5	31.0	31.5	32.0	32.5	33.0	33.5	34.0
3.1	666	696	726	759	793	828	865	903	943	985	1,029	1,075	1,123
3.2	680	710	742	774	809	844	882	921	961	1,004	1,048	1,094	1,143
3.3	695	725	757	790	825	861	899	938	979	1,022	1,067	1,114	1,163
3.4	710	740	773	806	841	878	916	956	998	1,041	1,087	1,134	1,183
3.5	725	756	789	823	858	896	934	975	1,017	1,061	1,107	1,154	1,204
3.6	740	772	805	840	876	913	953	993	1,036	1,080	1,127	1,175	1,226
3.7	756	788	822	857	893	931	971	1,012	1,056	1,101	1,147	1,196	1,247
3.8	772	805	839	874	911	950	990	1,032	1,076	1,121	1,168	1,218	1,269
3.9	789	822	856	892	930	969	1,009	1,052	1,096	1,142	1,190	1,240	1,292
4.0	806	839	874	911	949	988	1,029	1,072	1,117	1,163	1,212	1,262	1,315
4.1	828	857	892	929	968	1,008	1,049	1,093	1,138	1,185	1,234	1,285	1,338
4.2	841	875	911	948	987	1,028	1,070	1,114	1,159	1,207	1,256	1,308	1,361
4.3	859	893	930	968	1,007	1,048	1,091	1,135	1,181	1,229	1,279	1,331	1,385
4.4	877	912	949	987	1,027	1,069	1,112	1,157	1,204	1,252	1,303	1,355	1,410
4.5	896	932	969	1,008	1,048	1,090	1,134	1,179	1,226	1,275	1,326	1,380	1,435
4.6	915	951	989	1,028	1,069	1,112	1,156	1,202	1,249	1,299	1,351	1,404	1,460
4.7	934	971	1,010	1,049	1,091	1,134	1,178	1,225	1,273	1,323	1,375	1,430	1,486
4.8	954	992	1,031	1,071	1,113	1,156	1,201	1,248	1,297	1,348	1,401	1,455	1,512
4.9	975	1,013	1,052	1,093	1,135	1,179	1,225	1,272	1,322	1,373	1,426	1,482	1,539
5.0	996	1,034	1,074	1,115	1,158	1,203	1,249	1,297	1,347	1,399	1,452	1,508	1,566
5.1	1,017	1,056	1,096	1,138	1,181	1,226	1,273	1,322	1,372	1,425	1,479	1,535	1,594
5.2	1,039	1,078	1,119	1,161	1,205	1,251	1,298	1,347	1,398	1,451	1,506	1,563	1,622
5.3	1,061	1,101	1,142	1,185	1,229	1,276	1,323	1,373	1,425	1,478	1,533	1,591	1,651
5.4	1,084	1,124	1,166	1,209	1,254	1,301	1,349	1,399	1,452	1,506	1,562	1,620	1,680
5.5	1,107	1,148	1,190	1,234	1,279	1,327	1,376	1,426	1,479	1,534	1,590	1,649	1,710
5.6	1,131	1,172	1,215	1,259	1,305	1,353	1,402	1,454	1,507	1,562	1,619	1,678	1,740
5.7	1,155	1,197	1,240	1,285	1,332	1,380	1,430	1,482	1,535	1,591	1,649	1,709	1,770
5.8	1,180	1,222	1,266	1,311	1,358	1,407	1,458	1,510	1,564	1,621	1,679	1,739	1,802
5.9	1,205	1,248	1,292	1,338	1,386	1,435	1,486	1,539	1,594	1,651	1,710	1,770	1,834
6.0	1,231	1,274	1,319	1,366	1,414	1,464	1,515	1,569	1,624	1,682	1,741	1,802	1,866
6.1	1,257	1,301	1,346	1,393	1,442	1,493	1,545	1,599	1,655	1,713	1,773	1,835	1,899
6.2	1,284	1,328	1,374	1,422	1,471	1,522	1,575	1,630	1,686	1,745	1,805	1,868	1,932
6.3	1,311	1,356	1,403	1,451	1,501	1,552	1,606	1,661	1,718	1,777	1,838	1,901	1,967
6.4	1,339	1,385	1,432	1,481	1,531	1,583	1,637	1,693	1,751	1,810	1,872	1,935	2,001
6.5	1,368	1,414	1,462	1,511	1,562	1,615	1,669	1,725	1,784	1,844	1,906	1,970	2,037
6.6	1,397	1,444	1,492	1,542	1,594	1,647	1,702	1,759	1,817	1,878	1,941	2,006	2,073
6.7	1,427	1,474	1,523	1,574	1,626	1,679	1,735	1,792	1,852	1,913	1,976	2,042	2,109
6.8	1,458	1,505	1,555	1,606	1,658	1,713	1,769	1,827	1,887	1,949	2,012	2,078	2,147
6.9	1,489	1,537	1,587	1,639	1,692	1,747	1,803	1,862	1,922	1,985	2,049	2,116	2,184
7.0	1,521	1,570	1,620	1,672	1,726	1,781	1,839	1,898	1,959	2,022	2,087	2,154	2,223
7.1	1,553	1,603	1,654	1,706	1,761	1,817	1,875	1,934	1,996	2,059	2,125	2,193	2,262
7.2	1,586	1,636	1,688	1,741	1,796	1,853	1,911	1,971	2,044	2,098	2,164	2,232	2,302
7.3	1,620	1,671	1,723	1,777	1,832	1,890	1,948	2,009	2,072	2,137	2,203	2,272	2,343
7.4	1,655	1,706	1,759	1,813	1,869	1,927	1,987	2,048	2,111	2,176	2,244	2,313	2,384
7.5	1,690	1,742	1,795	1,850	1,907	1,965	2,025	2,087	2,151	2,217	2,265	2,354	2,426
7.6	1,727	1,779	1,833	1,888	1,945	2,004	2,065	2,127	2,192	2,258	2,326	2,397	2,469
7.7	1,764	1,816	1,871	1,927	1,985	2,044	2,105	2,168	2,233	2,300	2,369	2,440	2,513
7.8	1,801	1,855	1,910	1,966	2,025	2,085	2,146	2,210	2,275	2,343	2,412	2,484	2,557
7.9	1,840	1,894	1,949	2,006	2,065	2,126	2,188	2,252	2,318	2,386	2,456	2,528	2,603
8.0	1,879	1,934	1,990	2,048	2,107	2,168	2,231	2,296	2,362	2,431	2,501	2,574	2,649
8.1	1,919	1,975	2,031	2,089	2,149	2,211	2,275	2,340	2,407	2,476	2,547	2,620	2,695
8.2	1,960	2,016	2,073	2,132	2,193	2,255	2,319	2,385	2,462	2,522	2,594	2,667	2,743
8.3	2,002	2,059	2,116	2,176	2,237	2,300	2,364	2,431	2,499	2,569	2,641	2,715	2,791
8.4	2,045	2,102	2,160	2,220	2,282	2,345	2,410	2,477	2,546	2,617	2,689	2,764	2,841
8.5	2,089	2,146	2,205	2,266	2,328	2,392	2,457	2,525	2,594	2,665	2,739	2,814	2,891
8.6	2,134	2,192	2,251	2,312	2,375	2,439	2,505	2,573	2,643	2,715	2,789	2,864	2,942
8.7	2,179	2,238	2,298	2,359	2,423	2,488	2,554	2,623	2,693	2,765	2,840	2,916	2,994
8.8	2,226	2,285	2,346	2,408	2,472	2,537	2,604	2,673	2,744	2,817	2,892	2,968	3,047
8.9	2,274	2,333	2,394	2,457	2,521	2,587	2,655	2,725	2,796	2,869	2,944	3,021	3,101
9.0	2,322	2,382	2,444	2,507	2,572	2,639	2,707	2,777	2,849	2,923	2,998	3,076	3,155
9.1	2,372	2,433	2,495	2,559	2,624	2,691	2,760	2,830	2,903	2,977	3,053	3,131	3,211
9.2	2,423	2,484	2,547	2,611	2,677	2,744	2,814	2,885	2,958	3,032	3,109	3,187	3,268
9.3	2,475	2,536	2,599	2,664	2,731	2,799	2,869	2,940	3,014	3,089	3,166	3,245	3,326
9.4	2,527	2,590	2,653	2,719	2,786	2,854	2,925	2,997	3,070	3,146	3,224	3,303	3,384
9.5	2,582	2,644	2,709	2,774	2,842	2,911	2,982	3,054	3,129	3,205	3,283	3,362	3,444
9.6	2,637	2,700	2,765	2,831	2,899	2,969	3,040	3,113	3,188	3,264	3,343	3,423	3,505
9.7	2,693	2,757	2,822	2,889	2,958	3,028	3,099	3,173	3,248	3,325	3,404	3,484	3,567
9.8	2,751	2,815	2,881	2,948	3,017	3,088	3,160	3,234	3,309	3,387	3,466	3,547	3,630
9.9	2,810	2,874	2,941	3,009	3,078	3,149	3,222	3,296	3,372	3,450	3,529	3,611	3,694
10.0	2,870	2,935	3,002	3,070	3,140	3,211	3,285	3,359	3,436	3,514	3,594	3,676	3,759

A–5. (*Continued*)

Biparietal Diameters	Abdominal Circumferences											
	34.5	35.0	35.5	36.0	36.5	37.0	37.5	38.0	38.5	39.0	39.5	40.0
3.1	1,173	1,225	1,279	1,336	1,396	1,458	1,523	1,591	1,661	1,735	1,812	1,893
3.2	1,193	1,246	1,301	1,358	1,418	1,481	1,546	1,615	1,686	1,761	1,838	1,920
3.3	1,214	1,267	1,323	1,381	1,441	1,504	1,570	1,639	1,711	1,786	1,865	1,946
3.4	1,235	1,289	1,345	1,403	1,464	1,528	1,595	1,664	1,737	1,812	1,891	1,973
3.5	1,256	1,311	1,367	1,426	1,488	1,552	1,619	1,689	1,762	1,839	1,918	2,001
3.6	1,278	1,333	1,390	1,450	1,512	1,577	1,645	1,715	1,789	1,865	1,945	2,029
3.7	1,300	1,356	1,413	1,474	1,536	1,602	1,670	1,741	1,815	1,893	1,973	2,057
3.8	1,323	1,379	1,437	1,498	1,561	1,627	1,696	1,768	1,842	1,920	2,001	2,086
3.9	1,346	1,402	1,461	1,523	1,586	1,653	1,722	1,794	1,870	1,948	2,030	2,115
4.0	1,369	1,426	1,486	1,548	1,612	1,679	1,749	1,822	1,898	1,977	2,059	2,145
4.1	1,393	1,451	1,511	1,573	1,638	1,706	1,776	1,849	1,926	2,005	2,088	2,174
4.2	1,417	1,475	1,536	1,599	1,664	1,733	1,804	1,878	1,954	2,035	2,118	2,205
4.3	1,442	1,500	1,562	1,625	1,691	1,760	1,832	1,906	1,984	2,064	2,148	2,236
4.4	1,467	1,526	1,588	1,652	1,718	1,788	1,860	1,935	2,013	2,094	2,179	2,267
4.5	1,492	1,552	1,614	1,679	1,746	1,816	1,889	1,964	2,043	2,125	2,210	2,298
4.6	1,518	1,579	1,641	1,706	1,774	1,845	1,918	1,994	2,073	2,156	2,241	2,330
4.7	1,545	1,605	1,669	1,734	1,803	1,874	1,948	2,024	2,104	2,187	2,273	2,363
4.8	1,571	1,633	1,697	1,763	1,832	1,904	1,978	2,055	2,136	2,219	2,306	2,396
4.9	1,599	1,661	1,725	1,792	1,861	1,934	2,009	2,086	2,167	2,251	2,339	2,429
5.0	1,626	1,689	1,754	1,821	1,891	1,964	2,040	2,118	2,200	2,284	2,372	2,463
5.1	1,655	1,718	1,783	1,851	1,922	1,995	2,071	2,150	2,232	2,317	2,406	2,498
5.2	1,683	1,747	1,813	1,882	1,953	2,027	2,103	2,183	2,266	2,351	2,440	2,532
5.3	1,713	1,777	1,843	1,913	1,984	2,059	2,136	2,216	2,299	2,386	2,475	2,568
5.4	1,742	1,807	1,874	1,944	2,016	2,091	2,169	2,250	2,333	2,420	2,510	2,604
5.5	1,773	1,838	1,906	1,976	2,049	2,124	2,203	2,284	2,368	2,456	2,546	2,640
5.6	1,803	1,869	1,938	2,008	2,082	2,158	2,237	2,319	2,403	2,491	2,582	2,677
5.7	1,835	1,901	1,970	2,041	2,115	2,192	2,272	2,354	2,439	2,528	2,619	2,714
5.8	1,866	1,934	2,003	2,075	2,150	2,227	2,307	2,390	2,475	2,564	2,657	2,752
5.9	1,899	1,966	2,037	2,109	2,184	2,262	2,342	2,426	2,512	2,602	2,694	2,790
6.0	1,932	2,000	2,071	2,144	2,219	2,298	2,379	2,463	2,550	2,640	2,733	2,829
6.1	1,965	2,034	2,105	2,179	2,255	2,334	2,416	2,500	2,588	2,678	2,772	2,869
6.2	1,999	2,069	2,140	2,215	2,291	2,371	2,453	2,538	2,626	2,717	2,811	2,909
6.3	2,034	2,104	2,176	2,251	2,328	2,408	2,491	2,577	2,665	2,757	2,851	2,949
6.4	2,069	2,140	2,213	2,288	2,366	2,446	2,530	2,616	2,705	2,797	2,892	2,991
6.5	2,105	2,176	2,250	2,326	2,404	2,485	2,569	2,656	2,745	2,838	2,933	3,032
6.6	2,142	2,213	2,287	2,364	2,443	2,524	2,609	2,696	2,786	2,879	2,975	3,075
6.7	2,179	2,251	2,326	2,403	2,482	2,564	2,649	2,737	2,827	2,921	3,018	3,117
6.8	2,217	2,290	2,365	2,442	2,522	2,605	2,690	2,778	2,869	2,964	3,061	3,161
6.9	2,255	2,329	2,404	2,482	2,563	2,646	2,732	2,821	2,912	3,007	3,104	3,205
7.0	2,295	2,368	2,444	2,523	2,604	2,688	2,774	2,863	2,955	3,050	3,149	3,250
7.1	2,334	2,409	2,485	2,564	2,646	2,730	2,817	2,907	2,999	3,095	3,193	3,295
7.2	2,375	2,450	2,527	2,607	2,689	2,773	2,861	2,951	3,044	3,140	3,239	3,341
7.3	2,416	2,491	2,569	2,649	2,732	2,817	2,905	2,996	3,089	3,186	3,285	3,388
7.4	2,458	2,534	2,612	2,693	2,776	2,862	2,950	3,041	3,135	3,232	3,332	3,435
7.5	2,501	2,577	2,656	2,737	2,821	2,907	2,996	3,088	3,182	3,279	3,380	3,483
7.6	2,544	2,621	2,700	2,782	2,866	2,953	3,042	3,134	3,229	3,327	3,428	3,531
7.7	2,588	2,666	2,746	2,828	2,912	3,000	3,090	3,182	3,277	3,376	3,477	3,581
7.8	2,633	2,711	2,792	2,874	2,959	3,047	3,137	3,230	3,326	3,425	3,526	3,631
7.9	2,679	2,757	2,838	2,921	3,007	3,095	3,186	3,279	3,376	3,475	3,576	3,681
8.0	2,725	2,804	2,886	2,969	3,056	3,144	3,235	3,329	3,426	3,525	3,627	3,733
8.1	2,773	2,852	2,934	3,018	3,105	3,194	3,286	3,380	3,477	3,577	3,679	3,785
8.2	2,821	2,901	2,983	3,068	3,155	3,244	3,336	3,431	3,529	3,629	3,732	3,838
8.3	2,870	2,950	3,033	3,118	3,206	3,296	3,388	3,483	3,581	3,682	3,785	3,891
8.4	2,920	3,001	3,084	3,169	3,257	3,348	3,441	3,536	3,634	3,735	3,839	3,945
8.5	2,970	3,052	3,135	3,221	3,310	3,401	3,494	3,590	3,688	3,790	3,894	4,000
8.6	3,022	3,104	3,188	3,274	3,363	3,454	3,548	3,644	3,743	3,845	3,949	4,056
8.7	3,074	3,157	3,241	3,328	3,417	3,509	3,603	3,700	3,799	3,901	4,005	4,113
8.8	3,128	3,210	3,295	3,383	3,472	3,565	3,659	3,756	3,855	3,958	4,063	4,170
8.9	3,182	3,265	3,351	3,438	3,528	3,621	3,716	3,813	3,913	4,015	4,120	4,228
9.0	3,237	3,321	3,407	3,495	3,585	3,678	3,773	3,871	3,971	4,074	4,179	4,287
9.1	3,293	3,377	3,464	3,552	3,643	3,736	3,832	3,930	4,030	4,133	4,239	4,347
9.2	3,350	3,435	3,522	3,611	3,702	3,795	3,891	3,989	4,090	4,193	4,299	4,408
9.3	3,409	3,494	3,581	3,670	3,761	3,855	3,951	4,050	4,151	4,254	4,361	4,469
9.4	3,468	3,553	3,641	3,738	3,822	3,916	4,013	4,111	4,213	4,316	4,423	4,532
9.5	3,528	3,614	3,701	3,791	3,884	3,978	4,075	4,174	4,275	4,379	4,486	4,595
9.6	3,589	3,675	3,763	3,854	3,946	4,041	4,138	4,237	4,339	4,443	4,550	4,659
9.7	3,651	3,738	3,826	3,917	4,010	4,105	4,202	4,302	4,404	4,508	4,615	4,724
9.8	3,715	3,802	3,890	3,981	4,074	4,170	4,267	4,367	4,469	4,573	4,680	4,790
9.9	3,779	3,866	3,956	4,047	4,140	4,236	4,333	4,433	4,536	4,640	4,747	4,857
10.0	3,845	3,932	4,022	4,113	4,207	4,303	4,400	4,501	4,603	4,708	4,815	4,924

Log (birth weight) = −1.7492 + 0.166(BPD) + 0.046(AC) − 2.646 (AC + BPD)1000

SD = ±106.0 g/kg of birth weight.

A–6. ESTIMATES OF FETAL WEIGHT (IN GRAMS) BASED ON ABDOMINAL CIRCUMFERENCE (AC) AND FEMUR LENGTH (FL)

FL (cm)	AC (cm) 20.0	20.5	21.0	21.5	22.0	22.5	23.0	23.5	24.0	24.5	25.0	25.5	26.0	26.5	27.0	27.5	28.0	28.5	29.0	29.5	30.0
4.0	663	691	720	751	783	816	851	887	925	964	1006	1048	1093	1139	1188	1239	1291	1346	1403	1463	1525
4.1	680	709	738	769	802	836	871	907	946	986	1027	1070	1115	1162	1211	1262	1315	1371	1429	1489	1551
4.2	697	726	757	788	821	855	891	928	967	1007	1049	1093	1138	1186	1235	1287	1340	1396	1454	1515	1578
4.3	715	745	776	808	841	875	912	949	988	1029	1071	1116	1162	1209	1259	1311	1365	1422	1480	1541	1605
4.4	734	764	795	827	861	896	933	971	1010	1051	1094	1139	1185	1234	1284	1336	1391	1448	1507	1568	1632
4.5	753	783	815	847	882	917	954	993	1033	1074	1118	1163	1210	1259	1309	1362	1417	1474	1534	1596	1660
4.6	772	803	835	868	903	939	976	1015	1056	1098	1142	1187	1235	1284	1335	1388	1444	1501	1561	1623	1688
4.7	792	823	856	889	924	961	999	1038	1079	1122	1166	1212	1260	1310	1361	1415	1471	1529	1589	1652	1717
4.8	812	844	877	911	947	984	1022	1062	1103	1146	1191	1237	1286	1336	1388	1442	1498	1557	1618	1681	1746
4.9	833	865	899	933	969	1007	1046	1086	1128	1171	1216	1263	1312	1363	1415	1470	1527	1585	1647	1710	1776
5.0	855	887	921	956	993	1031	1070	1111	1153	1197	1243	1290	1339	1390	1443	1498	1555	1615	1676	1740	1806
5.1	877	910	944	980	1016	1055	1095	1136	1179	1223	1269	1317	1367	1418	1471	1527	1584	1644	1706	1770	1837
5.2	899	933	967	1004	1041	1080	1120	1162	1205	1250	1296	1344	1395	1447	1500	1556	1614	1674	1737	1801	1868
5.3	922	956	992	1028	1066	1105	1146	1188	1232	1277	1324	1373	1423	1476	1530	1586	1645	1705	1768	1833	1900
5.4	946	981	1016	1053	1091	1131	1172	1215	1259	1305	1352	1401	1452	1505	1560	1617	1675	1736	1799	1865	1933
5.5	971	1005	1041	1079	1118	1158	1199	1242	1287	1333	1381	1431	1482	1535	1591	1648	1707	1768	1832	1897	1966
5.6	995	1031	1067	1105	1144	1185	1227	1271	1316	1362	1411	1461	1513	1566	1622	1679	1739	1801	1864	1931	1999
5.7	1021	1057	1094	1132	1172	1213	1255	1299	1345	1392	1441	1491	1544	1598	1654	1712	1772	1834	1898	1964	2033
5.8	1047	1084	1121	1160	1200	1242	1285	1329	1375	1422	1472	1523	1575	1630	1686	1744	1805	1867	1932	1999	2068
5.9	1074	1111	1149	1188	1229	1271	1314	1359	1406	1454	1503	1555	1608	1663	1719	1778	1839	1902	1966	2034	2103
6.0	1102	1139	1178	1217	1258	1301	1345	1390	1437	1485	1535	1587	1641	1696	1753	1812	1873	1936	2002	2069	2139
6.1	1130	1168	1207	1247	1289	1331	1376	1421	1469	1518	1568	1620	1674	1730	1788	1847	1908	1972	2038	2105	2175
6.2	1160	1198	1237	1278	1319	1363	1408	1454	1501	1551	1602	1654	1709	1765	1823	1882	1944	2008	2074	2142	2212
6.3	1189	1228	1268	1309	1351	1395	1440	1487	1535	1585	1636	1689	1744	1800	1858	1919	1981	2045	2111	2180	2250
6.4	1220	1259	1299	1341	1384	1428	1473	1520	1569	1619	1671	1724	1779	1836	1895	1956	2018	2082	2149	2218	2289
6.5	1251	1291	1332	1373	1417	1461	1507	1555	1604	1655	1707	1760	1816	1873	1932	1993	2056	2121	2188	2256	2328
6.6	1284	1324	1365	1407	1451	1496	1542	1590	1640	1691	1743	1797	1853	1911	1970	2031	2094	2160	2227	2296	2367
6.7	1317	1357	1399	1441	1486	1531	1578	1626	1676	1728	1780	1835	1891	1949	2009	2070	2134	2199	2267	2336	2408
6.8	1351	1391	1433	1477	1521	1567	1615	1663	1713	1765	1819	1873	1930	1988	2048	2110	2174	2240	2307	2377	2449
6.9	1385	1427	1469	1513	1558	1604	1652	1701	1752	1804	1857	1913	1970	2028	2089	2151	2215	2281	2348	2418	2490
7.0	1421	1463	1506	1550	1595	1642	1690	1740	1791	1843	1897	1953	2010	2069	2130	2192	2256	2322	2391	2461	2533
7.1	1458	1500	1543	1588	1633	1681	1729	1779	1830	1883	1938	1994	2051	2110	2171	2234	2299	2365	2433	2504	2576
7.2	1495	1538	1581	1626	1673	1720	1769	1819	1871	1924	1979	2035	2093	2153	2214	2277	2342	2408	2477	2547	2620
7.3	1534	1577	1621	1666	1713	1761	1810	1861	1913	1966	2021	2078	2136	2196	2258	2321	2386	2453	2521	2592	2665
7.4	1573	1616	1661	1707	1754	1802	1852	1903	1955	2009	2065	2122	2180	2240	2302	2365	2431	2498	2566	2637	2710
7.5	1614	1657	1702	1749	1796	1845	1895	1946	1999	2053	2109	2166	2225	2285	2347	2411	2476	2543	2612	2683	2756
7.6	1655	1699	1745	1791	1839	1888	1939	1990	2043	2098	2154	2211	2270	2331	2393	2457	2523	2590	2659	2730	2803
7.7	1698	1742	1788	1835	1883	1933	1983	2035	2089	2144	2200	2258	2317	2378	2440	2504	2570	2638	2707	2778	2851
7.8	1741	1786	1833	1880	1928	1978	2029	2082	2135	2191	2247	2305	2365	2426	2488	2553	2618	2686	2755	2827	2899
7.9	1786	1832	1878	1926	1975	2025	2076	2129	2183	2238	2295	2353	2413	2474	2537	2602	2668	2735	2805	2876	2949
8.0	1832	1878	1925	1973	2022	2073	2124	2177	2232	2287	2344	2403	2463	2524	2587	2652	2718	2785	2855	2926	2999
8.1	1879	1926	1973	2021	2071	2121	2173	2227	2281	2337	2394	2453	2513	2575	2638	2702	2769	2837	2906	2977	3050
8.2	1928	1974	2022	2070	2120	2171	2224	2277	2332	2388	2446	2504	2565	2626	2690	2754	2821	2889	2958	3029	3102
8.3	1978	2024	2072	2121	2171	2223	2275	2329	2384	2440	2498	2557	2617	2679	2743	2807	2874	2942	3011	3082	3155

FL (cm)	30.5	31.0	31.5	32.0	32.5	33.0	33.5	34.0	34.5	35.0	35.5	36.0	36.5	37.0	37.5	38.0	38.5	39.0	39.5	40.0
												AC (cm)								
4.0	1590	1658	1729	1802	1879	1959	2042	2129	2220	2314	2413	2515	2622	2734	2850	2972	3098	3230	3367	3511
4.1	1617	1685	1756	1830	1907	1987	2071	2158	2249	2344	2442	2545	2652	2764	2880	3002	3128	3260	3397	3540
4.2	1644	1712	1783	1858	1935	2016	2100	2187	2279	2373	2472	2575	2683	2794	2911	3032	3159	3290	3427	3570
4.3	1671	1740	1812	1886	1964	2045	2129	2217	2308	2404	2503	2606	2713	2825	2942	3063	3189	3321	3458	3600
4.4	1699	1768	1840	1915	1993	2075	2159	2247	2339	2434	2533	2637	2744	2856	2973	3094	3220	3352	3488	3630
4.5	1727	1797	1869	1944	2023	2105	2189	2278	2370	2465	2565	2668	2776	2888	3004	3125	3251	3383	3519	3661
4.6	1756	1826	1898	1974	2053	2135	2220	2309	2401	2497	2596	2700	2807	2919	3036	3157	3283	3414	3550	3692
4.7	1785	1855	1928	2004	2083	2166	2251	2340	2432	2528	2628	2732	2840	2952	3068	3189	3315	3446	3582	3723
4.8	1814	1885	1959	2035	2115	2197	2283	2372	2464	2560	2660	2764	2872	2984	3100	3221	3347	3478	3613	3754
4.9	1845	1916	1990	2066	2146	2229	2315	2404	2497	2593	2693	2797	2905	3017	3133	3254	3380	3510	3645	3786
5.0	1875	1947	2021	2098	2178	2261	2347	2437	2530	2626	2726	2830	2938	3050	3166	3287	3412	3542	3677	3818
5.1	1906	1978	2053	2130	2210	2294	2380	2470	2563	2659	2760	2864	2972	3084	3200	3320	3445	3575	3710	3850
5.2	1938	2010	2085	2163	2243	2327	2413	2503	2597	2693	2794	2898	3006	3117	3234	3354	3479	3608	3743	3882
5.3	1970	2043	2118	2196	2277	2360	2447	2537	2631	2728	2828	2932	3040	3152	3268	3388	3513	3642	3776	3915
5.4	2003	2076	2151	2229	2311	2395	2482	2572	2665	2762	2863	2967	3075	3186	3302	3422	3547	3676	3809	3948
5.5	2036	2109	2185	2264	2345	2429	2516	2607	2700	2797	2898	3002	3110	3221	3337	3457	3581	3710	3843	3981
5.6	2070	2143	2220	2298	2380	2464	2552	2642	2736	2833	2933	3038	3145	3257	3372	3492	3616	3744	3877	4015
5.7	2104	2178	2254	2333	2415	2500	2587	2678	2772	2869	2970	3074	3181	3293	3408	3527	3651	3779	3911	4048
5.8	2139	2213	2290	2369	2451	2536	2624	2714	2808	2905	3006	3110	3218	3329	3444	3563	3686	3814	3946	4082
5.9	2175	2249	2326	2405	2488	2573	2660	2751	2845	2942	3043	3147	3254	3366	3480	3599	3722	3849	3981	4117
6.0	2211	2286	2363	2442	2525	2610	2698	2789	2883	2980	3080	3184	3292	3403	3517	3636	3758	3885	4016	4151
6.1	2248	2323	2400	2480	2562	2647	2736	2827	2921	3018	3118	3222	3329	3440	3554	3673	3795	3921	4052	4186
6.2	2285	2360	2438	2518	2600	2686	2774	2865	2959	3056	3157	3260	3367	3478	3592	3710	3832	3957	4087	4222
6.3	2323	2398	2476	2556	2639	2725	2813	2904	2998	3095	3195	3299	3406	3516	3630	3747	3869	3994	4124	4257
6.4	2362	2437	2515	2595	2678	2764	2852	2943	3037	3134	3235	3338	3445	3555	3668	3785	3906	4031	4160	4293
6.5	2401	2477	2555	2635	2718	2804	2892	2983	3077	3174	3274	3378	3484	3594	3707	3824	3944	4069	4197	4329
6.6	2441	2517	2595	2675	2759	2844	2933	3024	3118	3215	3315	3418	3524	3633	3746	3863	3983	4106	4234	4366
6.7	2481	2557	2636	2716	2800	2885	2974	3065	3159	3256	3355	3458	3564	3673	3786	3902	4021	4144	4271	4402
6.8	2523	2599	2677	2758	2841	2927	3016	3107	3200	3297	3397	3499	3605	3714	3826	3941	4060	4183	4309	4439
6.9	2564	2641	2719	2800	2884	2969	3058	3149	3242	3339	3438	3541	3646	3754	3866	3981	4100	4222	4347	4477
7.0	2607	2683	2762	2843	2927	3012	3101	3192	3285	3381	3481	3583	3688	3796	3907	4022	4140	4261	4386	4514
7.1	2650	2727	2806	2887	2970	3056	3144	3235	3328	3424	3523	3625	3730	3838	3948	4062	4180	4300	4425	4552
7.2	2694	2771	2850	2931	3014	3100	3188	3279	3372	3468	3567	3668	3772	3880	3990	4104	4220	4340	4464	4591
7.3	2739	2816	2895	2976	3059	3145	3233	3323	3416	3512	3610	3712	3816	3922	4032	4145	4261	4381	4503	4629
7.4	2785	2861	2940	3021	3105	3190	3278	3369	3461	3557	3655	3756	3859	3966	4075	4187	4303	4421	4543	4668
7.5	2831	2908	2987	3068	3151	3236	3324	3414	3507	3602	3700	3800	3903	4009	4118	4230	4344	4462	4583	4708
7.6	2878	2955	3034	3115	3198	3283	3371	3461	3553	3648	3745	3845	3948	4053	4161	4272	4387	4504	4624	4747
7.7	2926	3003	3081	3162	3245	3331	3418	3508	3600	3694	3791	3891	3993	4098	4205	4316	4429	4545	4665	4787
7.8	2974	3051	3130	3211	3294	3379	3466	3555	3647	3741	3838	3937	4039	4143	4250	4360	4472	4588	4706	4827
7.9	3024	3100	3179	3260	3343	3427	3514	3604	3695	3789	3885	3984	4085	4188	4295	4404	4515	4630	4748	4868
8.0	3074	3151	3229	3310	3392	3477	3564	3653	3744	3837	3933	4031	4131	4234	4340	4448	4559	4673	4790	4909
8.1	3125	3202	3280	3360	3443	3527	3614	3702	3793	3886	3981	4079	4179	4281	4386	4493	4604	4716	4832	4950
8.2	3177	3253	3332	3412	3494	3578	3664	3752	3843	3935	4030	4127	4226	4328	4432	4539	4648	4760	4875	4992
8.3	3230	3306	3384	3464	3546	3630	3716	3803	3893	3985	4080	4176	4275	4376	4479	4585	4693	4804	4918	5034

A–7. GROWTH OF ESTIMATED FETAL WEIGHT ALONG GESTATIONAL AGE

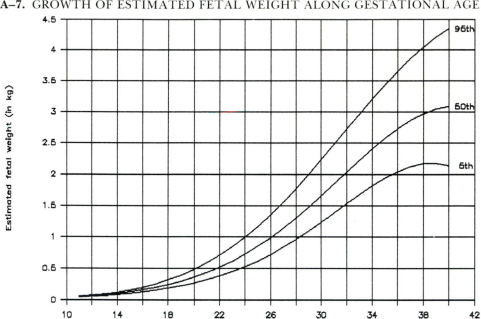

A–8. FETAL BIOMETRY NOMOGRAMS*

Cranial Biometry
Lateral ventricular width vs. gestational age, 4, 5
Lateral ventricle hemispheric width ratio vs. biparietal diameter, 4, 5
Biparietal diameter vs. gestational age, 9, 10, 11
Occipitofrontal diameter vs. gestational age, 11, 12
Transverse cerebellar diameter vs. gestational age, 14
Head perimeter vs. gestational age, 56
Femur length vs. head circumference, 57
Head to abdomen ratio, 58

Ocular Biometry
Ocular, interocular, and binocular measurements vs. gestational age, 83
Ocular diameter vs. gestational age, 84
Interocular distance vs. gestational age, 84
Ocular diameter vs. biparietal diameter, 85
Binocular distance vs. gestational age, 85
Interocular distance vs. biparietal diameter, 86
Binocular distance vs. biparietal diameter, 86

Cardiac Biometry
Left ventricle dimensions vs. gestational age, 134
Right ventricle dimensions vs. gestational age, 134
Interventricular septum dimensions vs. gestational age, 134
Aortic root dimensions vs. gestational age, 135
Left atrium dimensions vs. gestational age, 135

Abdominal Biometry
Spleen perimeter vs. gestational age, 247
Fetal spleen diameter, volume, and perimeter vs. gestational age, 247
Growth of spleen volume with gestational age, 248
Liver vertical dimensions vs. gestational age, 250

Stomach diameter vs. gestational age, 254
Colon diameter vs. gestational age, 254
Kidney biometry vs. gestational age, 256
Kidney length vs. gestational age, 257
Kidney thickness vs. gestational age, 257
Kidney width vs. gestational age, 258
Kidney volume vs. gestational age, 258
Kidney perimeter vs. abdominal perimeter, 259
Adrenal gland size vs. gestational age, 296

Skeletal Biometry
Humerus vs. gestational age, 318, 319
Radius vs. gestational age, 320
Ulna vs. gestational age, 320
Clavicle vs. gestational age, 321, 367
Femur vs. gestational age, 321
Tibia vs. gestational age, 322
Fibula vs. gestational age, 322
Long bones of the upper extremity, 323
Long bones of the lower extremity, 324
Head perimeter vs. femur, 324
Head perimeter vs. humerus, 325
Ulna vs. humerus, 326
Tibia vs. femur, 326
Thoracic circumference vs. gestational age, 330

Umbilical Cord Biometry
Umbilical vein diameter, 386

Estimated Fetal Weight
Based on biparietal diameter and abdominal circumference, 442–445
Based on femur length and abdominal circumference, 446–447
Estimated fetal weight vs. gestational age, 448

*This index provides specific page references to the nomograms contained within this text.

Index